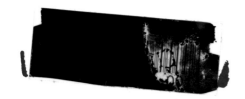

‖‖ ‖ ‖‖ ‖‖‖‖ ‖‖ ‖‖‖ ‖‖‖ ‖‖ ‖‖‖ ‖‖
D1570185

Social Psychophysiology

SOCIAL PSYCHOPHYSIOLOGY

A SOURCEBOOK

EDITED BY

John T. Cacioppo
University of Iowa

AND

Richard E. Petty
University of Missouri Columbia

FOREWORD BY
David Shapiro

THE GUILFORD PRESS
New York • London

Library of Congress Cataloging in Publication Data
Main entry under title:
Social psychophysiology.

Bibliography: p.
Includes index.
1. Psychology, Physiological.   2. Social medicine.   I. Cacioppo, John T.   II. Petty,
Richard E. [DNLM: 1. Psychology, Social.   2. Psychophysiology. WL 103 S678]
QP360.S6 1983   152   82-15575
ISBN 0-89862-626-9

To our spouses

Barbara L. Cacioppo
and
Lynn L. Petty

CONTRIBUTORS

Robert S. Baron, PhD, Department of Psychology, University of Iowa, Iowa City, Iowa

C. Daniel Batson, PhD, Department of Psychology, University of Kansas, Lawrence, Kansas

Jim Blascovich, PhD, Departments of Health Education Professions and Psychology, State University of New York at Buffalo, Buffalo, New York

Donn Byrne, PhD, Department of Psychology, State University of New York at Albany, Albany, New York

John T. Cacioppo, PhD, Department of Psychology, University of Iowa, Iowa City, Iowa

Charles S. Carver, PhD, Department of Psychology, University of Miami, Coral Gables, Florida

Michael Clark, PhD, Psychology Service, VA Medical Center, Chillicothe, Ohio

Jay S. Coke, PhD, U.S. Army Research Institute, Fort Sill, Oklahoma

Joel Cooper, PhD, Department of Psychology, Princeton University, Princeton, New Jersey

Andrew Crider, PhD, Department of Psychology, Williams College, Williamstown, Massachusetts

Paul Ekman, PhD, Human Interaction Laboratory, Department of Psychiatry, University of California–San Francisco, San Francisco, California

Russell H. Fazio, PhD, Department of Psychology, Indiana University, Bloomington, Indiana

Alan J. Fridlund, PhD, Psychology Service, Martinez VA Medical Center, Martinez, California, and CSPP–Berkeley, Berkeley, California

Russell G. Geen, PhD, Department of Psychology, University of Missouri–Columbia, Columbia, Missouri

Isidore Gormezano, PhD, Department of Psychology, University of Iowa, Iowa City, Iowa

Ruben C. Gur, PhD, Department of Neurology and Cerebrovascular Research Center, University of Pennsylvania, Philadelphia, Pennsylvania

Joseph C. Hager, Department of Psychiatry, University of California–San Francisco, San Francisco, California

Richard Hirschman, DMD, PhD, Department of Psychology, Kent State University, Kent, Ohio

Carroll E. Izard, PhD, Department of Psychology, University of Delaware, Newark, Delaware

Larry D. Jamner, Department of Psychology, State University of New York at Stony Brook, Stony Brook, New York

Edward S. Katkin, PhD, Department of Psychology, State University of New York at Buffalo, Buffalo, New York

Kathryn Kelley, PhD, Department of Psychology, State University of New York at Albany, Albany, New York

John T. Lanzetta, PhD, Department of Psychology, Dartmouth College, Hanover, New Hampshire

Howard Leventhal, PhD, Department of Psychology, University of Wisconsin–Madison, Madison, Wisconsin

Beverly S. Marshall-Goodell, PhD, Department of Psychology, University of Iowa, Iowa City, Iowa

Karen A. Matthews, PhD, Department of Psychiatry, University of Pittsburgh, Pittsburgh, Pennsylvania

F. J. McGuigan, PhD, Performance Research Laboratory, University of Louisville, Louisville, Kentucky

Gregory J. McHugo, PhD, Department of Psychology, Dartmouth College, Hanover, New Hampshire

Danny L. Moore, PhD, Marketing Department, College of Business Administration, University of Florida, Gainesville, Florida

Peter A. Mosbach, MS, Department of Psychology, University of Wisconsin-Madison, Madison, Wisconsin

James W. Pennebaker, PhD, Department of Psychology, Southern Methodist University, Dallas, Texas

Richard E. Petty, PhD, Department of Psychology, University of Missouri–Columbia, Columbia, Missouri

Judith Rodin, PhD, Department of Psychology, Yale University, New Haven, Connecticut

Ronald W. Rogers, PhD, Department of Psychology, University of Alabama, University, Alabama

Harold A. Sackeim, PhD, Department of Psychology, New York University, New York, New York, and Department of Biological Psychiatry, New York State Psychiatric Institute, New York, New York

Michael F. Scheier, PhD, Department of Psychology, Carnegie-Mellon University, Pittsburgh, Pennsylvania

Gary E. Schwartz, PhD, Department of Psychology, Yale University, New Haven, Connecticut

Lynn Spitzer, MS, Department of Psychology, Yale University, New Haven, Connecticut

Bernard Tursky, Department of Political Science, State University of New York at Stony Brook, Stony Brook, New York

Dolf Zillmann, PhD, Institute for Communication Research, Indiana University, Bloomington, Indiana

FOREWORD

In the study of behavior, we are in an age of compound science in which behavioral and biological concepts and methods are commonly merged together. Examples are numerous—psychobiology, biobehavioral sciences, sociobiology, and so on. It has also become fashionable to use "behavioral" or "bio" as combining terms, for example, behavioral physiology, behavioral neurology, behavioral medicine, biopolitics, and biosociology. Sometimes three fields are put together, as in sociopsychopharmacology, behavioral neurobiology, and psychoneuroimmunology. It is as if we are moving away from strict disciplinary concerns and single professional identities toward some kind of holistic behavioral science. Each compound has its own peculiar origin and history, and it is not always apparent what kinds of theoretical, empirical, or practical issues are addressed in each. In some cases the compound has its beginnings in unique research of a single investigator in which the specific combination of concepts or techniques were dominant. What ensues depends on the findings and their promise as well as the readiness of the established scientific community to follow the lead. In other cases, the compound seems to emerge as a full-blown specialty.

Sociopharmacology may serve as a representative case study of one compounding process, a field recently reviewed by McGuire, Raleigh, and Brammer (1982). Sociopharmacology grew out of observations suggesting that the effects of pharmacological agents on the behavior and feelings of individuals depend on the social setting and other social variables. An important direction in this endeavor occurred when systematic studies were carried out on the effects of drugs on animals (typically monkeys) of different social status. In this research, status-related behavioral responses were observed to equivalent doses of selected drugs. These studies also suggested that status differences were associated with distinct physiological and biochemical profiles. In their review, McGuire *et al.* distinguish three sets of major variables—biochemical–physiological–anatomical, pharmacological, social behavior–physical environment—and they point up the need for investigators to examine different "routes" of influence to show how one set of variables affects another and thereby to arrive at a more coherent picture of reciprocal effects. To find one's way along these routes requires knowledge and experience with diverse concepts and techniques. The task can be facilitated by interdisciplinary communication, cooperation, and collaboration. As in any scientific endeavor, humble observations and curiosity set the stage for what follows. On the practical level, socio-pharmacology has led some to consider whether psychotropic medications should be prescribed according to the patient's social status or other social attributes. One may wonder whether other nonpsychotropic medications are similarly affected.

This volume concerns the merger of social psychology and psycho-physiology. Psychophysiology is itself an earlier compound of behavioral sciences, physiology, psychiatry, and biomedical engineering. Although it lay in the shadow of physiological psychology for a long time, it has come unto its own in the past 15 to 20 years with its unique focus on relations between central and peripheral nervous system responses and behavior, cognition, and emotion in human beings. Although one may point to various concrete origins and earlier preoccupations, psychophysiology is now quite diversified. Current topics of investigation include: Pavlovian conditioning; biofeedback and operant conditioning of autonomic re-sponses; attention, orienting, and habituation; behavioral regulation of the cardiovascular system; individual differences in physiological functioning; relations between cognitive and physiological processes; emotion and hemisphere specialization; and others. Although earlier research in this field emphasized only selected physiological measures (e.g., heart rate, electrodermal activity, and electroencephalograms), there is greater di-versity in current studies (e.g., blood pressure, respiration, event-related potentials, pupil response, and blood volume).

Why the current merger of psychophysiology and social psychology? Previous attempts at integration have occurred throughout this century (see Chapters 1 and 2). One major earlier focus of activity involved studies of interpersonal interaction, concerned mainly with the evaluation of psychotherapeutic process and outcome (see Lacey, 1959) and subsequently with group processes more generally (e.g., Kaplan, Burch, Bloom, & Edelberg, 1963; Shapiro & Leiderman, 1967). This research was unique in that simultaneous physiological recordings were made in several people while they were engaged in some kind of social interaction. Another major center of activity in the 1960s derived its major impetus from the work of Stanley Schachter and associates concerning cognitive, physiological, and social determinants of emotional state (Schachter & Singer, 1962). The study of emotion is a classic issue in psychology (and physiology), and this research brought new vigor to the topic in the form of theoretical and methodological ingenuity.

In this volume it is clear that no single specific area of study, experi-mental procedure, or theoretical orientation is dominant, with the possible exception of modern thinking and research on emotion (see Plutchik & Kellerman, 1980). It may seem that the bits and pieces left behind by previous writers and researchers on social psychophysiology have been reassembled under the banner of social psychology. It is much more than that. As can be seen from the contents of this volume, this is a major commitment on the part of social psychologists "to study relationships between actual or perceived physiological events and the verbal and/or behavioral effects of human association" (Cacioppo & Petty, Chapter 1). It is supported by many excellent contributions characterized by theoretical depth and methodological rigor. From the gamut of topics and issues discussed in these chapters, it is clear that whatever faltering steps social psychophysiology may have taken in the past, the foundations are now well laid out and the field is here to stay.

Some comments are in order on reductionism, an issue often raised in response to attempts such as this to introduce physiological approaches into the study of complex behaviors and cognitions. In my view, when psychologists turn to biological concepts and methods, they are not reducing their phenomena but adducing considerations relevant to problems in hand. Although the study of social behavior, cognition, and feelings can proceed without getting under the skin, no one can deny the significance of internal bodily processes for behavior. It is equally foolish to deny the role of social variables in the study of bodily processes. Whether we talk of behavior, thoughts, and emotional experience on the one hand, or of brain potentials and visceral actions on the other, both have the same reality in my view. What we need is biobehavioral synthesis and not biological determinism, and that synthesis is well demonstrated in the contributions to this book.

Now that the foundations of social psychophysiology have been set down in this book, much work lies ahead in conceptual refinement, empirical demonstration, and critical experimentation. Inevitably, this will also entail further experience and education on the part of the scientists involved in this field. The simplifying assumptions and viewpoints, whether about social behavior or physiology, so necessary at this stage of development, will be pushed aside, and more realistic and valid assumptions will replace them. Social psychophysiology will also be strengthened by developments in related fields of inquiry. For example, sociobiology has focused on the biological adaptiveness of social behavior in an evolutionary context, suggesting in addition that neural and other physiological processes are associated with this process of adaptation and selection. Whether hypotheses and speculations derived from sociobiology can be applied effectively to human social behaviors remains to be determined. Other developments in research on neuroendocrine functions and brain peptides may suggest other integrative efforts. At the same time, social psychophysiology will gather strength through practical application of its concepts and methods to problems of health and disease, communication processes, politics, and education. We can only guess what new and fascinating compound sciences are on the horizon.

David Shapiro, PhD
University of California, Los Angeles

REFERENCES

Kaplan, H. B., Burch, N. R., Bloom, S. W., & Edelberg, R.   Affective orientation in physiological activity (GSR) in small peer groups. *Psychosomatic Medicine*, 1963, *25*, 242–252.

Lacey, J. I.   Psychophysiological approaches to the evaluation of psychotherapeutic process and outcome. In E. A. Rubinstein & M. B. Parloff (Eds.), *Research in psychotherapy*. Washington, D.C.: American Psychological Association, 1959.

McGuire, M. T., Raleigh, M. J., & Brammer, G. L.   Annual review of sociopharmacology. *Annual Reviews: Pharmacology and Toxicology*, 1982, *22*, 635–653.

Plutchik, R., & Kellerman, H.   *Emotion: Theory, research, and experience*. New York: Academic, 1980.

Schachter, S., & Singer, J. E.   Cognitive, social and physiological determinants of emotional state. *Psychological Review*, 1962, *69*, 379–399.

Shapiro, D., & Leiderman, P. H.   Arousal correlates of task role and group setting. *Journal of Personality and Social Psychology*, 1967, *5*, 103–107.

PREFACE

Research in social psychology has for many years focused on the situational determinants of social cognition and behavior largely to the exclusion of psychophysiological determinants. An inspection of any introductory social psychology textbook quickly reveals that little is said about the physiological reactions (whether perceptible or not) arising within people's bodies. Coverage of the early theorizing by Schachter and Singer (1962) can be found, but Schachter and Singer's theory of the cognitive and physiological determinants of emotional states is now being roundly criticized by social psychologists (e.g., Marshall & Zimbardo, 1979; Maslach, 1979; Zillmann, 1978) and psychophysiologists alike (e.g., Lang, Rice, & Sternbach, 1972; Plutchik & Ax, 1967). Thus, even this sparse coverage is in jeopardy. Moreover, although the second edition of *The Handbook of Social Psychology* contained an excellent chapter by Shapiro and Crider (1969) entitled "Psychophysiological Approaches to Social Psychology," and a chapter entitled "Psychophysiological Contributions to Social Psychology" (Shapiro & Schwartz, 1970) appeared in the *Annual Review of Psychology* the following year, few social psychologists or psychophysiologists pursued the potential of this interdisciplinary approach. Neither the third edition of *The Handbook of Social Psychology* (Lindzey & Aronson, in press) nor the initial version of the *Handbook of Psychophysiology* (Greenfield & Sternbach, 1972) contains a chapter representing perspectives on the role of bodily processes in social psychology. Also, the *Annual Review of Psychology* has not broached the topic since the appearance of Shapiro and Schwartz's (1970) original review.

This should not be taken as evidence that the physiological accoutrements of social cognition and behavior are silent regarding conceptual issues in social psychology, or that the most interesting or theoretically important behaviors are those in which only trivial physiological reactions arise. We believe that the strong emphasis by social psychologists on the situational determinants of social cognition and behavior is not so much due to any disagreement about the value of a psychophysiological perspective, but rather to the complexity and breadth of the methodologies and issues that social psychologists must master when simply considering situational factors (e.g., see Carlsmith, Ellsworth, & Aronson, 1976; Cook & Campbell, 1976; Crano & Brewer, 1973; Selltiz, Wrightsman, & Cook, 1976; Campbell & Stanley, 1963; Webb, Campbell, Schwartz, & Sechrest, 1966).

Similarly, the processes traditionally investigated by social psychologists, and the heuristics that have emerged from these investigations, often bear directly on issues in psychophysiology (e.g., see Cacioppo & Petty, 1981, 1982). Psychophysiologists, however, have a demanding task in trying to outline the effects of simpler, nonsocial factors on physiological responding. Volumes have been written in psychophysiology on techniques and instrumentation (e.g., Brown, 1967; Martin & Venables, 1980; McGuigan, 1979; Stern, Ray, & Davis, 1980; Venables & Martin, 1967), and formal, distinctively psychophysiological theories are still sparse. Consequently, social factors have generally been viewed as sources of artifacts or error variance rather than as objects of study.

This book, which grew out of two symposia that we organized for the 88th Annual Meeting of the American Psychological Association (APA), provides strong evidence for the utility of a *social psychophysiological* approach to human behavior. Our design initially was to identify laboratories that brought a psychophysiological perspective to social psychological issues, "compare notes" on problems and advances encumbered by pursuing this perspective, and improve the dialogue among investigators at the various laboratories. The programs of important research that we located quickly exceeded the time available to us at APA. Indeed, the number of research programs that, knowingly or not, dealt with social psychophysiological issues easily exceeded the space available in any single volume, such as the present. Hence, we developed this oversized sourcebook of social psychophysiological theory, method, and research by obtaining contributions that provide a representative rather than a comprehensive picture of the field. We hope the fact that this book stands as an initial rather than final word on social psychophysiology proves as exciting to readers as it did to us.

The book is organized into four major sections: Overview of Social Psychophysiology, Basic Social Psychophysiological Research, Methods of Social Psychophysiology, and Epilogue. The section on Basic Social Psychophysiological Research is easily the longest and has been partitioned into components on Attitudes and Social Cognition, Affect and Emotions, Interpersonal Processes, and Contributions to Health.

We are indebted to a large number of people and groups. First, we owe a great thanks to David Shapiro for his seminal work in this area (Leiderman & Shapiro, 1964; Schwartz & Shapiro, 1973; Shapiro & Crider, 1969; Shapiro & Schwartz, 1970), his helpful suggestions to us regarding this volume, and his kind consent to preparing the foreword to this volume. We are also grateful to the special research support provided to us by our universities (University of Iowa Faculty Scholar Award, Old Gold Fellowship, University of Missouri Research Council Grant), the National Science Foundation (BNS 78-18667, BNS 80-23589, and BNS 82-15734), and the National Institutes of Health (UI-BRSG, 31798-01). Their generous support has enabled us to develop this project and devote attention to detail.

We owe a tremendous debt of thanks to our authors for their yeoman service in the preparation of this sourcebook. All are accomplished in their own programs of research, and they graciously extended their work to entertain new ideas, observations, and approaches. We greatly enjoyed our interactions with the authors and can only hope that they might feel the same. In any case, readers should benefit from the authors' achievements in expressing complex ideas simply and conveying their own enthusiasm about social psychophysiology.

We especially wish to thank Gary E. Schwartz and Seymour Weingarten for their help and suggestions in developing this volume. A number of colleagues also provided very helpful comments, suggestions, and support, including Barbara Andersen, Curt Sandman, Isidore Gormezano, John Harvey, Charles Snyder, and many of the contributors to this volume. Our students (especially Leo Quintanar, Charlotte Lowell, Kathy McCann, Larry Gant, Kathy Morris, Mary Losch, Hai Sook Kim, Chuan Feng Kao, and Greg Bovee) and our secretaries (Gertrude Nath and Lenore Hizer) made valuable contributions to the book as well. Finally, thanks are due to our wives (Barbara and Lynn) and parents (Cyrus, Mary Katherine, Edmund, and JoAnne) for filling our working environments with love and joy.

John T. Cacioppo
Richard E. Petty

REFERENCES

Brown, C. C. *Methods in psychophysiology*. Baltimore: Williams & Wilkins, 1967.

Cacioppo, J. T., & Petty, R. E. Electromyograms as measures of extent and affectivity of information processing. *American Psychologist*, 1981, *36*, 441–456.

Cacioppo, J. T., & Petty, R. E. A biosocial model of attitude change: Signs, symptoms, and undetected physiological responses. In J. T. Cacioppo & R. E. Petty (Eds.), *Perspectives in cardiovascular psychophysiology*. New York: Guilford, 1982.

Campbell, D. T., & Stanley, J. C. *Experimental and quasi-experimental designs for research*. Chicago: Rand McNally, 1963.

Carlsmith, J. M., Ellsworth, P. C., & Aronson, E. *Methods of research in social psychology*. Reading, Mass.: Addison-Wesley, 1976.

Cook, T. D., & Campbell. D. T. The design and conduct of quasi-experiments and true experiments in field settings. In M. Dunnette (Ed.), *Handbook of industrial and organizational psychology*. Chicago: Rand McNally, 1976.

Crano, W. D., & Brewer, M. B. *Principles of research in social psychology*. New York: McGraw-Hill, 1973.

Greenfield, N. S., & Sternbach, R. A. *Handbook of psychophysiology*. New York: Holt, Rinehart & Winston, 1972.

Lang, P. J., Rice, D. G., & Sternbach, R. A. The psychophysiology of emotion. In N. S. Greenfield & R. A. Sternbach (Eds.), *Handbook of psychophysiology*. New York: Holt, Rinehart & Winston, 1972.

Leiderman, P. H., & Shapiro, D. (Eds.). *Psychobiological approaches to social behavior*. Stanford, Calif.: Stanford University Press, 1964.

Lindzey, G., & Aronson, E. *The handbook of social psychology* (3rd ed.) Reading, Mass.: Addison-Wesley, in press.

Marshall, G. D., & Zimbardo, P. G. Affective consequences of inadequately explained physiological arousal. *Journal of Personality and Social Psychology*, 1979, *37*, 970–988.

Martin, I., & Venables, P. H. *Techniques in psychophysiology*. Chichester: Wiley, 1980.

Maslach, C. Negative emotional biasing of unexplained arousal. *Journal of Personality and Social Psychology*, 1979, *37*, 953–969.

McGuigan, F. J. *Psychophysiological measurement of covert behavior: A guide for the laboratory*. New York: Wiley, 1979.

Plutchik, R., & Ax, A. F. A critique of determinants of emotional state of Schachter and Singer (1962). *Psychophysiology*, 1967, *4*, 79–82.

Schachter, S., & Singer, J. E. Cognitive, social, and physiological determinants of emotional state. *Psychological Review*, 1962, *69*, 379–399.

Schwartz, G. E., & Shapiro, D. Social psychophysiology. In W. F. Prokasy & D. C. Raskin (Eds.), *Electrodermal activity in psychological research*. New York: Academic, 1973.

Selltiz, C., Wrightsman, L. S., & Cook, S. W. *Research methods in social relations* (3rd ed.). New York: Holt, Rinehart & Winston, 1976.

Shapiro, D., & Crider, A. Psychophysiological approaches to social psychology. In G. Lindzey & E. Aronson (Eds.), *The handbook of social psychology* (2nd ed., Vol. 3). Reading, Mass.: Addison-Wesley, 1969.

Shapiro, D., & Schwartz, G. E. Psychophysiological contributions to social psychology. *Annual Review of Psychology*, 1970, *21*, 87–112.

Stern, R. M., Ray, W. J., & Davis, C. M. *Psychophysiological recording*. New York: Oxford University Press, 1980.

Venables, P. H., & Martin, I. *A manual of psychophysiological methods*. Amsterdam: North-Holland, 1967.

Webb, E., Campbell, D. T., Schwartz, R. D., & Sechrest, L. *Unobtrusive measures: Nonreactive research in the social sciences*. Chicago: Rand McNally, 1966.

Zillmann, D. Attribution and misattribution of excitatory reactions. In J. H. Harvey, W. Ickes, & R. F. Kidd (Eds.), *New directions in attribution research* (Vol. 2). Hillsdale, N.J.: Erlbaum, 1978.

CONTENTS

B. Affect and Emotions

III. METHODS OF SOCIAL PSYCHOPHYSIOLOGY

IV. EPILOGUE

Social Psychophysiology

OVERVIEW
OF
SOCIAL
PSYCHOPHYSIOLOGY

CHAPTER 1

Foundations of
Social Psychophysiology

John T. Cacioppo
University of Iowa
Richard E. Petty
University of Missouri–Columbia

INTRODUCTION

> It is often said that science progresses as new means are found to observe,
> measure, and quantify the phenomena of interest. . . . Social psychology,
> concerned with human behavior in a social context, is one of several
> disciplines . . . that has been turning to psychophysiology as a way of
> augmenting its tools of investigation. (Shapiro & Schwartz, 1970, p. 87)

Social psychophysiology can be characterized by the use of noninvasive
procedures to study the relationships between actual or perceived physiological events and the verbal or behavioral effects of human association.
This emerging field represents the intersection of the disciplines of social
psychology and psychophysiology and is surprisingly comprehensive and
vigorous given two parental disciplines so disparately focused. Social psychology, the older of the two spawning disciplines, is directed toward
understanding the phenomenological and behavioral effects of human
association (past, present, and future). Psychophysiology, on the other
hand, employs noninvasive procedures to study the interrelationships
between physiological events and a person's reportable and/or overt behavior. Social psychology is partitioned into conceptual areas of research
(e.g., attitudes and persuasion, interpersonal attraction, aggression, altruism) and is replete with abstract theories (e.g., Deutsch & Krauss, 1965;
Shaw & Costanzo, 1970; West & Wicklund, 1980). Psychophysiology, in
contrast, is more often partitioned into anatomical areas of research (e.g.,
cardiovascular system, gastrointestinal system) and is laden with tech-
nically sophisticated preparations and instrumentation (e.g., Greenfield &
Sternbach, 1972; Hassett, 1978; Stern, Ray, & Davis, 1980).

Recent research has shown that the differences between these disciplines can be complementing rather than defeating. For example, advances

have been made by employing social psychophysiological procedures in studies of attitudes (see Cacioppo & Sandman, 1981), aggression (e.g., Zillmann, Johnson, & Day, 1974), sexual arousal (e.g., Cantor, Zillmann, & Bryant, 1975; Geer, 1975), dissonance arousal (e.g., Fazio, Zanna, & Cooper, 1977; see Kiesler & Pallak, 1976), social facilitation (see Geen & Gange, 1977), persuasion (e.g., Cacioppo & Petty, 1979), decision making (e.g., Blascovich, Nash, & Ginsburg, 1978; Gerard, 1967), and other areas. Moreover, these and the advances reported in this book may mark only the beginning, since research in which physiological, verbal, and behavioral assessments are all made within a single experiment is becoming increasingly common (see Cacioppo & Petty, in press-b; Schwartz & Shapiro, 1973).

Social psychophysiological research that has employed electrophysiological procedures has already explored a wide variety of response systems (see Schwartz, 1982). These include electrodermal (EDA) (Cooper, 1959; Mewborn & Rogers, 1979), electromyographic (EMG) (Cacioppo & Petty, 1981a, 1981b), pupillographic (Collins, Ellsworth, & Helmreich, 1967; Hess, 1965), vasomotor (Gerard, 1967), differential electroencephalographic (EEG) (Cacioppo, Petty, & Quintanar, 1982), and cardiac (Buckout, 1966; Cacioppo, Sandman, & Walker, 1978) activity. The physiological measures are generally obtained continuously throughout an experimental session, whereas data relevant to the sequence of reportable and behavioral states, although occasionally monitored continuously, are generally collected at discrete intervals during or following the experimental treatment(s) (see Cacioppo & Petty, 1981a).

Social psychophysiological research has historically been defined by the collection of electrophysiological measures, and it most often has meant recording galvanic skin responses (GSRs) during what in all other respects would be regarded as a traditional social psychological experiment (Schwartz & Shapiro, 1973, review and critique a number of these studies). Social psychophysiological research, however, can no longer be characterized by any single measure or methodology (e.g., electrophysiological recording), as the relationship between social psychological variables and bodily states has now been studied using misattributional procedures (e.g., Zanna & Cooper, 1976; Zillmann, 1978), drugs (e.g., Cooper, Zanna, & Taves, 1978; Schachter & Singer, 1962), hypnosis (Maslach, 1979), cardiac pacemakers (Cacioppo, 1979), exercise (Pennebaker & Lightner, 1980), and operant training procedures for shaping physiological activity (Cacioppo et al., 1978). This broader conception of the field of social psychophysiology is reflected in the succeeding chapters.

The contributions to this book provide evidence for the notion that, although a social psychophysiological perspective harbors no privileged pathway to social psychological or psychophysiological processes, it does offer a host of advantages when used to complement the traditional approaches in the parental disciplines (cf. Cacioppo & Petty, in press-a). What are some of these advantages? First, social psychophysiological research can help to advance our understanding of the determinants of people's physiological responses and the operation of physiological mechanisms by expanding the set of independent and dependent variables in psychophysiology to include powerful social factors. Second, a social psychophysiological viewpoint can lead to the discovery and ultimately the explanation of instances of complex human behavior that are shaped by a combination of social, dispositional, and physiological factors. Third, psychophysiological procedures can provide means for assessing the construct validity of theoretical concepts in social psychology. Fourth, a social psychophysiological orientation can lead to refinements (e.g., greater specification) of existing theories, and to the development of new theories, of social processes when the extant abstract formulations within social psychology are found to be incompatible with the present state of knowledge about the structure and function of physiological systems. Fifth, a social psychophysiological approach can bring about refinements in or extensions of existing theories, and the development of new heuristics and theories, bearing on psychophysiological data. Finally, a general, social psychophysiological perspective can lead to important discoveries in applied areas such as behavioral medicine since the regulation (or deregulation) of the human organism is viewed within a broader social context. You will find these benefits illustrated in many of the chapters comprising this book. Our goal in the remainder of this introductory chapter is to review briefly the historical roots of social psychophysiology (see also Cacioppo & Petty, in press-a; Crider, Chapter 2, this volume), some of the fundamental concepts of psychophysiology that are of particular interest to social psychologists, and outline the general organization and contents of the remainder of the book.

BRIEF HISTORY

Evolution of a Perspective

In an early study, Kaplan, Burch, Bloom, and Edelberg (1963) investigated whether a strong affective relationship between members of a small group was reflected in more correlated social behavior and electrodermal activity (amplitude of EDA and number of spontaneous skin conductance responses). Medical students served as subjects in four-member groups, which were organized to represent affectively positive, affectively negative, and affectively neutral interpersonal relationships among group members. Each group met for five 45-minute discussions, during which time each participant's social behavior and EDA were recorded. Kaplan *et al.* (1963) observed that the social behavior and EDA of persons who initially either liked or disliked each other were more correlated than the behavior and EDA of persons who initially felt neutrally toward one another. Although it is not clear from this study whether the observed differences in overt behavior contributed to or accounted for the patterns of EDA that were obtained (a point to which we will return), the study is notable in its attempt to address the relationship between physiological and social psychological processes (see also Smith, 1936, described in Crider, Chapter 2).

The *earliest* writings reflecting an interest in the relationship between physiological and psychological processes appear to date back to the time of the ancient Greeks (e.g., about 500 B.C. in Plato's *Theatetus*). Plato conceived of the intellectual, emotional, and instinctual aspects of human behavior as being located in the head, heart and spinal marrow, and lower spinal cord and liver, respectively. Galen (a Roman physician of about A.D. 150) and Erastratos (a physician during the reign of Alexander the Great) were apparently among the first to use *psychophysiological* observations (e.g., the initiation of an irregular pulse beat when one's lover's name was mentioned) to isolate the *social* cause of a person's distress (i.e., "lovesickness"—see Mesulam & Perry, 1972).

Empirical research, even in the general area of psychophysiology, is still fairly recent, though, having begun only about 100 years ago (e.g., Angell & Thompson, 1899, provide an interesting review of some of this early research). Stern *et al.* (1980) suggest that the influential Platonic belief that empirical research was misleading because our senses deceived us, deflected scholarly efforts to acquire knowledge about the interrelationships between psychological processes and physiological events from scientific inquiry and into philosophical argument. Following the Renaissance and with the onset of the Age of Reason, this Platonic belief and occult superstitions that had developed began to give way to scientific thought about and studies of psychophysiological relationships. Still, prior to the development of the oscillograph (polygraph), the emergence of this research perspective was mired by technical problems in obtaining measures of gross physiological events that were reasonably free of artifacts and that were amenable to psychological interpretation (see Hoff, 1936). Hence, the coagulation of the scientific study of psychophysiology was closely coupled with the development and refinement of the oscillograph (Sternbach, 1966). In addition, the measures from early instrumentation were insensitive unless the investigator was particularly skillful. Consequently, much of the early research was characterized by the use of powerful experimental treatments that allowed an investigator to observe event-related physiological responses despite his or her somewhat noisy measures. Chester Darrow (1929), for instance, once used an unexpected gunshot to elicit a startle response. This research tactic, of course, seriously limited the utility of psychophysiological methods for studying subtle physiological events and syndromes, which theoretically were imbued with information regarding specific psychological states and processes (e.g., Darwin, 1872/1904; James, 1884).

In the 1940s, technical advances in electronics set the stage for the emergence of and improvements in the oscillograph, which allowed researchers to measure a variety of subtle electrical and physical forces within a person. In the 1960s, a pair of influential books on techniques in psychophysiology appeared (Brown, 1967; Venables & Martin, 1967), and for the first time the state of the art of sensing, amplifying, recording, and quantifying gross physiological responses in intact humans was widely available to researchers in other disciplines.

It is pertinent to note that almost all of the chapters in these early books centered on discussions of the physiological events being sought and the proper use of polygraphic instrumentation for monitoring these events. This meant that issues dealing with sensing and amplifying bioelectrical events subsumed most of the discussion, and issues surrounding the quantification of the data and the experimental context were paid little heed (cf. Martin & Venables, 1980, p. 2).

However, physiological variables, as Shapiro and Crider (1969) noted, are measures of nothing but themselves and cannot be taken as intrinsically more revealing indicators of psychological constructs than overt behaviors. "A response measure, whether of overt or covert functioning, has meaning only in the context of observation" (Shapiro & Crider, 1969, p. 3). As instrumentation and issues surrounding the proper use of the polygraph were more or less resolved (e.g., Jennings, Berg, Hutcheson, Obrist, Porges, & Turpin, 1981), important and troublesome issues regarding data quantification, analysis, and interpretation came to the forefront. For instance, there is a developing consensus that a physiological response must not only be interpreted within the context of other physiological events (e.g., see Schwartz, 1982), but also within the experimental and subjective (phenomenological) contexts in which it occurs (e.g., Cacioppo & Petty, 1982a; Shapiro & Reeves, 1982). As a consequence, the questions asked in early social psychophysiological research are being reconsidered with increasing sophistication and scientific yields (see Fridlund & Izard, Chapter 9, this volume).

In sum, the standardization and modernization of recording procedures have raised the likelihood that reliable, comparable, and valid measurements of physiological events can be collected by researchers with relatively brief training and access to technical consultants. The sophistication of equipment has increased over the years, but subjects are being made ever less aware of the (potentially) intimidating apparatus involved in much of this research. The experimental treatments to which subjects are now commonly exposed need not be nearly as traumatizing as was the case several decades ago, and the sample and sensitivity of the electrophysiological measures are greatly improved. Finally, the use of an oscillograph is no longer a defining attribute of research in social psychophysiology (or psychophysiology in general—see Martin & Venables, 1980, p. 2), as new instrumentation (e.g., laboratory computers) and innovative methodologies (e.g., rating photographic composites, misattribution procedures) yield important findings bearing on the interdependence of physiological processes and social stimuli.

Research Strategies: Illustration of Correlational and Experimental Approaches

Perhaps the major guiding conception held by psychophysiologists is that physiological and psychological events occur within the same biological system and constitute interdependent aspects of the same process. This does not mean that information from these domains is redundant, or that one field of inquiry can profitably be reduced to the other (cf. Cacioppo, 1982; Furedy, 1981; Lang, 1971; O'Connor, 1981). In the preceding section, we alluded briefly to a number of ways that the relationships between physiological and social psychological processes have been studied. (A more detailed discussion of this issue is provided by Crider, Chapter 2, this volume.) In this section we review the two most common design strategies employed, correlational and experimental studies, as they apply to current research in social psychophysiology.

The oldest and least demanding of the two research strategies is based on the simple view that behavioral and physiological events are strictly covariants (Porges & Coles, 1976). Often the motive for studies employing a correlative approach is that knowledge of a physiological event will serve as an index for an emotional state or behavioral predisposition. Cooper (1959), in an article in *Science* entitled "Emotion and Prejudice," for instance, argued that an individual's prejudice could be gauged by monitoring the size of the momentary change in EDA following his or her exposure to the attitude object or issue (but see Cacioppo & Sandman, 1981; Petty & Cacioppo, Chapter 3, this volume). Although investigators have not always heeded the interpretive limitations of correlational studies, no assertion regarding the influence of one event (e.g., the accessing of a prejudice) on another (e.g., increased EDA) is justified.

One task in social psychophysiology stimulated by this analytic approach is the specification of *which* significant social and physiological events covary. Perfect covariation is theoretically not to be found since covert and overt responses are also thought to contain unique information about the underlying mechanisms of each (see Schwartz, 1982). Hence, a second, complementing task is to specify the psychological significance of *failures* to find covariation between these classes of events. For example, Tursky, Lodge, and Reeder (1979) conducted a cross-modal (psychophysical and psychophysiological) study to determine the race-relatedness of political words and phrases. Psychophysical measures included category and magnitude scaling, whereas the psychophysiological measure was skin conductance responses (SCRs) following the classical conditioning of these responses (i.e., they served previously as conditioned responses) to black-related and white-related words and phrases (e.g., "slavery" and "Caucasian" served as the conditioned stimuli, whereas 1-second white-noise blasts served as the unconditioned stimulus). As expected, the psychophysical and psychophysiological measures both yielded gradients of race-relatedness when test words were presented in the second part of the experiment. However, there were differences in both the order and amplitude of the responses obtained from these psychophysical and psychophysiological measures. Although no definitive evidence was provided, Tursky *et al.* (1979) suggested that "it is possible that the automatic response properties of the autonomic nervous system override the intellectual or social desirability properties which produced the similar judgmental responses (on the psychophysical tasks)" (p. 461; for more details, see Tursky & Jamner, Chapter 4, this volume).

The explanation of associations and dissociations between psychophysiological and social events is best evaluated using the more powerful, experimental research strategy. Often the guiding assumption in studies employing this approach is that if a manipulation of one (e.g., social) event leads to an increase or decrease in the magnitude of another (e.g., psychophysiological) event, then the former is causally related to the latter. One problem with this line of reasoning, however, is in specifying what exactly constitutes a social event. For instance, in the Kaplan *et al.* (1963) study on affective relationships and EDA reviewed above, the manipulation of the intensity of the interpersonal attachments were confounded with the intensity (i.e., amount of physical and cognitive activity) of the social interactions. This made it impossible to determine whether the cognitive, conative, or affective component of the social interactions was responsible for the observed differences in EDA.

A second problem involves specifying exactly what constitutes a "physiological event." For instance, a wetness of the palms may correlate with intense concentration, muscular exertion, or a warm environment. The single physiological response, palmar sweating, does not constitute the most appropriate physiological response to study if one wants to understand these various events. Although the output at the palms may appear the same, the antecedent physiological processes and the output at various other physiological effectors[1] (e.g., the heart) may differ among these conditions (e.g., see Fowles, 1982; Schwartz, 1982). For example, heart rate

---

1. The term "effector" refers to the smooth muscle cells of the viscera and the blood vessels, striated skeletal-muscular cells, and glandular cells that are innervated by (i.e., receive neural signals from) efferent (outwardly traveling) neurons.

may decrease during intense attention, increase during muscular exertion, and remain fairly constant when the ambient temperature rises slightly— while palmar sweating may increase in each instance (e.g., see B. C. Lacey & Lacey, 1974). For this reason, the *pattern* of physiological responses, rather than the intensity of the output of any single physiological effector, is in many instances regarded as the most informative "physiological response" for study.

The problems regarding the interpretation of experimental studies in social psychophysiology are by no means limited to this field, but are illustrated briefly here because of the relative novelty of their form. More detailed discussion of experimental psychophysiological methods are provided in the chapters by McGuigan (Chapter 22), McHugo and Lanzetta (Chapter 23), and Cacioppo, Marshall-Goodell, and Gormezano (Chapter 24). In the following section, selected concepts, heuristics, and principles from the field of psychophysiology that will be encountered throughout this book are surveyed.

OVERVIEW OF SELECTED CONCEPTS

The human organism possesses two major systems for biological control and communication. The fastest is the nervous system with its nerve cells spanning the distances between the brain and internal or peripheral receptors and effectors. The endocrine system, which operates through the release of chemical hormones from glands into the blood, is slower and generally more diffuse acting (at least when the hormones are released outside the brain) than the nervous system. Although increasing attention is being directed by psychophysiologists toward the endocrine system (e.g., see Christie & Woodman, 1980), by far most work in social psychophysiology concerns physiological events associated directly with the functioning of the human nervous system. For that reason, the contributions comprising this book are slanted toward discussions of the human nervous system rather than the endocrine system. The endocrine system *is* described briefly in this chapter to familiarize the reader with a potentially important domain for future study.

The Nervous System

The human nervous system serves to transmit quickly information concerning the external (i.e., physical) and internal (i.e., biological) environments to reflexive response mechanisms (e.g, the simple reflex arc of the knee) and/or to integrative neural structures in the brain. These neural structures are, in turn, the source of decisions and instructions to the skeletal muscles to act (or inhibit action) on the external environment and to the viscera and glands to act (or inhibit action) on the internal environment. The incoming information travels along *afferent* or sensory neural

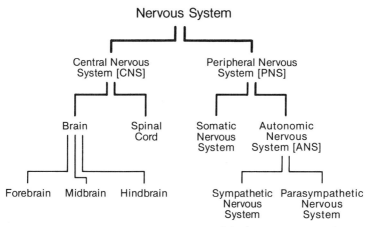

FIGURE 1-1. Classification of the divisions of the human nervous system.

pathways, whereas the instructions travel along *efferent* or commandatory neural pathways.

The human nervous system can be divided anatomically into distinct segments (see Figure 1-1). The *central nervous system* (CNS) represents the majority of the neural fibers in the body and is comprised of the brain and spinal cord located within the vertebral column and the cranium. The portion of the nervous system that extends from the CNS to the outlaying areas of the body is termed the *peripheral nervous system* (PNS) and is comprised of the somatic and autonomic nervous systems. Simply speaking, the primary function of the PNS is to detect internal and external environmental changes, transmit this information to the CNS in temporally and spatially summated afferent volleys,[2] and carry the consequent instructions to the appropriate effector organs. The CNS primarily serves to integrate the incoming information, store or alter the storage of the detected events, and initiate preparatory or compensatory actions. Not all of the information that impinges on sensory receptors is transmitted to the CNS (e.g., sensory receptors are not stimulated by X rays), and not all of the information that is received by the CNS is reportable even when this information affects behavior (e.g., we cannot typically report the sensory information used to maintain various postures). (These and other points regarding bodily sensation and perception are discussed below.)

2. Afferent volleys refer to the sensory information traveling to the CNS. These afferent signals consist of the firing of neurons that are oriented in such a manner as to link a receptor to the CNS. Any single neuron either fires (depolarizes) or not, depending on such factors as the intensity of the stimulus and the prestimulus state of the neuron. Unique trains of afferent signals can derive from a single neuron firing at various frequencies (called temporal summation) and/or from multiple neurons spread across an area of the body firing nearly simultaneously (called spatial summation).

The PNS can be further divided into the *somatic nervous system* and the *autonomic nervous system*. The somatic system carries information to and from the external sense receptors (exteroceptors, which includes teleceptors such as the eyes), skeletal muscles (e.g., biceps), and somatic receptors (proprioceptors, providing information about muscle tension) and regulates the bodily processes commonly thought to be controlled voluntarily (e.g., muscle movements). The autonomic nervous system traditionally is considered only an output system. The autonomic nervous system carries information to glands (e.g., thymus) and smooth muscles (e.g., stomach), and regulates the bodily processes over which it is generally more difficult to exert direct, voluntary control (e.g., heart rate). Feedback from these effectors travels along visceral afferents which are distinguished by definition from the autonomic nervous system. Obviously, however, the signals traveling along the visceral afferents are a function of autonomic activity.

The autonomic nervous system functions primarily to maintain equilibrium (i.e., homeostasis) in the internal environment and can be further subdivided into the *sympathetic* and *parasympathetic nervous systems* because of their anatomical, neurochemical, and functional distinctions (Van Toller, 1979). The sympathetic system consists of nerve fibers that originate in the thoracic and lumbar portions of the spinal cord, between the cervical (neck) and sacral (lower spinal) regions (see Figure 1-2). The sympathetic system tends (though not invariantly) to act as a unit and in a manner that excites the organs and glands to which it travels. These effects are depicted graphically in Figure 1-2.

The parasympathetic branch of the autonomic nervous system consists of nerve fibers originating in the areas of the cranium and spinal cord above and below the sympathetic branch (i.e., cranial and sacral regions). Unlike the sympathetic branch, the parasympathetic branch tends to act in a specific fashion, affecting one organ at a time, and usually in a manner that quiets or decreases activity. There are important exceptions to the principle that sympathetic and parasympathetic activity are antagonistic, some of which are evident by an inspection of Figure 1-2. More detailed discussions of this topic can be found in Gardner (1975) and Van Toller (1979).

The brain occupies the crowning and ruling position in the human nervous system. The brain can be broken down into three gross components: hindbrain, midbrain, and forebrain. Although a comprehensive review of brain structures and functions is well beyond the scope of this chapter or book, the rudimentary nature of the brain, the most complex and powerful integration center in the body, can be obtained from this gross categorization.

The brain, now accepted as the nesting place of cognitive processes (see Hassett & Danforth, 1982, and Uttal, 1975, for historical views), emerges from the spinal cord as the *hindbrain* (see Figures 1-3 and 1-4). The

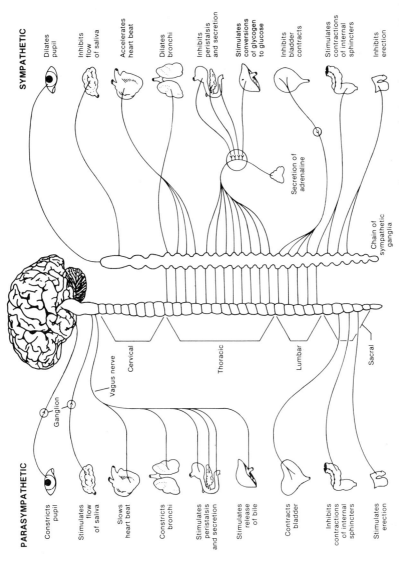

FIGURE 1-2. Divisions of the autonomic nervous system, and the influences of the sympathetic and parasympathetic branches. Adapted from Netter (1974).

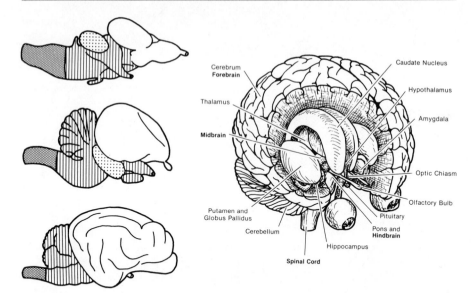

FIGURE 1-3. The central nervous system (CNS) can be subdivided into smaller segments according to gross appearance, embryology, or cellular organization. In the left panel (adapted from Nauta & Karten, 1970) are pictured schematics of the CNS of the frog (top-left panel), pigeon (middle-left panel), and cat (bottom-left panel). The human brain is depicted in the right panel (adapted from Nauta & Feirtag, 1979). Note that the drawings are made on very different scales.

hindbrain is the most primitive component of the human brain and maintains the general tubular structure of the spinal cord. As is apparent in Figures 1-3 and 1-4, the hindbrain includes the subcortical neural structures called the medulla and the pons. The medulla is the port for most (7 of 12) of the cranial nerves and contains specific nuclei (clusters of neural cell bodies) that are associated with the autonomic nervous system, specifically the life-sustaining functions of cardiac, respiratory, and gastrointestinal activity. The pons is located just above the medulla and (the pons proper) bridges between the cerebrum and cerebellum. The pons also serves as a relay for motor fibers connecting the cortex and the spinal cord (e.g., actions in nuclei in the pons can inhibit or facilitate movement and respiratory activity).

The *midbrain*, which appears to have evolved after and above the hindbrain, is located just above the pons and retains the basic tubular form of the spinal cord. The lower portion of the midbrain houses nuclei important in the control of eye movement and neural tracts interconnecting the upper and lower portions of the brain. The upper portion of the midbrain, which is bounded at the top by the thalamus and hypothalamus, houses nuclei that act as important relays for the auditory and visual systems (see Figures 1-3 and 1-4).

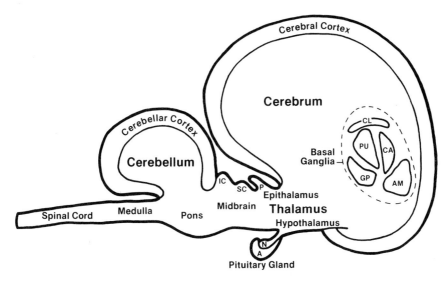

FIGURE 1-4. Highly schematized representation of some major structures of the mammalian central nervous system. The spinal cord, as it enters the cranium, becomes the medulla, pons, midbrain, and thalamus. These are somewhat arbitrary divisions (they have no specific "functions" except as improperly designated in classical texts), and the portion inside the cranium (the medulla, pons, midbrain, and thalamus) is known as the brainstem. Pairs of cranial nerves (to and from the brainstem) and pairs of spinal nerves (to and from the spinal cord) form the segments of the CNS. Usually, the number of cranial nerves is considered to be 12, and the number of spinal nerves depends on the species (humans have 31). Thus, 43 pairs (left and right) of nerves constitute the peripheral nervous system (somatic and autonomic—see Figure 1-1) of humans. Superimposed on the brainstem are the two suprasegmental structures, the cerebellum and the cerebrum. The major link to the cerebrum is the thalamus and the major links to the cerebellum are the pons and medulla. However, all parts are interconnected: There are approximately 10^{11} units (the neurons), and each unit makes about 10^{4} connections, yielding 10^{15} interconnections within the brain (DeFeudis & DeFeudis, 1977). The outer layer of the cerebellum and the cerebrum consists of cell bodies of neurons and are called the cerebellar and cerebral cortex, respectively. Another dense collection of cell bodies is found in the cerebrum, the basal ganglia (caudate, putamen, globus pallidus, amygdala, claustrum). There are glandular structures attached to the thalamus called the pineal gland and the pituitary gland. The pineal gland produces melatonin, an anti-gonadal substance, and the pituitary produces at least 10 substances which control peripheral endocrine glands, reproductive physiology, milk production and milk let-down, and other metabolic processes. Abbreviations: P,pineal gland; IC,inferior colliculus, SC,superior colliculus (both forming the roof of the midbrain); N,neurohypophysis, A,adenohypophysis (both forming the pituitary gland); AM,amygdala, CA,caudate, PU,putamen, GP,globus pallidus, CL,claustrum (forming the basal ganglia). Figure and description courtesy Walter L. Randall.

Also pervasive in the hindbrain and midbrain is a network of cell bodies, fibers, and nuclei extending from the spinal cord to the thalamus known as the reticular formation. The reticular formation has been suggested as serving the function of controlling the level of cortical excitation or general physiological arousal (e.g., Lindsley, 1951):

> In terms of evolution it is probable that, at a certain period of time in nervous tissue development, an animal existed having an internal vegetative nervous system and a brain that was little more than a hindbrain with a general activating role. This system would roughly correspond to what we now understand as the reticular activating system. Thus, we might expect to find a special and close relationship between the reticular activating system and the autonomic nervous system arising from an earlier evolutionary stage. (Van Toller, 1979, p. 43)

As Van Toller (1979) notes, however, this statement is speculative. More recently, disputes about the specificity of the actions of the reticular formation have emerged (e.g., see Grossman, 1973). As Van Toller (1979) notes, the reticular activating system is not a simple homogeneous structure, but rather "complex aggregations of nuclei and neuronal pathways that can be shown to have specific effects" (p. 85).

Perhaps the simplest illustration of the orchestrated actions of the hindbrain and midbrain (including the reticular formation) comes from animal (e.g., cat) studies in which all brain tissue above the midbrain is removed. These animals can continue to live for extended periods of time. The vast repertoires of behavior that these animals normally display are lost; nevertheless, these animals are more than simply "aroused or not." They can walk and sleep, eat and vocalize, move about, and in notably simple forms, express emotion and display learning (e.g., Norman, Buchwald, & Villablanca, 1977). It should not be surprising that people are generally unaware of the activities transpiring under the "control" of the hindbrain and midbrain and yet are influenced substantially by bodily processes occurring here that are more complex than subcortical arousal.

The most recent evolutionary development, the *forebrain*, is the focus of most investigations in mental processes such as perception, voluntary movements, thinking, learning, and memory. The forebrain, although anatomically distinct (it no longer is characterized in form by the tubular structure of the spinal cord), operates in conjunction with the hindbrain and midbrain, and ascriptions of "functions" to specific loci in the brain are oversimplifications (adopted here for didactic purposes only). With this cavaet, we proceed to outline briefly the actions in which the following components of the forebrain appear to be influential: thalamus, hypothalamus, limbic system, and cerebral cortex.

The thalamus, which you may recall is located just above the midbrain, serves as a sensory relay station. Nuclei within the thalamus receive neural signals from afferent pathways and channel them to specific regions in the cerebral cortex (e.g., the somatic sensory, visual, or auditory cortex). The thalamus appears to be among the systems of nuclei that modulate the EEG activity of the cortex.

A cluster of nuclei just above the midbrain and beneath the thalamus (just above the top of the mouth) is called the hypothalamus, which, through its influence on the endocrine system (via the pineal gland), is related to feeding, fighting, fleeing, sexual behavior, sleeping, drinking, and regulating body temperature. The hypothalamus is also part of a wide-ranging set of neural structures called the limbic system. Like the lower portions of the brain, the limbic system appears to be related to the regulation of the autonomic nervous system, although these influences are not necessarily redundant. The limbic system is also interconnected with regions in the cerebral cortex, most notably with regions in the temporal and frontal cortex. The limbic system has been said to suppress the activities of the more primitive hindbrain and midbrain (Isaacson, 1974), interpret the total sensory input as pleasant or unpleasant and thereby contribute to somatovisceral approach–avoidance actions (Watts, 1975), and regulate the expression of emotion and motivation (Thompson, 1967—see Van Toller, 1979).

Finally, the uppermost portion of the human brain is the cerebral cortex. The major divisions of the cortex are the frontal, temporal, parietal, and occipital lobes. Although oversimplified, you might find it useful to think of visual percepts arising from a portion of the occipital cortex, skin, and muscle percepts arising from the forward portion of the parietal lobe, auditory percepts arising from parts of the temporal cortex, and the control of voluntary movements emanating from a strip of cortex separating the frontal and parietal lobes. The remaining portions of the cortex are called association areas since these areas are presumably involved in more complex associative processes. For instance, association areas within the frontal lobe are related to planning and temporal ordering, and association areas within the temporal lobes are involved in language and spatial processes. The specificity in form and function that exists in the human nervous system serves well the vast and flexible behavioral repertoires of humans. It also calls into question the overreliance on or simplistic notions of physiological arousal.

Physiological Arousal

Physiological arousal, which has been an important heuristic in social psychology as well as psychophysiology, refers to the intensity of physiological functioning. Physiological arousal has typically been defined as the degree of general or diffuse physiological responding (e.g., speed of heart rate, amount of EDA), and synonyms have included activation, excitation, and energy mobilization.

Although there are subtle distinctions among some of the early arousal theories (Duffy, 1957; Lindsley, 1951; Malmo, 1959), the major points of these theories can be stated simply (see Shapiro & Crider, 1969): Behavioral processes are viewed as consisting of a directional component, which represents the orientation of the person toward a goal, and an intensive component, which specifies the concomitant degree of energy expenditure. The intensive component is viewed as being synonymous with the level of neural activity in the CNS and as exerting an effect on performance. According to arousal theory, behavioral efficiency increases as arousal increases to some optimal level, after which point behavioral efficiency decreases as arousal continues to increase. Malmo (1959), for instance, monitored the heart rate and bar-pressing activities of rats across 72 hours of food deprivation. He found that the heart rate of the rats increased steadily across the 72-hour period, whereas bar pressing for water increased for the first 36 hours and then decreased in frequency. Hebb (1955) proposed that the brain arousal system is the neural basis of generalized motivational states, or drive; Hebb's notion of the brain arousal system was based on Lindsley's (1951) suggestion that the EEG reflected the neural substrates of behavioral arousal.

As theoretically appealing as the concept of arousal has been for social psychologists and psychophysiologists, matters regarding this concept are more complicated than are typically acknowledged. The finding and mapping of the reticular formation (Moruzzi & Magoun, 1949), which initially appeared to serve as a general arousal mechanism for the brain, for a time provided a physiological locus for the construct of arousal. But as noted above, the reticular formation is not as homogeneous as was first believed. Apparently, it is a collection of nuclei that can have specific effects depending on the site of stimulation as well as divergent effects depending on the intensity of stimulation (see Grossman, 1973; Van Toller, 1979). This suggests that even if a noninvasive measure of reticular activation was feasible, it might be an insufficient index of a general and diffuse state of physiological, reportable, and behavioral arousal.

In addition, in the last several decades of research, specific conceptual problems have been raised regarding arousal notions. The basic assumption regarding the measurement of physiological arousal has been that, although some general measure of the level of excitation characterizing the CNS would be best, *any* measure of the extent that the sympathetic dominated the parasympathetic nervous system would serve as a valid and sensitive measure. For instance, the degree of activation of an autonomic (e.g., heart rate) *or* somatic (e.g., general muscle tonus) measure could serve as a convenient indirect measure of arousal within the CNS (Duffy, 1957). Still other researchers suggested that the EEG be used to index physiological arousal more directly (e.g., Lindsley, 1957). They point out that during sleep, EEG activity is typically slow. During waking, thinking states, EEG activity is much faster and asynchronous. Finally, since these various physiological processes were presumed to covary (Cannon, 1939), it was not considered crucial which peripheral measure of physiological arousal was used; all were believed to yield approximately the same information regarding the excitation of the CNS. It was, therefore, an influential criticism of the conceptualization of physiological arousal when J.I. Lacey (1967) indicated that this basic assumption was incorrect; that electrocortical, autonomic, somatic, and behavioral measures do not tend to covary. Indeed, Lacey has argued that even the physiological responses obtained from effectors within a single system (e.g., the autonomic nervous system) are not highly correlated. J. I. Lacey, Kagan, Lacey, and Moss (1963), for example, found that when subjects performed a task that required them to monitor flashing lights, the subjects' heart rate decreased while electrodermal activity increased. This *directional fractionation* of physiological responding across and within physiological systems constitutes an important problem for arousal theory: Are the subjects more aroused (as, e.g., their electrodermal activity might indicate) or less aroused (as their heart rate might suggest) during than before the task?

A second issue that has emerged concerns the relationship between physiological arousal and reportable arousal. Mackay (1980) has suggested that a person's self-report of arousal may be a good or better measure of actual physiological arousal than any one physiological measure. This suggestion, however, ignores the empirical independence that has been found to exist among physiological, reportable, and behavioral states (e.g., Lang, 1971; Lazarus, Averill, & Opton, 1970) and the work indicating that felt (reportable) arousal subsides more quickly than do the increases in heart rate and blood pressure that follow exercise (Zillmann, 1978; see Zillmann, Chapter 8, this volume). It would seem to be more useful *at this stage* not to assume that general physiological arousal, reportable levels of felt physiological arousal, and overt behavioral arousal necessarily covary (see Cacioppo & Petty, 1982a). Treatment of these constructs as being independent may allow a speedier identification of suitable operationalizations of each, what factors lead to their convergence (e.g., following dramatic events such as a near accident—see Lang, 1971; Mewborn & Rogers, 1979), and the relationship between each and social behavior (e.g., see Kelley & Byrne, Chapter 16, this volume).

In sum, although the concept of arousal has been important in psychophysiology and social psychology, the existing data still support Shapiro and Crider's (1969) conclusion that "the major contribution of arousal theory has been to provide a unifying hypothesis for encouraging . . . research rather than its ability to organize the data so obtained" (p. 25). The evidence that a single physiological measure cannot be used to gauge the state of general physiological arousal suggests that aggregates of physiological measures of CNS excitation (see McHugo & Lanzetta, Chapter 23, this volume) or changes in hormonal levels (see Mason, 1972) may serve as the best index, while analyses of the profiles of multiple physiological responses may harbor yet additional information about social psychological processes (e.g., see Fridlund & Izard, Chapter 9). It is to the issue of physiological response patterning that we turn next.

Response Patterns

It is useful to think of any single physiological response as the result of multiple influences operating on a physiological mechanism at any one moment in time. Physiological arousal may be one of these influences, but certainly it is not the only or most influential one. Five other influences that are described in this section are individual response stereotypy, stimulus response stereotypy, cognitive sets, the orienting response, and the defense response.

Individual Response Stereotypy (IRS)

IRS represents the tendency for the same person to display the same profile of physiological response to a wide variety of eliciting situations and stimuli. This characteristic manifests as a *response hierarchy*. This means that, for any one individual, stimuli consistently elicit the greatest change in responding from one effector (e.g., a change in heart rate), the second greatest change in responding from some other effector (e.g., electrodermal changes), and so on. Thus, which effector responds most, second most, and so forth, to stimuli varies across individuals. The ordering of which effector responds most, second most, and so on, constitutes the individual's response hierarchy. Differences among people in their response hierarchies constitute the notion of IRS (J. I. Lacey, 1959; J. I. Lacey & Lacey, 1958).

Stimulus Response Stereotypy (SRS)

SRS represents the tendency for a situation or stimulus to elicit a common pattern or profile of responses from various people. A horrific picture (e.g., a photograph of an autopsy), for instance, tends to elicit a slowing of heart rate and an increase in electrodermal activity in almost everyone (e.g., Cacioppo & Sandman, 1978; Hare, Wood, Britain, & Shadman, 1971). In other words, SRS refers to the inclination for the same physiological pattern to be evinced by most individuals when confronted by a particular situation or stimulus (J. I. Lacey, 1959; J. I. Lacey et al., 1963). These response profiles may serve as useful indices of social psychological constructs within particular contexts (e.g., see Chapter 3); in addition, the Laceys (1974) have suggested that they reflect different reciprocal transactions between the person and the environment.

Cognitive Sets

Another influence on physiological responding is termed cognitive set (Sternbach, 1966). This refers to the effect on physiology of a person's expectations or interpretations of a stimulus. It is this influence that has been the focus of much of the research on psychosomatic disorders. This concept is illustrated in psychophysiology by the finding that people who believe they are being touched by the leaves of a tree to which they are allergic display an allergic reaction even when they are, in fact, being touched by harmless leaves (Ikemi & Nakagawa, 1962). That is, their physiological responses are influenced as much by their subjective interpretation of the stimulation as by the objective attributes of the stimulus (see also O'Connor, 1981).

Orienting Response (OR)

The notion of an orienting or "what-is-it" response emerged from Pavlov's (1927) studies of classical conditioning in dogs. Pavlov observed that a dog's conditioned response to a stimulus would fail to appear if some unexpected event occurred:

> It is this reflex [the OR] which brings about the immediate response in men and animals to the slightest changes in the world around them, so that they immediately orientate their appropriate receptor organ in accordance with the perceptible quality in the agent bringing about the change, making a full investigation of it. The biological significance of this reflex is obvious. (Pavlov, 1927, p. 12)

An OR occurs in response to a novel stimulus to facilitate a possible adaptive behavioral response to the stimulus (Sokolov, 1963). Lynn (1966) has summarized the physiological profile of an OR as: decreased heart rate, increased sensitivity of the sense organs, increased skin conductance and general muscle tonus (but a decrease in irrelevant muscle activity), pupil dilation, vasoconstriction in the limbs and vasodilation in the head, and more asynchronous, low-voltage EEG activity.

Defense Response (DR)

Stimuli that would normally elicit an OR, if extremely intense, would elicit a DR instead. Thus, the DR appears to be the complement of the OR and functions to protect an organism from intense stimulation. For instance, there is a decrease rather than an increase in the sensitivity of sense organs, vasoconstriction occurs in both the limbs and head, heart rate increases, and postural shifts are away from rather than toward the stimulus (see Lynn, 1966).

Interestingly, whether a stimulus elicits a DR or OR can be affected by an individual's cognitive set. An interesting study illustrating this point is reported by Hare (1973). Subjects were shown slides of spiders and of more neutral content (e.g., landscapes). Hare (1973) found that subjects who were very afraid of spiders evinced the physiological pattern of a DR to the slides of spiders, whereas subjects who were not afraid of spiders exhibited the physiological pattern of an OR to these slides.

In sum, there are subtle distinctions among the concepts of physiological arousal, stimulus and individual response stereotypies, cognitive sets, and orienting and defense responses that are important to consider when interpreting psychophysiological data. Each concept refers to a different form of influence on psychophysiological relationships, and several of these influences can coexist within the organism at any one moment in time.

Law of Initial Values

Thus far we have discussed topics including the intensity (arousal) and direction of physiological responses as they are affected by the stimulus (stimulus response stereotypy), the individual's physiological response hierarchy (individual response stereotypy), the individual's interpretation of or subjective response to the stimulus (cognitive set) and the individual's orienting or defensive responses to stimuli. It should be obvious now why observing one or two physiological responses provides equivocal information regarding the "arousal" of the organism. Another factor influencing the direction and intensity of physiological responses (and thus the pattern of activity and the meaning of any single response) is the degree to which the output at the effector is elevated (or reduced) from the homeostatic level *prior* to the presentation of a stimulus. Consider two people standing quietly when a passing car backfires unexpectedly. These people are likely to display quite a change in their level of activity. Their facial expressions might change quite drastically, and they might jump away from the source of the noise. But now consider these same two people jogging instead of standing in this area. Their muscles are already tense and active. When the car backfires, the intensity and perhaps even the direction of the *change* in muscle activity (i.e., the "event-related responses") may be different in the persons when jogging than when simply standing calmly.

Any evoked, short-term physiological response may be determined in part by the prestimulus level of activity. This possible relationship has been described as the "law of initial values" (Benjamin, 1963; Wilder, 1931/1976). According to this "law," the response to a stimulus is smaller (and eventually, inverted) the higher the prestimulus level of activity in the effector (e.g., cardiovascular) system. The implication of this principle is that the relationship between covert and overt responses may appear in one of a variety of forms, depending on the initial level of physiological activity.[3] Thus, the pattern of physiological responses may vary slightly if a person is calm or anxious when the experimental stimuli are introduced.

To circumvent this problem, most psychophysiological investigations involve persons who display a fairly calm and quiet physiological state prior to the introduction of any experimental manipulation. This feat is accomplished most often by having subjects sit quietly in (i.e., "adapt to") the laboratory for several minutes prior to the introduction of any experimental stimuli. Sometimes, subjects are also given a tour of the laboratory and explanation of the experimental procedure a week or so before they participate in the study (see Cacioppo *et al.*, Chapter 24, this volume). The generalizability of the associations that are found using these procedures to more active environments is, of course, uncertain at present. The development of telemetric measures (compact electrophysiological recording devices that allow a person to move freely) and alternative procedures to electrophysiological measures should be especially informative in this regard.

Habituation

Thus far we have described various contributors to bodily events evoked by a stimulus. The next concept that is discussed is *habituation*, which is a process that complements the process of evoked physiological responding. When the same stimulus is presented repeatedly, there is a diminution of physiological responding (e.g., ORs) to it. This decrement in evoked physiological responsivity is called habituation. Habituation occurs more slowly when, for some reason, the stimulus is attention getting or meaningful. If the stimulus is novel, unique, or complex, physiological responses to it will habituate more slowly than if it is boring or indistinctive. Intense, infrequent, and irregular presentations of a stimulus also slow habituation. Unless the stimulus is extremely intense, however, repeated presentation of the stimulus will eventually cease to be accompanied by (i.e., will fail to evoke) these physiological responses (see also Geen, Chapter 13, this volume).

Depending on the focus of one's study, habituation can be an aid or a hinderance. Researchers typically are not interested in subjects' physiological responses to the laboratory setting per se. Hence, experiments are generally preceded by an "adaptation" period, which is included to allow the subject's physiological responses evoked by the laboratory setting per se to subside. To facilitate this adaptation, the subjects' chambers are

3. This "problem" is not as pervasive as it once seemed. For instance, the law of initial values appears to apply to changes in skin resistance but not substantially to heart rate (see Martin & Venables, 1980; Tursky & Jamner, 1982).

usually characterized by familiar, soothing colors, sound-attenuating walls, ambient temperatures, and a minimum of novel or intimidating-looking furniture and equipment. In other words, precautions are taken to reduce the likelihood that ORs or DRs are elicited by the laboratory (see Chapters 23 and 24). On the other hand, when the independent variable is presented repeatedly, the person *may* habituate to it, too, which can make obtaining a stable-appearing measure of event-related bodily events more difficult. Procedures for securing valid, reliable, and sensitive measures of evoked physiological responses or profiles of responses are discussed in detail in Section III.

Interactive Effects

One characteristic of social psychophysiology is that the object of study is the natural functioning human system in a social context rather than a dissected component or animal model of that system. Interactive effects refer to the characteristics or output of an operating system that could not be predicted additively from knowledge about the characteristics of the components or parts of the system (e.g., see Schwartz, 1982).

A psychophysiological study illustrating this point was reported by Schwartz, Davidson, and Pugash (1976). They taught individuals how to control the EEG activity of the right and left hemispheres of the brain. When the subjects quickened the activity of the right hemisphere of their brain, they reported experiencing an increase in spatial types of thoughts and images. When the subjects activated the left hemisphere, they reported an increase in the frequency of verbal or numerical thoughts. But when both sides of the brain were activated, subjects reported feeling a state of concentration, an effect not predictable by applying an additive model to the previous results. Several chapters in this book contain reports of other instances in which interactive effects have revealed surprising findings with implications for social psychologists and psychophysiologists.

Bodily Sensation and Perception

Although the study of actual physiological responses is unquestionably interesting in its own right and empirically fruitful for advances in social psychology, focus on this information alone yields an incomplete picture of social psychophysiological processes. The physiological responses may be detected by the person, or they may not. If they *are* detected, the physiological reactions may be detected internally as symptoms (i.e., felt bodily sensations) or they may be detected externally as signs (e.g., discoloration of the skin). We suggested this tripartite of bodily responses as a heuristic for interpreting psychophysiological effects in a recent review of attitude change (Cacioppo & Petty, 1982a). For instance, the role of bodily responses in social psychological processes could be considered after classifying the bodily response as a "symptom" (i.e., detected proprioceptively or interoceptively), "sign" (i.e., detected exteroceptively), or undetected. This tripartite yields categories of bodily response that are surprisingly similar to the distinctions drawn in the field of applied pathologic physiology. For instance, MacBryde and Blacklow (1970), in their opening comments in *Signs and Symptoms*, explained:

> As broadly and generally employed, the word *symptom* is used to name any manifestation of disease. Strictly speaking, symptoms are subjective, apparent only to the affected person. *Signs* are detectable by another person and sometimes by the patient himself. Pain and itching are symptoms; jaundice, swollen joints, cardiac murmurs, etc., are physical signs. Some phenomena, like fever, are both signs and symptoms. (p. 1)

In the tripartite applicable to social psychophysiological studies, signs and symptoms are partially overlapping categories of physiological responding, whereas these categories do not overlap with undetected physiological responses. Symptoms refer to the subjective component of a physiological reaction (whether that reaction is constituted by changes in a single effector system or several such systems and whether or not there are identifiable physiological concomitants of the perception), but the physiological reaction need not refer to manifestation of disease. Hence, our use of the term "symptom" is compatible with, but more general than, that characterizing the field of applied pathologic physiology. Signs in the present tripartite refer to the objective component of a physiological reaction that the affected person detects himself or herself. Thus, signs are physiological reactions that are verifiable by others and about which the person learns through an objective procedure, perhaps with the aid of sophisticated instrumentation. As with symptoms, it is not necessary that the "objective" signs have actual physiological manifestations. Thus, bogus feedback (e.g., a faulty thermometer) would be considered a sign. Signs differ from symptoms in that the former is open to public verification or disconfirmation, whereas the latter is not. Signs differ from *undetected* physiological responses *not* in each's potential for being quantified, but rather in the person's awareness that a change in physiological functioning has occurred. For instance, a slight speeding of the heartbeat might be detected by an investigator using an electrocardiogram but go undetected by the individual whose heart rate is being monitored. This response would be termed an undetected response. If the investigator provided feedback to the individual about his or her heart rate, however, the physiological response would act as a sign to the individual even if the feedback is unveridical. Finally, if the individual felt a "speeding" of his or her heart beat, possible because of its association with a concomitant increase in stroke volume, the feeling of a speeding heart beat would serve as a symptom even if this perception were inaccurate.

Given that these distinctions among bodily responses may be important, it is necessary to address the basis of people's sensations and perceptions of bodily events. Traditionally, investigators in sensation and perception have focused on "long-range" senses such as vision and hearing. Fortunately, the search for lawful relationships between physiological events acting as stimuli on humans and the reportable states and overt behaviors they evoke is now being assumed by psychophysiologists (e.g., see Brener, 1977) and social psychologists (see Pennebaker, Chapter 19; Blascovich & Katkin, Chapter 17). In this section, issues and terminology from the area of sensation and perception are surveyed.

Sensation and perception occur only when a stimulus is appropriate and intense enough to activate a particular sense receptor. A physical stimulus can have a substantial influence on an organism without being sensed (e.g., we can be burned by ultraviolet light), but a physical stimulus that *does* lead to a sensation can then be characterized along four dimensions: (1) the *quality* or kind of physical energy that evoked the sensation (e.g., eyes respond to electromagnetic light); (2) the *intensity* of the physical stimulation, which is nonlinearly related to the sensation; (3) the *duration* of the sensation; and (4) the *extent* or area of the stimulation (e.g., localized versus diffuse tactile stimulation).

No one of these dimensions is preeminent. For instance, the electromagnetic waves to which people's eyes respond can vary in length from 380 to 780 nm (a nanometer is one-billionth of a meter). People are exposed, however, to electromagnetic waves that vary from about 10-trillionths of an inch in the case of cosmic rays to several miles in the case of radio waves. This illustrates that people can perceive only a very small segment of the spectrum of physical stimulation even when the quality of the stimulation is appropriate for the receptor mechanism. Similarly, a burst of electromagnetic energy within the range 380 to 780 nm that lasts for a fraction of a millisecond does not lead to the perception of light, even though other necessary characteristics of the stimulus are present (e.g., quality, intensity). In other words, there are *segments* of each of the four dimensions of physical stimulation described above that are necessary preconditions for a percept to be evoked. As is illustrated in Figure 1-5 and in chapters by Scheier, Carver, and Matthews (Chapter 18), Zillmann (Chapter 8), Blascovich and Katkin (Chapter 17), and Pennebaker (Chapter 19), even these factors are necessary but not sufficient for the recognition of a bodily response.

There are three functional classifications for receptors (Schmidt, 1978). *Exteroceptors* transmit information on the immediate environment and include the skin receptors associated with tactile events and the long-

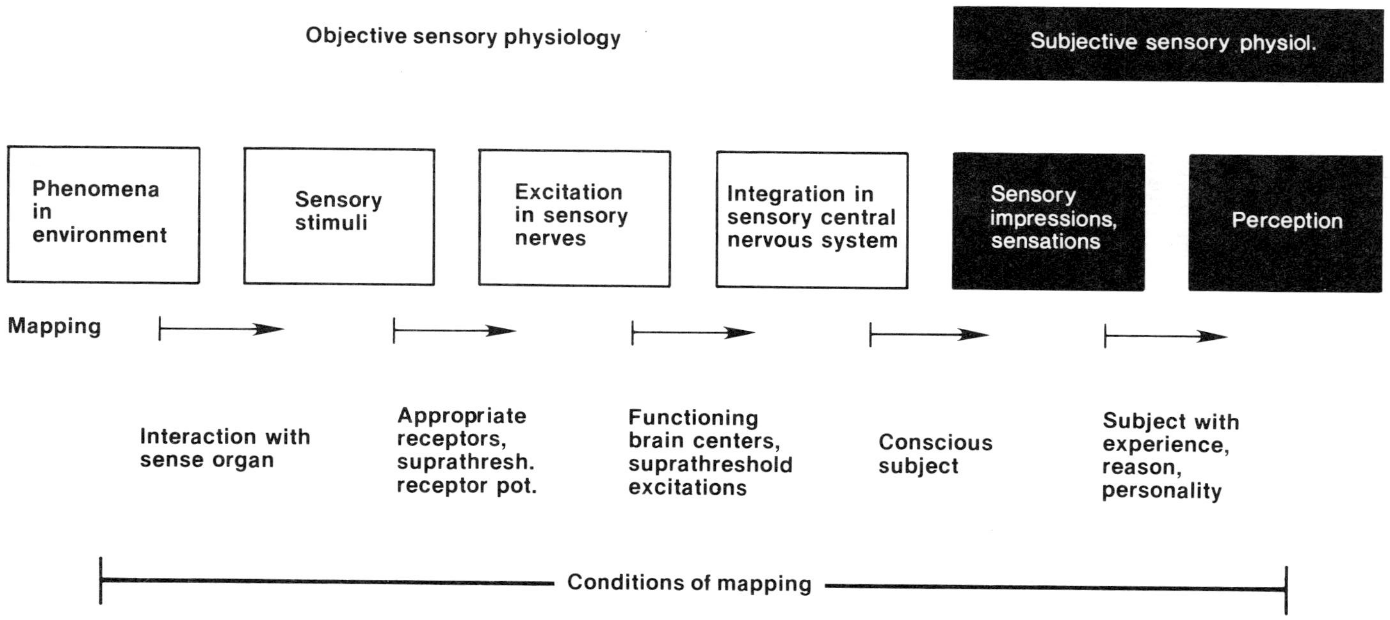

Objective sensory physiology

| Phenomena in environment | Sensory stimuli | Excitation in sensory nerves | Integration in sensory central nervous system |

Subjective sensory physiol.

| Sensory impressions, sensations | Perception |

Mapping

Interaction with sense organ — Appropriate receptors, suprathresh. receptor pot. — Functioning brain centers, suprathreshold excitations — Conscious subject — Subject with experience, reason, personality

Conditions of mapping

FIGURE 1-5. The words in the boxes denote basic phenomena of sensory physiology, and the arrows between them indicate the "mapping" of sensory physiology. Below the basic phenomena, the conditions for mapping are shown. From **Fundamentals of sensory physiology** by R. F. Schmidt, New York: Springer-Verlag, 1978, p. 6. Copyright 1978 by Springer-Verlag, Inc. Reprinted by permission.

27

distance receptors ("teleceptors" such as ears) that transmit information about the distant environment. *Proprioceptors* furnish information about the orientation and position of the body in space and include receptors in the muscles, tendons, and joints. Proprioception, the sensory information traveling to the CNS from proprioceptors, enables people to know when they are smiling, distending their stomach, or pointing their finger. Proprioception also facilitates fine motor movements (e.g., balancing a pencil on a finger) and overlearned movements and motor adjustments (e.g., riding a bicycle). Finally, *interoceptors* provide information about the events that occur in the viscera (internal organs). Interoception, the sensory information traveling to the CNS from interoceptors, enables a person to feel hunger and thus know to eat; and bladder pressure and thus know to excrete. Interoceptors are less localized than other sensory receptors and hence lead to more diffuse or inaccurately localized sensations. For example, the sensation of pain in the abdomen and back may indicate an inflammation of the pancreas (i.e., pancreatitis) or an erosion of an area on the stomach (i.e., a peptic ulcer—see Wasson, Walsh, Sox, & Tomkins, 1975). For the most part, various contributors to this book focus on interoceptive and/or proprioceptive processes and influences.

The Endocrine System

Physiological reactions, and the perceptions of physiological reactions, are influenced by hormonal as well as direct CNS instructions. Since the study of social psychophysiological events is destined to be incomplete until consideration is given to the integrated actions of the nervous and endocrine systems, some highlights in this area are reviewed in this section (see Spitzer & Rodin, Chapter 20, this volume, for one instance). For more detail, the interested reader may wish to consult Mason (1972), Van Toller (1979), or Christie and Woodman (1980).

There are two types of glands in the human body: the *exocrine glands*, which secrete either onto the surface of the body (e.g., sweat or tear glands) or into a cavity within the body (e.g., digestive or salivary glands), and the *endocrine glands*, which secrete their chemical products directly into the bloodstream. Figure 1-6 displays the location of endocrine glands in the human body. Two endocrine mechanisms are described in this section to illustrate their potential interest to social psychologists. These are the sympathetic–adrenomedullary and pituitary–adrenocortical complexes (see Figure 1-6).

The integrated actions of the nervous and endocrine systems are suggested immediately in a survey of the sympathetic–adrenomedullary system. The sympathetic nervous system (via the splanchnics) directly stimulates the medullary cells of the adrenal gland, causing the release of

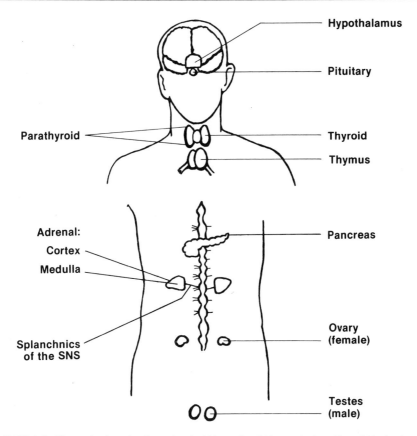

FIGURE 1-6. The endocrine glands are located throughout the central portion of the body and secrete their chemical messengers directly into the bloodstream. The hypothalamus exerts an influence over the pituitary gland, which in turn affects the other endocrine glands.

the catecholamine hormones, epinephrine and norepinephrine. Cannon (1929) believed that the sympathetic–adrenomedullary system was activated primarily during emergency (fight-or-flight) responses and played a role in maintaining homeostasis within the body and adapting to environmental and psychological stressors (see Mason, 1972; Van Toller, 1979).

The actions of the sympathetic–adrenomedullary mechanisms are attributable primarily to epinephrine. These physiological actions include an increase in muscular efficiency (accomplished by reducing muscular tonicity *and* the threshold for firing), increased arterial blood pressure in the muscles and cardiovascular system, and release of glycogen reserves ("animal starch" that the body breaks down to a simple sugar for energy).

Because of differences in the receptors in the arterial walls, catecholamines cause vasodilation within the internal organs (e.g., the brain, heart) and vasoconstriction in the periphery (e.g., at the surface of the skin, in the fingers and hands). This pattern of perfusion has adaptive utility: In emergencies, the CNS and muscles need more blood to mobilize and cope with the situation; the constriction of peripheral areas not only facilitates the rapid redistribution of blood within the body, but also minimizes the loss of blood should an injury be incurred. The physiological effects of norepinephrine (the neurotransmitter of the sympathetic nervous system), although not as general or as powerful as those of epinephrine, are important in regulating cardiovascular and sympathetic tone, thereby allowing blood to be channeled to needed organs and areas. Finally, with the presence of pressure-sensitive receptors in the arterial walls (e.g., Bonvallet & Allen, 1963), circulatory changes initiated by the release of epinephrine and norepinephrine can feed back and alter the activity of the human nervous system.

Since the sympathetic–adrenomedullary system is directly innervated by the sympathetic nervous system, it may respond more quickly than the pituitary–adrenocortical system to stressors. The latter, however, has more general effects, since the pituitary gland serves as a kind of "master gland" in the endocrine system. Briefly, a release of a hormone (adrenocorticotrophic hormone, or ACTH) from the pituitary can be initiated from the hypothalamus and causes the adrenal gland to secrete carbohydrate-active steroids that have wide-ranging effects on the body's metabolism (see Figure 1-6). Selye (1936, 1956) demonstrated that physical stressors resulted in morphological changes in the adrenal cortex, and Mason (1972) indicated that psychological stressors could also elevate the actions of the pituitary–adrenal cortex system. The pituitary–adrenal cortex system now seems to be one of the important physiological mechanisms underlying what Selye termed the "general adaptation syndrome" (GAS) to stress. The initial physiological reaction in the GAS is an emergency fight-or-flight response believed to be, in most instances, adaptive. If ineffective behavioral coping results, additional compensatory actions occur, such as increased and sustained secretions of steroids and decreased secretions of catecholamines (epinephrine and norepinephrine), which result in altered homeostatic levels for a number of physiological systems (e.g., water retention, circulatory pressure). If the stress continues for a protracted period without relief, the physiological coping mechanisms may not be able to prevent permanent physiological damage to organs or the demise of the organism. Although social psychologists have generally not examined the endocrinological effects of social factors, a recent review of stress and cancer suggests that social factors, such as housing conditions, can have profound hormonal, neural, and immunological effects (Sklar & Anisman, 1981).

ADUMBRATION

Social psychophysiology is a young field, diverse in both its theoretical focus and methodologies. You can anticipate open disagreements among contributors regarding the proper methodological approach to a question and the interpretation of empirical data. Where appropriate, we have asked these contributors to consider explicitly what appears in related chapters. Our aim was to make the exchanges more meaningful to readers rather than to promote one point of view over another.

You can also expect to be informed about a wide variety of issues emerging from the field. To facilitate this, we have partitioned the book into four major sections: Overview of Social Psychophysiology, Basic Social Psychophysiological Research, Methods of Social Psychophysiology, and Epilogue. In addition, the section on Basic Social Psychophysiological Research, which is the most wide-ranging component of the book, has been partitioned into the areas of Attitudes and Social Cognition, Affect and Emotions, Interpersonal Processes, and Contributions to Health.

The overview consists of two chapters designed to provide a brief history of the field and a discussion of the perspectives that now characterize the field. Together, these chapters should provide a broad survey of research and orientations in social psychophysiology.

The second section deals with a number of basic theoretical issues in social psychology. The many successful applications that are illustrated in this portion of the book underscore the value of the study of bodily processes, both as independent and dependent variables, and both through electrophysiological and nonelectrophysiological methods. In the first set of chapters, authors consider various aspects of attitudes and social cognition. Following these chapters is a subsection containing descriptions of research on the determinants and communication of affect and emotion. Several of the chapters detail research programs that are enjoying currency in other areas of psychology, but for one or another reason have escaped the perusings of many social psychologists. A third clustering of chapters deals with a number of classic issues pertaining to individual differences and group processes. The final subsection of chapters deals with applications of social psychophysiological research to the field of health. Social psychophysiology itself is rather new as a distinct and recognized approach, but its applications to real-world issues, particularly to health-related concerns, is straighforward and fruitful. The chapters in this section alert the reader to new directions that are emerging.

The third section on the methods of social psychophysiology is designed to make it possible for interested readers to adopt a psychophysiological perspective in their own studies of social psychological phenomena. An effort has been made to caution readers about common types of methodological pitfalls and misinterpretations. Laboratory issues are discussed, and inexpensive microcomputer-based data acquisition systems are described. The discussion of methods is not confined to psychophysiological recording techniques, however, as a number of important advancements in the field have grown out of alternative procedures, such as misattribution and drug ingestion.

The final section consists of an epilogue chapter designed to provide a retrospective on the various contributions of this book. A brief and selective review of Soviet psychophysiological research is used to highlight the unique perspective adopted by the contributors to this volume.

ACKNOWLEDGMENTS

The authors wish to thank Walter Randall for his comments on our sections dealing with the human nervous and endocrine systems, and David Shapiro, Barbara L. Andersen, and Gertrude Nath for comments on earlier drafts of this chapter. Preparation of the chapter was facilitated by National Science Foundation Grant 80-23589 and a University Faculty Scholar Award.

REFERENCES

Angell, J. R., & Thompson, H. B.   A study of the relations between certain organic processes and consciousness. *Psychological Review*, 1899, *6*, 32–69.

Benjamin, L. S.   Statistical treatment of the law of initial values (LIV) in autonomic research: A review and recommendation. *Psychosomatic Medicine*, 1963, *25*, 556–566.

Blascovich, J., Nash, R. F., & Ginsburg, G. P.   Heart rate and competitive decision making. *Personality and Social Psychology Bulletin*, 1978, *4*, 111–118.

Bonvallet, M., & Allen, M. B.   Prolonged spontaneous and evolved reticular activation following discrete bulbar lesions. *Electroencephalography and Clinical Neurophysiology*, 1963, *15*, 969–988.

Brener, J.   Visceral perception. In J. Beatty & J. Legewie (Eds.), *Biofeedback and behavior*. New York: Plenum, 1977.

Brown, C.C.   *Methods in psychophysiology*. Baltimore: Williams & Wilkins, 1967.

Buckout, R.   Changes in heart rate accompanying attitude change. *Journal of Personality and Social Psychology*, 1966, *4*, 695–699.

Cacioppo, J. T.   The effects of exogenous changes in heart rate on facilitation of thought and resistance to persuasion. *Journal of Personality and Social Psychology*, 1979, *37*, 487–496.

Cacioppo, J. T.   Social psychophysiology: A classic and contemporary approach. *Psychophysiology*, 1982, *19*, 241–251.

Cacioppo, J. T., & Petty, R. E.   Attitudes and cognitive responses: An electrophysiological approach. *Journal of Personality and Social Psychology*, 1979, *37*, 2181–2199.

Cacioppo, J. T., & Petty, R. E.   Electromyograms as measures of extent and affectivity of information processing. *American Psychologist*, 1981, *36*, 441–456. (a)

Cacioppo, J. T., & Petty, R. E.   Electromyographic specificity during covert information processing. *Psychophysiology*, 1981, *18*, 518–523. (b)

Cacioppo, J. T., & Petty, R. E.   A biosocial model of attitude change. In J. T. Cacioppo & R. E. Petty (Eds.), *Perspectives in cardiovascular psychophysiology*. New York: Guilford, 1982. (a)

Cacioppo, J. T., & Petty, R. E. (Eds.).   *Perspectives in cardiovascular psychophysiology*. New York: Guilford, 1982. (b)

Cacioppo, J. T. & Petty, R. E.   Social processes. In M. G. H. Coles, E. Donchin, & S. W. Porges (Eds.), *Handbook of psychophysiology*. New York: Guilford, in press. (a)

Cacioppo, J. T., & Petty, R. E.   Social psychophysiology. In L. Stegagano (Ed.), *Psychophysiology*. Turin: Boringhieri, in press. (b)

Cacioppo, J. T., Petty, R. E., & Quintanar, L. R.   Individual differences in relative hemispheric alpha abundance and cognitive responses to persuasive communications. *Journal of Personality and Social Psychology*, 1982, *43*, 623–636.

Cacioppo, J. T., & Sandman, C. A.   Physiological differentiation of sensory and cognitive tasks as a function of warning, processing demands, and unpleasantness. *Biological Psychology*, 1978, *6*, 181–192.

Cacioppo, J. T., & Sandman, C. A.   Psychophysiological functioning, cognitive responding, and attitudes. In R. E. Petty, T. M. Ostrom, & T. C. Brock (Eds.), *Cognitive responses to persuasion*. Hillsdale, N.J.: Erlbaum, 1981.

Cacioppo, J. T., Sandman, C. A., & Walker, B. B.   The effects of operant heart rate conditioning on cognitive elaboration and attitude change. *Psychophysiology*, 1978, *15*, 330–338.

Cannon, W. B.   *Bodily changes in pain, hunger, fear, and rage*. New York: Appleton-Century, 1929.

Cannon, W. B.   Homeostasis in senescence. *Journal of the Mount Sinai Hospital*, 1939, *5*, 598–606.

Cantor, J. R., Zillmann, D., & Bryant, J.   Enhancement of experienced sexual arousal in response to erotic stimuli through misattribution of unrelated residual excitation. *Journal of Personality and Social Psychology*, 1975, *32*, 69–75.

Christie, M. J., & Woodman, D. D.   Biochemical methods. In I. Martin & P. H. Venables (Eds.), *Techniques in psychophysiology*. Chichester: Wiley, 1980.

Collins, B. E., Ellsworth, P. C., & Helmreich, R. L.   Correlations between pupil size and semantic differential: An experimental paradigm in pilot study. *Psychonomic Science*, 1967, *9*, 627–628.

Cooper, J. B.   Emotion and prejudice. *Science*, 1959, *130*, 314–318.

Cooper, J., Zanna, M. P., & Taves, P. A.   Arousal as a necessary condition for attitude change following induced compliance. *Journal of Personality and Social Psychology*, 1978, *36*, 1101–1106.

Darrow, C. W.   Electrical and circulatory responses to brief sensory and ideational stimuli. *Journal of Experimental Psychology*, 1929, *12*, 267–300.

Darwin, C.   *The expression of the emotions in man and animals*. London: Murray, 1904. (Originally published, 1872.)

DeFeudis, F. V., & DeFeudis, P. A. F.   *Elements of the behavioral code*. New York: Academic, 1977.

Deutsch, M., & Krauss, R. M.   *Theories in social psychology*. New York: Basic Books, 1965.

Duffy, E.   The psychological significance of the concept "arousal" or "activation." *Psychological Review*, 1957, *64*, 265–275.

Fazio, R. H., Zanna, M. P., & Cooper, J.   Dissonance and self-perception: An integrative view of each theory's proper domain of application. *Journal of Experimental Social Psychology*, 1977, *13*, 464–479.

Fowles, D. C.   Heart rate as an index of anxiety: Failure of a hypothesis. In J. T. Cacioppo & R. E. Petty (Eds.), *Perspectives in cardiovascular psychophysiology*. New York: Guilford, 1982.

Furedy, J. J.   Cognitive and response processes in psychophysiology: Definitions and illustrations from human Pavlovian autonomic conditioning. *Psychophysiology*, 1981, *18*, 167. (Abstract)

Gardner, E.   *Fundamentals of neurology* (6th ed.). Philadelphia: Saunders, 1975.

Geen, R. G., & Gange, J. J.   Drive theory of social facilitation: Twelve years of theory and research. *Psychological Bulletin*, 1977, *84*, 1267–1288.

Geer, J. H.   Direct measurement of genital responding. *American Psychologist*, 1975, *30*, 415–418.

Gerard, H. B.   Choice difficulty, dissonance, and the decision sequence. *Journal of Personality*, 1967, *35*, 91–108.

Greenfield, N. S., & Sternbach, R. A.   *Handbook of psychophysiology*. New York: Holt, Rinehart & Winston, 1972.

Grossman, S. P.   *Essentials of physiological psychology.* New York: Wiley, 1973.

Hare, R. D.   Orienting and defensive responses to visual stimuli. *Psychophysiology*, 1973, *10*, 453–464.

Hare, R. D., Wood, K., Britain, S., & Shadman, J.   Autonomic responses to affective visual stimulation. *Psychophysiology*, 1971, *7*, 408–417.

Hassett, J.   *A primer of psychophysiology.* San Francisco: W. H. Freeman, 1978.

Hassett, J., & Danforth, D.   An introduction to the cardiovascular system. In J. T. Cacioppo & R. E. Petty (Eds.), *Perspectives in cardiovascular psychophysiology.* New York: Guilford, 1982.

Hebb, D. O.   Drives and the C.N.S. (conceptual nervous system). *Psychological Review*, 1955, *62*, 243–254.

Hess, E. H.   Attitude and pupil size. *Scientific American*, 1965, *212*, 46–54.

Hoff, H.   Galvani and the pre-Galvanian electrophysiologists. *Annals of Science*, 1936, *1*, 147–172.

Ikemi, Y., & Nakagawa, S.   A psychosomatic study of contagious dermititus. *Kyushu Journal of Medical Science*, 1962, *13*, 335–350.

Isaacson, R. L.   *The limbic system.* New York: Plenum, 1974.

James, W.   What is emotion? *Mind*, 1884, *9*, 188–204.

Jennings, J. R., Berg, W. K., Hutcheson, J. S., Obrist, P., Porges, S., & Turpin, G.   Publication guidelines for heart rate studies in man. *Psychophysiology*, 1981, *18*, 226–231.

Kaplan, H. B., Burch, N. R., Bloom, S. W., & Edelberg, R.   Affective orientation in physiological activity (GSR) in small peer groups. *Psychosomatic Medicine*, 1963, *25*, 242–252. ·

Kiesler, C. A., & Pallak, M. S.   Arousal properties of dissonance manipulations. *Psychological Bulletin*, 1976, *83*, 1014–1025.

Lacey, B. C., & Lacey, J. I.   Studies of heart rate and other bodily processes in sensory motor behavior. In P. A. Obrist, A. H. Black, J. Brener, & L. V. DiCara (Eds.), *Cardiovascular psychophysiology.* Chicago: Aldine, 1974.

Lacey, J. I.   Psychophysiological approaches to the evaluation of psychotherapeutic process and outcome. In E. A. Rubinstein & M. B. Parloff (Eds.), *Research in psychotherapy.* Washington, D.C.: American Psychological Association, 1959.

Lacey, J. I.   Somatic response patterning and stress: Some revisions of activation theory. In M. H. Appley & R. Trumbull (Eds.), *Psychological stress: Issues in research.* New York: Appleton-Century-Crofts, 1967.

Lacey, J. I., Kagan, J., Lacey, B., & Moss, H. A.   The visceral level: Situational determinants and behavioral correlates of autonomic response patterns. In P. H. Knapp (Ed.), *Expression of the emotions in man.* New York: International Universities Press, 1963.

Lacey, J. I., & Lacey, B. C.   Verification and extension of the principle of autonomic response stereotypy. *American Journal of Psychology*, 1958, *71*, 50–73.

Lang, P. J.   The application of psychophysiological methods to the study of psychotherapy and behavior modification. In A. E. Bergin & S. L. Garfield (Eds.), *Handbook of psychotherapy and behavior change: An empirical analysis.* New York: Wiley, 1971.

Lazarus, R. S., Averill, J. R., & Opton, E. M.   Towards a cognitive theory of emotion. In M. Arnold (Ed.), *Feelings and emotion.* New York: Academic, 1970.

Lindsley, D. B.   Emotion. In S. S. Stevens (Ed.), *Handbook of experimental psychology.* New York: Wiley, 1951.

Lindsley, D. B.   Psychophysiology and motivation. In M. R. Jones (Ed.), *Nebraska Symposium on Motivation* (Vol. 5). Lincoln: University of Nebraska Press, 1957.

Lynn, R.   *Attention, arousal and the orientation reaction.* Oxford: Pergamon, 1966.

MacBryde, C. M., & Blacklow, R. S.   *Signs and symptoms: Applied pathologic physiology and clinical interpretation* (5th ed.). Philadelphia: Lippincott, 1970.

Mackay, C. J.   The measurement of mood and psychophysiological activity using self-report techniques. In I. Martin & P. H. Venables (Eds.), *Techniques in psychophysiology.* Chichester: Wiley, 1980.

Malmo, R. B.   Activation: A neuropsychological dimension. *Psychiatric Research Reports*, 1959, *11*, 86–109.

Martin, I., & Venables, P. H. (Eds.). *Techniques in psychophysiology*. Chichester: Wiley, 1980.

Maslach, C.   Negative emotional biasing of unexplained arousal. *Journal of Personality and Social Psychology*, 1979, *37*, 953–969.

Mason, J. W.   Organization of psychoendocrine mechanisms: A review and reconsideration of research. In N. S. Greenfield & R. A. Sternbach (Eds.), *Handbook of psychophysiology*. New York: Holt, Rinehart & Winston, 1972.

Mesulam, M., & Perry, J.   The diagnosis of lovesickness: Experimental psychophysiology without the polygraph. *Psychophysiology*, 1972, *9*, 546–551.

Mewborn, C. R., & Rogers, R. W.   Affects of threatening and reassuring components of fear appeals and physiological and verbal measures of emotion and attitudes. *Journal of Experimental Social Psychology*, 1979, *15*, 242–253.

Moruzzi, G., & Magoun, H. W.   Brainstem reticular formation and activation of the EEG. *Electroencephalography and Clinical Neurophysiology*, 1949, *1*, 455–473.

Nauta, W. J. H., & Feirtag, M.   The organization of the brain. *Scientific American*, 1979.

Nauta, W. J. H., & Karten, H. J.   A general profile of the vertebrate brain, with sidelights on the ancestry of the cerebral cortex. In F. O. Schmitt (Ed.), *The neurosciences: Second study program*. New York: Rockefeller University Press, 1970.

Netter, F. H.   *The CIBA collection of medical illustrations* (Vol. 1). Summit, N.J.: CIBA, 1974.

Norman, R. F., Buchwald, J. S., & Villablanca, J. R.   Classical conditioning with auditory discrimination of the eye blink in decerebrate cats. *Science*, 1977, *196*, 551–553.

O'Connor, K. P.   The intentional paradigm and cognitive psychophysiology. *Psychophysiology*, 1981, *18*, 121–128.

Pavlov, I. P.   *Conditioned reflexes*. New York: Oxford University Press, 1927.

Pennebaker, J. W., & Lightner, J. M.   Competition of internal and external information in an exercise setting. *Journal of Personality and Social Psychology*, 1980, *39*, 165–174.

Porges, S. W., & Coles, M. G. H.   *Psychophysiology*. Stroudsbourg, Pa.: Dowden, Hutchinson & Ross, 1976.

Schachter, S., & Singer, J. E.   Cognitive, social and physiological determinants of emotional state. *Psychological Review*, 1962, *69*, 379–399.

Schmidt, R. F.   *Fundamentals of sensory physiology*. New York: Springer-Verlag, 1978.

Schwartz, G. E.   Cardiovascular psychophysiology: A systems perspective. In J. T. Cacioppo & R. E. Petty (Eds.), *Perspectives in cardiovascular psychophysiology*. New York: Guilford, 1982.

Schwartz, G. E., Davidson, R. J., & Pugash, E.   Voluntary control of patterns of EEG parietal asymmetry: Cognitive concomitants. *Psychophysiology*, 1976, *13*, 498–504.

Schwartz, G. E., & Shapiro, D.   Social psychophysiology. In W. F. Prokasy & D. C. Raskin (Eds.), *Electrodermal activity in psychological research*. New York: Academic, 1973.

Selye, H.   A syndrome produced by diverse nocuous agents. *Nature*, 1936, *138*, 32.

Selye, H.   *The stress of life*. New York: McGraw-Hill, 1956.

Shapiro, D., & Crider, A.   Psychophysiological approaches in social psychology. In G. Lindzey & E. Aronson (Eds.), *The handbook of social psychology* (2nd ed., Vol. 3). Reading, Mass.: Addison-Wesley, 1969.

Shapiro, D., & Reeves, J. L. II.   Modification of physiological and subjective responses to stress through heart rate biofeedback. In J. T. Cacioppo & R. E. Petty (Eds.), *Perspectives in cardiovascular psychophysiology*. New York: Guilford, 1982.

Shapiro, D., & Schwartz, G. E.   Psychophysiological contributions to social psychology. *Annual Review of Psychology*, 1970, *21*, 87–112.

Shaw, M. E., & Costanzo, P. R.   *Theories in social psychology*. New York: McGraw-Hill, 1970.

Sklar, L. S., & Anisman, H.   Stress and cancer. *Psychological Bulletin*, 1981, *89*, 369–406.

Smith, C. E.   A study of the autonomic excitation resulting from the interaction of the individual opinion and group opinion. *Journal of Abnormal and Social Psychology*, 1936, *30*, 138–164.

Sokolov, A. N.   *Perception and a conditioned reflex*. Oxford: Pergamon, 1963.

Stern, R. M., Ray, W. J., & Davis, C. M.   *Psychophysiological recording*. New York: Oxford University Press, 1980.

Sternbach, R. A. *Principles of psychophysiology*. New York: Academic, 1966.

Thompson, R. F. *Foundations of physiological psychology*. New York: Harper & Row, 1967.

Tursky, B., & Jamner, L. Measurement of cardiovascular functioning. In J. T. Cacioppo & R. E. Petty (Eds.), *Perspectives in cardiovascular psychophysiology*. New York: Guilford, 1982.

Tursky, B., Lodge, M., & Reeder, R. Psychophysical and psychophysiological evaluation of the direction, intensity, and meaning of race-related stimuli. *Psychophysiology*, 1979, *16*, 452–462.

Uttal, W. R. *Cellular neurophysiology and integration*. Hillsdale, N.J.: Erlbaum, 1975.

Van Toller, C. *The nervous body*. Chichester: Wiley, 1979.

Venables, P. H., & Martin, I. *A manual of psychophysiological methods*. Amsterdam: North-Holland, 1967.

Wasson, J., Walsh, B. T., Sox, H., & Tomkins, R. *The common symptom guide*. New York: McGraw-Hill, 1975.

Watts, G. O. *Dynamic neuroscience: Its application to brain disorders*. New York: Harper & Row, 1975.

West, S. G., & Wicklund, R. A. *A primer of social psychological theories*. Monterey, Calif.: Brooks/Cole, 1980.

Wilder, J. The "law of initial values," a neglected biological law and its significance for research and practice (1931). In S. W. Porges & M. G. H. Coles (Eds.), *Psychophysiology*. Stroudsburg, Pa.: Dowden, Hutchinson & Ross, 1976.

Zanna, M. P., & Cooper, J. Dissonance and the attribution process. In J. H. Harvey, J. W. Ickes, & R. F. Kidd (Eds.), *New directions in attribution research*. Hillsdale, N.J.: Erlbaum, 1976.

Zillmann, D. Attribution and misattribution of excitatory reactions. In J. H. Harvey, J. W. Ickes, & R. F. Kidd (Eds.), *New directions in attribution research* (Vol. 2). Hillsdale, N.J.: Erlbaum, 1978.

Zillmann, D., Johnson, R. C., & Day, K. D. Attribution of apparent arousal and proficiency of recovery from sympathetic activation affecting excitation transfer to aggressive behavior. *Journal of Experimental Social Psychology*, 1974, *10*, 503–515.

CHAPTER 2

The Promise of Social Psychophysiology

Andrew Crider
Williams College

INTRODUCTION

Social psychophysiology combines the questions and experimental paradigms of the social psychologist with the procedures, recording technology, and empirical generalizations of the psychophysiologist. Psychophysiology is itself a hybrid discipline that developed when experimental psychologists and psychiatrists began to adapt various electrophysiological methods to laboratory studies with human subjects. In the following, I will try to show why the melding of social psychological and psychophysiological research traditions into a feasible social psychophysiology is not only eminently reasonable but stands to benefit both parties.

A PROTOTYPICAL EXAMPLE

Social psychophysiology has a novel ring to it, but its roots can be traced back almost a half-century to a study by Carl E. Smith (1936), which was probably the first experiment explicitly to combine social psychological and psychophysiological methodologies. The experiment was conducted at Henry Murray's Harvard research center and was entitled "A Study of the Autonomic Excitation Resulting from the Interaction of Individual Opinion and Group Opinion." Smith's study is worth describing in some detail because it so nicely illustrates the nature and advantages of the social psychophysiological approach.

Smith began by asking a group of undergraduate volunteers to indicate their agreement or disagreement—as well as their degree of conviction on a 6-point scale—to 20 controversial statements. Some examples were: "The taxation of large incomes should be increased," "The Soviet experiment in government should be encouraged," and "Divorce should be

37

granted only in the case of grave offense." Several weeks later subjects were individually tested in a laboratory setting, where a continuous recording of the palmar skin resistance response [galvanic skin response (GSR)] was made. A fictitious majority attitude on each of the 20 statements was first read to each subject. Half of the fictitious attitudes agreed with the subject at the same levels of conviction, while half disagreed at the same levels of conviction. After each fictitious attitude was read, the subjects were asked to restate their original attitude, at which point the resulting GSR was observed.

The major findings appear in Figure 2-1, which plots GSR amplitude in standard deviation units as a function of the degree of conviction expressed in agreeing with or disagreeing with the majority. Two major effects are apparent. Attitudes held against the majority tended to elicit larger GSRs than attitudes held with the majority, and more strongly held

FIGURE 2-1. GSR amplitude elicited by the expression of attitudes held with or against a peer group majority as a function of attitude strength. Redrawn from "A study of the autonomic excitation resulting from the interaction of individual opinion and group opinion" by C. E. Smith, **Journal of Abnormal and Social Psychology**, 1936, **30**, 138–164.

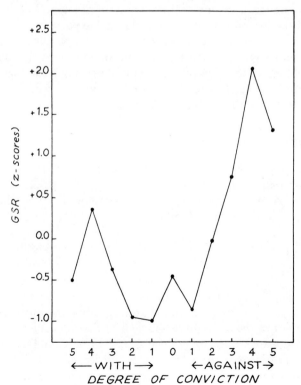

attitudes tended to elicit larger responses than those less strongly held. A notable exception to the latter effect occurred at the highest level of conviction, where the GSR was smaller than at lower levels of conviction.

Smith discussed these results in remarkably contemporary terms. He suggested that two processes—"assertional conflict" and "decisional conflict"—jointly determined GSR amplitude on any trial. According to Smith, assertional conflict occurs with the public affirmation of an attitude held against peer norms and is due to the threat of countervailing social pressures being brought to bear against the deviant. This process is seen in the greater GSR activity accompanying the expression of attitudes held against the majority than of those held with the majority. Decisional conflict, on the other hand, is an internally generated state of arousal produced by the balance between an expressed attitude and potential counterarguments. The degree of decisional conflict varies in curvilinear fashion with the strength of attitudinal conviction. At low levels of conviction, decisional conflict is minimal because the individual is relatively indifferent to the attitude expressed and therefore not threatened by counterarguments. Decisional conflict increases at higher levels of conviction as counterarguments increasingly threaten more strongly held attitudes. At the highest level of conviction, decisional conflict is abruptly reduced because firmly held attitudes may not be susceptible to counterargumentation. Or, in Smith's words: "Absolutism indicates a complete victory, at least consciously, of one conflicting component, and a complete rout of the other" (p. 161). The similarity of Smith's account of decisional conflict to Festinger's (1957) later concept of cognitive dissonance will be readily apparent to contemporary social psychologists.

Following the Smith study, a modest but respectable body of research using psychophysiological recordings in social contexts appeared in the 1940s and 1950s. This work was reviewed by Lacey (1959) and, more recently, by Shapiro and Crider (1969). This tradition slackened somewhat following the appearance of the highly influential Schachter and Singer (1962) study, which embodied a novel approach to social psychophysiology in the context of a theory of emotion. The key hypothesis of Schachter and Singer was that an unexplained and diffuse surge of autonomic arousal will lead people to search the social environment for an appropriate emotional label to explain their arousal.

Schachter and Singer (1962) tested this hypothesis by injecting subjects with the sympathomimetic drug epinephrine. Some subjects were fully informed that the injection would cause them to feel aroused, whereas other subjects were not. Subjects were then placed individually in a room with another person who, unbeknownst to them, was a confederate of the experimenter. The experimenter introduced the confederate as another subject and asked both individuals to complete questionnaires. At approximately the time that the drug began to take effect, the confederate acted as if filling out the questionnaires were making him or her either very angry or very euphoric. According to Schachter and Singer's hypothesis, subjects who knew that their arousal was due to the injection should not be affected by the confederate's behavior, but subjects who experienced an unexplained surge of arousal should use the confederate's behavior to define their own emotional state. As expected by this reasoning, subjects who were paired with an "angry" confederate and who did not know that the injection was causing them to feel aroused believed themselves to be more angry than subjects paired with an "angry" confederate and who knew the injection was causing them to feel aroused. Contrary to Schachter and Singer's line of reasoning, however, subjects paired with a "euphoric" confederate were generally unaffected by information about the possible side effects of the injection. The latter result suggests that a sudden onset of unexplained arousal may not be experienced as neutral but rather as generally dysphoric (Maslach, 1979). Moreover, problems in the methodology and type of analysis performed by Schachter and Singer, together with recent failures to replicate the original findings, have raised serious questions as to the adequacy of their model (e.g., Marshall & Zimbardo, 1979; Rogers & Deckner, 1975).

The apparent dissolution of the 20-year consensus regarding the Schachter and Singer (1962) hypothesis among social psychologists has rekindled interest in the older social psychophysiological tradition inaugurated by Smith (1936). The present volume testifies to the current vitality of this field. The following comments outline some mutually beneficial interactions between social psychological and psychophysiological research that underlie the promise of a thoroughgoing social psychophysiology.

PSYCHOPHYSIOLOGICAL ANALYSIS IN SOCIAL PSYCHOLOGICAL CONTEXTS

Smith's (1936) pioneering study exemplifies certain distinct advantages of psychophysiological approaches in social psychological experiments.

First, psychophysiological recordings provide a relatively unobtrusive and continuous means of assessing the impact of experimental events on the individual. After a brief period of adaptation to the presence of recording sensors, subjects are relatively unencumbered in carrying out the requirements of the experimental protocol. The need to break into the flow of the experiment to ask for self-reports, either verbally or with rating methods, is reduced or eliminated. Moreover, the continuous nature of psychophysiological recordings provides a wealth of information impossible to duplicate with discrete self-reports. Changes in activity levels can be monitored and analyzed in accord with experimental hypotheses. In some cases this may call for the analysis of phasic responses to discrete events, as in Smith's study. In other cases the analysis may call for an assessment of increases or decreases in tonic levels of activity over relatively lengthy time periods or for a comparison of activity levels among experimental conditions lasting several minutes or more. In sum, psychophysiological recordings allow the experimenter to time-lock individual reactions to experimental manipulations with a precision difficult or impossible to duplicate with other methods.

A second advantage is that psychophysiological recordings can often serve as a validity check on the impact of experimental manipulations on the individual. This function is fulfilled when the experimental treatment produces a physiological difference from some control condition. This is somewhat different from using psychophysiological recordings to test hypotheses, in that it does not require a *directional* difference between conditions. For example, Smith confirmed his hypothesis that attitudes held contrary to the majority elicit larger amplitude electrodermal responses than conforming attitudes. Yet the validity of his "fictitious majority" manipulation would have been confirmed by differences in any direction between attitudes that agreed and disagreed with majority opinion. Consider also the similar example provided by Rogers, Chapter 6, this volume. Rogers was unable to confirm previous findings suggesting that attitudes toward smoking are changed after fear appeals. Was it possible that this disconfirmation was due to an ineffective induction of fear in his own work? Rogers was able to eliminate this possibility by showing that psychophysiological recordings clearly differentiated high- and low-fear inductions and also covaried with a self-report anxiety measure.

A third, and more substantive advantage of psychophysiological recordings lies in their all-too-frequent ability to disconfirm our expectations and thus prompt the search for a more adequate theoretical understanding of our subject matter. Consider Smith's unanticipated finding that opinions held with absolute conviction elicited smaller GSRs than attitudes held with lesser conviction. Had Smith not found this response decrement at the absolute level of conviction, he probably would have concluded that electrodermal arousal is a linear function of attitude strength. This is a highly plausible, though fairly trivial, extension of the law of stimulus intensity in psychophysiology. But because this did not occur, Smith was obliged to develop a more complex and interesting analysis of the shifting balance between dissonant cognitions as a function of attitude strength.

This last point deserves some elaboration. Physiological data will tend to disconfirm our hypotheses to the extent that the latter are naively generated. It is always tempting to regard physiological data as operational measures of psychological constructs. We "need a measure" of anxiety, anger, arousal, or some other psychological state and for no very precise reason define a readily recorded physiological variable as an index of this state. Yet as Shapiro and Crider (1969) pointed out, the labeling of physiological variables is too often determined by the demands of particular psychological hypotheses, often doing an injustice to the simplicity of the function measured and forcing it to carry a larger significance than is warranted by its biopsychological properties. In the most concrete sense, physiological variables are indices of nothing but their own intrinsic activity and thus cannot be considered ready-made measures of psychological constructs.

The solution to disconfirmations generated by an overly-hasty operationalism lies somewhere between a reductionistic flight into physiology on the one hand and a complete disavowal of interest in physiological measures on the other. It may be the case that many social psychologists could benefit from a more thorough understanding of contemporary concepts of neural organization and peripheral physiology, as suggested in a recent monograph by Van Toller (1979). On the other hand, psychologically meaningful concepts do not spring from the mere contemplation of physiological structure and function. Such concepts must necessarily be derived from the rich corpus of method and theory available to social psychologists qua psychologists. But there must be corresponding willingness to modify these concepts when confronted by the challenge of physiological data that do not behave as expected. Meeting this challenge requires that physiological data be dealt with in the context of contemporary biopsychology, rather than appropriated as convenient indices of hypothetical constructs.

SOCIAL PSYCHOLOGICAL ANALYSIS
IN PSYCHOPHYSIOLOGICAL CONTEXTS

If psychophysiological methods and approaches can be used to advantage in social psychology, the obverse is at least equally true. Social psychological thinking and experimental paradigms have the potential to extend and enrich the discipline of psychophysiology. This potential is tacitly acknowledged in psychophysiology by the convention of employing experimental settings designed to *exclude* the operation of social factors. The typical psychophysiological experiment is conducted with a single subject who performs a relatively undemanding task while isolated in an environmentally controlled chamber. All forms of social interaction, including communication with the experimenter, are tightly controlled or confined to periods before and after the experiment proper.

The simplification of psychophysiological environments is, in many respects, good science. It has paid off in replicated findings and in a number of important empirical generalizations, sometimes known as "principles" of psychophysiology. Yet the artificiality of psychophysiological settings has contributed to a certain conceptual aridity in psychophysiology, which tends to be long on methodology but short on theory. This point can easily be confirmed by a perusal of texts in psychophysiology, such as those by Andreassi (1980), Grings and Dawson (1978), Hassett (1978), and Stern,

Ray, and Davis (1980). Social psychology is relatively rich, both conceptually and in terms of experimental procedures for the controlled investigation of social interaction. The broadening of psychophysiological investigations to include social psychological approaches can lend a vitality that is often missing in such investigations.

The promise of a thoroughgoing social psychophysiology derives from repeated demonstrations of the transmuting effects of social influence on individual psychophysiological response. An example is found in a series of case studies by Horsley Gantt and his colleagues of the "effects of person" on cardiovascular arousal in dogs undergoing classical aversive conditioning (Gantt, Newton, Royer, & Stephens, 1966; Lynch, 1977). The typical effect observed was a marked reduction in tonic heart rate and blood pressure levels during conditioning when an experimenter was present in the chamber with the animal and an ever greater reduction when the animal was petted during the procedure. A more systematic study by Lynch and McCarthy (1967) found that the typical 50- to 100-beat-per-minute heart rate acceleration to a conditioned stimulus seen in isolated dogs could be eliminated or, in some cases, converted into a deceleration if the experimenter petted the animal during each conditioning trial. These demonstrations provide an interesting social psychophysiological analogue to repeated findings on the human level of the importance of social support in protecting individuals from the deleterious consequences of stressful life events (Caplan, 1981; Cobb, 1976).

Under nonstressful conditions, social psychological factors often potentiate individual psychophysiological reactions to experimental tasks. A study by Tursky, Schwartz, and Crider (1970) demonstrated how a simple social psychological manipulation can convert a weak psychophysiological effect into a more robust one. The study was designed to investigate skin resistance and heart rate concomitants of mental effort. The experimental procedure is depicted in Figure 2-2. On each of several trials, subjects first listened to a series of four tape-recorded digits at the segment marked *Hear*. After a 5-second pause, they were given instructions during the *Task* segment. This involved the instruction to repeat the digits in an "easy" condition or the instruction to add a specific number to each digit in a "hard" condition. Following another pause, subjects were asked to read out their digit series in synchrony with one-per-second clicks during the *Response* segment. On half the trials the subjects were signaled to respond privately by repeating the digit series to themselves ("think" condition). On the remaining trials they responded publicly by writing out their series on a sheet of paper ("write" condition). The public response condition can be considered a simple form of social communication between subject and experimenter.

The lower two curves of Figure 2-2 show the effects of private mental effort on skin resistance: There was a slightly arousing effect that was

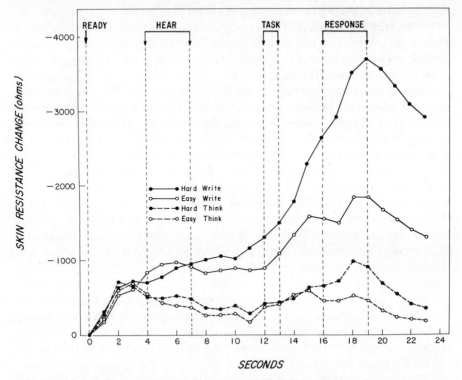

FIGURE 2-2. Second-by-second skin resistance changes during a mental task as a function of task difficulty (**Easy** vs **Hard**) and response mode (**Think** vs. **Write**). From "Differential patterns of heart rate and skin resistance during a digit transformation task" by B. Tursky, G. E. Schwartz, & A. Crider, *Journal of Experimental Psychology*, 1970, 83, 451–457. Copyright 1970 by the American Psychological Association. Reprinted by permission.

larger for the more difficult task. The upper two curves show a marked enhancement of these effects in the conditions calling for a communication. Not only was the overall effect of mental effort more pronounced, but there was also a greater differentiation between the "easy" and "hard" tasks. Similar but somewhat more complex effects were also found in the analysis of heart rate responses in the four conditions.

Both this study and those from Gantt's laboratory demonstrate the considerable impact of even rudimentary social psychological manipulations on psychophysiological activity. Unlike the Smith (1936) study described above, however, these demonstrations represent effects in search of theoretical interpretation. An important task for social psychophysiology is to harness such effects with the more sophisticated modes of analysis and experimental procedures available in contemporary social psychology.

MELDING SOCIAL PSYCHOLOGY
AND PSYCHOPHYSIOLOGY

Smith's (1936) study illustrates the sophistication necessary for a thorough-going social psychophysiology. Another fine example is a recent study by Cacioppo, Sandman, and Walker (1978). The point of departure for the latter study was the Lacey "directional fractionation" hypothesis of auto-nomic arousal (Lacey, 1967; Lacey & Lacey, 1970). On an empirical level, directional fractionation refers to an observed dissociation between heart rate and electrodermal activity in certain situations. That is, the normal sympathetic-like covariation between these two systems is at times re-placed by concomitant increases in electrodermal activity and decreases in heart rate. On a more theoretical level, the hypothesis holds that heart rate deceleration accompanied by sympathetic arousal will occur in settings calling for selective attention to environmental features, while heart rate acceleration accompanied by sympathetic arousal will occur in settings calling for the cognitive elaboration of information. On a third and more speculative level, the hypothesis holds that the direction of heart rate change in fact supports either selective attention or cognitive elaboration by means of feedback from blood pressure receptors to central nervous system structures involved in these two forms of activity. This bold hypothesis is at once an important organizing notion in psychophysiology and a source of continuing controversy (Obrist, Black, Brener, & DiCara, 1974). One reason for its controversial status is that its supporting evidence is primarily correlational. Although the directionality of heart rate change does generally differentiate cognitive processing tasks from selective at-tention tasks, few attempts have been made to manipulate heart rate independently of task demands.

Cacioppo et al. (1978) dealt with the correlational problem by using an operant conditioning procedure to train subjects either to accelerate or to decelerate heart rate in response to discriminative stimuli. They then devised a novel testing procedure. Previous work had shown that counter-attitudinal statements prompt the cognitive elaboration of counterargu-ments to such statements (Petty & Cacioppo, 1977). Cacioppo et al. reasoned that counterattitudinal statements presented during periods of accelerated heart rate should result in greater elaboration of counterarguments and increased resistance to persuasion than similar statements presented during periods of decelerated heart rate. Their test of this formulation was essen-tially positive: During heart rate acceleration trials, subjects generated more counterarguments and were more resistant to attitude change than during heart rate deceleration and baseline trials. These results significantly support and extend the directional fractionation hypothesis.

Note that the Cacioppo et al. study blurs the disciplinary boundaries between psychophysiology on the one hand and social psychology on the other. In one respect, the study builds on and extends a sizable psycho-physiological literature on the directional fractionation hypothesis. In another respect it is a social psychological experiment that investigates factors associated with resistance to persuasion. Yet the methods used to test the Lacey hypothesis could only have been devised by investigators versed in social psychology, while the manipulation of heart rate levels required an expert understanding of contemporary psychophysiology. In other words, the Cacioppo *et al.* study, like the prototypical Smith (1936) study, melds two experimental traditions to create a third form of investigation properly called social psychophysiology.

SUMMARY

In summary, the pieces appear to be in place for a concerted development of social psychophysiology. First, social psychophysiology has a respectable history, marked by a growing corpus of experiments and demonstrations. Second, psychophysiological recording technology is readily appropriated by social psychologists. This technology offers several methodological advantages and at the same time prompts conceptual innovation. Finally, the impact of social psychological factors on individual physiological activity is indisputable. A refined understanding of this impact requires the theoretical and experimental tools of social psychology. The melding of social psychology and psychophysiology creates a distinct discipline with a promising future.

REFERENCES

Andreassi, J. L. *Psychophysiology*. New York: Oxford University Press, 1980.
Cacioppo, J. T., Sandman, C. A., & Walker, B. B. The effects of operant heart rate conditioning on cognitive elaboration and attitude change. *Psychophysiology*, 1978, *15*, 330–337.
Caplan, G. Mastery of stress: Psychosocial aspects. *American Journal of Psychiatry*, 1981, *138*, 413–420.
Cobb, S. Social support as a moderator of life stress. *Psychosomatic Medicine*, 1976, *38*, 300–314.
Festinger, L. *A theory of cognitive dissonance*. Evanston, Ill.: Row, Peterson, 1957.
Gantt, W. H., Newton, J. E. O., Royer, F. L., & Stephens, J. H. Effect of person. *Conditional Reflex*, 1966, *1*, 18–35.
Grings, W. W., & Dawson, M. E. *Emotions and bodily responses*. New York: Academic, 1978.
Hassett, J. *A primer of psychophysiology*. San Francisco: W. H. Freeman, 1978.
Lacey, J. I. Psychophysiological approaches to the evaluation of psychotherapeutic process and outcome. In E. A. Rubinstein & M. B. Parloff (Eds.), *Research in psychotherapy*. Washington, D.C.: American Psychological Association, 1959.
Lacey, J. I. Somatic response patterning and stress: Some revisions of activation theory. In M. H. Appley & R. Trumbull (Eds.), *Psychological stress*. New York: Appleton-Century-Crofts, 1967.

Lacey, J. I., & Lacey, B. C. Some autonomic–central nervous system relationships. In P. Black (Ed.), *Physiological correlates of emotion*. New York: Academic, 1970.

Lynch, J. J. *The broken heart*. New York: Basic Books, 1977.

Lynch, J. J., & McCarthy, J. F. The effect of petting on a classically conditioned emotional response. *Behaviour Research and Therapy*, 1967, 5, 55–62.

Marshall, G. D., & Zimbardo, P. G. Affective consequences of inadequately explained physiological arousal. *Journal of Personality and Social Psychology*, 1979, 37, 970–988.

Maslach, C. Negative emotional biasing of unexplained arousal. *Journal of Personality and Social Psychology*, 1979, 37, 953–969.

Obrist, P. A., Black, A. H., Brener, J., & DiCara, L. V. *Cardiovascular psychophysiology: Current issues in response mechanisms, biofeedback and methodology*. Chicago: Aldine, 1974.

Petty, R. E., & Cacioppo, J. T. Forewarning, cognitive responding, and resistance to persuasion. *Journal of Personality and Social Psychology*, 1977, 35, 645–655.

Rogers, R. W., & Deckner, C. W. Effects of fear appeals and physiological arousal upon emotion, attitudes, and cigarette smoking. *Journal of Personality and Social Psychology*, 1975, 32, 222–230.

Schachter, S., & Singer, J. Cognitive, social, and physiological determinants of emotional state. *Psychological Review*, 1962, 69, 379–399.

Shapiro, D., & Crider, A. Psychophysiological approaches in social psychology. In G. Lindzey & E. Aronson (Eds.), *The handbook of social psychology* (2nd ed., Vol. 3). Reading, Mass.: Addison-Wesley, 1969.

Smith, C. E. A study of the autonomic excitation resulting from the interaction of individual opinion and group opinion. *Journal of Abnormal and Social Psychology*, 1936, 30, 138–164.

Stern, R. M., Ray, W. J., & Davis, C. M. *Psychophysiological recording*. New York: Oxford University Press, 1980.

Tursky, B., Schwartz, G. E., & Crider, A. Differential patterns of heart rate and skin resistance during a digit-transformation task. *Journal of Experimental Psychology*, 1970, 83, 451–457.

Van Toller, C. *The nervous body*. New York: Wiley, 1979.

BASIC SOCIAL PSYCHOPHYSIOLOGICAL RESEARCH

A · ATTITUDES AND SOCIAL COGNITION

CHAPTER 3

The Role
of Bodily Responses
in Attitude Measurement
and Change

Richard E. Petty
University of Missouri–Columbia
John T. Cacioppo
University of Iowa

INTRODUCTION

You are delivering a speech on the importance of controlling nuclear weapons. As you speak you notice that many members of the audience have pleasant expressions on their faces, and others are nodding their heads up and down. You become more confident as you speak since you infer that the audience agrees with what you are saying.

You are sitting in a crowded cafeteria when a highly attractive member of the opposite sex sits down beside you. You start to feel your heart beating faster and faster and you begin to think that you are really attracted to the person sharing your table.

Each of the situations above deals with attitudes—one's positive or negative feelings about people, objects, or issues. The situations clearly indicate that people sometimes infer the attitudes of other people as well as their own attitudes on the basis of signals emitted from the body. In fact, when cues from the body conflict with the verbal statements of others or one's own previous beliefs, the bodily cues may be given greater credence. For example, if a person claimed that she liked you, but she stood distant from you and continually frowned in your presence, you might come to seriously question her verbal statements. Similarly, if you believed that you liked a person, but got an uncomfortable feeling in your stomach whenever he approached, you might similarly put more faith in the negative implications of your bodily responses. Our goal in this chapter is to outline the many approaches researchers have taken in an attempt to link bodily responses to attitudes. Most of our discussion focuses on the utility of bodily responses in measuring a person's attitudes and attitude-relevant processes, but at the end of the chapter we present a model that outlines the role of bodily responses in producing attitude changes.

BODILY RESPONSES AND THE MEASUREMENT OF ATTITUDES AND ATTITUDE PROCESSES

The measurement of bodily responses has generally served two purposes in research on attitudes and persuasion, and we have therefore divided our discussion of measurement into two major parts. First, we discuss the wide variety of attempts to use bodily response measures to assess a person's attitude toward a particular stimulus. Next, we discuss research in which bodily response measures are used to provide evidence for a particular process that is thought to mediate attitude formation or change.

Bodily Responses and Attitude Measurement

There are many reasons why researchers have sought a way to assess attitudes by observing bodily responses rather than by directly asking people to provide self-reports of their feelings. Perhaps the most obvious and important reason is that researchers cannot always rely on people to report their true feelings. People may not report their true attitudes either because they are not aware of how they really feel (e.g., a person who has a repressed hatred of his brother), or because although they are aware of their true feelings, they are motivated to hide them (e.g., a student who is afraid to admit to the experimenter that he dislikes members of another racial group; see Cook & Selltiz, 1964). We have divided the attempts to measure attitudes by using bodily responses into four categories: (1) an attempt is made to relate a naturally occurring overt (observable) bodily response to attitudes, (2) an attempt is made to relate a naturally occurring covert (hidden) bodily response to attitudes, (3) an attempt is made to condition a bodily response to indicate an attitude, and (4) researchers give people the false impression that bodily responses are being monitored in an effort to convince subjects to be truthful in their verbal reports.

Natural Overt Responses

The link between the attitude concept and observable bodily responses goes back at least to the eighteenth century, when the term "attitude" was used primarily to refer to the posture or bodily orientation of a statue or figure in a painting. This definitional link between attitudes and bodily orientation is gone today, but the image remains in such sayings as: "What is your *position* on capital punishment?" or "Where do you *stand* on the new tax proposal?" In the nineteenth century, Charles Darwin used the term "attitude" to refer to the physical expression of an emotion (e.g., a scowling face indicated a hostile attitude). Thus, the first definitions of attitude had to do with observable bodily responses (see Allport, 1935; Fleming, 1967; Petty, Ostrom, & Brock, 1981).

One of the earliest hints that bodily responses could be used to gauge positive or negative feelings (today's definition of attitude) can be found in Galton's paper on the measurement of character in 1884. Galton wrote:

> When two persons have an "inclination" to one another, they visibly incline or slope together when sitting side by side, as at a dinner table, and they then throw the stress of their weights on the near legs of their chairs. It does not require much ingenuity to arrange a pressure gauge with an index and dial to indicate changes in stress. . . . I have made some crude experiments, but being busy with other matters, have not carried them on. (p. 184)

When conceptually similar studies actually were carried out nearly a century later, considerable evidence emerged that a person's observable bodily responses could be used as an index of attitude (see Mehrabian, 1981). For example, Byrne, Ervin, and Lamberth (1970) reported a significant negative correlation between verbally reported liking for another and how close two people stood together—the greater the liking, the smaller the distance separating them when they were unobtrusively observed. Similarly, one's body position (leaning toward or away from another person; Mehrabian, 1968), and the amount of interpersonal eye contact (Argyle, 1967) have also been employed successfully as attitude measures.

In a study more specifically related to persuasion, Wells and Petty (1980) surreptitiously made videotapes of college students as they listened to a speech that was either consistent with their initial attitude (tuition should be lowered) or inconsistent (tuition should be raised). Independent raters, blind to message content, subsequently scored the videotapes for spontaneous horizontal and vertical head movements. For students hearing the proattitudinal message 73% of the head movements were vertical, whereas for students hearing the counterattitudinal message only 47% were vertical ($p < .05$). Additionally, subjects' head movement scores (proportion of vertical movements) were correlated with their postmessage opinions about tuition. For subjects hearing the counterattitudinal message the correlation was .42 ($p < .05$; the greater the proportion of vertical head movements, the larger subjects thought the tuition should be), and for subjects hearing the proattitudinal message the correlation was −.28 (not significant; the greater the proportion of vertical head movements, the smaller subjects thought the tuition should be). Thus, in both the experimental and correlational analyses, subjects' naturally occurring and observable head movements provided some indication of the extent of agreement with the communication.

Perhaps the most obvious overt response to monitor in order to assess attitudes would be facial expressions. As we noted earlier, Darwin (1872) linked attitudes directly to facial expressions and argued that different facial expressions were biologically tied to different emotions. Ekman (1971) has provided convincing evidence that at least six different emotions can be linked to unique facial expressions across a wide variety of cultures: happiness, sadness, anger, fear, surprise, and disgust. When these emotions are strong and spontaneously expressed, they are easily observable. However, overt facial expressions have not proven useful in predicting the more subtle attitudinal responses that result from exposue to persuasive communications (Love, 1972). These more subtle facial expressions may only be observed in photographs and videotapes where repeated inspection and slow-motion observation are possible (see Hager & Ekman, Chapter 10, this volume), or may not be detected at all unless magnified with electrophysiological procedures (Cacioppo & Petty, 1979a). In the next section we assess the utility of a variety of covert bodily responses as measures of attitudes, including covert facial expressions.

Natural Covert Responses

One potential problem with using overt responses to assess attitudes is that if people know they are being observed, it is relatively easy for them to control the bodily cues that they emit. For example, people can easily choose to smile when they are unhappy, stand apart from those they love, and nod yes when they are thinking no. Thus, the major advantage of using bodily response measures over direct verbal reports of attitudes may be lost unless the observations are made surreptitiously or people are unaware of the natural connection between an overt bodily response and their feelings (e.g., people may not be aware of the tendency to lean toward those they like). In order to solve the problem of a person's control over observable bodily responses, some investigators have advocated measuring covert physiological responses (McGuire, 1966; Shapiro & Crider, 1969). In this section we discuss the utility of four physiological measures for assessing attitudes: electrodermal activity, pupillary responses, facial electromyographic activity, and measures of hemispheric asymmetry. All of these measures can, to some extent, be monitored overtly (e.g., a person may be sweating so much as to result in visible perspiration), but the research that we will highlight focuses on changes small enough that without appropriate magnification would be undetectable to the naked eye.

Electrodermal Activity.   Although there are a wide variety of possible electrodermal measures, the most frequently employed in social psychophysiological studies of attitudes is the skin resistance response (SRR), the change in the ability of the skin to conduct electricity. This response is induced by differential activity of the sweat glands which are under the control of the sympathetic nervous system (see Venables & Christie, 1980, for further details). In social psychophysiological studies, changes in skin resistance are typically measured by applying a small electrical current across two electrodes that are attached to the palm of the hand. Changes in the resistance of the skin may occur spontaneously or in direct response to an external stimulus.[1] Schwartz and Shapiro (1973) suggest that SRRs became a favorite in social psychophysiological studies because the measure had a long history; it was relatively easy and inexpensive to record; with appropriate equipment, changes could be easily detected with the eye; and the measure had a direct link to sweating, which common sense indicated was related to such subjective experiences as stress and emotionality.

One of the earliest areas of research relevant to electrodermal activity and attitudes concerned the physiological effects of presenting different kinds of words to people. For example, Syz (1926–1927) found that a group of medical students showed enhanced SRRs to emotion-laden words such as "prostitute" (see also W. Smith, 1922). Similarly, Dysinger (1931; reported in McCurdy, 1950) monitored skin resistance as subjects were presented with words that varied in their rated pleasantness. Dysinger found that the SRRs were significantly correlated with the extremity of the words ($r = .85$), but could not predict whether the words were rated as pleasant or unpleasant.

In a second body of studies, subjects were presented with complete attitude statements rather than individual words while electrodermal activity was monitored. A major finding of these studies has been that exposure to inconsistent opinion statements elicits greater SRRs than exposure to consistent statements. Dickson and McGinnies (1966), for example, exposed students who scored either prochurch, antichurch, or neutral on a Likert-type attitude scale to 12 statements adapted from Thurstone and Chave's (1929) list of opinions about the church. Average SRRs to each type of statement were calculated for each group. A significant interaction indicated that prochurch students showed the highest electrodermal responses to the antichurch statements, whereas antichurch students showed the highest responses to the prochurch statements (see also Cooper & Singer, 1956; Gerard, 1961; Katz, Cadoret, Hughes, & Abbey, 1965; McGinnies & Aiba, 1965; C. A. Smith, 1936).

A third area of research on electrodermal activity and attitudes has investigated people's reactions to other people. In one early study, Rankin and Campbell (1955) measured skin resistance from a subject's right hand

---

1. Although skin resistance is typically measured, most current researchers transform the data to skin conductance (the reciprocal of resistance). The conductance measure is preferred because it is linearly related to sweat secretion (see Darrow, 1964) and tends to be more normally distributed, facilitating statistical analysis (Hassett, 1978).

while they were exposed to a free association task with such words as "flunk" and "mother" as the stimuli. The experimental manipulation involved having a black and a white experimental assistant adjust the electrodes on the subject's left hand. Following each adjustment, average skin conductance responses to the word associations were calculated. Rankin and Campbell reported that regardless of a subject's level of prejudice toward blacks, skin conductance responses to the word associations were higher following the adjustments made by the black assistant than those made by the white assistant. On the other hand, the average correlation (over all groups and orders of attitude assessment) between the direct measure of attitudes toward blacks and the difference in skin conductance between the black and white assistants was .42—the more negative the attitude toward blacks, the greater the relative skin conductance response to the black over the white assistant.[2] Although this study did not find a very strong link between prejudiced attitudes and electrodermal activity, subsequent studies have provided further support for a link. For example, later investigators have demonstrated that people with negative attitudes toward blacks show larger electrodermal responses to pictures of blacks than do people with more favorable attitudes (see Vidulich & Krevanick, 1966; Westie & DeFleur, 1959).

What does the accumulated research suggest about the utility of using the skin resistance response as a measure of attitudes? In a recent review of this literature, Cacioppo and Sandman (1981) argued that the skin resistance responses observed in the studies just described might be better viewed as indicants of orienting reactions than of attitudes. Recall from Chapter 1 that the SRR is one component of a physiological pattern labeled the orienting reflex (Pavlov, 1927; Sokolov, 1963) which occurs to a wide variety of novel, unexpected, and attention-getting stimuli. Thus, the SRRs elicited by emotional words may not be reflecting a positive or negative attitudinal reaction, but instead may represent a subject's surprise at hearing such emotional or taboo words in the experimental setting (see also Hassett, 1978). Similarly, attitudinally inconsistent opinion statements may elicit SRRs because "this inconsistency may be seen as a source of novelty, incongruity, or violation of expectancy" (Shapiro & Crider, 1969, p. 22). Finally, even the studies of prejudice may be susceptible to the orienting interpretation. As Cacioppo and Sandman (1981) noted: "A black experimenter may have been more novel to a prejudiced person than to a person not prejudiced; similarly 10 to 20 years ago, photographs of blacks may have been more novel or unexpected for prejudiced than for un-

2. The correlation collapsed across conditions was computed and reported initially by Schwartz and Shapiro (1973). One important problem with the study is that only one black (age 32, height 5 feet 11 inches, weight 192 pounds) and one white (age 23, 5 feet 9 inches, 155 pounds) assistant were used. Thus, many other variables are confounded with the black–white difference.

prejudiced persons" (p. 86). Therefore, until further research is conducted in which novelty is carefully controlled, it would be inappropriate to conclude that the reliable electrodermal activity elicited by some attitudinal stimuli reflects an underlying emotional feeling about them.

Pupillary Responses.   Unlike the skin resistance response, which is unidirectional, the pupils of the eye are capable of a bidirectional response. Specifically, the pupils dilate naturally in response to dark stimuli and constrict in response to light stimuli in order to maximize visual acuity. Pupillary dilation is under the control of the sympathetic nervous system, whereas constriction is controlled by the parasympathetic. In this section we address the question of whether or not the pupils can provide an index of attitudes. In the typical study on pupillary responses to stimuli, the pupil is photographed with infrared movie film and subsequently projected on a screen, where the enlarged image can be measured with a ruler or mechanical devices (see Young & Sheena, 1975, for a description of several more recent procedures).

In a widely cited paper in the journal *Science*, Hess and Polt (1960) argued that pupil size was related to the "interest value of visual stimuli" (p. 349). In this early study, four male and two female subjects were exposed to five different pictures alternated with a control pattern (which was not described). The subjects' pupils were photographed 20 times during the 10-second exposure to each test stimulus and control stimulus. The change in mean pupil size from the preceding control stimulus to the subsequent test picture served as the dependent measure. The data revealed a striking sex difference in response to the pictures, with males showing greater dilation to the picture that would presumably be of greater interest to men (the female pinup figure), and females showing the greatest dilation to pictures that would stereotypically be of greater interest to women (e.g., male pinup figure, mother and baby).

In later papers, Hess expanded his claims for the pupillary measure. For example, in 1965 Hess wrote: "It is always difficult to elicit from someone information that involves private attitudes toward some person, concept, or thing. The pupil response technique can measure just such attitudes . . . [and] may yield more accurate representations of an attitude than can be obtained with even a well drawn questionnaire" (p. 53). Hess provided a variety of new evidence for this claim. For example, in one study subjects were exposed to pictures of food. People who were deprived of food for 4 to 5 hours showed dilation that was more than 2.5 times larger than subjects who had eaten within an hour of being tested. Hess interpreted this effect as being due to different attitudes about the food.

The most intriguing aspect of the follow-up work was Hess's claim that "constriction is as characteristic in the case of certain aversive stimuli as dilation is in the case of interesting or pleasant pictures." For example,

Hess reported that female subjects tended to show constriction to pictures of sharks. Not all of Hess's results were consistent with the hypothesis, however. For example, he reported that tasting both pleasant and unpleasant liquids induced dilation compared to tasting water; and that viewing the presumably unpleasant pictures of dead soldiers and corpses produced initial dilation in some subjects. Hess (1972) explained the latter finding by arguing that for some subjects, the initial dilation is a result of a "shock" (orienting) reaction that shifts to constriction upon repeated presentation. Inconsistent data were occasionally still reported, however, when the pupillary results were averaged across repeated stimulus presentations. For example, in a recent study Metalis and Hess (1982) found that although female subjects showed constriction to slides of female nudes, male subjects showed dilation to slides of male nudes.

A large number of attempts to validate Hess's hypothesis have produced a conflicting pattern of results. A few studies appear to be highly confirmatory, but many others are highly contradictory. For example, Barlow (1969) reported that politically liberal subjects showed dilation to a picture of a politically liberal presidential candidate, but constriction to a picture of a political conservative. Politically conservative subjects showed the opposite pattern (see also Atwood & Howell, 1971; Hicks & LaPage, 1976). However, most of the replication studies have failed to show both dilation to positive and constriction to negative stimuli even when the stimuli are repeatedly presented (Collins, Ellsworth, & Helmreich, 1967; Janisse, 1974; Peavler & McLaughlin, 1967; White & Maltzman, 1978; Woodmansee, 1970).

There have been two lines of attack on the idea that the pupils can measure attitudes. One line of attack has been primarily methodological. Some critics have noted that most experiments have not been conducted carefully enough to allow a proper test of the attitude–pupil size relationship (e.g., pupillary responses have not been permitted to return to baseline prior to assessment; inadequate control stimuli have been employed), and that many factors that are nonpsychological in nature can affect pupil size (e.g., the sequence of stimulus presentation, the wavelength of visual stimuli; see Janisse, 1977; Peavler, 1975; Tryon, 1975). Perhaps the most telling critique has been that Hess's crucial aversion–constriction hypothesis has only been demonstated with pictoral stimuli (in a minority of studies), and it is extremely difficult to control the numerous light-reflex-related variables that can confound such studies (Goldwater, 1972; Janisse & Peavler, 1974; Mueller, 1970).

A second line of attack has argued that the pupils may reflect a psychological state, but that the state is not an attitudinal or evaluative one. A variety of possibilities have been suggested (e.g., fatigue: Lowenstein & Lowenfeld, 1951; sexual arousal: Bernick, Kling, & Borowitz, 1971; stress: Arima & Wilson, 1972; and others), but most interest has focused on the following two. First, pupillary dilation is part of the general orienting reflex (Sokolov, 1963), and thus the pupillary response, much like the SRR described earlier, may be used to assess attentiveness or perceptual orienting (see Cacioppo & Sandman, 1981; Woodmansee, 1970). This is especially true on the initial presentation of a stimulus (Libby, Lacey, & Lacey, 1973). Second, the pupillary response has been associated with thinking or mental effort (Kahneman, 1973). We discuss this possibility further later in the chapter. At present we can conclude that despite some initial promise, the pupillary response has not proven to be a useful measure of attitudes or qualitatively different affective states.

Facial EMG Activity. The contraction of muscle fibers is accompanied by electrical potentials that can be measured by determining the voltage from two electrodes placed on the surface of the skin over a particular muscle group. Typically, the electrical potentials are summed so that the total amount of electrical activity over a particular muscle group in a given period of time is recorded. In the type of nonstrenuous situation encountered in most attitude experiments, total muscular contraction is reasonably reflected by this summary (see Goldstein, 1972). Unlike the two physiological measures that we have previously discussed, skeletal muscles are not innervated by the autonomic nervous system (see Cacioppo & Petty, Chapter 1, this volume); rather, the facial muscles are innervated by the central nervous system and the bodily muscles are innervated by the somatic system. The electrode placement sites for the major facial muscles involved in affective responses are depicted in Figure 9-1, this volume (p. 254).

Earlier in this chapter we noted how Darwin (1872) linked different emotions to unique facial expressions. Based on this and the contemporary research and theory of Ekman (1971; Ekman & Friesen, 1975), Tomkins (1962, 1963, 1981), and Izard (1971, 1976), Schwartz reasoned that different affective states should be identifiable in the pattern of covert contractions of the facial muscles. In one study, for instance, Schwartz and his colleagues (Schwartz, Fair, Salt, Mandel, & Klerman, 1976) asked people to imagine positive or negative events in their lives while electromyographic (EMG) activity over the corrugator, zygomatic, and depressor muscle sites was recorded. The results indicated that when imagining happy events, people generally showed more EMG activity in the zygomatic (smiling) and less activity in the corrugator (frowning) muscles than when imagining sad events (see also Schwartz, Ahern, & Brown, 1979; Sirota & Schwartz, 1982). More details about facial expressions and emotion can be found in the chapters in this volume by Fridlund and Izard (Chapter 9) and by Hager and Ekman (Chapter 10).

In a recent study we have attempted to determine if these unique facial muscle patterns could also distinguish positive from negative reactions to a persuasive communication (Cacioppo & Petty, 1979a, Experiment 2). In this study we recorded facial EMG activity from the corrugator, depressor, and zygomatic sites while college students anticipated receiving (warning interval) and actually listened to (message interval) an involving proattitudinal (e.g., advocating more lenient visitation hours in dormitory rooms) or an involving counterattitudinal (e.g., advocating more strict visitation hours) communication. A control group was forewarned only that they would hear a message (without learning the topic) and actually heard what we believed would be a relatively neutral speech about an archeological expedition. The results of this study are presented in Figure 3-1. In the right panel, EMG responses during the message presentation are depicted. As would be expected from previous research, subjects who heard the counterattitudinal message showed significantly less zygomatic activity than subjects exposed to the proattitudinal message. Subjects exposed to the counterattitudinal message also tended to show more corrugator and less depressor activity than proattitudinal subjects. The neutral message was rated by subjects as being relatively pleasant and it is interesting to note that the EMG pattern elicited by this message more closely matches the pro than the counterattitudinal communication. In the left panel of Figure 3-1, the EMG responses elicited after the warning but

FIGURE 3-1. Median change from prewarning baseline for corrugator (C), zygomatic (Z), and depressor (D) electromyographic (EMG) activity during the postwarning–premessage (left panel) and message (right panel) intervals. The data are displayed separately for subjects in the neutral, proattitudinal, and counterattitudinal groups. From "Attitudes and cognitive response. An electrophysiological approach" by J. T. Cacioppo & R. E. Petty, **Journal of Personality and Social Psychology**, 1979, **37**, 2181–2199. Copyright 1979 by the American Psychological Association. Reprinted by permission.

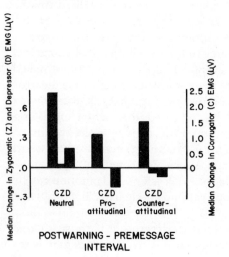

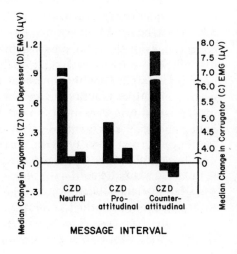

before the message are presented. These data generally mirror in a weaker form the patterns elicited during message presentation. It is especially interesting to note that a marginally significant difference in the magnitude of corrugator activity was found between the pro- and counterattitudinal forewarnings, which is consistent with the view that subjects spontaneously generate negative cognitive responses (counterarguments) or at least feel more negatively when they are about to be presented with a counter-attitudinal message on an involving topic (Petty & Cacioppo, 1977). The utility of corrugator EMG activity as an index of negative responses was also demonstrated by Teasdale and Rezin (1978), who reported a correlation of .81 between corrugator region EMG activity and the frequency of negative thoughts.

In summary, it appears that subtle facial muscle patterns that are not detectable to the naked eye can be used to distinguish positive from negative affective states, including states that are induced by the kinds of persuasive messages that are typical of those employed in many persuasion studies. It is up to future research to reveal if the patterns of facial EMG activity identified in the cited research will prove useful in determining the intensity as well as the direction of feeling, and also the processes underlying changes in affective states.

Hemispheric Asymmetry.   Finally, we briefly note an emerging area of research that is potentially relevant to the assessment of different affective states. Considerable evidence now exists that the two hemispheres of the brain have specialized to take on different functions. Although there is considerable agreement that for right-handed males, at least, the left hemisphere is concerned with linguistic logical thinking, whereas the right hemisphere tends toward spatial intuitive thinking (e.g., Ornstein, 1972), there is less agreement about other specialized functions. Nevertheless, recent evidence has suggested that negative affect is mediated to a greater extent by the right hemisphere and positive affect by the left hemisphere.

The evidence suggesting this conclusion comes from a variety of sources and measures. For example, in one study Ahern and Schwartz (1979) found that right-handers tend to move their eyes to the left following negative emotional questions and to be right following positive emotional questions. Given contralateral control of eye movements (Kinsbourne, 1972), this is consistent with the view that the left hemisphere is more concerned with positive emotions and the right hemisphere more concerned with negative emotions.

Using a unique contact-lens system that permitted showing stimuli to visual half-fields, Dimond, Farrington, and Johnson (1976) found that stimuli presented to the left half-fields (right hemisphere) were rated more negatively than stimuli presented to the right half-fields (left hemisphere). Sackeim and Gur (1978; Sackeim, Gur, & Saucy, 1978) found that when raters judged left and right composite pictures, for all emotions except happiness, the left-side composite was judged as being more intense in its degree of emotional expression than the right-side composite. Again, assuming contralateral control of muscles in the lower two-thirds of the face, this finding is consistent with the view that the left hemisphere is more positively oriented than the right (see Sackeim & Gur, Chapter 11, this volume, for further details).

Finally, two studies have measured electroencephalographic (EEG) activity and have found that reflection on positive events is associated with relative activation in the left frontal lobes, whereas reflection on negative events is associated with relative activation in the right frontal lobes (Davidson, Schwartz, Saron, Bennett, & Goleman, 1979; Tucker, Stenslie, Roth, & Shearer, 1981). Interestingly, these hemispheric differences do not occur on measures taken in the parietal area (Cacioppo, Petty, & Quintanar, 1982; Davidson *et al.*, 1979) nor in the central or occipital regions (Tucker *et al.*, 1981). (We discuss hemispheric asymmetry in the parietal area later in this chapter in the section on cognitive elaboration.)

Although there is considerable disagreement and speculation among the various researchers about why these effects occur, most view the data as indicating that the right hemisphere contributes more to negative affect and the left contributes more to positive affect (Tucker, 1981). Considerably more research needs to be done, but the present data indicate that measures of hemispheric asymmetry may hold some future promise for distinguishing positive from negative reactions to attitudinal stimuli.[3]

Classically Conditioned Responses

In the preceding two sections we saw how researchers have attempted to measure attitudes by observing bodily responses that are the natural result of exposure to attitude-relevant stimuli. Some of these responses were easily observable (e.g., overt head movements), whereas others required the use of sophisticated psychophysiological equipment (e.g., facial

---

3. In addition to the four categories of measures discussed in the section on covert responses, some researchers have argued that heart rate might relate to positive and negative feelings. For example, one review of early research by Rihl (1926; cited in J. I. Lacey, 1967) concluded that pleasant stimuli produced cardiac deceleration, whereas unpleasant stimuli produced cardiac acceleration. However, other investigators have found that "pictures that were rated as unpleasant and bad evoked more deceleration than those rated as pleasant and good" (Libby, Lacey, & Lacey, 1973, p. 284). Still others (e.g., Katz, Cadoret, Hughes, & Abbey, 1965) have found that the presentation of both acceptable (pleasant) and unacceptable (unpleasant) attitude statements enhanced heart rate over neutral statements. Of course, there are many methodological and substantive differences among these studies that could account for the conflicting relationships. In any case, the relationship between heart rate and the direction of affect has not been resolved at present (for further discussion, see Obrist, 1982; Shapiro & Reeves, 1982). There is, however, some agreement as to how heart rate reflects non-affect-laden cognitive activity (see footnote 4).

EMG activity). An alternative measurement approach is to classically condition some bodily response to indicate an attitude. This approach is based on a phenomenon called "semantic generalization" (see Creelman, 1966; Feather, 1965). In an early demonstration of semantic generalization, Razran (1939) showed that once a conditioned stimulus word (CS) reliably elicited a conditioned response (CR), words similar in meaning to the initial CS would also elicit the CR, although in a weaker form.

The first attempt to use the principle of semantic generalization to assess attitudes physiologically was reported by a Soviet investigator, Volkova (1953; cited in Razran, 1961). Using cranberry sauce as the unconditioned stimulus (UCS), Volkova reported conditioning the salivary responses of a young boy to the Russian word for "good." Because of semantic generalization, the boy was expected to salivate to statements that he thought were good, but not to statements that he thought were bad. Apparently, the procedure was successful. For example, upon testing the boy is reported to have salivated 2 drops to the "bad" statement "The pupil broke the glass," but to have salivated 23 drops to the "good" statement "The pioneer helps his comrades" (see Cacioppo & Petty, Chapter 25, this volume, for further details and other research on Soviet contributions to the psychophysiology of attitude measurement and change). A successful conceptual replication of Volkova's observations was reported by Acker and Edwards (1964), who conditioned a vasomotor response (constriction of the blood vessels in the left index finger) to the word "good" or "bad." In the subsequent test phase, these investigators obtained the appropriate generalization to words that were previously rated as good or bad on a semantic differential scale.

Relatively few studies have used the classical conditioning approach to assess attitudes (e.g., Tursky, Lodge, & Reeder, 1979), but it is already clear that this approach is not completely free of problems. For example, Tognacci and Cook (1975), using electric shock as the UCS, conditioned SRRs to the visual presentation of sentences that depicted something bad (e.g., The old Irishman poisoned the little boy's dog). Statements that described something good (e.g., The young Japanese boy helped the old woman up when she fell on the ice) were not followed by shock. Following the conditioning trials, SRRs were monitored as subjects were presented with a combination of nonprejudicial (e.g., The Negro family moved into a house in a fine all-white neighborhood), and prejudicial (e.g., The real estate agent only showed the Negro buyer houses in Negro neighborhoods) statements.

The data provided partial support for the utility of the classical conditioning approach. Unprejudiced subjects, as assessed by an attitude scale that was administered earlier, showed greater SRRs to the prejudicial than to the unprejudicial statements (since they presumably thought these statements were bad). Prejudiced subjects, however, did not show differential SRRs to the two kinds of statements. To account for this unexpected finding, Tognacci and Cook suggested that perhaps the prejudiced college students in their sample "were not sufficiently prejudiced to view many of our (unprejudicial) statements as bad, and hence, failed to show the expected generalization to these sentences" (p. 144). Alternatively, perhaps the prejudiced subjects were more nervous throughout the testing phase (because of a fear of being found out). This would make it more difficult to detect the required changes in skin resistance for these subjects. If true, then the classical conditioning approach using SRRs may only be effective for subjects who have socially desirable attitudes, or when subjects do not suspect that the study has to do with attitude assessment. One way to avoid these problems might be to employ physiological responses that are less susceptible to influence by cognitive factors than are skin resistance responses (see Tursky & Jamner, Chapter 4, this volume, for a discussion of the assessment of beliefs and belief structures with the classical conditioning approach).

Bogus Physiological Responses

In the last approach to attitude measurement that we address, an attempt is made to convince subjects that their physiological responses are being measured, and that these responses provide a true indication of their attitudes. The rationale for this procedure, known as the "bogus pipeline," was stated succinctly by Jones and Sigall when they introduced it in 1971:

> The paradigm is based on the simple premise that no one wants to be second guessed by a machine. If a person could be convinced that we do have a machine that precisely measures attitudinal direction and intensity, we assume that he would be motivated to predict accurately what the machine is saying about him. (p. 349)

Gerard (1960; cited in Gerard, 1964) may have been the first contemporary social psychologist to convince subjects that he could measure their true response tendencies with a polygraph. In Gerard's study, the subject's task was to make a choice by pressing one of two buttons with either the left or right index finger. All subjects had EMG electrodes attached to their right and left forearms and they were told (falsely) that the highly sensitive electromyographic equipment would register their initial tendencies to press either the right or the left button.

Jones and Sigall (1971) made the important contribution of noting that the false physiological feedback procedure introduced by Gerard might be modified and used to obtain a more veridical report of subjects' attitudes. In a demonstration and test of the bogus pipeline procedure, Sigall and Page (1971) had some subjects make judgments on standard rating scales, and others made their judgments under bogus pipeline conditions. Subjects in the pipeline conditions were told to hold onto a steering wheel connected to a pointer; turning the wheel allowed the pointer to move from 0 to any point on the attached −3 to +3 rating scale. Electrodes were attached to subjects' forearms and they were told that the EMG recordings could predict how far in either direction they would turn the wheel. A few practice trials were conducted in which the EMG data were shown to predict subjects' true responses (this was accomplished because unknown to the subjects, the investigator had access to their opinions from a previous questionnaire). Subjects were even asked to try to fool the EMG on one trial, and found that they could not. Once the subjects were convinced that the EMG could read their minds, the ratings of interest were made. Half of the subjects, all of whom were white females, were asked to judge whether or not certain trait adjectives (e.g., honest) were characteristic of "Americans," and half were asked if they were characteristic of blacks. In the pipeline conditions, subjects were asked to "predict" what the EMG data would show (i.e., would they show a tendency to turn the wheel in the "characteristic" or "uncharacteristic" direction and how far). In the nonpipeline conditions, these judgments were made on standard rating scales. The results were relatively straightforward. "Americans" received more favorable evaluations under the bogus pipeline than under the rating conditions, but blacks received more favorable evaluations under the rating than under the bogus pipeline conditions.

Of course, in this study and others on the bogus pipeline (e.g., Arkin, Appelman, & Burger, 1980; Jones, Bell, & Aronson, 1971) it is impossible to tell which set of judgments is more valid (rating or bogus pipeline) because the investigators really do not have unique access to the truth. Quigley-Fernandez and Tedeschi (1978) solved this problem by experimentally creating beliefs in subjects. Specifically, subjects were first wrongly informed about how to perform well on an experimental test. They were later given a chance to "cheat" on the test and were subsequently asked if they possessed any prior information about the test. Subjects questioned under the bogus pipeline conditions "confessed" more often than those who were not. Thus, the accumulated studies do suggest that the bogus pipeline procedure may be effective in getting people to reveal socially undesirable attitudes or information about themselves. One possible problem with the pipeline measure, however, is that the procedure itself apparently induces a negative arousal in subjects (Gaes, Kalle, & Tedeschi, 1978). This unfortunate feature might render the measure inappropriate in certain contexts (e.g., in dissonance studies, where it might serve as a misattribution cue). Also, as the procedure becomes more widely known (and with the continued public controversy over the use of the polygraph in lie detection), it may become increasingly difficult to convince people that the physiological equipment can measure their attitudes.

Bodily Assessment of Attitude-Relevant Processes

Different theories of attitudes and persuasion postulate different intervening processes between initial exposure to an attitude-relevant stimulus
(e.g., a persuasive communication) and the subsequent attitudinal response
(e.g., boomerang, resistance, or yielding). Some theories rely on processes
that might be assessed with bodily response measures, and we address
three such processes in this section: fear, dissonance, and cognitive elaboration.

Fear

Arousing fear in a communication was initially thought to be an effective
persuasion technique because people would be motivated to reduce the
fear by adopting the recommendations in the message (see Janis, 1967).
Can fear be distinguished physiologically from other emotions? In a study
that has since become a classic, Ax (1953) demonstrated that fear was
accompanied by a unique pattern of physiological responses. In his study,
a variety of electrodes were attached to subjects and the subjects were told
to lie down quietly as a nurse took their blood pressures once each minute
(subjects believed that they were participating in research on hypertension).
After an appropriate baseline period of observation, the operator of the
physiological equipment began acting in an obnoxious and arrogant manner.
The nurse was criticized, the subject was roughly treated, insulted, and
blamed for not cooperating. This act proceeded for about 5 minutes and
was designed to elicit "anger" in subjects. Finally, the equipment operator
left and the nurse apologized for his behavior. After a rest period, an
attempt was made to induce "fear" in the subjects. To accomplish this, a
gradually increasing shock was administered to the subject's finger; the
experimenter acted alarmed and cautioned the subject to remain still, and
at one point pressed a button that caused sparks to emerge from the
equipment to which the subjects were attached. Of the 14 physiological
measures taken, 7 were significantly different between the anger and fear
conditions. For example, anger induced greater diastolic blood pressure
increases and heart rate decreases than fear, but muscle tension responses
were greater during fear than anger. Additionally, skin conductance level
was more responsive to anger, whereas spontaneous skin conductance
responses were more indicative of fear. In any case, this early study (and
subsequent conceptual replications; cf. Weerts & Roberts, 1976) suggest
that fear can be distinguished by a unique pattern of physiological responses.

In the typical study of fear and persuasion, however, it is relatively
uncommon to take physiological measures (Beck & Frankel, 1981). Nevertheless, studies that have employed even a modest number of physiological
measures (e.g., Mewborn & Rogers, 1979) have led to a rejection of the
initial aversive arousal reduction model of the effects of fear on persuasion

(Janis, 1967). It appears today that physiological changes are neither directly responsible nor necessary for the effectiveness of fear appeals. Cognitive coping and appraisal processes are much more important (Leventhal, 1970; Rogers & Mewborn, 1976). For a complete discussion of fear, physiological responses, and persuasion, consult Rogers (Chapter 6, this volume).

Dissonance

The one theory of attitude change linked to physiological activity that has generated the most research is Festinger's (1957) theory of cognitive dissonance. Dissonance occurs when a person feels responsible for bringing about a foreseeable negative consequence (cf. Wicklund & Brehm, 1976). In various accounts, the state of dissonance has been described using such terms as "drive-like," "arousing," "unpleasantly tense," and others. One way of reducing dissonance is to change one's attitude to make it more consistent with the behavior that triggered the dissonance. For example, if for a meager $10 incentive you were to recommend that a friend buy a car that you knew to be in bad repair, the ensuing dissonance could be resolved by coming to view the car more positively, thereby justifying your recommendation.

A number of other theories in social psychology have purported to be able to explain dissonance-like effects, and many experiments have been conducted to try to resolve the theoretical controversy (e.g., Fazio, Zanna, & Cooper, 1977). Since dissonance theory postulates something about a person's internal bodily responses, a number of investigators have sought a physiological measure of the "arousal" or "tenseness" presumably induced by dissonant behavior. These attempts have ranged from measuring vaso-constriction in the fingers following a dissonance-inducing choice (blood vessel constriction is a sign of stress; see Gerard, 1967), to measuring the abundance of occipital alpha electroencephalographic (EEG) activity after giving subjects a sufficient or insufficient justification for participating in an experiment (the presence of alpha activity generally indicates relaxation; see McMillen & Geiselman, 1974). None of these studies, however, has provided definitive evidence for a bodily response correlate of cognitive dissonance (Kiesler & Pallak, 1976).

Considerably more progress has been made in identifying whether or not dissonance induces unique feelings in a person regardless of whether or not there are any actual physiological correlates of these feelings. The most common procedure in these investigations involves a "misattribu-tion" paradigm (see Zillmann, Chapter 8, this volume). The basic idea of the misattribution studies (e.g., Zanna & Cooper, 1974) is that when subjects can be induced to misattribute their feelings of discomfort to an appropriate external stimulus (e.g., a pill that is said to produce tenseness as a side effect), no attitude change should result from the discrepant behavior. The fact that this misattribution procedure works suggests that regardless of the actual physiological changes produced by dissonant behavior, such behavior does induce a feeling of tenseness. For a thorough review of research relevant to dissonance and bodily responses, both real and perceived, consult Fazio and Cooper (Chapter 5, this volume).

Cognitive Elaboration

The 1970s brought a remarkable consensus among persuasion researchers around the idea that people are active information processors rather than passive recipients of persuasive communications. This consensus shifted researchers away from a focus on how well people learned and then subsequently recalled the arguments presented in a message (e.g., Miller & Campbell, 1959) to what people's thoughts were as they anticipated, scrutinized, and reflected on a message (see Greenwald, 1968; Petty *et al.*, 1981). A variety of procedures developed to assess the amount of thinking that people were doing about a message (see the review by Cacioppo & Petty, 1981c), although most techniques required people to report their thoughts either during or after message exposure (e.g., Brock, 1967). This self-report procedure, of course, raises the same kinds of problems that were involved in the direct verbal reports of attitudes. For example: Are people reporting their true thoughts? Are people making up thoughts merely to appear as if they have carefully scrutinized the message? (See Miller & Baron, 1973.) Not surprisingly, then, a direct concomitant physiological measure of cognitive elaboration would prove highly useful.

In persuasion research emphasizing cognitive elaboration, two questions about message elaboration have proven important. One question concerns the *extent* of elaboration. Are people doing a great deal of effortful thinking about the content of the message (e.g., relating the message to their own lives), or are they simply focusing on various cues in the persuasion situation (e.g., how loud the message is or how fast the speaker is talking). The first kind of task is presumably more difficult and requires more cognitive effort than the latter. The second question concerns the *nature* of the elaboration. Are the thoughts generated all on one side of the issue (i.e., affectively polarized), or are they more balanced? Current research suggests that the nature of the thoughts generated has important implications for the amount and direction of attitude change that results, and the extent of elaboration has important implications for the persistence of persuasion (greater elaboration results in greater persistence) (see the reviews by Cialdini, Petty, & Cacioppo, 1981; Petty & Cacioppo, in press). In the next two sections we address potential psychophysiological measures of the extent and nature of cognitive elaboration.

Extent of Elaboration.   Two psychophysiological measures have shown considerable relevance for assessing the amount of cognitive effort associated with a task. The first, pupillary dilation, is one that we discussed previously. Recall that Hess (1972; Hess & Polt, 1960) initially proposed that the pupils might be a useful indicant of a person's attitude, but that subsequent research seriously questioned this view. Interestingly, Hess and Polt (1964) also proposed that pupil size could "be used as a direct measure of mental activity" (p. 1190; for much earlier suggestions of this connection in the French and German psychological literature, see Mentz, 1895; Roubinovitch, 1901). In the Hess and Polt investigation, subjects were presented with four multiplication problems of increasing difficulty. Although no statistical analyses were reported, the mean change in pupil diameter from baseline to peak generally increased with the increasing difficulty of the problems.

Subsequent to the Hess and Polt study, a large number of experiments have indicated that pupillary dilation is positively associated with the difficulty of cognitive tasks and thus might serve as an index of cognitive effort (see Kahneman, 1973; Paivio, 1973). For example, pupil size has been shown to increase as the number of digits that subjects are asked to repeat is increased (Kahneman & Beatty, 1966), as an imagining task moves from concrete to abstract concepts (Paivio & Simpson, 1966), and as division problems become more complex (Bradshaw, 1968). In one interesting study, Stanners, Headley, and Clark (1972) told subjects that they would either have to paraphrase or memorize different sentences. The results of this study indicated that when subjects were listening to a sentence, pupil size was larger in the memorize than in the paraphrase condition, but in the period immediately after the presentation of the sentence, pupil size was larger if subjects thought that they would have to paraphrase the sentence rather than repeat it verbatim. This finding may suggest that memorization requires considerable cognitive effort during the presentation of the sentence, but less afterward. On the other hand, paraphrasing requires greater cognitive effort after the sentence has been heard (when subjects must presumably generate a new sentence with the same meaning as the old). In sum, the accumulated evidence is consistent with the view that pupillary dilation may reflect the cognitive requirements of a task (see Beatty, 1982, and Janisse, 1977, for reviews). To date, however, no experiment has investigated the pupillary measure in a persuasion situation, and thus it cannot yet be determined if the measure can provide a useful indicant of the cognitive effort associated with thinking about a message. In investigating this question, of course, researchers must be careful to control for other features of the persuasive message that could affect pupillary responses (e.g., message complexity, difficulty in understanding, novelty).

In addition to the literature on pupillary responses, a second body of research suggests that the activity of the perioral musculature may reflect the processing induced by a variety of cognitive tasks. For example, Sokolov (1969, 1972) reported a series of experiments in which covert oral (lip and tongue) EMG activity was elevated during the initial performance of tasks requiring cognitive effort (e.g., mental arithmetic; generating a title for a story, etc.). However, when the tasks were no longer cognitively effortful (because they had been practiced sufficiently to become relatively automatic), the EMG activity returned to baseline levels (see Cacioppo & Petty, Chapter 25, this volume, for further information on Sokolov's work; see also the reviews of oral EMG research by Garrity, 1977, and McGuigan, 1970, 1978).

We attempted to provide a relatively straightforward test of whether or not covert oral EMG activity could be used to index the extent or depth of processing. To make this test we selected the well-researched orienting-task paradigm developed by cognitive psychologists for studying encoding operations (see Cermak & Craik, 1978; Craik & Lockhart, 1972). In this paradigm, a subject is instructed by a cue question to focus on a specific feature of a stimulus to solve the problem posed by the cue question. For example, when people are asked to determine if a trait adjective (e.g., friendly) is self-descriptive, they are more likely to remember the word in a later test than if they are asked to determine if the word is printed in lowercase letters. The more durable memory trace produced by the first encoding task is thought to be due to the more distinctive and elaborate linguistic analyses that are required to perform the task. Thus, in the former case the adjective might be related to a wide variety of other information already stored in memory, whereas in the latter case only the sensory features of the word need be examined.

In an initial experiment (Cacioppo & Petty, 1979c), subjects were asked in half of the trials to judge whether or not a trait adjective was self-descriptive, and in the other half to judge whether the trait was printed in uppercase letters. Following each cue question, subjects saw a trait adjective that was printed in either upper- or lowercase letters, and was either self-descriptive or not (determined from subjects' pretests 10 days earlier). The adjectives were presented for about 2 seconds, at which time subjects were to respond to the cue question by pressing one of two buttons labeled "yes" and "no." During the task, EMG recordings were made from sensors placed over the nonpreferred forearm and adjacent to the lips (see Fridlund & Izard, Chapter 9, this volume, for further details on recording covert oral EMG activity). Finally, subjects were tested for their ability to recall the trait adjectives employed in the study. The recall measure showed that subjects were better able to recall the adjectives processed in response to the self-reference than the orthographic cue question. More interesting, however, was the fact that the incipient EMG activity monitored over the lip muscle region was greater during the self-reference than during the orthographic task, but the EMG activity monitored over the nonpreferred forearm (control) site did not differentiate the two tasks.

In order to provide a more stringent test of the hypothesis that covert oral EMG activity could index extent or depth of information processing, we conducted a second study (Cacioppo & Petty, 1981b). In this study, five rather than two orienting tasks were used, and a number of methodological refinements were made (e.g., stimulus presentations were aural rather than visual; subject-determined rather than fixed processing intervals were employed; etc.). In addition to again measuring lip and nonpreferred forearm EMG activity during the tasks, a test of recognition confidence was administered as a test of memory for the trait adjectives presented. The results from the study are presented in Figure 3-2. First, note the ordering of encoding efficiency presented in the left panel. The self-reference and evaluation encoding tasks led to the highest recognition confidence ratings (presumably resulting from a high degree of semantic elaboration), the volume discrimination and rhyme tasks led to the lowest (presumably resulting from a low degree of semantic elaboration), and the association task fell in between. Given this pattern of results, it is particularly important to note that the pattern of EMG activity over the lip

FIGURE 3-2. Mean recognition confidence (left panel) and median change from prestimulus levels for electromyographic activity during the processing interval for lip (middle panel) and nonpreferred forearm (right panel) as a function of orienting task. Abbreviations: VD, volume discrimination (Is the following word spoken louder than this question?); RH, rhyme (Does the following word rhyme with ____?); AS, association (Is the following word similar in meaning to ____?); EV, evaluation (Is the following word "good"?); SR, self-reference (Is the following word self-descriptive?). Data from Cacioppo and Petty (1981b).

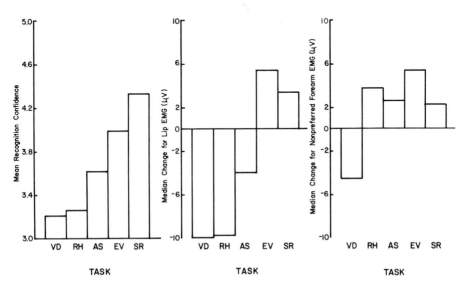

muscle region (middle panel) parallels this quite nicely. Interestingly, several of the low-elaboration tasks actually resulted in a decrease in EMG activity over the prestimulus baseline. One possible explanation for this is that the cognitive operations required for the simple tasks actually involved less extensive cognitive processing than that which occurred spontaneously during the brief pauses between tasks. Finally, in the right panel, it is once again clear that the nonpreferred forearm (control) EMG data were unrelated to the type of cognitive task performed. The two studies together provide rather strong support for the view that covert oral EMG responses can reflect the extent of semantic processing.[4]

In two additional studies we attempted to see if oral EMG responses could be used to reflect cognitive effort in a persuasion paradigm. In order to provide a maximally sensitive and interpretable test of the utility of this measure, we chose not to assess EMG responses during the presentation of a message, but rather after a forewarning of message presentation (Freedman & Sears, 1965). If we had measured and observed an increase in oral EMG responses during the presentation of a message, we would not be able to tell if the enhanced responses represented the passive rehearsal of the message or the active process of evaluating and elaborating the message. In the forewarning paradigm, message rehearsal is not a problem. Since previous research suggests that the motivation to think about a message is strongest when the topic is personally involving (Petty & Cacioppo, 1979b) and counterattitudinal (Cacioppo & Petty, 1979b), in our initial investigation (Cacioppo & Petty, 1979a, Experiment 1) we forewarned subjects that they would soon be hearing messages on six involving counterattitudinal issues (e.g., that their university was considering raising tuition by $90 a quarter). In an earlier study (Petty & Cacioppo, 1977) employing the thought-listing procedure, we demonstrated that subjects engaged in anticipatory counterarguing in the period after the forewarning but prior to the message (see also Brock, 1967). Electromyographic activity in relevant (lip, chin, and throat) and irrelevant (trapezius or back) areas was monitored during the minute preceding each forewarning (during which time subjects were asked to sit quietly), and during the minute

---

4. Other physiological measures have also been related to the cognitive requirements of a task. For example, the Laceys (1974) have argued and provided evidence for the view that heart rate acceleration is associated with cognitive elaboration and manipulation, whereas heart rate deceleration is associated with sensory intake and attention. Thus, heart rate acceleration accompanies such tasks as spelling words backward and mental arithmetic, whereas deceleration accompanies such tasks as watching light flashes (see Cacioppo & Sandman, 1978; J. I. Lacey, Kagan, Lacey, & Moss, 1963; Tursky, Schwartz, & Crider 1970). The Laceys' hypothesis stems from the view that increases in heart rate lead to baroreceptor feedback that can affect cortical excitability (see J. I. Lacey, 1967). We recorded heart rate in our orienting task studies, but it failed to differentiate the tasks. Thus, the oral EMG measure may be a more sensitive index of linguistic elaboration.

following each forewarning (during which time they were asked to collect their thoughts on the issue). Skeletomuscular responses during the "collect thoughts" interval revealed that oral EMG activity increased, whereas irrelevant EMG remained constant and quiescent compared to the preforewarning period.

Armed with this evidence, we conducted a second study (Cacioppo & Petty, 1979a, Experiment 2) to determine whether covert oral EMG activity (presumably reflecting cognitive activity) would occur spontaneously while people anticipated receiving an involving counterattitudinal communication. Two other conditions were also run. Some subjects anticipated receiving a proattitudinal communication, and others anticipated receiving simply an unidentified message. These groups were not expected to show any cognitive preparation in anticipation of the message (because the message posed no threat), and were included in part to rule out a number of possible artifacts (e.g., that any instruction might cause people to repeat the instruction silently to themselves until the onset of the message). Some of the results of this study (facial muscles) were presented in Figure 3-1. The oral (mentalis) EMG data indicated that subjects who expected to hear a proattitudinal or unidentified message failed to display any reliable increase in muscle activity during the postwarning–premessage period, whereas subjects who expected to hear the involving counterattitudinal message showed significant increases in the magnitude of oral EMG responses. All subjects, regardless of the type of message, exhibited elevated oral EMG activity during the actual presentation of the message. The EMG data from the forewarning period suggest that anticipating a counterattitudinal message results in more extensive cognitive preparation than anticipating a proattitudinal one. This effort is probably attributable to the relative importance of defending one's attitudes and beliefs on an involving issue from attack. Collectively our program of research on covert oral EMG suggests that the magnitude of this response may reflect covert linguistic processing (see Cacioppo & Petty, 1981a). Thus, in appropriate contexts, oral EMG may provide an important supplement to verbal reports of cognitive activity.

Nature of Elaboration. Earlier in this chapter we noted that recent research has indicated that the two hemispheres of the brain differ in their specialized functions. Thus, we reported that EEG measures from the frontal lobes suggested that the hemispheres might differ in their affective tone (Davidson et al., 1979; Tucker et al., 1981). We also noted that EEG measures from other brain areas did not demonstrate this pattern. For example, in the Davidson et al. (1979) study, EEG measures taken from the right and left parietal areas indicated that the right hemisphere was relatively more active during both positive and negative emotion. This finding is consistent with the views of some that while the left hemisphere is relatively logical and analytical, the right is more emotional (see the review by Tucker, 1981). If true, then people who display relative right-hemispheric activation during the presentation of a communication might also generate cognitive responses that are more affectively polarized than subjects who display relative left activation. Another view of the two hemispheres is provided by Corballis (1980), who argues that the left hemisphere is more specialized for abstract representation, whereas the right tends to maintain "representations that are isomorphic with reality" (p. 288). This formulation also suggests that the relative activation of the right hemisphere might be associated with more polarized cognitive responses. If a message was clearly proattitudinal, then with relative right-hemispheric involvement, a person's thoughts should polarize toward favorability (since this would best represent the subjective "reality" of the message), but if the message was clearly counterattitudinal, thoughts should polarize toward unfavorability. In a series of exploratory studies, we sought to investigate the relationship between hemispheric asymmetry and the nature of the cognitive responses elicited by the anticipation and presentation of a persuasive communication.

In our initial study (Cacioppo *et al.*, 1982, Experiment 1), 40 right-handed men anticipated and received either a pro- or a counterattitudinal message while EEG activity (alpha) was monitored over the left and right parietal areas. The specific sequence of events included a 60-second initial baseline period and then a 195-second communication period. The message subjects heard contained a mixture of strong and weak arguments (this was done to increase the likelihood that an analytical style of processing would result in a balanced profile of thoughts, and that subjective reality would be defined more by a person's own attitude than by argument quality). Following exposure to the message, subjects were given 2.5 minutes to list the thoughts and ideas that occurred to them during the communication period. Subjects then rated their thoughts as being favorable, unfavorable, or neutral toward the advocacy. A measure of the affective polarization of cognitive responses was calculated by subtracting the number of favorable from unfavorable thoughts for the counterattitudinal issue, and the reverse for the proattitudinal one. A second measure was employed to assess the simple total of affect-laden thoughts about the issue and was calculated by summing the number of favorable and unfavorable thoughts listed.

Prior to analysis of the cognitive response data, a median split was calculated on the basis of the differential hemispheric alpha abundance evinced during the pretreatment baseline, and another was performed on the basis of the EEG data collected during the communication period. A blocking factor for relative hemispheric activation was then used in the analyses of the cognitive response data. The analyses revealed that the individual differences in hemispheric activation during the baseline period did not account for a significant portion of the variance in either of the cognitive response measures. However, individual differences in hemispheric activation during the communication period showed the expected relationship to the affective polarization index. Subjects who showed relative activation of the right hemisphere during the communication period produced a more polarized profile of thoughts ($M = 2.2$) than did subjects who showed relative activation of the left hemisphere ($M = .15$). Differences in relative hemispheric activation during the communication period did not show a significant relationship to the total number of favorable and unfavorable thoughts listed.

In a second experiment (Cacioppo *et al.*, 1982, Experiment 2), a conceptual replication of the first study was undertaken to assess the reliability of the effect. Three major changes in procedure were made:

1. Communications on new topics were prepared.
2. We partitioned the EEG sampling epoch into four distinct periods: forewarning (15 seconds), postwarning–premessage period of silence (45 seconds), persuasive message (60 seconds), and postmessage period of silence (15 seconds).
3. Each subject was exposed to both pro- and counterattitudinal communications (with the order determined randomly for each subject).

Separate median splits and analyses were performed on the basis of the relative hemispheric alpha abundance obtained during each distinct period. As in the first study, subjects characterized by relative right-hemispheric activation generated more polarized (one-sided) thoughts regarding the attitude issue compared to subjects characterized by relative left-hemispheric activation. This effect emerged regardless of the communication period used to calculate the alpha ratio (all p's $< .05$). Again, for none of the sampling periods did the EEG ratios relate to the total number of favorable and unfavorable thoughts listed.

The data from these studies suggest one quite reliable effect: Individuals producing a relatively polarized profile of cognitive responses to a persuasive communication also demonstrate relative right-hemispheric EEG activation as assessed in the parietal lobes.[5] If the EEG ratio is used in

5. In a third study (Cacioppo, Petty, & Quintanar, 1982, Experiment 3) we obtained some evidence consistent with a causal explanation for the obtained relationship between hemispheric asymmetry and the affective polarization of cognitive responses. Employing a modification of Tesser's (1978) time-to-think paradigm (in which he finds that attitudes and thoughts polarize in the direction of their initial tendency with increased thinking), we manipulated the amount of time subjects had to think about an issue (20 vs. 90 seconds) and found that as individuals thought longer about an issue, a shifting of relative hemispheric activation toward the right hemisphere occurred. In a reanalysis of data collected by Appel, Weinstein, and Weinstein (1979), Krugman (1980) reported a conceptually similar effect. As repetitions of an advertisement increased (allowing more thought), subjects showed a shifting of relative activation from the left to the right hemisphere.

combination with the covert oral EMG measure described in the preceding section and the facial EMG profile of measures noted earlier in the chapter, it might be possible to index not only the extent of thinking, but also its affective intensity and its direction. For example, a relatively high score on oral EMG activity might indicate that a person was doing a lot of thinking about an issue, but it wound not indicate the nature of the thoughts. If, in addition, a pattern of relative right-hemispheric activation was present, it might be concluded that the extensive thinking was relatively one-sided. By including measures of facial muscle EMG (e.g., corrugator, zygomatic) as well, it might also be possible to detect the direction of the polarized thinking.

A BIOSOCIAL PERSPECTIVE ON ATTITUDE CHANGE

The major part of this chapter has been devoted to discussing and evaluating the circumstances under which bodily responses might be useful in measuring either attitudes or attitude-relevant processes. In the final part of this chapter we address the relationship between bodily responses and changes in attitude.

The bodily cues that affect attitudes can emanate from a communicator or from the target of an influence attempt. A communicator's bodily cues can influence attitudes in a variety of ways. For example, Mehrabian and Williams (1969) found that the degree of persuasive intent of a communicator could be correctly rated by judges who were only able to rely on postural cues for their decisions. The perception of persuasive intent generally leads to reduced persuasion (Petty & Cacioppo, 1979a). Other bodily cues can affect persuasion by signaling that the communicator either likes or dislikes the recipient, is of high or low status, or is of high or low credibility (McGuire, 1969). For example, increased eye contact can make a communicator more likable (Ellsworth & Carlsmith, 1968) and the speed (Miller, Maruyama, Beaber, & Valone, 1976) and style (Lind & O'Barr, 1979) of a communicator's speech can affect perceptions of credibility and honesty. Among the bodily cues that people perceive to indicate dishonesty are postural shifting, reductions in smiling and gazing, and slower, more hesitant speech (see the review by Zuckerman, DePaulo, & Rosenthal, 1981). Interestingly, some people are better at detecting and decoding bodily cues than others (Hall, 1978), and the effects of a particular cue may be quite different for good and poor decoders. For example, Hall (1980) found that people who were generally good at detecting the emotions of others were more influenced by a communicator who spoke in a warm, expressive tone, but that people who were poor at detecting emotions in others were more influenced by a communicator who spoke in a stiff, business-like tone. Hall suggests that poor decoders may find the emotional cues emitted by others aversive since they have difficulty understanding their meaning.

Most researchers have focused on the relationship between an individual's own bodily responses and attitude change. Our discussion of this issue will be presented in two parts. We first address bodily responses of which the person is or becomes aware, and then we address bodily responses that may affect attitudes even though the person is not aware of them. Any given bodily response may be detected or not. For example, a covert bodily response such as an elevated heart rate may be detected either by a person who feels a racing heart or by a nurse who takes the person's pulse. On the other hand, elevations in heart rate may remain completely undetected. Similarly, a person may be aware or unaware of a change in an overt bodily response. For example, a person may deliberately smile to provide encouragement to another, or may smile without realizing it. If no obvious reason for a detected bodily response is apparent (i.e., the response is unexpected), the person will probably be motivated to explain the response to his or her satisfaction. Under the appropriate circumstances, this search for an explanation may result in an attitude change. If the bodily response is not detected, however, it will probably have an influence on attitudes only by affecting some attitude-relevant process of which the person is unaware.[6]

Detected Bodily Responses

A person can experience a change in a bodily response in two ways. Some responses are "felt" directly, whereas other responses are pointed out to us by other people or by instrumentation. In Chapter 1 we noted that bodily responses of which a person is aware are analogous to "symptoms" in medical terminology, and the observable (verifiable) manifestations of bodily responses are analogous to medical "signs." Any given bodily response can serve as either a sign or a symptom. For example, an increase in body temperature can be detected either when a person feels hot (symptom) or when a thermometer registers 100 degrees (sign). Figure 3-3 presents an elaboration of part of our biosocial model of attitude change (see Cacioppo & Petty, 1982). The portion of the model that we first consider diagrams the potential attitudinal consequences of signs and symptoms. The model is presented as a series of questions. We do not mean to imply that persons necessarily are conscious of asking these questions of themselves, but rather that the processes by which detected bodily responses influence attitude change are outlined by these questions.

---

6. See Zillmann (Chapter 8, this volume) for a discussion of how residual physiological responses that are undetected can combine with subsequent physiological responses that are detected to enhance the subjective experience of affect or emotion.

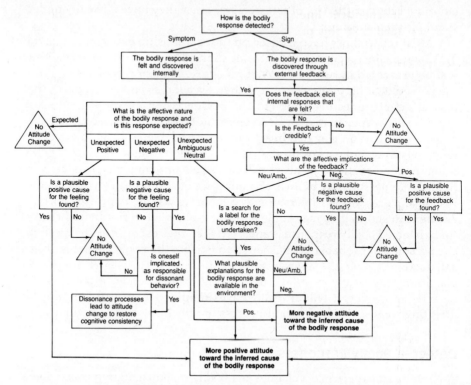

FIGURE 3-3. Biosocial model of attitude change.

Whether these questions are consciously posed or can be reported by a subject is doubtful, at least for some of these questions. For example, the first question in the model is: How is the bodily response detected? It seems more likely that people experience bodily responses as signs and/or concomitant symptoms than as answers to this question. With this distinction noted, we now consider the possible consequences of this "question."

Felt Bodily Responses

Interest in the role of felt bodily responses on attitude change stems primarily from Schachter and Singer's (1962, 1979) well-known two-factor theory of emotion. Schachter and Singer proposed that the felt sensation of physiological arousal could be labeled differently (misattributed) depending on the situational cues that were present. Thus, a person who felt "aroused" in the presence of an attractive member of the opposite sex might infer that this person was liked very much, but a person who felt aroused in the presence of an unattractive individual might infer that this person was disliked very much (see White, Fishbein, & Rustein, 1981).

Several independent lines of evidence have emerged that question the generalizability of this process. Zajonc (1980) argues that primitive affective (i.e., positive/neutral/negative) reactions sometimes precede cognitive reactions such as recognition and encoding. Similarly, we have suggested that the proprioceptive or interoceptive detection of bodily reactions may yield an affective response as part of the symptom experienced (Cacioppo & Petty, 1982; see also Pennebaker, Chapter 19, this volume). Finally, Maslach (1979) provides tentative evidence that the sudden and unexpected onset of sympathetic activation is experienced as an unpleasant rather than a neutral change in bodily state. Hence, a general affective reaction may be part and parcel of the detection of a symptom. This affective tone of the symptom is important for, as we shall see, it can determine the nature and extent of attitude change.

What occurs if the symptom was expected? Although Schachter (1964) spoke specifically about arousal rather than symptoms, his observations regarding this question are informative. Schachter proposed that: "Given a state of physiological arousal for which an individual has a completely appropriate explanation, no evaluative needs will arise, and the individual is unlikely to label his feelings in terms of the subjective cognitions available" (p. 53). Others, however, have proposed that felt arousal (or a symptom) could be misattributed to a source even when the actual source of the felt bodily response was obvious and expected (cf. Dutton & Aron, 1974). In four studies testing this extension of Schachter and Singer's two-factor theory, Kenrick, Cialdini, and Linder (1979) found no support for it. In their studies, male students were led to believe that they were either going to receive a painful electric shock (high felt arousal) or a mildly distracting noise (no felt arousal). While waiting for the stimuli to be presented, subjects were introduced to an attractive confederate (the nature of the interaction varied across the four studies), and they were asked to rate the confederate on a variety of first impression scales (e.g., liking, desire to date). Although physiological and self-report measures supported the effectiveness of the manipulation of felt bodily state, the manipulation had no effect on the ratings of the attractive confederate. Consistent with Schachter's (1964) notions, the authors concluded that if perceived arousal is to affect attraction, "it is most likely to do so where arousal is of ambiguous origin and not where the highly salient aversive stimuli are present" (p. 332). Thus, the model in Figure 3-3 depicts a question regarding the expectedness of the positive, neutral, or negative symptom that arose. Feelings that have obvious explanations are unlikely to elicit further thought that can result in misattribution and attitude change. For example, if you already knew that you were in love with someone, expected to feel sexually aroused in the presence of this person, and did, no change in attitude toward the person would occur as a result of the felt bodily response.

If there is no obvious explanation for the felt bodily response, there is a higher likelihood that the individual will search for a plausible cause, and this search will be biased by the affective as well as the informational features of the symptom. If the response is pleasant, the person searches the environment for a plausible explanation for the positive feeling. If a plausible cause for the positive feeling is found, it is likely that the person will adopt a more positive attitude toward the inferred cause of the positive feeling. For example, if a person detected unexpected sexual arousal (see Kelley & Byrne, Chapter 16, this volume) in the presence of a stranger, and the stranger was a plausible cause for the arousal, a more positive attitude toward the person would be likely than if no feeling of positive arousal was present. If the felt bodily response was negative (e.g., nausea), however, and the other person was a plausible cause for this feeling, a more negative attitude would probably be induced.[7]

One negative feeling that can arise in an attitude situation is cognitive dissonance. As we noted earlier, the accumulated research on dissonance theory indicates that if a person freely engages in discrepant behavior that results in foreseeable negative consequences, this behavior will elicit feelings of "tenseness" and "unpleasantness" (cf. Higgins, Rhodewalt, & Zanna, 1979; Shaffer, 1975; Fazio & Cooper, Chapter 5, this volume) that can be reduced through attitude change. If, however, the person who has engaged in dissonant behavior is given (or discovers) a plausible explanation for feeling uncomfortable (e.g., a pill that they have taken; Zanna & Cooper, 1974), no attitude change toward the object of the discrepant behavior occurs. Instead, subjects presumably become more negatively disposed toward the inferred cause of their discomfort (i.e., the pill). If no plausible external cause is provided for the unpleasant feeling, and the person feels responsible for engaging in the dissonant behavior, the person's attitude becomes more positive toward the discrepant behavior. Therefore, dissonance theory provides the interesting case of where negative feelings can result in more favorable attitudes toward an initially disliked stimulus. The more favorable attitude results from the person's attempt to justify (and therefore feel more positively about) the dissonant act.

Finally, the feelings arising from one's body may be neither particularly positive nor negative. Schachter and Singer, in fact, proposed that many cues from the body were of this ambiguous nature, and that under such circumstances the person would search the environment in order to evaluate and "label" the feelings. If the most plausible cues in the environment

---

7. Although these attitude changes might result from the attributional process described (cf. Bem, 1972), these attitude changes might also be due at least in part to classical or instrumental conditioning (cf. Byrne & Clore, 1970; Lott & Lott, 1968; Staats & Staats, 1958).

suggested a positive emotion, more favorable feelings would be induced by the arousal, but if the most plausible cues in the environment suggested a negative emotion, more unfavorable feelings would be induced. The classic Schachter and Singer (1962) study testing this view was described by Crider in Chapter 2. Recall that subjects were injected with a small amount of epinephrine. Some subjects were told that the injection would make them aroused, whereas others were not. Subjects were then placed in a room with a confederate who began to act in an angry or happy manner. The results of this study indicated that subjects who were paired with the angry confederate rated themselves as more angry when they were uninformed as to the arousing effects of the epinephrine than when they were informed.[8] Contrary to Schachter and Singer's expectations, however, subjects' self-reports of emotions were not affected when they were paired with the happy confederate. This result is consistent with the view that a sudden onset of unexplained arousal may not be experienced as neutral (and thus amenable to both positive and negative explanations), but may be perceived as distressful and unpleasant (Marshall & Zimbardo, 1979; Maslach, 1979), and thus only amenable to explanation by a plausible negative cause (see Cacioppo & Petty, in press, and Cotton, 1981, for recent reviews and critiques of the varied uses of Schachter and Singer's two-factor theory of emotion in social psychology).

Geen, Rakosky, and Pigg (1972) induced a state of ambiguous arousal by having subjects read a literary passage that was sexually arousing at the same time that a confederate presumably freely chose to deliver eight noxious shocks to the subject. In this situation, subjects were probably not sure if their felt arousal was due primarily to the sexual passage or to anger at the confederate. In order to guide subjects' inferences about their felt arousal, Geen *et al*, attached electrodes to subjects' forearms and fingertips and provided them with bogus physiological feedback from two voltmeters. One meter was said to register sexual arousal, and the other to register arousal due to the electric shock. Some subjects were led to believe that they were primarily sexually aroused as they read the passage and received shock, whereas others were led to believe that they were aroused primarily because of the shock. After this, subjects rated their emotional state and were given an opportunity to deliver shock to the confederate as he read a literary passage. When the voltmeter indicated that the arousal was due to the shock, subjects reported feeling significantly more "angry," and delivered more and higher-intensity shocks to the confederate than when the voltmeter indicated that their arousal was primarily sexual.

8. Presumably, if the confederate had insulted the subject rather than the experimenter's questionnaire in order to induce anger, he would probably have been liked less in the uninformed than in the informed conditions, as the perceived sensations would probably have been attributed to the confederate's insult.

In summary, the available data are generally consistent with the model presented in Figure 3-3. When a person perceives bodily sensations that arise from an uncertain origin, a search of the immediate environment is made to find an explanation for the sensations. If the sensations are pleasant, the search is for an explanation that is consistent with feeling positive. If the sensations are unpleasant, the search is biased in the negative direction. If a plausible explanation is found that is consistent with the bodily sensations, attitudes may change in the appropriate direction (dissonance theory providing an intriguing exception to this; see Figure 3-3). If the bodily sensations are neutral or ambiguous, the search is unconstrained and either positive or negative attitude changes may result, depending on whether the most plausible explanation in the immediate environment favors a positive or a negative cause of the bodily responses.

Externally Discovered Bodily Responses

If the person does not directly feel a bodily response, another means of detecting such responses is to have the response pointed out by another person or via instrumentation. In social psychology, subjects have typically "discovered" their bodily responses externally through false physiological feedback. Recall from our earlier discussion of the bogus pipeline procedure for measuring attitudes that the earliest use of bogus physiological feedback in social psychology was to convince people that the investigator already knew their specific belief or attitudinal tendencies (cf. Gerard, 1960). Therefore, the meaning of the bogus feedback in these studies was clearly specified. For example, in an ethically controversial study, Bramel (1962) used false physiological feedback to convince male subjects that they were showing "homosexual arousal" to pictures of men in various states of undress. Bramel reports that careful efforts were made to convince the subjects that the galvanometer to which they were exposed did not measure general anxiety and that the procedure was designed to be "so impressive to the subject that denial of the fact that homosexual arousal was being indicated would be very difficult" (p. 123). Most current research on bogus feedback, however, has followed Valins's (1966) procedure of providing ambiguous physiological information and leaving the interpretation of the feedback to the subject. Valins's ambiguous false-feedback paradigm was developed to test his belief that contrary to Schachter and Singer's notions, people do not actually have to *feel* any physiological activation for emotional experiences to be initiated.

Given the research that we discussed earlier on bodily responses that are felt, one important question about bogus physiological feedback is: Does the feedback elicit internal responses that are felt? Several studies have suggested that bogus physiological feedback may alter actual physiological activity (e.g., Hirschman & Hawk, 1978; Kerber & Coles, 1978), although investigators have typically not assessed if this activity is perceived by subjects. If the physiological activity is perceived, it is quite possible that people will follow the information search process for felt bodily responses outlined in the preceding section. In most instances, however, the modest physiological changes that are induced are probably not perceived accurately by subjects (see Blascovich & Katkin, Chapter 17, this volume). In any case, the accumulated research clearly indicates that actual physiological reactions are not necessary for bogus physiological feedback to affect attitudinal responses to stimuli (see the review by Liebhart, 1979).

If the bogus feedback does not correspond to any physiological sensations that are perceived, one important question about the feedback becomes: Is the feedback credible? If subjects do not experience anything subjectively, they will need to have a high degree of confidence in the investigator and the feedback equipment if the false information is to be believed. For example, in one study, Detweiler and Zanna (1976) told subjects that increased feedback (e.g., heart rate) indicated a negative emotional response to the stimuli presented (the names of countries) and that decreased feedback indicated a positive emotional response. As part of the cover story introducing the feedback equipment, however, the investigator made the subjects wait because of "equipment trouble," and subsequently subjects were taken on a tour of the control room where the experimenter's polygraph was described as "very old and working improperly." Even though the subjects' feedback was described as coming from different equipment borrowed from another lab that the "fellows from the electronics shop wired," subjects may have lost confidence in the entire procedure (i.e., if the fellows from the electronics shop could not get the experimenter's equipment to work properly, why should they trust the wiring on the other equipment?) Detweiler and Zanna found that the positive and negative feedback manipulation failed to differentially affect subjects' attitudes toward the nations, suggesting that the experimenter-provided labeling of the feedback may not have been believed.

If the bogus feedback is credible, the question becomes: What are the affective implications of the feedback? As we noted above, some feedback is designed to make subjects believe that they are experiencing positive arousal to some stimulus, whereas other feedback is designed to make the subjects believe that they are experiencing negative arousal. For example, in the relevant conditions of one study, Pittman, Cooper, and Smith (1977) exposed subjects to bogus arousal feedback which they were told indicated either interest in the game that they were playing, or interest in a monetary incentive provided for playing the game. When the subjects were told that their bodily responses reflected interest in the game, reported enjoyment of the game was enhanced over conditions where the arousal was said to reflect interest in the money.

In the Pittman *et al.* study and in others that have found similar effects (Brehm & Behar, 1966), the false feedback provided to subjects was clearly specified so that subjects would have no trouble deciding the cause of their externally detected bodily responses. Sometimes, however, the positive or negative feedback may not be specifically tied to a particular cause by the investigator. Under these conditions subjects might, for example, attribute the positive or negative feedback to their own daydreaming rather than to the stimuli in the experiment. If this were to happen, the investigator would observe no change on a measure of attitude toward the experimental stimuli. In other cases, the subjects' inferences about the positive or negative feedback may produce indirect effects on attitudes toward the experimental stimuli. For example, Giesen and Hendrick (1974) exposed subjects to a persuasive message on the problems of pesticides. In two of the conditions of this study subjects learned that they displayed either a low or a high amount of "unpleasant arousal" during the message. Post-message assessment of agreement with the message indicated that subjects in the high-unpleasant-arousal condition had more favorable attitudes toward the message than subjects in the low-unpleasant-arousal condition. Thus, feedback of unpleasant arousal was associated with more favorable attitudes toward the experimental stimuli (the message). How can this occur? Since the investigators did not explicitly state that the unpleasant-ness meter indicated that subjects disliked (disagreed with) the message, subjects may have inferred that the unpleasantness resulted from the fact that the arguments were so powerful that they induced fear or concern over the use of pesticides. Thus, feedback of unpleasant arousal may have led to more negative feelings about pesticides (consistent with the biosocial model), but more favorable feelings about the message, which expressed serious concern over the continued use of pesticides. In sum, if the specific cause of the positive or negative false feedback is not clearly provided by the experimenter, subjects may draw a number of possibly unintended inferences that may yield no attitude change toward the experimental stimuli or only indirect attitude effects.

In most studies on false feedback, neither the cause nor the affective nature of the feedback is provided by the investigator, and subjects are therefore free to draw a wide variety of inferences. In these situations, where neither affective nor causal label is provided for the false feedback, the major question is: Is a search for a label undertaken? When a person actually feels unexpected bodily sensations that are ambiguous, it is highly likely that a cognitive search will be undertaken, but when the sensations are not felt (i.e., they are only registered on a meter), a person may be less likely to engage in an extensive search for a label. Liebhart (1979) suggests that a search for an explanation for an unfelt bodily response may occur only when the feedback is particularly interesting or unexpected (creating some uncertainty), uncertainty reduction is important, and there is suffi-cient opportunity (time) for the search to occur. If the person is not motivated and able to engage in a search for an explanation for the bodily response, no attitude change will result.

If a search is undertaken, however, the important question, just as it was for felt bodily responses that were ambiguous is: What plausible explanations for the bodily response are salient in the environment? If the most plausible explanations available are positive, more favorable attitudes toward the inferred cause of the bodily response will result; but if the most plausible explanations available are negative, more unfavorable attitudes toward the inferred cause of the bodily response will result. Thus, when the salient stimuli in the environment are pleasant (e.g., nudes of the opposite sex), ambiguous bogus feedback will result in more favorable attitudes (cf. Valins, 1966), but when the salient stimuli in the environment are unpleasant (e.g., pictures of accident victims), ambiguous bogus feedback will result in less favorable attitudes (cf. Hirschman, 1975; see Hirschman & Clark, Chapter 7, this volume, for an extensive review of studies using a bogus physiological feedback procedure).[9]

In summary, if a credible externally originated indication of bodily response is detected, the cognitive processes that ensue are nearly identical to the processes that occur for felt bodily responses. If the bogus feedback is clearly labeled and tied to a specific stimulus, subjects will make the appropriate inferences about that stimulus. If the bogus feedback is ambiguous, a search of the environment is made for plausible explanations. Depending on the affective nature of the stimuli in the surrounding environment, either positive or negative attitude changes may result.

Undetected Bodily Responses

In the preceding section we argued that bodily responses that were detected influenced attitudes primarily by affecting the inferences that people made

9. Some investigators have proposed that the effects of ambiguous bogus feedback do not depend on subjects believing that the feedback represents their own bodily responses. For example, Parkinson and Manstead (1981) exposed subjects to pulsed sounds that they were told either represented their own heart rates or were simply electronic bleeps. When subjects were instructed to pay attention to the sounds, visual stimuli (slides of skin diseases) associated with acceleration of the pulsed sounds were rated as more unpleasant than stimuli associated with no change in the sounds. This effect occurred regardless of the meaning assigned to the sounds, and can be interpreted in a variety of ways. One possibility is that the feedback (whether it is labeled as heart rate or bleeps) may produce felt bodily sensations that lead to a search for a label. Another possibility is that any unusual feedback that draws attention to the stimulus induces further thought about the stimulus and attitude polarization in the direction of one's initial tendency (cf. Tesser, 1978). Finally, it should be noted that just because another kind of stimulus (unusual noises to which subjects are instructed to pay attention) produces the same attitudinal effects as false physiological feedback of bodily responses, this does not necessarily indicate that the two manipulations affect attitudes via the same underlying process.

about the causes of their bodily symptoms and signs. Bodily responses of which people are unaware, on the other hand, may affect attitudes by changing the manner in which an attitudinal stimulus is processed. Recent research suggests that undetected bodily responses can affect stimulus processing in either a relatively objective or a relatively biased manner.

Objective Influence

Based on the accumulated evidence for the hypothesis that phasic heart rate deceleration is associated with increased sensory sensitivity and phasic heart rate acceleration is associated with cognitive effort (B. C. Lacey & Lacey, 1974; J. I. Lacey, Kagan, Lacey, & Moss, 1973), Cacioppo, Sandman, and Walker (1978) proposed that transient and specific heart rate acceleration could facilitate the processing of a persuasive communication. Over a 5-day period, subjects were operantly conditioned momentarily to accelerate and decelerate their heart rates without altering their respiratory or somatic activity. After successful training, subjects were presented with brief counterattitudinal messages during periods of cardiac acceleration, deceleration, and basal heart rate. Attitudes toward the recommendations were obtained after each persuasive message, and retrospective reports of subjects' thoughts during the messages were obtained. The major result of this study was that cardiac acceleration was associated with the increased production of counterarguments and reduced agreement with the messages compared to the deceleration and basal heart rate conditions. Although the results of this study are consistent with the view that momentary and specific heart rate acceleration facilitates the generation of negative thoughts about a counterattitudinal message, since subjects were aware of their heart rate responses (because of the feedback provided), alternative explanations are possible for the data (e.g., subjects confronted with accelerated heart rate feedback may have inferred that they were upset with the message).

In order to provide more definitive support for the hypothesis, Cacioppo (1979) conducted two additional experiments in a cardiology clinic using fully informed outpatients who had implanted cardiac pacemakers. In these studies heart rate was varied exogenously (without the subject's knowledge) by placing a magnet over a reed in the subject's pacemaker. The patients' pacemakers were "demand type," so called because they paced the heart at a constant rate (72 beats per minute) when natural pacing produced a rate below the set level. The pacemaker level could be accelerated to and maintained at a rate of 88 beats per minute when an uncapped magnet was placed appropriately over the pacemaker. In the first pacemaker study, subjects were asked to generate sentences (cf. J. I. Lacey et al., 1963) and take a reading comprehension test (cf. Spence, Lugo, & Youdin, 1972) under accelerated and basal heart rate trials. Accelerated relative to basal heart rate significantly improved reading comprehension and tended to improve performance on the sentence generation task.

In a second pacemaker study (Cacioppo, 1979, Experiment 2), 22 elderly subjects read counterattitudinal communications on two involving issues (e.g., that all social security and medicare programs be eliminated). The order in which heart rate was varied (basal or acceleration first) served as a between-subjects factor, whereas paced heart rate (basal vs. accelerated) served as a within-subjects factor. The two messages were always presented in the same order. Each subject read each message at his or her own rate under the appropriate heart rate condition. Following each message, subjects were asked to report all their thoughts about the message into a tape recorder and give their attitudes on the issue. The thoughts were subsequently transcribed and scored by judges who were blind to the experimental conditions. The major result of the study was that subjects generated signifcantly more counterarguments when the message was read under accelerated than under basal heart rate conditions. On an individual subject basis, 13 of the subjects generated more counterarguments to the message read under accelerated than under basal heart rate conditions, 3 generated fewer, and 6 generated the same number. Although attitudes were not affected significantly by the heart rate manipulation (probably because of a ceiling effect; 59% of the subjects responded with the most extreme disagreement possible), attitudes showed a significant negative correlation with the number of counterarguments generated ($r = -.46, p < .05$).

The results of the pacemaker studies, of course, are not susceptible to the same kind of alternative explanations as were possible for the operant conditioning study and more clearly suggest that a transient and specific acceleration of heart rate is associated with enhanced cognitive elaboration.[10] Nevertheless, in both studies on heart rate and influenceability, the persuasive messages employed elicited primarily counterarguments, and elevated heart rate was shown to increase negative cognitive responses. To provide more definitive support for the view that elevated heart rate enhances message processing in general (and not counterarguing in particular), a study employing a message that elicits predominantly favorable thoughts should be conducted. For example, if a person has a greater ability to process a message with strong arguments due to accelerated heart rate, enhanced production of favorable thoughts and increased persuasion should result.

10. It is important to note that manipulations that produce nonspecific or tonic changes in heart rate would not be expected to have the same effects. For example, the elevated heart rate associated with a standing over a reclining posture has not been found to facilitate message comprehension (Cacioppo, 1979). In fact, the greater distractions associated with the standing over the reclining posture appear to reduce the likelihood of message elaboration in some contexts (Petty, Wells, Heesacker, Brock, & Cacioppo, 1983).

Biased Influence

Based on the emerging research showing that manipulations of overt bodily responses such as facial expressions can influence affective responses[11] (see Buck, 1980), Wells and Petty (1980) tested the hypothesis that affectively relevant bodily movements could influence agreement with a persuasive communication. In this study, subjects were led to believe that they were participating in consumer research on the sound quality of stereo headphones. They were told that the manufacturer was interested in how the headphones tested (as to sound quality, comfort, etc.) when listeners were engaged in movement (e.g., dancing, jogging). Three experimental conditions were created. Some subjects were told that they should move their heads up and down (vertical movement condition) about once per second to test the headphones, whereas others were told to move their heads from side to side. A final group of subjects was told that they were controls and heard no specific statements about head movements.

Head movements were chosen for study because of their strong association with agreeing and disagreeing responses in a wide variety of cultures (Eibl-Eibesfeldt, 1972). Darwin (1872), in fact, suggested that head shaking has a universal negative meaning that originated from food refusal. The interesting question was whether or not these movements would bias responses to a persuasive communication. After subjects were given their instructions, a tape from a purported campus radio program was played. The tape began with music, and then the disc jockey introduced a station editorial. Subjects either heard an editorial in favor of raising tuition at their university (this message elicited primarily counterarguments in a pretest), or one in favor of reducing tuition (this message elicited primarily favorable thoughts in a pretest). Following the radio broadcast, subjects rated the headphones on a variety of dimensions, and gave their opinions about the music and editorial. The key attitude measure asked subjects what they thought the appropriate semester tuition should be. These data are graphed in Figure 3-4. Two significant effects emerged: a message main effect (subjects advocated greater tuition after the raise than after the lower-tuition message), and a message × head movement interac-

---

11. For example, Rhodewalt and Comer (1979) found that relative to people who wrote a counterattitudinal essay with their faces in a neutral position, subjects whose faces were subtly manipulated into a frown reported a more negative mood and changed their attitudes significantly more toward the position taken in their essays, whereas subjects whose faces were subtly manipulated into a smile reported a more positive mood and changed their attitudes significantly less. Presumably, the overt but undetected facial expression facilitated or inhibited the experience of cognitive dissonance with the expected ramifications for attitude change [see the chapters by Fridlund & Izard (Chapter 9), Hager & Ekman (Chapter 10), Sackeim & Gur (Chapter 11), and Leventhal & Mosbach (Chapter 12), this volume, for more on the effects of facial feedback on the experience of emotion].

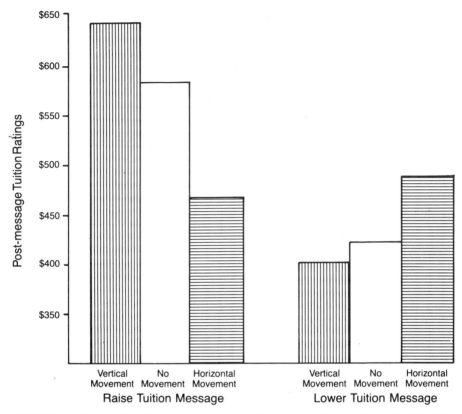

FIGURE 3-4. Effects of overt head movement on attitudes toward pro- and counterattitudinal messages. Data from Wells and Petty (1980).

tion. The interaction indicated that vertical-head-movement subjects advocated more tuition than horizontal-head-movement subjects in response to the raise-tuition message, but vertical-head-movement subjects advocated less tuition than did horizontal-head-movement subjects in response to the reduce-tuition message. In other words, vertical head movements led to greater agreement with the message in both cases than did horizontal head movements. The no-movement control group fell in between for both messages.

Postexperimental questioning of subjects indicated that they were not aware of the experimental hypotheses or of the effect of the head movements on their attitudes. Therefore, it is unlikely that the effect is due to "demand characteristics" or to an attributional process similar to that described for bodily responses that are detected. Two other possibilities remain, however. One possibility is that the head movements directly produce either positive or negative affect. According to this explanation, the positive feelings induced by the vertical head movements would translate into more positive evaluations of the message, and the negative feelings induced by the horizontal head movements would translate into more negative evaluations of the message (Zajonc & Markus, 1982). Alternatively, vertical head movements might be compatible with and therefore facilitate the generation of favorable thoughts to a message, and be incompatible with and therefore inhibit the generation of message counterarguments. The opposite would be the case for horizontal head movements. This explanation contends that head movements affect attitudes indirectly by biasing the cognitive processing of the persuasive message. Whichever explanation proves correct, it is clear that overt bodily responses can exert an influence on the amount and direction of persuasion.

The Nature of Attitude Changes Induced via Bodily Responses

Most of the research on bodily responses and persuasion has centered on the question of whether or not the detection or manipulation of bodily responses can induce attitude change, but research has generally ignored the nature of the changes induced through bodily responses. Elsewhere we have proposed a general model of attitude change that proposes that there are basically two routes to persuasion (Petty & Cacioppo, 1981, in press). One, called the central route, views attitude change as resulting from the diligent consideration and elaboration of issue-relevant arguments (or object-relevant attributes). The other, called the peripheral route, views attitude change as resulting from the application of simple decision rules or the association of the attitude issue or object with either positive or negative cues. These decision rules (e.g., the more arguments, the better) and cues (e.g., external rewards, an attractive message source) may shape attitudes without the need for engaging in extensive issue- or object-relevant thought.

We have argued that the two routes to persuasion occur under different antecedent conditions and that they have different consequences. The central route to persuasion is most likely when a message recipient is highly motivated and able to think about the issue-relevant arguments or object-relevant attributes presented. Thus, issue-relevant thought has been found to be an important determinant of persuasion when the persuasion situation facilitates thinking (e.g., the issue is personally involving, few distractions are present, the message is repeated; Cacioppo & Petty, 1979b; Petty, Cacioppo, & Heesacker, 1981). The peripheral route is more likely when these conditions are absent. For example, in one study we manipulated the personal relevance of the issue presented to subjects together with the expertise of the source of the message and the strength of the arguments used to support the position (Petty, Cacioppo, &

Goldman, 1981). When the issue was of low importance, attitudes were affected by the expertise manipulation but not by argument strength (peripheral route). On the other hand, when the issue was of high personal importance, attitudes were affected by the quality of the arguments presented but not by the expertise of the source (central route). Current research indicates that the route to persuasion may be an important determinant of the persistence of induced attitude changes and the attitude behavior link (see Petty & Cacioppo, 1983).

What kind of attitude change is produced by the detection of bodily responses? Although this issue has not been addressed specifically in research, we believe that the detection of a bodily response can lead to attitude change by either route. Once an inference is made about the cause of a bodily response ("That picture seems to be making me excited!"), one of two things may happen. In some situations (e.g., low involvement and low prior knowledge about the stimulus), the labeling process (if it takes place at all) may stop with a simple attitudinal inference ("That picture must appeal to me") (Chaiken & Baldwin, 1981; Taylor, 1975). In this case the detected bodily response serves as a positive cue for one's attitude (the peripheral route). In other situations, however, the person may engage in considerable thought about *why* the picture seems appealing. This may involve extensive cognitive processing of the attributes of the picture. If the picture is generally pleasant, for example, scrutiny of the picture may elicit a number of favorable cognitive responses that produce attitude polarization (cf. Liebhart, 1979; Tesser, 1978). If this occurs, the central route to persuasion has been followed. In any given study, depending on the nature of the stimuli employed (e.g., involving or not), the type of bodily response detected (symptoms, because they are felt, probably induce more thinking than signs), the amount of time provided to think (the more time, the more thought), and other factors, the attitude change induced may be either central or peripheral. Central changes are likely to be enduring and predictive of subsequent behavior, whereas peripheral changes are not.

CONCLUSION

In this chapter we have reviewed a wide variety of ways in which bodily responses are related to attitude measurement and change. In the first part of the chapter we noted that researchers have long sought a reliable and valid bodily response measure of attitudes. Our review indicated that although various natural *overt* bodily response measures appeared to have validity in some contexts, the search for a naturally occurring *covert* bodily response to indicate attitudes has been more frustrating. Studies have typically measured only one bodily response (e.g., SRR or pupillary dilation) and these studies have been vulnerable to the criticism that the attention or interest value of stimuli were being measured rather than positive or negative feelings (evaluations). The most promising covert measure appears to reside in the pattern of facial EMG activity. Although this measure has great potential, to date it has been tested in only one persuasion study. Also, although the measure appears to provide a clear discrimination of positive from negative affective states (an essential feature of any useful covert measure), it is not yet apparent if the measure will prove useful in distinguishing important subtle differences in degree of attitude favorability.

The classical conditioning approach, wherein a covert bodily response is trained to indicate an attitude, has been only partially successful. The major problem with this measure is that sophisticated subjects may exert voluntary control over their bodily responses, negating the purpose of the conditioning. One of the most interesting uses of bodily responses in attitude measurement does not require bodily responses to be measured at all. Through the bogus pipeline procedure, subjects may be convinced that their attitudes actually can be measured and therefore they may decide to report their true feelings more honestly. Two serious drawbacks of this procedure, however, are that it appears to induce negative affect, and its continued usefulness is dependent on a naive public.

Given some of the problems encountered in using covert bodily respones to measure attitudes directly, a promising direction for future research may be to use covert respones to assess the processes underlying attitude change. We reviewed some evidence suggesting that physiological measures might profitably be employed in this regard. For example, the persuasion process is typically viewed as encompassing several sequential steps (e.g., attention, elaboration). The physiological measures that we have reviewed may prove better measures of some of these underlying processes than of the attitudes themselves (e.g., SRRs for attention/interest; oral EMG for elaboration).

In the second part of the chapter we saw that just as researchers have sought to use bodily responses to measure people's attitudes, under appropriate conditions people naturally use the physiological feedback from their own bodies (whether real or bogus) to infer their own attitudes. The major finding was that people generally formed positive attitudes toward causes that they believe have made them feel good, and negative attitudes toward causes that they believe have made them feel bad. When the bodily response detected was of ambiguous affectivity, attribution to a positive cause produced more favorable attitudes and attribution to a negative cause produced less favorable attitudes. Although these attitudinal results have been observed in a wide variety of studies, the underlying processes are not completely clear. In fact, we have suggested that two distinct routes to persuasion may underlie these changes.

Finally, we reviewed some recent research suggesting that manipulations of bodily responses could affect attitudes indirectly by changing the extent or the affectivity of the information-processing activity preceding the change. Perhaps the most important conclusion to be drawn from our review of the role of bodily responses in attitude measurement and change is that although bodily response measures and manipulations have some utility in regard to measuring and influencing attitudes directly, even greater utility may be found in measuring and influencing the underlying *processes* of persuasion.

R E F E R E N C E S

Acker, I. E., & Edwards, A. E.   Transfer of vasoconstriction over a bipolar meaning dimension. *Journal of Experimental Psychology*, 1964, 67, 1–6.

Ahern, G. L., & Schwartz, G. E.   Differential lateralization for positive versus negative emotion. *Neuropsychologia*, 1979, 17, 693–697.

Allport, G. W.   Attitudes. In C. Murchison (Ed.), *Handbook of social psychology* (Vol. 2). Worcester, Mass.: Clark University Press, 1935.

Appel, V., Weinstein, S., & Weinstein, C.   Brain activity and recall of TV advertising. *Journal of Advertising Research*, 1979, 19, 7–15.

Argyle, M.   *The psychology of interpersonal behavior*. Baltimore: Penguin Books, 1967.

Arima, J. K., & Wilson, G. E.   Situational stress, anxiety, and the pupillary response. *Proceedings of the 80th Annual Convention of the American Psychological Association*, 1972, 7, 269–270.

Arkin, R. M., Appelman, A. J., & Burger, J. M.   Social anxiety, self-presentation, and the self-serving bias in causal attribution. *Journal of Personality and Social Psychology*, 1980, 38, 23–35.

Atwood, R. W., & Howell, R. J.   Pupilometric and personality test score differences of female aggressing pedophiliacs and normals. *Psychonomic Science*, 1971, 22, 115–116.

Ax, A. F.   The physiological differentiation between anger and fear in humans. *Psychosomatic Medicine*, 1953, 15, 433–442.

Barlow, J. D.   Pupillary size as an index of preference in political candidates. *Perceptual and Motor Skills*, 1969, 28, 587–590.

Beatty, J.   Task-evoked pupillary responses, processing load, and the structure of processing resources. *Psychological Bulletin*, 1982, 91, 276–292.

Beck, K. H., & Frankel, A.   A conceptualization of threat communications and protective health behavior. *Social Psychology Quarterly*, 1981, 44, 204–217.

Bem, D. J.   Self-perception theory. In L. Berkowitz (Ed.), *Advances in experimental social psychology* (Vol. 6). New York: Academic, 1972.

Bernick, N., Kling, A., & Borowitz, G.   Physiologic differentiation of sexual arousal and anxiety. *Psychosomatic Medicine*, 1971, 33, 341–352.

Bradshaw, J. L.   Pupil size and problem solving. *Quarterly Journal of Experimental Psychology*, 1968, 20, 116–122.

Bramel, D.   A dissonance theory approach to defensive projection. *Journal of Abnormal and Social Psychology*, 1962, 64, 121–129.

Brehm, J. W., & Behar, L. B.   Sexual arousal, defensiveness, and sex preferences in affiliation. *Journal of Experimental Research in Personality*, 1966, 1, 195–200.

Brock, T. C.   Communication discrepancy and intent to persuade as determinants of counterargument production. *Journal of Experimental Social Psychology*, 1967, 3, 269–309.

Buck, R.   Nonverbal behavior and the theory of emotion: The facial feedback hypothesis. *Journal of Personality and Social Psychology*, 1980, 38, 811–824.

Byrne, D., & Clore, G.   A reinforcement model of evaluative responses. *Personality: An International Journal*, 1970, 1, 103–128.

Byrne, D., Ervin, C. R., & Lamberth, J.   Continuity between the experimental study of attraction and "real life" computer dating. *Journal of Personality and Social Psychology*, 1970, *16*, 157–165.

Cacioppo, J. T.   The effects of exogenous changes in heart rate on the facilitation of thought and resistance to persuasion. *Journal of Personality and Social Psycholgoy*, 1979, *37*, 487–496.

Cacioppo, J. T., & Petty, R. E.   Attitudes and cognitive response: An electrophysiological approach. *Journal of Personality and Social Psychology*, 1979, *37*, 2181–2199. (a)

Cacioppo, J. T., & Petty, R. E.   Effects of message repetition and position on cognitive response, recall, and persuasion. *Journal of Personality and Social Psychology*, 1979, *37*, 97–109. (b)

Cacioppo, J. T., & Petty, R. E.   Lip and nonpreferred forearm EMG activity as a function of orienting task. *Journal of Biological Psychology*, 1979, *9*, 103–113. (c)

Cacioppo, J. T., & Petty, R. E.   Electromyograms as measures of extent and affectivity of information processing. *American Psychologist*, 1981, *36*, 441–456. (a)

Cacioppo, J. T., & Petty, R. E.   Electromyographic specificity during covert information processing. *Psychophysiology*, 1981, *18*, 518–523. (b)

Cacioppo, J. T., & Petty, R. E.   Social psychological procedures for cognitive response assessment: The thought listing technique. In T. V. Merluzzi, C. R. Glass, & M. Genest (Eds.), *Cognitive assessment*. New York: Guilford, 1981. (c)

Cacioppo, J. T., & Petty, R. E.   A biosocial model of attitude change. In J. T. Cacioppo & R. E. Petty (Eds.), *Perspectives in cardiovascular psychophysiology*. New York: Guilford, 1982.

Cacioppo, J. T., & Petty, R. E.   Social psychophysiology. In L. Stegagno (Ed.), *Psychophysiology*. Turin: Boringhieri, in press.

Cacioppo, J. T., Petty, R. E., & Quintanar, L.   Individual differences in relative hemispheric alpha abundance and cognitive responses to persuasive communications. *Journal of Personality and Social Psychology*, 1982, *43*, 623–636.

Cacioppo, J. T., & Sandman, C. A.   Physiological differentiation of sensory and cognitive tasks as a function of warning, processing demands, and reported unpleasantness. *Journal of Biological Psychology*, 1978, *6*, 181–192.

Cacioppo, J. T., & Sandman, C. A.   Psychophysiological functioning, cognitive responding, and attitudes. In R. E. Petty, T. M. Ostrom, & T. C. Brock (Eds.), *Cognitive responses in persuasion*. Hillsdale, N.J.: Erlbaum, 1981.

Cacioppo, J. T., Sandman, C. A., & Walker, B. B.   The effects of operant heart rate conditioning on cognitive elaboration and attitude change. *Psychophysiology*, 1978, *15*, 330–338.

Cermak, L. S., & Craik, F. I. M. (Eds.).   *Levels of processing in human memory*. Hillsdale, N.J.: Erlbaum, 1978.

Chaiken, S., & Baldwin, M. W.   Affective–cognitive consistency and the effect of salient behavioral information on the self-perception of attitudes. *Journal of Personality and Social Psychology*, 1981, *41*, 1–12.

Cialdini, R. B., Petty, R. E., & Cacioppo, J. T.   Attitude and attitude change. *Annual Review of Psychology*, 1981, *32*, 357–404.

Collins, B. E., Ellsworth, P. C., & Helmreich, R. L.   Correlations between pupil size and the semantic differential: An experimental paradigm and pilot study. *Psychonomic Science*, 1967, *9*, 627–628.

Cook, S. W., & Selltiz, C. A.   A multiple indicator approach to attitude measurement. *Psychological Bulletin*, 1964, *62*, 36–55.

Cooper, J. B., & Singer, D. N.   The role of emotion in prejudice. *Journal of Social Psychology*, 1956, *44*, 241–247.

Corballis, M. C.   Laterality and myth. *American Psychologist*, 1980, *35*, 284–295.

Cotton, J. L.   A review of research on Schachter's theory of emotion and the misattribution of arousal. *European Journal of Social Psychology*, 1981, *11*, 365–397.

Craik, F. I. M., & Lockhart, R. S.   Levels of processing: A framework for memory research. *Journal of Verbal Learning and Verbal Behavior*, 1972, *11*, 671–684.

Creelman, M. B. *The experimental investigation of meaning.* New York: Springer, 1966.

Darrow, C. W. The rationale for treating the change in galvanic skin response as a change in conductance. *Psychophysiology,* 1964, *1,* 31–38.

Darwin, C. *The expression of the emotions in man and animals.* London: Murray, 1872.

Davidson, R. J., Schwartz, G. E., Saron, C., Bennett, J., & Goleman, D. J. Frontal versus parietal EEG asymmetry during positive and negative affect. *Psychophysiology,* 1979, *16,* 202–203. (Abstract)

Detweiler, R. A., & Zanna, M. P. On the physiological mediation of attitudinal responses. *Journal of Personality and Social Psychology,* 1976, *33,* 107–116.

Dickson, H. W., & McGinnies, E. Affectivity in the arousal of attitudes as measured by galvanic skin response. *American Journal of Psychology,* 1966, *79,* 584–587.

Dimond, S. J., Farrington, L., & Johnson, P. Differing emotional response from right and left hemispheres. *Nature,* 1976, *261,* 690–692.

Dutton, D., & Aron, A. Some evidence for heightened sexual attraction under conditions of high anxiety. *Journal of Personality and Social Psychology,* 1974, *30,* 510–517.

Dysinger, D. W. A comparative study of affective responses by means of the impressive and expressive methods. *Psychological Monographs,* 1931, *41,* 14–31.

Eibl-Eibesfeldt, I. Similarities and differences between cultures in expressive movement. In R. A. Hinde (Ed.), *Nonverbal communication.* Cambridge: Cambridge University Press, 1972.

Ekman, P. Universals and cultural differences in facial expressions of emotion. In J. K. Cole (Ed.), *Nebraska Symposium on Motivation* (Vol. 19). Lincoln: University of Nebraska Press, 1971.

Ekman, P., & Friesen, W. V. *Unmasking the face.* Englewood Cliffs, N.J.: Prentice-Hall, 1975.

Ellsworth, P., & Carlsmith, J. Effects of eye contact and verbal content on affective response to a dyadic interaction. *Journal of Personality and Social Psychology,* 1968, *10,* 15–20.

Fazio, R. H., Zanna, M. P., & Cooper, J. Dissonance and self-perception: An integrative view of each theory's proper domain of application. *Journal of Experimental Social Psychology,* 1977, *13,* 464–479.

Feather, B. Semantic generalization of classically conditioned responses: A review. *Psychological Bulletin,* 1965, *63,* 425–441.

Festinger, L. *A theory of cognitive dissonance.* Stanford, Calif.: Stanford University Press, 1957.

Fleming, D. Attitude: The history of a concept. *Perspectives in American History,* 1967, *1,* 287–365.

Freedman, J. L., & Sears, D. O. Warning, distraction, and resistance to influence. *Journal of Personality and Social Psychology,* 1965, *1,* 262–266.

Gaes, G. G., Kalle, R. J., & Tedeschi, J. T. Impression management in the forced compliance situation. *Journal of Experimental Social Psychology,* 1978, *14,* 493–510.

Galton, F. Measurement of character. *Fortnightly Review,* 1884, *42,* 179–185.

Garrity, L. Electromyography: A review of the current status of subvocal speech research. *Memory & Cognition,* 1977, *5,* 615–622.

Geen, R. G., Rakosky, J. J., & Pigg, R. Awareness of arousal and its relation to aggression. *British Journal of Social and Clinical Psychology,* 1972, *11,* 115–121.

Gerard, H. B. Acts, attitudes, and conformity. *Symposia Study Series No. 4,* The National Institute of Social and Behavioral Science, September 1960.

Gerard, H. B. Disagreement with others, their credibility, and experienced stress. *Journal of Abnormal and Social Psychology,* 1961, *62,* 559–564.

Gerard, H. B. Physiological measurement in social psychological research. In P. H. Leiderman & D. Shapiro (Eds.), *Psychobiological approaches to social behavior.* Stanford, Calif.: Stanford University Press, 1964.

Gerard, H. B. Choice difficulty, dissonance, and the decision sequence. *Journal of Personality,* 1967, *35,* 91–108.

Giesen, M., & Hendrick, C. Effects of false positive and negative arousal feedback on persuasion. *Journal of Personality and Social Psychology,* 1974, *30,* 449–457.

Goldstein, I. B.   Electromyography: A measure of skeletal muscle response. In N. S. Greenfield & R. A. Sternbach (Eds.), *Handbook of psychophysiology*. New York: Holt, Rinehart &
Winston, 1972.

Goldwater, B. C.   Psychological significance of pupillary movements. *Psychological Bulletin*,
1972, *77*, 340–355.

Greenwald, A. G.   Cognitive learning, cognitive response to persuasion, and attitude change.
In A. G. Greenwald, T. C. Brock, & T. M. Ostrom (Eds.), *Psychological foundations of attitudes*.
New York: Academic, 1968.

Hall, J. A.   Gender effects in decoding nonverbal cues. *Psychological Bulletin*, 1978, *85*, 845–857.

Hall, J. A.   Voice tone and persuasion. *Journal of Personality and Social Psychology*, 1980, *38*,
924–934.

Hassett, J.   *A primer of psychophysiology*. San Francisco: W. H. Freeman, 1978.

Hess, E. H.   Attitude and pupil size. *Scientific American*, 1965, *212*, 46–54.

Hess, E. H.   Pupillometrics. In N. S. Greenfield & R. A. Sternbach (Eds.), *Handbook of psychophysiology*. New York: Holt, Rinehart & Winston, 1972.

Hess, E. H., & Polt, J. M.   Pupil size as related to interest value of visual stimuli. *Science*,
1960, *132*, 349–350.

Hess, E. H., & Polt, J. M.   Pupil size in relation to mental activity during simple problem
solving. *Science*, 1964, *143*, 1190–1192.

Hicks, R. A., & LaPage, S.   *A pupillometric test of the bidirectional hypothesis*. Paper presented at the
meeting of the Western Psychological Association, Los Angeles, April 1976.

Higgins, E. T., Rhodewalt, F., & Zanna, M.   Dissonance motivation: Its nature, persistence,
and reinstatement. *Journal of Experimental Social Psychology*, 1979, *15*, 16–34.

Hirschman, R.   Cross modal effects of anticipatory bogus heart rate feedback in a negative
emotional context. *Journal of Personality and Social Psychology*, 1975, *31*, 13–19.

Hirschman, R., & Hawk, G.   Emotional responsivity to nonveridical heart rate feedback as a
function of anxiety. *Journal of Research in Personality*, 1978, *12*, 235–242.

Izard, C. E.   *The face of emotion*. New York: Appleton-Century-Crofts, 1971.

Izard, C. E.   *Human emotions*. New York: Plenum, 1976.

Janis, I. L.   Effects of fear arousal on attitude change: Recent developments in theory and
experimental research. In L. Berkowitz (Ed.), *Advances in experimental social psychology* (Vol. 3).
New York: Academic, 1967.

Janisse, M. P.   Pupil size, affect, and frequency of exposure. *Social Behavior and Personality*,
1974, *2*, 125–146.

Janisse, M. P.   *Pupillometry: The psychology of the pupillary response*. Washington, D.C.: Hemisphere,
1977.

Janisse, M. P., & Peavler, J. S.   Pupillary research today: Emotion in the eye. *Psychology Today*,
1974, *7*, 60–63.

Jones, E. E., Bell, L., & Aronson, E.   The reciprocation of attraction from similar and
dissimilar others. In C. C. McClintock (Ed.), *Experimental social psychology*. New York: Holt,
Rinehart & Winston, 1971.

Jones, E. E., & Sigall, H.   The bogus pipeline: A new paradigm for measuring affect and
attitude. *Psychological Bulletin*, 1971, *76*, 349–364.

Kahneman, D.   *Attention and effort*. Englewood Cliffs, N.J.: Prentice-Hall, 1973.

Kahneman, D., & Beatty, J.   Pupil diameter and load on memory. *Science*, 1966, *154*,
1583–1585.

Katz, H., Cadoret, R. J., Hughes, K. R., & Abbey, D. S.   Physiological correlates of acceptable
and unacceptable attitude statements. *Psychological Reports*, 1965, *17*, 78.

Kenrick, D. T., Cialdini, R. B., & Linder, D. E.   Misattribution under fear-producing circumstances: Four failures to replicate. *Personality and Social Psychology Bulletin*, 1979, *5*,
329–334.

Kerber, K. W., & Coles, M. G.   The role of perceived physiological activity in affective judgments. *Journal of Experimental Social Psychology*, 1978, *14*, 419–433.

Kiesler, C. A., & Pallak, M. S.   Arousal properties of dissonance manipulations. *Psychological Bulletin*, 1976, *83*, 1014–1025.

Kinsbourne, M.   Eye and head turning indicates cerebral lateralization. *Science*, 1972, *176*, 539–541.

Krugman, H. E.   Point of view: Sustained viewing of television. *Journal of Advertising Research*, 1980, *20*, 65–68.

Lacey, B. C., & Lacey, J. I.   Studies of heart rate and other bodily processes in sensorimotor behavior. In P. A. Obrist, A. H. Black, J. Brener, & L. V. DiCara (Eds.), *Cardiovascular psychophysiology*. Chicago: Aldine, 1974.

Lacey, J. I.   Somatic response patterning and stress: Some revisions of activation theory. In M. H. Appley & R. Trumbull (Eds.), *Psychological stress: Issues in research*. New York: Appleton-Century-Crofts, 1967.

Lacey, J. I., Kagan, J., Lacey, B., & Moss, H. A.   The visceral level: Situational determinants and behavioral correlates of autonomic response patterns. In P. H. Knapp (Ed.), *Expression of the emotions in man*. New York: International Universities Press, 1963.

Leventhal, H.   Findings and theory in the study of fear communications. In L. Berkowitz (Ed.), *Advances in experimental social psychology* (Vol. 5). New York: Academic, 1970.

Libby, W. L., Lacey, B. C., & Lacey, J. I.   Pupillary and cardiac activity during visual attention. *Psychophysiology*, 1973, *10*, 270–294.

Liebhart, E. H.   Information search and attribution: Cognitive processes mediating the effect of false autonomic feedback. *European Journal of Social Psychology*, 1979, *9*, 19–37.

Lind, E. A., & O'Barr, W. M.   The social significance of speech in the courtroom. In H. Giles & R. St. Clair (Eds.), *Language and social psychology*. Oxford: Blackwell, 1979.

Lott, A. J., & Lott, B. E.   A learning theory approach to interpersonal attitudes. In A. G. Greenwald, T. C. Brock, & T. M. Ostrom (Eds.), *Psychological foundations of attitudes*. New York: Academic, 1968.

Love, R. E.   *Unobtrusive measurement of cognitive reactions to persuasive communications.* Unpublished doctoral dissertation, Ohio State University, 1972.

Lowenstein, O., & Lowenfeld, I. E.   Types of central autonomic innervation and fatigue. *Archives of Neurology and Psychiatry*, 1951, *66*, 581–599.

Marshall, G. D., & Zimbardo, P. G.   Affective consequences of inadequately explained physiological arousal. *Journal of Personality and Social Psychology*, 1979, *37*, 970–988.

Maslach, C.   Negative emotional biasing of unexplained arousal. *Journal of Personality and Social Psychology*, 1979, *37*, 953–969.

McCurdy, H. G.   Consciousness and the galvanometer. *Psychological Review*, 1950, *57*, 322–327.

McGinnies, E., & Aiba, H.   Persuasion and emotional response: A cross cultural study. *Psychological Reports*, 1965, *16*, 503–510.

McGuigan, F. J.   Covert oral behavior during the silent performance of language tasks. *Psychological Bulletin*, 1970, *74*, 309–326.

McGuigan, F. J.   *Cognitive psychophysiology: Principles of covert behavior.* New York: Appleton-Century-Crofts, 1978.

McGuire, W. J.   Attitudes and opinions. *Annual Review of Psychology*, 1966, *17*, 475–514.

McGuire, W. J.   The nature of attitudes and attitude change. In G. Lindzey & E. Aronson (Eds.), *The handbook of social psychology* (2nd ed., Vol. 3). Reading, Mass.: Addison-Wesley, 1969.

McMillen, D. L., & Geiselman, J. H.   Effect of cognitive dissonance on alpha frequency activity. *Personality and Social Psychology Bulletin*, 1974, *1*, 150–151.

Mehrabian, A.   Relationship of attitude to seated posture, orientation, and distance. *Journal of Personality and Social Psychology*, 1968, *10*, 26–30.

Mehrabian, A.   *Silent messages: Implicit communication of emotions and attitudes* (2nd ed.). Belmont, Calif.: Wadsworth, 1981.

Mehrabian, A., & Williams, M.   Nonverbal concomitants of perceived and intended persuasiveness. *Journal of Personality and Social Psychology*, 1969, *13*, 37–58.

Mentz, P.   Die wirkung akustischer sinnesreize auf Puls und Athmung. *Philosophische Studien*, 1895, *11*, 61–124; 371–393; 562–602.

Metalis, S. A., & Hess, E. H.   Pupillary response/semantic differential scale relationships. *Journal of Research in Personality*, 1982, *16*, 201–216.

Mewborn, C., & Rogers, R. W.   Effects of threatening and reassuring components of fear appeals on physiological and verbal measures of emotion and attitudes. *Journal of Personality and Social Psychology*, 1979, *37*, 242–253.

Miller, N., & Baron, R. S.   On measuring counterarguing. *Journal for the Theory of Social Behavior*, 1973, *3*, 101–118.

Miller, N., & Campbell, D. T.   Recency and primacy in persuasion as a function of the timing of speeches and measurements. *Journal of Abnormal and Social Psychology*, 1959, *59*, 1–9.

Miller, N., Maruyama, G., Beaber, R., & Valone, K.   Speed of speech and persuasion. *Journal of Personality and Social Psychology*, 1976, *34*, 615–625.

Mueller, D. J.   Physiological techniques of attitude measurement. In G. A. Summers (Ed.), *Attitude measurement*. Chicago: Rand McNally, 1970.

Obrist, P. A.   Cardiac–behavioral interactions: A critical appraisal. In J. T. Cacioppo & R. E. Petty (Eds.), *Perspectives in cardiovascular psychophysiology*. New York: Guilford, 1982.

Ornstein, R. E.   *The psychology of consciousness*. San Francisco: W. H. Freeman, 1972.

Paivio, A.   Psychophysiological correlates of imagery. In F. McGuigan & R. Schoonover (Eds.), *The psychophysiology of thinking: Studies of covert processes*. New York: Academic, 1973.

Paivio, A., & Simpson, H. M.   The effect of word abstractness and pleasantness on pupil size during an imagery task. *Psychonomic Science*, 1966, *5*, 55–56.

Parkinson, B., & Manstead, A. S. R.   An examination of the roles played by meaning of feedback and attention to feedback in the "Valins effect." *Journal of Personality and Social Psychology*, 1981, *40*, 239–245.

Pavlov, I. P.   *Conditioned reflexes*. New York: Oxford University Press, 1927.

Peavler, J. S.   A reply to Hamel. *Journal of Psychology*, 1975, *90*, 113–114.

Peavler, J. S., & McLaughlin, J. P.   The question of stimulus content and pupil size. *Psychonomic Science*, 1967, *8*, 505–506.

Petty, R. E., & Cacioppo, J. T.   Forewarning, cognitive responding, and resistance to persuasion. *Journal of Personality and Social Psychology*, 1977, *35*, 645–655.

Petty, R. E., & Cacioppo, J. T.   Effects of forewarning of persuasive intent and involvement on cognitive responses and persuasion. *Personality and Social Psychology Bulletin*, 1979, *5*, 173–176. (a)

Petty, R. E., & Cacioppo, J. T.   Issue involvement can increase or decrease persuasion by enhancing message-relevant cognitive responses. *Journal of Personality and Social Psychology*, 1979, *37*, 1915–1926. (b)

Petty, R. E., & Cacioppo, J. T.   *Attitudes and persuasion: Classic and contemporary approaches*. Dubuque, Iowa: Wm. C. Brown, 1981.

Petty, R. E., & Cacioppo, J. T.   Central and peripheral routes to persuasion. Application to advertising. In L. Percy & A. Woodside (Eds.), *Advertising and consumer psychology*. Lexington, Mass.: Lexington Books, 1983.

Petty, R. E., & Cacioppo, J. T.   *Attitude change: Central and peripheral routes to persuasion*. New York: Springer-Verlag, in press.

Petty, R. E., Cacioppo, J. T., & Goldman, R.   Personal involvement as a determinant of argument based persuasion. *Journal of Personality and Social Psychology*, 1981, *41*, 847–855.

Petty, R. E., Cacioppo, J. T., & Heesacker, M.   Effects of rhetorical questions on persuasion: A cognitive response analysis. *Journal of Personality and Social Psychology*, 1981, *40*, 432–440.

Petty, R. E., Ostrom, T. M., & Brock, T. C.   Historical foundations of the cognitive response approach to attitudes and persuasion. In R. E. Petty, T. M. Ostrom, & T. C. Brock (Eds.), *Cognitive responses in persuasion*. Hillsdale, N.J.: Erlbaum, 1981.

Petty, R. E., Wells, G. L., Heesacker, M., Brock, T. C., & Cacioppo, J. T.   The effects of recipient posture on persuasion: A cognitive response analysis. *Personality and Social Psychology Bulletin*, 1983.

Pittman, T. S., Cooper, E. E., & Smith, T. W.   Attribution of causality and the overjustification effect. *Personality and Social Psychology Bulletin*, 1977, *3*, 280–283.

Quigley-Fernandez, B., & Tedeschi, J. T.   The bogus pipeline as lie detector: Two validity studies. *Journal of Personality and Social Psychology*, 1978, *36*, 247–256.

Rankin, R. E., & Campbell, D. T.   Galvanic skin response to Negro and white experimenters. *Journal of Abnormal and Social Psychology*, 1955, *51*, 30–33.

Razran, G.   A quantitative study of meaning by conditioned salivary technique (semantic conditioning). *Science*, 1939, *90*, 89–91.

Razran, G.   The observable unconscious and the inferable conscious in current Soviet psychophysiology. *Psychological Review*, 1961, *68*, 81–147.

Rhodewalt, F., & Comer, R.   Induced-compliance attitude change: Once more with feeling. *Journal of Experimental Social Psychology*, 1979, *15*, 35–47.

Rihl, J.   Die Frequenz des Herzschlages. In A. V. Bethe, G. Bergmann, G. Embden, & A. Ellinger (Eds.), *Handbuch der Normalen und pathologischen Physiologie, 7-1 (Blutzikulation)*. Berlin: Julius Springer, 1926.

Rogers, R., & Mewborn, C.   Fear appeals and attitude change. Effects of a threat's noxiousness, probability of occurrence, and the efficacy of coping responses. *Journal of Personality and Social Psychology*, 1976, *34*, 54–61.

Roubinovitch, J.   Des variations du diamètre pupillaire en rapport avec l'effort intellectuel. In P. Janet (Ed.), *Quatrième congrès international de psychologie 1900*. Paris: Alcan, 1901.

Sackeim, H. A., & Gur, R. C.   Lateral asymmetry in intensity of emotional expression. *Neuropsychologia*, 1978, *16*, 473–481.

Sackeim, H. A., Gur, R. C., & Saucy, M. C.   Emotions are expressed more intensely on the left side of the face. *Science*, 1978, *202*, 434–436.

Schachter, S.   The interaction of cognitive and physiological determinants of emotional state. In L. Berkowitz (Ed.), *Advances in experimental social psychology* (Vol. 1). New York: Academic, 1964.

Schachter, S., & Singer, J. E.   Cognitive, social, and physiological determinants of emotional state. *Psychological Review*, 1962, *69*, 379–399.

Schachter, S., & Singer, J. E.   Comments on the Maslach and Marshall–Zimbardo experiments. *Journal of Personality and Social Psychology*, 1979, *37*, 989–995.

Schwartz, G. E., Ahern, G. L., & Brown, S. L.   Lateralized facial muscle response to positive versus negative emotional stimuli. *Psychophysiology*, 1979, *16*, 561–571.

Schwartz, G. E., Fair, P. L., Salt, P., Mandel, M. R., & Klerman, G. L.   Facial muscle patterning to affective imagery in depressed and nondepressed subjects. *Science*, 1976, *192*, 489–491.

Schwartz, G. E., & Shapiro, D.   Social psychophysiology. In W. F. Prokasy & D. C. Raskin (Eds.), *Electrodermal activity in psychological research*. New York: Academic, 1973.

Shaffer, D. R.   Some effects of consonant and dissonant attitudinal advocacy on initial attitude salience and attitude change. *Journal of Personality and Social Psychology*, 1975, *32*, 160–168.

Shapiro, D., & Crider, A.   Psychophysiological approaches in social psychology. In G. Lindzey & E. Aronson (Eds.), *The handbook of social psychology* (2nd ed., Vol. 3). Reading, Mass.: Addison-Wesley, 1969.

Shapiro, D., & Reeves, J. L. II   Modification of physiological and subjective responses to stress through heart rate biofeedback. In J. T. Cacioppo & R. E. Petty (Eds.), *Perspectives in cardiovascular psychophysiology*. New York: Guilford, 1982.

Sigall, H., & Page, R.   Current stereotypes: A little fading, a little faking. *Journal of Personality and Social Psychology*, 1971, *18*, 247–255.

Sirota, A. D., & Schwartz, G. E.   Facial muscle patterning and lateralization during elation and depression imagery. *Journal of Abnormal Psychology*, 1982, *91*, 25–34.

Smith, C. A.   A study of the autonomic excitation resulting from the interaction of individual opinion and group opinion. *Journal of Abnormal and Social Psychology*, 1936, *31*, 138–164.

Smith, W.   *The measurement of emotion*. London: Paul, 1922.

Sokolov, A. N.   *Perception and the conditioned reflex*. Oxford: Pergamon, 1963.

Sokolov, A. N.   Studies of the speech mechanisms of thinking. In M. Cole & I. Maltzman (Eds.), *A handbook of contemporary Soviet psychology*. New York: Basic Books, 1969.

Sokolov, A. N.   *Inner speech and thought*. New York: Plenum, 1972.

Spence, D. P., Lugo, M., & Youdin, R.   Cardiac change as a function of attention to and awareness of continuous verbal text. *Science*, 1972, *176*, 1344–1346.

Staats, A. W., & Staats, C. K.   Attitudes established by classical conditioning. *Journal of Abnormal and Social Psychology*, 1958, *57*, 37–40.

Stanners, R. F., Headley, D. B., & Clark, W. R.   The pupillary response to sentences: Influences of listening set and deep structure. *Journal of Verbal Learning and Verbal Behavior*, 1972, *11*, 257–263.

Syz, H.   Observations on unreliability of subjective reports of emotional reactions. *British Journal of Psychology*, 1926–1927, *17*, 119–126.

Taylor, S.   On inferring one's attitudes from one's behavior: Some delimiting conditions. *Journal of Personality and Social Psychology*, 1975, *31*, 126–131.

Teasdale, J. D., & Rezin, V.   Effect of thought stopping on thoughts, mood, and corrugator EMG in depressed patients. *Behaviour Research and Therapy*, 1978, *16*, 97–102.

Tesser, A.   Self-generated attitude change. *Advances in Experimental Social Psychology*, 1978, *11*, 289–338.

Thurstone, L. L., & Chave, E. J.   *The measurement of attitude*. Chicago: University of Chicago Press, 1929.

Tognacci, L., & Cook, S.   Conditioned autonomic responses as bidirectional indicators of racial attitude. *Journal of Personality and Social Psychology*, 1975, *31*, 137–144.

Tomkins, S. S.   *Affect, imagery, consciousness* (Vol. 1). *The positive affects*. New York: Springer, 1962.

Tomkins, S. S.   *Affect, imagery, consciousness* (Vol. 2). *The negative affects*. New York: Springer, 1963.

Tomkins, S. S.   The quest for primary motives: Biography and autobiography of an idea. *Journal of Personality and Social Psychology*, 1981, *41*, 306–329.

Tryon, W. W.   Pupillometry: A survey of sources of variation. *Psychophysiology*, 1975, *12*, 90–93.

Tucker, D. M.   Lateral brain function, emotion, and conceptualization. *Psychological Bulletin*, 1981, *89*, 19–46.

Tucker, D. M., Stenslie, C. E., Roth, R. S., & Shearer, S. L.   Right frontal lobe activation and right hemisphere performance decrement during a depressed mood. *Archives of General Psychiatry*, 1981, *38*, 169–174.

Tursky, B., Lodge, M., & Reeder, R.   Psychophysical and psychophysiological evaluation of the direction, intensity, and meaning of race-related stimuli. *Psychophysiology*, 1979, *16*, 452–462.

Tursky, B., Schwartz, G., & Crider A.   Differential patterns of heart rate and skin resistance during a digit transformation task. *Journal of Experimental Psychology*, 1970, *83*, 451–457.

Valins, S.   Cognitive effects of false heart rate feedback. *Journal of Personality and Social Psychology*, 1966, *4*, 400–408.

Venables, P. H., & Christie, M. J.   Electrodermal activity. In I. Martin & P. Venables (Eds.), *Techniques in psychophysiology*. New York: Wiley, 1980.

Vidulich, R. N., & Krevanick, F. W.   Racial attitudes and emotional response to visual representations of the Negro. *Journal of Social Psychology*, 1966, *68*, 85–93.

Volkova, B. C.   Some characteristics of the conditioned reflex formation to verbal stimuli in children. *Sechenov Physiological Journal of the USSR*, 1953, *39*, 540–548.

Weerts, T. C., & Roberts, R.   The physiological effects of imagining anger-provoking and fear-provoking scenes. *Psychophysiology*, 1976, *13*, 174. (Abstract)

Wells, G. L., & Petty, R. E.   The effects of overt head-movements on persuasion: Compatibility and incompatibility of responses. *Basic and Applied Social Psychology*, 1980, *1*, 219–230.

Westie, F. R., & DeFleur, M. L.   Autonomic responses and their relationship to race attitudes. *Journal of Abnormal and Social Psychology*, 1959, *58*, 340–347.

White, G. L., Fishbein, S., & Rustein, J.   Passionate love and the misattribution of arousal. *Journal of Personality and Social Psychology*, 1981, *41*, 56–62.

White, G. L., & Maltzman, I.   Pupillary activity while listening to verbal passages. *Journal of Research in Personality*, 1978, *12*, 361–369.

Wicklund, R. A., & Brehm, J. W.   *Perspectives on cognitive dissonance*. Hillsdale, N.J.: Erlbaum, 1976.

Woodmansee, J. J.   The pupil response as a measure of social attitudes. In G. F. Summers (Ed.), *Attitude measurement*. Chicago: Rand McNally, 1970.

Young, F. A., & Sheena, D.   Eye-movement measurement techniques. *American Psychologist*, 1975, *30*, 315–330.

Zajonc, R. B.   Feeling and thinking: Preferences need no inferences. *American Psychologist*, 1980, *35*, 151–175.

Zajonc, R. B., & Markus, H.   Affective and cognitive factors in preferences. *Journal of Consumer Research*, 1982, *9*, 123–131.

Zanna, M. P., & Cooper, J.   Dissonance and the pill: An attribution approach to studying the arousal properties of dissonance. *Journal of Personality and Social Psychology*, 1974, *29*, 703–709.

Zuckerman, M., DePaulo, B. M., & Rosenthal, R.   Verbal and nonverbal communication of deception. *Advances in Experimental Social Psychology*, 1981, *14*, 1–59.

CHAPTER 4

Evaluation of Social and Political Beliefs: A Psychophysiological Approach

Bernard Tursky
State University of New York at Stony Brook

Larry D. Jamner
State University of New York at Stony Brook

INTRODUCTION

The goals of any science and the true understanding of any phenomenon may be reflected in the ability of the scientist to explain, predict, and control the phenomenon under investigation (Myers, 1980). The social scientist in general and the political scientist in particular has been continuously interested in evaluating the direction, intensity, and meaning of stimuli, beliefs, and attitudes related to social and political issues and behavior. In this quest these scientists have relied primarily on self-report measures as the major mode of obtaining information and establishing construct validity (Summers, 1970; Wahlke, 1979).

It has been estimated that as much as 90% of social science research is dependent on the interview and questionnaire (Webb, Campbell, Schwartz, & Sechrest, 1966). More recently, Wahlke (1979), sampling from *The American Political Science Review*, found that 70% of the analyses reported were based on self-report measures. Wahlke and Lodge (1972), in their discussion of the problems associated with the use of surveys in political science, state: "No research technique is more intimately associated with the development of modern behavioral political science than the mass survey—it has been commonly viewed by many political scientists as the most distinctive methodology of their trade." Thus, much of what political scientists believe about public beliefs, political attitudes, and individual or micropolitical behavior stems from a population's verbal responses to a set of semantic stimuli. Moreover, this reliance on one modality of response behavior (what people say to what other people ask) may weaken correlations across measures of opinion, or between opinions and behavior.

If this is true, then in terms of previously stated goals of scientific inquiry (explanation, prediction, and control), we are left with a method that delivers weak predictions, is lacking in explanatory powers, and does not enhance the investigator's ability to control the phenomena under investigation. Some of the problems inherent in the overreliance on self-report measures of beliefs and attitudes were noted in Chapter 3. To overcome these problems, social scientists must alter their research behavior along several dimensions.

They must (1) acknowledge the multidimensional properties of beliefs and attitudes, (2) adopt a cross-modal multiple indicator approach to attitude and belief measurement, and (3) increase the precision of their measures of stimulus and response characteristics (Tursky, Lodge, & Cross, 1976). These steps can best be accomplished in the behavioral research laboratory, where the use of advanced psychophysical and psychophysiological techniques can provide the methodology to study social beliefs, attitudes, and behavior experimentally rather than by the use of post facto observation or impressionistic methods (Lodge & Tursky, 1973).

In Chapter 3, Petty and Cacioppo described the utility of a psychophysiological approach to the assessment of social attitudes and attitude change. The major aim of the present chapter is to provide an overview and rationale for the use of psychophysiological techniques in the assessment of social and political beliefs and belief structures. In addition, we discuss and provide evidence for the utility of supplementing psychophysiological procedures with sophisticated verbal and psychophysical techniques in a "cross-modal" multiple indicator approach.[1]

CROSS-MODAL MULTIPLE INDICATOR ANALYSIS OF ATTITUDES AND BELIEFS

The failure of self-report scales to account for major portions of the variance of human sociopsychological behavior may be the result of neglecting the complexity and multidimensionality of social and political attitudes and beliefs. This failure suggests that social scientists must utilize a cross-modal multiple indicator assessment technique that takes into account the multidimensional properties of the attitude construct (Cook & Selltiz, 1964). A "cross-modal multiple indicator" approach entails systematic multiple measurements *across* several response components (verbal, physical, and physiological) by means of more than one instrument, scale, or indicator within each response component. What is suggested by this model goes beyond the simple correlations of multiple measurements within and across independent modes of response; rather, this approach

1. For detailed information on the use of magnitude scaling and a comprehensive comparison of magnitude and category scaling, we refer you to Lodge (1981) and Lodge and Tursky (1981).

relies on theory-derived measurements of responses with known, predictable interrelationships. Figure 4-1 illustrates the cross-modal approach.

The use of selected indicators from each response component allows for the formulation of a "composite" evaluation, which serves to improve the measurements of beliefs and attitude. Major improvements in verbal and survey response measures have been achieved by utilizing sophisticated psychophysical measurement techniques in the evaluation of social stimuli (Dawson & Brinker, 1971; Lodge, 1981; Lodge, Cross, Tursky, & Tanenhaus, 1975; Stevens, 1966). These techniques range from multidimensional scaling (Kruskal, 1964) and functional measurement (Anderson, 1974) to advanced cross-modality matching psychophysical scaling procedures (Lodge & Tursky, 1981).[2] Although it has been demonstrated that cross-modality matching improves the measurement of attitudinal direction and intensity (Lodge & Tursky, 1979), and that multidimensional scaling may help to define the attitude structure (Feger, 1982), none of these measures provide an unambiguous indication of which meaning of the complex social or political stimulus is eliciting the response. What is required is a methodology that will provide the investigator with unambiguous responses that provide information about the meaning–response relationship of complex political stimuli.

PSYCHOPHYSIOLOGY IN THE STUDY OF ATTITUDES AND BELIEFS

Advantages and Disadvantages

One of the features that clearly differentiates psychophysiological response measures from verbal or motor response measures is the involuntary nature of the physiological response. This characteristic reduces the vulnerability of these measures to manipulation of the biases that affect most voluntary verbal and motor responses. For example, the question–answer format employed in most survey instruments may promote an intellectual response bias (Lazarus, Opton, Monikos, & Rankin, 1965; Lazarus, Speisman, Mordkoff, & Davison, 1962) and may generate rationalizations in the respondent about the political world (Crespi, 1971). Thus, information derived from verbal measures tends to indicate attitude structures that may be inappropriately rationalistic and, with the partial exception of routinized behaviors (i.e., voting), cannot reliably predict overt political behaviors (Wahlke & Lodge, 1972).

It must be made clear that psychophysiological measures may also be subject to biases produced by cognitive set (Lazarus *et al.*, 1965), experi-

---

2. For detailed information on various types of psychophysical measurement of social and political attitudes, we refer the reader to *Social Attitudes and Psychophysical Measurement* (Wegener, 1982).

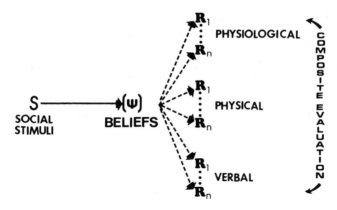

FIGURE 4-1. Cross-modal multiple indicator measurement model.

mental demands (Orne, 1962), or individual response stereotopy (Lacey, 1967; Sternbach, 1966). However, these response tendencies and biases can be controlled by rigorous research design. Given adequate experimental controls, psychophysiological techniques and measures can provide objective, relatively bias free indices of human reaction. Tursky *et al.* (1976) outlined several of the major advantages of employing psychophysiological methods in the study of political behavior. These were: (1) the measuring devices, once properly applied, do not require experimenter intervention or direct observation, thereby eliminating a major source of bias; (2) physiological measurements are stable, in that variations in responses are a function of changes in the subject, not the measuring instrument, thereby alleviating the problem of reproducibility; (3) physiological measurements may be derived from subjects while they are engaged in other tasks, such as decision making, social interaction, and self-rating scales; (4) because they may be recorded independently of the subject's voluntary response system or more commonly in conjunction with other measures (e.g., subvocal speech, self-report, performance in a task or a social behavior), physiological measures may provide multiple indicator data for the analysis of consistencies and incongruities in human reaction; and (5) since much behavior is probably immediate and automatic, physiological measurements may be used to indicate the presence of persistent but habituated involuntary reactions to stimuli.

The efforts of electro- and psychophysiologists have provided considerable evidence of predictable relationships between various cognitive processes and central and autonomic nervous system activity that may be of significant utility in the study and measurement of social and political attitudes and concepts and beliefs. Other chapters in this volume describe and reference social/psychological studies that employ psychophysiological measures in the evaluation of the direction and strength of attitudes. Thus, we will not review that material here.

Psychophysiological Assessment of Political Attitudes and Beliefs

Although social scientists have clearly demonstrated the utility of psychophysiological measures in the study of psychological and social attitudes and behavior, these measures have not often been utilized in political science research. Recently, a growth in interest in a biobehavioral approach to the study of political attitudes and behavior (Somit, Peterson, Richardson, & Goldfisher, 1980) has aroused an interest in the use of psychophysiological measures by political scientists. Barlow (1969), for example, monitored the pupillary dilation of subjects classified as either liberal or conservative in response to slides of three political leaders (Lyndon Johnson, George Wallace, and Martin Luther King). Barlow reported that liberals demonstrated a dilatory response to the slides of Johnson and King and pupillary constriction to the slide of Wallace, whereas conservative subjects demonstrated the opposite pattern.

Watts and Sumi (1979) attempted to demonstrate that psychophysiological measures could be utilized to validate attitude scales related to violence and aggression. Watts and Sumi conducted two experiments to test several general hypotheses: (1) that higher acceptance of violence, greater traditionalism, and greater machiavellianism would be negatively associated with autonomic arousal (as measured by skin conductance), and (2) that subjects scoring high on the MACH IV, violence ideology, and traditionalism scales would tend to demonstrate heart rate decelerations when presented with models of interpersonal aggression, whereas subjects scoring low on each of these scales would tend to respond to models of interpersonal aggression with an acceleration in heart rate.

Watts and Sumi reported findings consistent with their hypotheses. In these studies skin conductance and heart rate responses were negatively correlated with scores on the attitude scales administered. The investigators conclude that the reported associations of the scales tested with the psychophysiological response data added to the scales' claims of validity, and more generally, that psychophysiological measures can serve in the validation of self-report scales.

Although psychophysiological measures have been successfully utilized in the assessment of attitudinal *intensity*, a critical question remains: *What is the respondent responding to?* Much of the difficulty with research in this area has been its failure to consider what specific *meaning* a stimulus has to a given subject (Edelberg, 1972). Much of the variability of physiological as well as verbal measures in response to complex semantic stimuli may simply reflect the fact that stimuli are interpreted differently by different subjects. The major methodological concern of the problem of meaning must be carefully addressed.

Classical Conditioning, Generalization, and Discrimination

Social stimuli are complex, carry multiple meanings, connotations, and associations which affect how stimulus information is interpreted, evaluated, and processed. This in turn can greatly affect an individual's verbal and physiological responses (Tursky, Lodge, & Reeder, 1979). A major concern of political science research which focuses on the individual's responses to the presentation of social or political stimuli is that the investigators, in most instances, do not know to what meaning of the stimulus the respondent is responding. This issue is of particular concern when psychophysiological measures are utilized because of the extreme sensitivity of these measures. Unless the investigator can gain some degree of control over the measurement of the meanings elicited by the social stimuli, useful interpretation of obtained results is problematic. What is required is a method that allows the investigator to identify the specific meaning of interest for each of the social stimuli and to utilize an experimental procedure that will guarantee the specificity of the elicited physiological response to that meaning. The principles of classical conditioning, generalization, and discrimination combined with psychophysiological measures readily offer a solution to the problem presented. Before tying together all the elements mentioned thus far, a brief review of the terminology utilized in classical conditioning is necessary.

Classical conditioning refers to a set of operations whose essential elements are: (1) an unconditioned stimulus (UCS), which reliably elicits a reflexive measurable unconditioned response (UCR); (2) a conditioned stimulus (CS), a previously neutral stimulus which did not originally elicit the UCR; and (3) repeated contiguous pairings of the CS with the UCS independent of the behavior of the organism. The specified temporal patterning between the UCS and CS results in the capability of the CS to elicit a response (similar to that of the UCR) referred to as the conditioned response (CR). After a conditioned response has been established, the phenomena of *stimulus generalization* may be observed in which stimuli similar to the CS can, to varying degrees, elicit the conditioned response. That is, a subject demonstrates stimulus generalization if after learning to respond to the CS he or she produces a comparable response to another stimulus that has similar properties. Conversely, *discrimination* refers to the process of the subject failing to respond to other stimuli after learning to respond to one particular stimulus.

Semantic Generalization

The rules that govern conditioning, generalization, and discrimination of simple physical stimuli can also apply to social and political stimuli (A. W. Staats, 1969). These more complex stimuli may derive their meanings through the same learning mechanisms and conditions that govern the acquisition of other behavioral responses. Examples of this assertion may be found in the substantive body of literature which demonstrates that it is possible to elicit a behavioral response to a conditioned stimulus consisting of either nonsense syllables (Razran, 1939), words (Lang, Geer, & Hnatiow, 1963; A. W. Staats, Staats, & Crawford, 1962), or attitudes (A. W. Staats & Staats, 1958; Tognacci & Cook, 1975; Tursky et al., 1979). In addition, the presentation of another stimulus which bears some semantic relationship to the CS results in the production of a generalized response. This process has been termed *semantic generalization*. Employing semantic generalization, C. K. Staats and Staats (1957) transferred the meanings of Osgood, Suci, and Tannenbaum's (1957) evaluative, potency, and activity scale to nonsense words. Using a counterbalanced design, each of six syllables (YOF, LAJ, XEH, WUH, GIW, QUG) was presented to subjects 18 times. Two syllables (YOF, XEH) were paired with different words that had either a negative or positive evaluative meaning, while the other syllables were paired with words with no systematic meaning. Following conditioning, subjects rated all six syllables along a 7-point semantic evaluative differential scale. Staats and Staats found that syllables paired with positive or negative evaluative words were rated more positive or negative, respectively, than were neutral syllables. In two similar experiments in the same study, Staats and Staats demonstrated that the meaning of the same two nonsense syllables could also be altered along the potency and activity dimensions.

In another study using the same classical conditioning paradigm, A. W. Staats and Staats (1958) were also able to demonstrate that evaluative attitudinal responses to socially significant objects, nationalities (German, Swedish, Italian, French, Dutch, Greek), and names (Harry, Tom, Jim, Ralph, Bill, and Bob) could be established and/or modified. Thus, it would appear that it is possible to utilize the classical conditioning paradigm to transfer components of meaning from one set of words to another, and to alter previously held attitudes toward sociopolitical stimuli.

A. W. Staats et al. (1962) demonstrated that physiological responses can be conditioned in a parallel manner. In this study, one word (large) out of 25 verbal stimuli served as the conditioned stimulus. The CS was paired with an aversive UCS (i.e., loud noise and electric shock) while skin conductance was recorded. Results indicated that the SCR was conditioned to the CS, and that for subjects who had been conditioned, the CS was rated as unpleasant on a 7-point semantic differential scale. More recently,

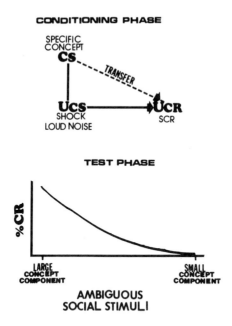

FIGURE 4-2. Diagram of classical conditioning and generalization to a specific concept.

Tognacci and Cook (1975) utilized some of the principles of semantic generalization and psychophysiological recording techniques to demonstrate both the direction and intensity of racial attitudes. Returning to the original point, the integration of these principles and procedures (i.e., classical conditioning, semantic generalization, parallel physiological conditioning) provide a means by which the investigator can gain control over the meanings elicited by ambiguous sociopolitical stimuli. That is, employing the classical conditioning paradigm, the investigator can transfer a physiological response (e.g., skin conductance or a set of responses) normally elicited by an aversive UCS (e.g., loud noise, electric shock) to the specific attitudinal meaning of a series of social stimuli. Once conditioning has been established, the elicitation and amplitude of the conditioned physiological response can serve as an involuntary measure of the degree to which a specific attitudinal meaning is generalized to other, more ambiguous sociopolitical stimuli (see Figure 4-2).

CLASSICAL CONDITIONING OF PSYCHOPHYSIOLOGICAL MEASURES OF BELIEFS

Tursky, Lodge, Foley, Reeder, and Foley (1976) employed a differential classical conditioning design to measure directly the extent to which a set of denotatively nonracial political issues could elicit a racially (black–white) associated physiological response. In their study, subjects categorically rated 60 words and phrases as to the degree to which each stimulus was related to black people and black problems. The 15 items judged to be most black related and the 15 items judged to be least black related were used as CSs. The test stimuli were 10 political issues, 5 of which were hypothesized to be differentially black related, and 5 hypothesized to be not black related Subjects were assigned to one of two groups: For one-half the subjects, black-related items were paired with a 100-dB white noise of 1-second duration (UCS). Thus, for this group the black-related items served as CS+ trials and the non-black-related items were CS− trials.[3] For the remaining half of the subjects, the non-black-related items were accompanied by the aversive noise; in this case the non-black-related items were designated as the CS+ trials. Thus, group 1 represents the black-conditioning group and group 2 the non-black-conditioning group. The stimuli were visually presented using a slide projector, and subjects' skin conductance response to each of the presented stimuli was recorded.

Figure 4-3 illustrates the difference in mean amplitude of skin conductance responses to black- and non-black-conditioned stimuli by both the group conditioned to respond to black-related items (black bars) and the group conditioned to respond to non-black-related items (white bars). The results clearly indicate successful differential conditioning, with each group demonstrating greater physiological responsivity to CS+ items than to CS− items.

Having "primed" a physiological response to a specific concept, either black or non-black relatedness, Tursky *et al.* then evaluated the extent to which subjects rated the 10 ambiguous political test items along a black–white-related continuum. Given the degree to which subjects associate the test items with the conditioned concept, one would expect a gradient of SCR responding. The greater the association between the political test items and the concept (black–white relatedness), the greater the magnitude of physiological responding. The test items employed in the study, all of which were denotatively nonracial, produced SCRs that seemed to reflect the strength of their association to the conditioned concept. As shown in Figure 4-4, in the black-related condition the magnitude of skin conductance response was greatest for test items such as civil rights, welfare, budget and crime in the street, issues that were hypothesized to be black related. For subjects in the non-black-related condition, greatest magnitude responding was elicited by the test items space program, women's rights, Watergate, defense budget, and NATO, all of which were hypothesized to be unrelated to black issues. In addition, the data give strong indications of

---

3. CS+ is a term used to designate a conditioned stimulus that is paired (associated) with a UCS. CS− is the term used to designate a presented stimulus that is never paired with a UCS.

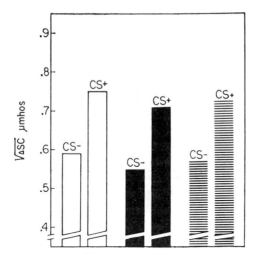

FIGURE 4-3. Comparison of mean amplitude of skin conductance (SC) responses to black- and non-black-conditioned stimuli (CS) by the group conditioned to respond to black-related stimuli (solid, or black, bars) and the group conditioned to respond to non-black-related stimuli (open, or white, bars). (Shaded, or striped, bars indicate the difference in mean SC response to CS+ and CS− trials for the combined black- and non-black-conditioning groups.) From "Evaluation of the cognitive component of political issues by the use of classical conditioning" by B. Tursky, M. Lodge, M. A. Foley, R. Reeder, & H. Foley, *Journal of Personality and Social Psychology*, 1976, **34**, 865–873. Copyright 1976 by the American Psychological Association. Reprinted by permission.

an orderly response continuum that relates response amplitude to degree of generalization. The left half of Figure 4-5 shows the average skin conductance response of subjects to one of the political test stimuli—crime in the streets. Note the large SCRs elicited from the group conditioned to black-related items compared with the responses produced by the group conditioned to non-black-related items. Conversely, in the right half the opposite pattern is evidenced for the test item Watergate.

In summary, the Tursky *et al.* study clearly demonstrated the utility of the conditioned skin conductance response in determining the degree to which ambiguous social stimuli are associated with a specific attitudinal concept.

CROSS-MODAL COMPARISON OF BELIEF ASSESSMENT

In a second study, Tursky *et al.* (1979) utilized the cross-modal approach to evaluate the direction, meaning, and intensity of race-related stimuli. In this study, psychophysical (category and magnitude scaling) and psychophysiological responses (classically conditioned SCRs) were generated to measure the race-related attributes of each of 32 stimuli (see Table 4-1).

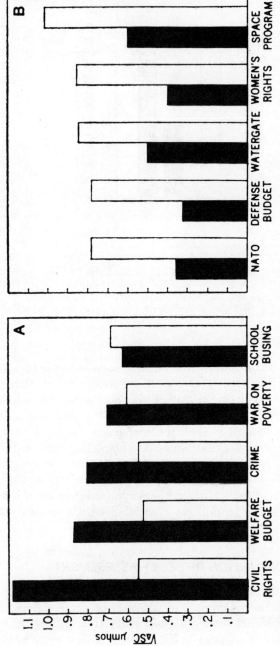

FIGURE 4-4. Comparison of the mean skin conductance (SC) response amplitude to each of the 10 political test stimuli for the black (solid, or black, bar)- and non-black (open, or white, bar)-conditioning groups. (Figure 4A shows t! e comparison of SC responses to the political black-related stimuli and Figure 4B shows the same comparison of responses to political non-black-related stimuli.) From "Evaluation of the cognitive component of political issues by the use of classical conditioning" by B. Tursky, M. Lodge, M. A. Foley, R. Reeder, & H. Foley, *Journal of Personality and Social Psychology*, 1976, **34**, 865–873. Copyright 1976 by the American Psychological Association. Reprinted by permission.

112

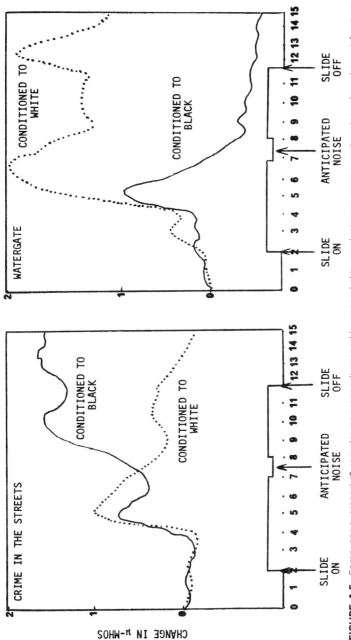

FIGURE 4-5. Computer-averaged (3 samples per second) second-by-second skin conductance responses (in micromhos change) for two representative and equaled test trials. One, crime in the streets, was paired with black-related CSs. The other, Watergate, was paired with white-related CSs. Seconds 7–8 (anticipated noise) is the interval during which the UCS had been presented in the CS+ trials. Both test trials show appropriate conditioned responses. From "Evaluation of the cognitive component of political issues by the use of classical conditioning" by B. Tursky, M. Lodge, M. A. Foley, R. Reeder, & H. Foley, *Journal of Personality and Social Psychology*, 1976, **34**, 865–873. Copyright 1976 by the American Psychological Association. Reprinted by permission.

113

TABLE 4-1. Stimuli Used in Psychophysical and Psychophysiological Experiments

BLACK-RELATED STIMULI	WHITE-RELATED STIMULI	POLITICAL TEST STIMULI
Negro	Israel	Civil rights
Harlem	Caucasian	Welfare budget
Slavery	Gerald Ford	Inflation
Ghetto	Watergate	Crime in the streets
Sickle-cell anemia	Iceland	Unemployment
Afro-American	Billie Jean King	Jobs
Martin Luther King	Suburbia	Defense budget
Angela Davis	Belfast	Abortion
NAACP	Polish-American	Gun control
Emancipation Proclamation	White-collar crime	Aid to cities
		Trust in government
		Tax reform

Note. From "Psychophysical and psychophysiological evaluation of the direction, intensity, and meaning of race-related stimuli" by B. Tursky, M. Lodge, & R. Reeder, *Psychophysiology*, 1979, *16*, 452–462. Copyright 1979 by The Society for Psychophysiological Research. Reprinted by permission.

Ten stimulus items had been previously judged to be clearly black related and 10 had been judged to be clearly white related; these stimuli were used as CS+ and control (CS−) items in the conditioning process. In addition, 12 denotatively nonracial political stimuli employed in the 1972–1976 Gallup and Harris opinion polls were selected as test items.

Using a differential classical conditioning procedure, 50% of the subject group were conditioned to respond to black-related items and 50% were conditioned to respond to white-related items. For the black-conditioned group some of the denotatively black related stimuli (CS+) were paired with a 1-second blast of 100-dB white noise (UCS). For the white-conditioned group, some of the denotatively white related stimuli (CS+) were paired with the noise. After three paired and unpaired trials, the 12 political test stimuli were presented in random order among the remaining 14 CS+ and CS− stimuli.

Skin conductance responses to each CS+, CS−, and test stimulus were evaluated as a standardized z score for each trial for each subject, to permit better comparison between subjects and groups.

The results of this study clearly demonstrated successful differential conditioning, with subjects in the black-conditioned group producing significantly greater SCRs to black-related items and subjects in the white-conditioned group producing significantly greater SCRs to white-related items. This demonstration of differential racial conditioning suggests that the SCRs to the denotatively nonracial test stimuli should produce a generalization response gradient that should indicate the group's racial associations for each test stimulus. Figure 4-6 illustrates the mean SCR to

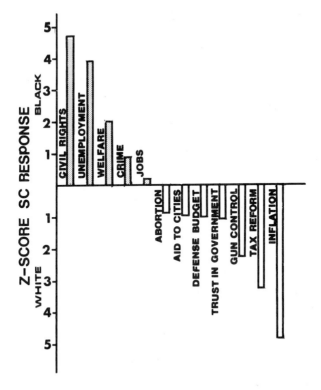

FIGURE 4-6. Comparison of mean skin conductance (z score) responses to individual test items. Each bar represents the skin conductance z-score difference between the white- and black-conditioned groups for the designated test stimulus. From "Psychophysical and psychophysiological evaluation of the direction, intensity, and meaning of race-related stimuli" by B. Tursky, M. Lodge, & R. Reeder, **Psychophysiology**, 1979, **16**, 452–462. Copyright 1979 by The Society for Psychophysiological Research. Reprinted by permission.

each individual test item. Each bar represents the z-score SC difference between the black- and white-conditioned groups for that item. The results demonstrate that two of the test items, civil rights and unemployment, were significantly reacted to as black items and three test stimuli, inflation, tax reform, and gun control, were significantly responded to as white items. However, all 12 items produced the predicted response generalization gradient.

Another phase of this study involved the psychophysical scaling of the race-relatedness of each of the 32 stimuli. Subjects participated in two psychophysical judgment tasks. One was a cross-modality matching procedure involving number and line production to scale the extent to which each stimulus was perceived as either black or white related; the other task involved judging the race-relatedness of all stimuli along a standard 7-point bipolar (black–white) category scale.

The design of this study generates multiple response indicators in two separate modalities (i.e., verbal and physiological) and thus permits a cross-modal evaluation in which the information derived from the "composite" evaluation may produce a more valid interpretation of the effect of race-relatedness on attitudes toward the sociopolitical issues employed. Figure 4-7 illustrates the "composite" evaluation generated from the use of the cross-modal approach. Category, magnitude, and skin conductance responses were compared on arbitrarily equated scales. Some of the major findings based on this composite evaluation include: (1) the superior evaluative power of both magnitude and physiological response scales in producing a continuous gradient of race-related responses; (2) the ability to assess differences in the judgmental and automatic properties of responses; (3) that in certain instances automatic response properties of the autonomic nervous system may override intellectual or social desirability, thus providing a more accurate representation of an attitude; and (4) that in situations where stimuli are not clearly defined by a physical dimension, multiple measures provide a validity check rather than being redundant information.

Although the results of this study focus on the sociophysiological concept of race-relatedness, the utility of such an approach to other sociopsychological dimensions is apparent. Research is under way to apply this technique to other concepts in political science (liberalism–conservatism). These multimodal procedures have also been utilized in evaluating and quantifying the different dimensions underlying the concept of pain (Tursky & Jamner, 1982; Tursky, Jamner, & Friedman, 1982).

In summary, the utility of psychophysiological measures in the assessment of the direction, intensity, and associative foundations of attitude has been advanced. The use of psychophysiological measures in conjunction with other techniques (i.e., classical conditioning, psychophysical scaling) can serve to improve our understanding of stimulus and response characteristics of beliefs, attitudes, and schemata and provide a validity check for other assessment procedures.

USE OF NONOBTRUSIVE MEASURES

This chapter has concentrated on the use of psychophysiological measures for the evaluation of social and political stimuli, beliefs, and attitudes. It has been demonstrated that psychophysiological responses can be related to a political schema of interest by the use of classical conditioning techniques. However, these procedures are restricted for the most part to laboratory use and to volunteer subjects. These restrictions introduce situational and subject biases that may limit the results and conclusions.

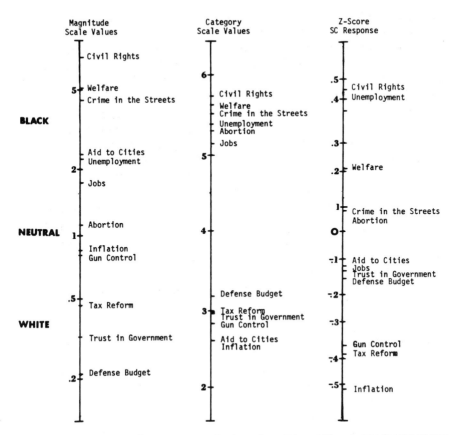

FIGURE 4-7. Comparison of category, magnitude, and conditioned SC responses for the 12 test items. The physical ranges of category and SC response measures were arbitrarily adjusted to be equal to the log-scale distance of the magnitude (ψ) scale values. From "Psychophysical and psychophysiological evaluation of the direction, intensity, and meaning of race-related stimuli" by B. Tursky, M. Lodge, & R. Reeder, *Psychophysiology*, 1979, **16**, 452–462. Copyright 1979 by The Society for Psychophysiological Research. Reprinted by permission.

Recently, attempts have been made to utilize nonobtrusive instruments in the form of the psychological stress evaluator (PSE) to obtain stress related measures in real-life situations. The PSE is an instrument that processes voice records of a speech or statement from audiotape recordings to produce information related to the psychological stress the subject is experiencing. The physiological principles that underlie this process are related to the subvocal vibrations produced by stress. Undetectable to the human ear, these patterns are discernable by the instrument independent of the loudness of the recording. The PSE has been utilized in measuring stress in voice records of actors to assess stage fright

(Brenner, 1974), in the evaluation of antianxiety drugs (Borgen & Goodman, 1976), and in lie detection (Barland, 1974; Podlesny & Raskin, 1977). In a recent study Brenner, Branscomb, and Schwartz (1979) failed to find PSE useful in detecting guilty knowledge but determined that this procedure was useful in evaluating stress due to task difficulty. Wiegele (1976, 1978) has attempted to utilize PSE to measure psychological stress in real-life voice recordings from crisis periods such as Truman's 1950 address regarding the invasion of South Korea, Kennedy's 1961 report on the Berlin crisis, Kennedy's 1962 report on the Cuban missile crisis, Johnson's 1964 speech on the Gulf of Tonkin attack, and Johnson's 1968 report on the *Pueblo* incident.

Statements were extracted from these tapes that dealt with a similar theme—that the United States was determined to see its way successfully through the crises even if it meant going to war. Although encouraged by the results of his research, Wiegele pointed out some of the problems of the use of PSE. He emphasized the need for careful controls and the role that meaning may play in the material being analyzed. He also commented on the need for good quality in the recording being used. Wiegele recommended further research in this promising area of evaluation.

CONCLUSIONS

Interest in a biobehavioral approach to the study of political beliefs, attitudes, and behavior has grown significantly in the last decade (Barner-Barry, 1979; Corning, Lasco, & Wiegele, 1981; Somit et al., 1980). This approach attempts to explain the relationship between biology and political science along several dimensions: (1) the ethological and sociobiological explanations of social and political behaviors; (2) the study of physiological, biological, and pharmacological influences on these behaviors; (3) the application of biological principles to the formulation of public policy; and (4) the implementation of psychophysiological techniques in political science research (Somit et al., 1980).

John Wahlke, in his presidential address to the 1978 convention of the American Political Science Association (Wahlke, 1979), argued that only a shift to (micro) behavior could provide true behavioral information.

Wahlke suggested that the political scientist must borrow methodology and concepts from the biological and behavioral sciences to study political behavior. He particularly advocates the use of a cross-modal (psychophysical–psychophysiological measures) approach in the study of individual political attitudes and behavior.

The major thrust of this chapter is to advocate the use of a cross-modal multiple indicator approach that utilizes psychophysiological and improved psychophysical response measures to evaluate political beliefs and attitudes. It is understandable that laboratory facilities may not be readily available to the political scientist, but it has been demonstrated that collaborative efforts between psychologists and political scientists are possible. Such efforts can produce the necessary research to enable political science to move toward a better understanding of political attitude and beliefs.

Albert Ax (1964), in a paper entitled "Goals and Methods of Psychophysiology," stated: "Scientific goals must be theoretically attainable by the methods at hand. Advancement of the state-of-the-art in these methods may open attainable new goals for a science. It is largely on the basis of advances in techniques that psychophysiology has raised its sights toward a more ambitious goal."

Almost two decades have passed since these words were written. The state of the art of psychophysiological methodology has advanced far beyond Ax's greatest expectations. Many psychophysiology laboratories are now computer controlled and physiological and behavioral data can be generated, processed, and analyzed with almost zero lag time (Andrus, 1982). These technical advances have made it possible for the behavioral scientist to conduct complex psychophysiological experiments in a fraction of the time required in the past. These improved techniques have resulted in the spread of the use of psychophysiology to other behavioral and clinical disciplines and the time is right for political scientists to utilize this methodology.

REFERENCES

Anderson, N. H. Cognitive algebra. In L. Berkowitz (Ed.), *Advances in experimental social psychology* (Vol. 7). New York: Academic, 1974.

Andrus, D. C. Research at Stony Brook: Political Science in a biobehavioral laboratory. *Politics and the Life Sciences*, 1982, *1*, 58–59.

Ax, A. Goals and methods of psychophysiology. *Psychophysiology*, 1964, *1*, 8–25.

Barland, G. H. Use of voice changes in the detection of deception. *Journal of the Acoustical Society of America*, 1974, *55*, 423. (Abstract)

Barlow, J. D. Pupillary size as an index of preference in political candidates. *Perceptual and Motor Skills*, 1969, *28*, 587–590.

Barner-Barry, C. *Psychophysiology and political behavior*. Roundtable discussion, annual meeting of the American Political Science Association, Washington, D.C., 1979.

Borgen, L. A., & Goodman, L. I. Voice print analysis of anxiolytic drug effects: Preliminary results. *Clinical Pharmacology and Therapeutics*, 1976, *19*, 104. (Abstract)

Brenner, M. *Stagefright and Stevens law*. Paper presented at the meeting of the Eastern Psychological Association, April 1974.

Brenner, M., Branscomb, H. H., & Schwartz, G. E. Psychological stress evaluator—two tests of a vocal measure. *Psychophysiology*, 1979, *16*, 351–357.

Cook, S. W., & Selltiz, C. A multiple-indicator approach to attitude measurement. *Psychological Bulletin*, 1964, *62*, 36–55.

Corning, P., Lasco, J., & Wiegele, T. C. Political science and the life sciences, *Political Science*, Summer 1981, 590–594.

Crespi, I.   What kinds of attitude measurements are predictive of behavior? *Public Opinion Quarterly*, 1971, *35*, 327–334.

Dawson, W. E., & Brinker, R. P.   Validation of ratio scales of opinion by multimodality matching. *Perception and Psychophysics*, 1971, *9*, 413–417.

Edelberg, R.   Electrical activity of the skin. In N. S. Greenfield & R. A. Sternbach (Eds.), *Handbook of psychophysiology*. New York: Holt, Rinehart & Winston, 1972.

Feger, H.   Multidimensional scaling of attitudes: Intra- and interindividual variations in preferences and cognitions. In B. Wegener (Ed.), *Social attitudes and psychophysical measurement*. Hillsdale, N.J.: Erlbaum, 1982.

Kruskal, J. B.   Multidimensional scaling by optimizing goodness of fit to a numeric hypothesis. *Psychometrika*, 1964, *29*, 1–27.

Lacey, J. I.   Somatic response patterning and stress: Some revisions of activation theory. In M. H. Appley & R. Trumbull (Eds.), *Psychological stress*. New York: Appleton-Century-Crofts, 1967.

Lang, P. J., Geer, J., & Hnatiow, M.   Semantic generalization of conditioned autonomic responses. *Journal of Experimental Psychology*, 1963, *65*, 552–558.

Lazarus, R. S., Opton, E. M., Monikos, M. S., & Rankin, N. O.   The principle of short circuiting of threat: Further evidence. *Journal of Personality*, 1965, *33*, 622–635.

Lazarus, R. S., Speisman, J. C., Mordkoff, A. M., & Davison, L. A.   A laboratory study of psychological stress produced by a motion picture film. *Psychological Monographs*, 1962, *76*, 553.

Lodge, M.   *Magnitude scaling: Quantitative measurement of opinions*. Sage University Paper Series on Quantitative Applications in the Social Sciences, Series No. 07-025. Beverly Hills, Calif.: Sage, 1981.

Lodge, M., & Tursky, B.   The analysis of political behavior: A bio-behavioral approach. *International Studies Newsletter*, 1973, pp. 58–63.

Lodge, M., & Tursky, B.   Comparisons between category and magnitude scaling of political opinion. *American Political Science Review*, 1979, *73*(1), 50–66.

Lodge, M., & Tursky, B.   Workshop on the magnitude scaling of political opinion. *American Journal of Political Science*, 1981, *25*(2), 376–419.

Lodge, M., Cross, D., Tursky, B., & Tanenhaus, J.   The psychophysical scaling and validation of a political support scale. *American Journal of Political Science*, 1975, *19*, 611–649.

Myers, A.   *Experimental psychology*. New York: D. Van Nostrand Co., 1980.

Orne, M. T.   On the social psychology of the psychological experiment. *American Psychologist*, 1962, *17*, 776–783.

Osgood, C. E., Suci, G. J., & Tannenbaum, P. H.   *The measurement of meaning*. Champaign, Ill.: University of Illinois Press, 1957.

Podlesny, J. A., & Raskin, D. C.   Physiological measures and the detection of deception. *Psychological Bulletin*, 1977, *84*, 782–799.

Razran, G.   A quantitative study of meaning by a conditioned salivary technique (semantic conditioning). *Science*, 1939, *90*, 89–90.

Somit, A., Peterson, S. A., Richardson, W. D., & Goldfisher, D. S.   *The literature of biopolitics*. De Kalb, Ill.: Center for Biopolitical Research, 1980.

Staats, A. W.   Experimental demand characteristics and the classical conditioning of attitudes. *Journal of Personality and Social Psychology*, 1969, *11*, 187–192.

Staats, A. W., & Staats, C. K.   Attitudes established by classical conditioning. *Journal of Abnormal and Social Psychology*, 1958, *57*, 37–40.

Staats, A. W., Staats, C. K., & Crawford, H. L.   First-order conditioning of meaning and paralleled conditioning of the GSR. *Journal of General Psychology*, 1962, *67*, 159–167.

Staats, C. K., & Staats, A. W.   Meaning established by classical conditioning. *Journal of Experimental Psychology*, 1957, *54*, 74–80.

Sternbach, R. A.   *Principles of psychophysiology: An introductory text and readings*. New York: Academic, 1966.

Stevens, S. S.   A metric for the social consensus. *Science*, 1966, *151*, 530–541.

Summers, G. F.   *Attitude measurement*. Chicago: Rand McNally, 1970.

Tognacci, L., & Cook, S.   Conditioned autonomic responses as bidirectional indicators of racial attitude. *Journal of Personality and Social Psychology*, 1975, *31*, 137–144.

Tursky, B., & Jamner, L.   The behavioral assessment of pain. In R. S. Surwit, R. B. Williams, Jr., A. Steptoe, & R. Biersner (Eds.), *Behavioral treatment of disease*. New York: Plenum, 1982.

Tursky, B., Jamner, L. D., & Friedman, R.   The pain perception profile: A psychophysical approach. *Behavior Therapy*, 1982, *13*, 376–394.

Tursky, B., Lodge, M., & Cross, D.   A bio-behavioral framework for the analysis of political behavior. In A. Somit (Ed.), *Biology and politics*. Paris: Mouton, 1976.

Tursky, B., Lodge, M., Foley, M. A., Reeder, R., & Foley, H.   Evaluation of the cognitive component of political issues by the use of classical conditioning. *Journal of Personality and Social Psychology*, 1976, *34*, 865–873.

Tursky, B., Lodge, M., & Reeder, R.   Psychophysical and psychophysiological evaluation of the direction, intensity, and meaning of race-related stimuli. *Psychophysiology*, 1979, *16*, 452–462.

Wahlke, J. C.   Pre-behaviorialism in political science. *The American Political Science Review*, 1979, *73*, 9–31.

Wahlke, J. C., & Lodge, M.   Psychophysiological measures of political attitudes and behavior. *Midwest Journal of Political Science*, 1972, *16*, 505–537.

Watts, M. W., & Sumi, D.   Studies in the physiological component of aggression-related social attitudes. *American Journal of Political Science*, 1979, *23*, 528–558.

Webb, E., Campbell, D. T., Schwartz, R. D., & Sechrest, L.   *Unobtrusive measures: Nonreactive research in the social sciences*. Chicago: Rand McNally, 1966.

Wegener, B.   *Social attitudes and psychophysical measurement*. Hillsdale, N. J.: Erlbaum, 1982.

Wiegele, T. C.   *Voice stress analysis: The application of a physiological measurement technique to the study of the Cuban missile crisis*. Paper prepared for delivery at the annual convention of the International Studies Association, Edinburgh, 1976.

Wiegele, T. C.   The psychophysiology of elite stress in five international crises. *International Studies Quarterly*, 1978, *22*, 467–511.

CHAPTER 5

Arousal in
the Dissonance Process

Russell H. Fazio
Indiana University
Joel Cooper
Princeton University

INTRODUCTION

In 1957, Leon Festinger proposed his theory of cognitive dissonance. For many years, the theory occupied the research activities of hosts of social psychologists and served a central role in the field's perspective on human behavior. With the rise of the cognitive perspective, this overwhelming attention has declined. Yet, over two decades after its conception, the theory continues to generate research, controversy (e.g., Greenwald & Ronis, 1978), and additional theoretical (e.g., Fazio, Zanna, & Cooper, 1977) and practical implications (e.g., Cooper, 1980).

The theory of cognitive dissonance concerns individuals' reactions to inconsistency. The perception of inconsistency among cognitions leads a person to alter one or more cognitions to bring them into consonance. When a behavior that a person undertakes, for example, is inconsistent with an attitude that he or she holds, the inconsistency is often observed to prompt a change in that attitude to bring it into line with the behavior. In the first "induced compliance" experiment, Festinger and Carlsmith (1959) asked college students to deceive an ostensible fellow participant into believing that an extremely dull experimental task was interesting and exciting. Psychological inconsistency was created between the attitude, "This task is dull!" and the behavior, "I just convinced someone that the task was interesting." Subjects' reactions to such inconsistency depended on the degree of monetary inducement they had received for attempting the deception. Subjects paid merely $1 to do so later reported valuing the task more than subjects paid $20. Given minimal external justification for having performed the counterattitudinal behavior, individuals modified their attitudes toward the direction implied by the behavior.

The Festinger and Carlsmith experiment demonstrated that inconsistency in and of itself is not sufficient to prompt attitude change. Merely telling someone that a dull task was interesting did not prompt an attitude change when the external justification was very high. Subsequent research has clarified the notion of cognitive dissonance and, in so doing, has further defined its scope. Research has shown that behaving in ways inconsistent with one's attitudes will prompt attitude change when the behavior was freely engaged in rather than coerced (Davis & Jones, 1960; Linder, Cooper, & Jones, 1967). The behavior itself must both be committing (Davis & Jones, 1960) and create unwanted, aversive consequences (Cooper & Worchel, 1970; Cooper, Zanna, & Goethals, 1974; Nel, Helmreich, & Aronson, 1969). Furthermore, the possibility of these aversive consequences arising must be foreseeable at the time of the individual's decision to perform the behavior (Cooper, 1971; Goethals, Cooper, & Naficy, 1979). These findings have served to clarify when compliance with a request to perform a counterattitudinal behavior produces attitude change. Only when an individual feels personally responsible for having committed himself or herself to perform a behavior that may foreseeably produce an aversive consequence does the individual display attitude change. Over the years, then, the theory of cognitive dissonance has become much more restricted than in the Festinger's original framework.

Despite such restriction, the theory remains enormously powerful. Not only does it explain attitude change as a consequence of induced compliance, but the theory has also spawned the development of additional research paradigms that together attest to its breadth and power. For example, cognitive dissonance theory explains individuals' tendencies to enhance the perceived value of a chosen alternative postdecisionally (e.g., Brehm, 1956; Knox & Inkster, 1968). In the Knox and Inkster experiment, bettors at the $2 window of a horse race track expressed more confidence in their selection after having placed their bets than similar bettors who had not yet bet but were in line to do so. The "effort justification" paradigm has illustrated how dissonance theory can account for individuals' increased attraction to a goal as a consequence of simply having chosen to "suffer" in order to attain the goal (e.g., Aronson & Mills, 1959; Gerard & Mathewson, 1966). Both of these experiments demonstrate that the more severe the initiation an individual is willing to undergo in order to attain membership in a group, the more the individual comes to value the group. Furthermore, dissonance theory provides a viable explanation of many other attitudinal phenomena, including reversals of normal communicator effects. Jones and Brehm (1967) demonstrated that sometimes the less attractive of two communicators produces greater attitude change. This reversal of the typical effect of communicator attractiveness occurred when an individual chose to listen to a communication known to be personally objectionable—a situation that produces psychological inconsistency between one's attitude toward the issue and one's decision.

In addition to its relevance to many basic research issues, dissonance theory has proven fruitful with regard to practical implications. Brehm and Cohen (1962), Worchel and Cooper (1979), and Cooper and Fazio (1979) each have discussed the relevance of the theory to racial integration. The theory, and the effort justification principle in particular, have been shown to be of relevance to the success of therapy. For example, Cooper (1980) has shown that improvement in snake phobics' ability to approach a snake can be brought about by an effortful, yet bogus therapy, provided that the individuals freely choose to engage in the therapeutic procedure. Similarly, assertiveness can be increased (Cooper, 1980), and weight loss induced (Axsom & Cooper, 1981), by judicious use of the effort justification principle. The theory also accounts for the relative success of participative budgeting (i.e., procedures by which the "workers" play a role in determining the production goals of the business unit rather than having a budget thrust upon them) in enhancing both workers' commitment to and satisfaction with the budget and their actual job performance (Tiller, 1980). The implications of the theory for the marketing of new products at introductory price discounts have also been investigated (Doob, Carlsmith, Freedman, Landauer, & Tom, 1969).

THE CONCEPT OF DISSONANCE

Cognitive dissonance theory has not rested unchallenged. Possibly because of the very breadth and power that makes the theory so attractive, numerous "competing" theories have been proposed. These explanations typically may provide valid alternative interpretations of, at least, some subset of the experiments relevant to dissonance theory (e.g., impression management: Tedeschi, Schlenker, & Bonoma, 1971; evaluation apprehension: Rosenberg, 1965). One "competing" explanation, Bem's self-perception theory (1967), has been even more successful in that it provides a seemingly plausible account of the many attitudinal effects observed in experiments related to dissonance theory.

Given these various alternative interpretations, it becomes all the more important and critical to have the capacity to detect when a given attitude change effect is the result of a dissonance process versus some other mechanism such as self-perception. Fortunately, dissonance theory posits a unique feature that sets it apart from the competing concepts. That feature is the state of dissonance itself. We will have much more to say about this state momentarily. Critical at this point, however, is the understanding that detection of the state of dissonance has the potential of serving to validate that a particular class of situations produces attitude change through the mechanism proposed by cognitive dissonance theory as opposed to the mechanisms suggested by various alternative theories (cf. Fazio *et al.*, 1977). For this reason it becomes important to be able to detect, directly or indirectly, the existence of the state of dissonance.

Unfortunately, Festinger's description of the state of dissonance in his original proposal is sparse and sketchy. Interestingly, in light of the later developments that were to occur, a close examination fails to reveal any definitive statements about the nature of the state on the part of Festinger (1957). The state of dissonance is described as "psychological discomfort" (p. 2) for which "one can substitute other notions similar in nature, such as 'hunger,' 'frustration,' or 'disequilibrium'" (p. 3). Furthermore, it is proposed that "dissonance acts in the same way as a state of drive or need or tension. The presence of dissonance leads to action to reduce it just as, for example, the presence of hunger leads to action to reduce the hunger" (p. 18). Thus, all Festinger did was to draw an analogy to drive states such as hunger. Whether dissonance is itself a drive is unclear from these statements. Also left open to interpretation is the issue of whether the state involves any *physiological* arousal. Is dissonance simply a desire for homeostasis or equilibrium, or is the state actual physiological arousal that can be reduced by attitudinal readjustment?

It was not until Brehm and Cohen's (1962) major restatement of cognitive dissonance theory that one finds explicit characterization of the state of dissonance as a drive and as an arousal state[1] (see Chapter 12 of their work, in particular). Brehm and Cohen distinguished general motives (i.e., chronic states) from "motivational or drive states" that "are tied to specific arousal" (p. 227) and explicitly classify dissonance as the latter. The implication is that dissonance is a learned drive acquired through childhood socialization which is aroused in the presence of a given set of stimuli.

Since the development of this learned drive has been discussed so little, a few speculative comments are in order. We would suggest that the state of dissonance arousal may be viewed as a conditioned emotional response. Pairing of a neutral stimulus with shock has been shown to produce conditioned fear in rats. That is, when only the previously neutral stimulus is presented, the rat displays evidence of "fear" (e.g., Kamin, 1969). Furthermore, the reduction of such conditioned arousal states is thought to be rewarding and may underlie organisms learning to avoid or escape the previously neutral stimuli (cf. Mowrer, 1947, 1960). As a result

---

1. Although some theorists (e.g., Spence, 1956) have been careful to deny any link between drive states and arousal, this distinction has become blurred over the years in the dissonance literature. Dissonance theorists have typically considered the dissonance to be an arousal state with drive properties. Consequently, we shall use the two terms somewhat loosely and interchangeably at this point. A distinction that we draw later in this chapter between dissonance arousal and dissonance motivation will help to clarify this issue.

of early experience, humans may learn that being personally responsible for the production of a negative consequence is often followed by some form of negative social sanctions. For example, parents or peers might be critical of a child for performing a behavior that has unwanted implications for both the child and them. Or, in teaching children that they must live with the consequences of their decisions, parents and educators may deny children the opportunity to select a second alternative from a variety of options. Eventually, negative reinforcement may come to be expected following the production of negative effects. Anticipation of such retribution may prompt the individual to become aroused. Given a sufficient number of such experiences, an arousal state may become conditioned to having engaged in any behavior that might potentially result in a negative consequence. This state can then be reduced by convincing oneself that the consequence is not actually negative, that is, by changing one's attitude.

A considerable body of research has been conducted over the last decade in order to document the postulated existence of dissonance as an arousal state. It is to a review of this evidence that we now address ourselves. We shall discuss first research indicating that the consequence of dissonance manipulations is a state that shares the properties of other arousal states: (1) like other such states it tends to energize dominant responses, and (2) like the arousal involved in emotions, the state needs to be interpreted and cognitively labeled in an appropriate manner for attitude change to occur. These two research enterprises approach the issue of arousal indirectly and allow us to infer the existence of a state of dissonance arousal from the effects that are observed. Attempts to measure dissonance arousal directly have been few in number, but we will then turn our attention to such research. Throughout, we shall attempt to point to issues that are in need of further research.

ENERGIZING PROPERTIES OF DISSONANCE AROUSAL

Arousal states typically energize dominant responses (Cottrell, Rittle, & Wack, 1967; Spence, Farber, & McFann, 1956). That is, the presence of arousal increases the likelihood that the organism will emit the strongest response in a hierarchy of response alternatives. Consequently, arousal typically facilitates performance on simple, well-learned tasks for which the dominant response is the correct response. On more complex and difficult tasks, arousal tends to inhibit performance because the dominant response is likely to be incorrect. This basic principle has been applied to the question of whether dissonance manipulations produce arousal. If they do so, the argument goes, subjects in a high-dissonance situation should demonstrate superior performance on a simple task and inferior performance on a complex task relative to subjects in a low-dissonance situation.

A variety of such experiments have been conducted. Since this research area has been reviewed in detail by both Kiesler and Pallak (1976) and Wicklund and Brehm (1976), we shall present only a single exemplary piece of research. Pallak and Pittman (1972) manipulated dissonance by committing subjects to performing a boring "pronunciation" task under conditions of high versus low choice. That is, half the subjects were given the opportunity to decline to participate in the boring task whereas the others were told that they were obliged to complete the task. Following the choice manipulation, all subjects participated in an ostensibly unrelated experiment involving a Stroop Color-Word Task. Two versions of this task were employed so as to manipulate simplicity of the task. The more difficult version consisted of trials on which color words ("green," "blue," "red") were printed in incongruent colored ink (e.g., "red" printed in green ink). The subject's task was to announce the color of the ink as opposed to the word. The simpler version consisted of words again printed in colored ink, but none of these words were associated with colors ("lot," "safe," "close"). This particular manipulation had proved sensitive enough to reveal effects of arousal produced by threat of electric shock in earlier research (Pallak, Pittman, Heller, & Munson, 1975). The number of errors made in terms of announcing the ink's color served as the performance measure. The results revealed the predicted choice by task complexity interaction. On the simpler version of the Stroop task, high-choice subjects performed better than low-choice subjects. The reverse was true on the more difficult Stroop task. This evidence is certainly consistent with the notion that dissonance arousal exists. Yet the measure intended to provide evidence of dissonance-produced attitude change with regard to perception of the boring task to which subjects had been committed failed to reveal any effects. Thus, it is not clear whether it was dissonance that was produced by the choice manipulation.[2]

Fortunately, a second experiment employing the same manipulation did reveal the predicted attitude change effect. This study involved only the more difficult version of the Stroop task and found (1) performance deficits in the high-choice condition relative to the low-choice condition, (2) more positive evaluation of the pronunciation task on the part of high-choice than on the part of low-choice subjects, and (3) that neither the performance nor the attitudinal effect occurred in conditions in which subjects had been provided with strong external justification for agreeing

2. As Pallak and Pittman (1972) note, the failure to find evidence of attitude change has been a recurring problem in research investigating the energizing properties of dissonance arousal. They suggest that the tasks the subjects are called on to perform following the dissonance manipulation may distract the subject from the dissonance-producing act. Such a suggestion is consistent with recent research by Zanna (1975) that indicates that distraction can weaken the typical induced compliance finding of attitude change.

to perform the pronunciation. This limiting effect of external justification is, of course, perfectly consistent with dissonance theory. Dissonance arousal would be minimal in the case of strong external justification for the behavior and, hence, neither performance effects nor attitude change are to be expected.

DISSONANCE AROUSAL AND THE SCHACHTER–SINGER MODEL OF EMOTIONS

A second indirect approach to the issue of dissonance arousal has been provided largely by Zanna and Cooper (1974, 1976). These investigators have noted a parallel between the concept of dissonance and the Schachter and Singer (1962) model of emotions. As proposed by Schachter and Singer, emotions involve a multiplicative function of arousal and cognitive labeling of the arousal. An undifferentiated state of arousal is interpreted and labeled in accord with the available situational cues. Both the arousal state and the appropriate label are necessary for a given emotion to occur. Zanna and Cooper (1974) suggested that the same may be true of dissonance. In order to experience pressure to change one's attitudes, one needs to experience an arousal state and interpret that state as resulting from one's having produced aversive consequences.

Misattribution of Dissonance Arousal

The Schachter and Singer proposal spawned a number of experiments demonstrating that the process of cognitive interpretation can result in the individual's misattributing the arousal he or she is experiencing to an improper source. That is, the individual may attribute the arousal to a potential source in the situation that is not, in fact, the source responsible for the arousal he or she is experiencing (e.g., Nisbett & Schachter, 1966; Ross, Rodin, & Zimbardo, 1969; Schachter & Singer, 1962; Storms & Nisbett, 1970). On the basis of such findings, Zanna and Cooper (1974) reasoned that if the state of dissonance does involve arousal, that arousal would also require interpretation. Hence, it may be attributed inappropriately to a source other than the negative consequence producing action. Such misattribution would be expected to occur only if the situational cues provided an alternative potential source of arousal. Yet, if misattribution were to occur, the individual would not experience any motivation to change his or her attitude so as to justify his or her action. Thus, misattribution should produce an attenuation of the typical attitude change effect observed in an induced compliance experiment.

In the experiment conducted by Zanna and Cooper (1974), subjects who were induced to behave in a manner inconsistent with their attitudes were also presented with a misattributional stimulus. The volunteers had agreed to participate in a study pertaining to the effect of an experimental drug on memory. After performing a free-recall task, subjects were given their capsule, assured that it was harmless, and were then given one of three sets of information designed to establish a possible misattribution for any arousal that the later manipulations might cause.

Although the capsule actually contained only powdered milk, subjects in the tension condition were told: "This . . . capsule contains chemical elements that are more soluble than other parts of the compound. In this form of the drug, these elements may produce a reaction of tenseness prior to the total absorption of the drug, 5 minutes after ingestion. The side effect will disappear within 30 minutes." In another set of conditions, the word "tenseness" was replaced with "relaxation." Finally, in a no-information condition, the subjects were told that the drug had no side effects.

While waiting for the drug to be totally absorbed, the subjects participated in what they believed would be a completely separate experiment. They believed that a prestigious interuniversity group was considering placing a ban on "inflammatory" speakers at college campuses. The subjects' task was to write a strong and forceful essay in favor of such a ban. This position was known to be discrepant from the subjects' true attitude. Half of the subjects were requested to write the essay and were constantly reassured that the decision to write such an essay was completely their own. The other half were merely told to write the essay. Subjects' attitudes toward the ban were then measured.

In the typical induced compliance study, writing attitude-discrepant essays under conditions of high choice produces greater opinion change than under conditions of low choice. In the no-information conditions of the Zanna and Cooper experiment, this typical finding was replicated, as can be seen in the center column of Table 5-1.

The findings of immediate interest are the results of the tension condition. It was expected that subjects who wrote counterattitudinal essays with high choice would experience arousal but would have the drug capsule to help them explain the meaning of their arousal. Therefore, there would be no need to change their attitudes. Indeed, the first column of Table 5-1 indicates that this is what occurred. The high-choice–tension condition did not differ from its low-choice counterpart nor from a control group that did not participate in the memory study but only had their attitudes assessed. Finally, the third column of Table 5-1 illustrates the exaggerated attitude-change finding for high-choice subjects in the relaxation condition. These subjects believed that they should have been relaxed by the drug. Still apparently feeling aroused by their attitude-discrepant behavior, they attributed even more tension to themselves and changed their attitudes more than any other group of subjects in the experiment.

TABLE 5-1. Mean Opinions toward Banning Speakers on Campus

DECISION FREEDOM	POTENTIAL SIDE EFFECT OF THE DRUG		
	TENSION	NO INFORMATION	RELAXATION
High	3.40_a	9.10_b	13.40_c
Low	3.50_a	4.50_a	4.70_a

Note. Cell $n = 10$. The larger the mean, the more agreement with the attitude-discrepant essay (control group $\bar{X} = 2.30_a$). Cells not sharing a common subscript differ at the .01 level by the Newman–Keuls procedure; cells showing a common subscript do not differ at the .05 level. From "Dissonance and the pill: An attribution approach to studying the arousal properties of dissonance" by M. P. Zanna & J. Cooper, *Journal of Personality and Social Psychology,* 1974, *29,* 703–409. Copyright 1974 by the American Psychological Association. Reprinted by permission.

The findings of Zanna and Cooper have been replicated in many similar situations. In addition to the attenuation of attitude change occurring after misattribution to an allegedly tension-producing pill (cf. Higgins, Rhodewalt, & Zanna, 1979; Zanna, Higgins, & Taves, 1976), dissonance has also been attributed to the threat of electric shock (Pittman, 1975), small soundproof booths in which one is seated (Fazio *et al.*, 1977), fluorescent lighting (Gonzalez & Cooper, 1976), and humorous cartoons (Cooper, Fazio, & Rhodewalt, 1978).

In sum, the misattribution approach suggested by Zanna and Cooper has succeeded in providing a means by which dissonance arousal can be detected. Unfortunately, the approach has proven somewhat less successful in clarifying further the nature of the state of dissonance. In particular, researchers have recently addressed the issue of whether the state that follows one's having freely produced an unwanted consequence is specifically aversive or a more general and labile heightened state of arousal. The misattribution approach has yielded evidence that, at least on the surface, appears inconsistent.

Employing the pill paradigm, both Zanna *et al.* (1976) and Higgins *et al.* (1979) manipulated the ostensible side effects of a pill that subjects ingested prior to induced compliance. The notion was that only side-effect descriptions that matched the subject's phenomenological experience would result in an attenuation of attitude change because only such descriptions provide an appropriate misattribution opportunity. Zanna *et al.* varyingly described the side effects as "tenseness" or "pleasant excitement" and found misattribution to occur only in the case of the pill that supposedly produced feelings of tension. Higgins *et al.* employed four different descriptions intended to represent each of the cells in a 2×2 matrix involving the presence or absence of arousal and pleasant or unpleasant feelings. The drug side effects were described as feelings of "pleasant excitement," "relaxation," "tenseness," or "unpleasant sedation." Each of the latter two terms, but not the former two, yielded misattribution of dissonance to the pill (as evidenced by the attitude-change data). Higgins *et al.* interpreted these findings as an indication that the state experienced following production of an unwanted consequence is phenomenologically one, not of arousal, but of discomfort.

Do these results imply that one necessarily experiences a specific state of discomfort following induced compliance? We tend to think not. The problem that arises in considering misattribution experiments of this sort is that we have no way of knowing the degree to which subjects engaged in any interpretation of their phenomenological states prior to misattribution to the pill. In particular, subjects may have experienced an immediate state of general, heightened arousal which they subsequently labeled as negative. Recall that subjects believed that they were taking an experimental pill that was still being tested and potentially produced side effects. Concerns about the experimental status of the pill may have provided a strong contextual cue for labeling any general arousal as a negative feeling. Once the state is judged to be aversive, this discomfort and not any accompanying arousal, may form the key feature whose cause subjects seek to understand. Having labeled the arousal as negative, subjects may be searching specifically for a potential source of discomfort. Thus, only side-effect descriptions involving some unpleasantness could serve as misattribution stimuli.

There is, in fact, some evidence consistent with the notion that the dissonance state can be misattributed to sources of positive arousal, implying that the state is more general and labile than suggested by the Zanna *et al.* and Higgins *et al.* findings. Cooper *et al.* (1978) found that under appropriate conditions, subjects who had been freely committed to performing a counterattitudinal behavior misattributed their arousal to a humorous cartoon. Specifically, subjects who were exposed to the cartoon immediately following the behavioral commitment and before completing a final attitude measure tended to find the cartoon relatively funnier and to change their attitudes less than subjects who were not exposed to the cartoon until they had completed the final attitude measure. Thus, given the appropriate timing, dissonance arousal was interpreted as humorous reaction to the cartoon. Consequently, pressure to change one's attitude was never experienced. These data, together with the earlier described findings concerning the energizing properties of dissonance arousal and some research that we will review in later sections of this chapter, suggest that dissonance is initially an undifferentiated state of heightened arousal.

The results of the many misattribution experiments imply that dissonance arousal occurs when one willingly performs an action that has the potential of producing aversive consequences. The findings also make it quite evident that "correct" interpretation of this arousal state is necessary for attitude change to occur. Moreover, the findings imply that it may be necessary to distinguish what we shall term dissonance arousal and dissonance motivation. We shall use the term "dissonance arousal" to refer to the undifferentiated state of physiological arousal that appears to occur when one feels personally responsible for the occurrence of a negative consequence. This arousal, like any other emotional arousal, is open to many varied interpretations and can be attributed to positive or negative sources of arousal. "Dissonance motivation," on the other hand, occurs only when the subject labels this arousal negatively and attributes it to his or her production of an aversive consequence. We shall use the term to refer to the psychological discomfort that motivates or "drives" the attitude-change process. Apparently, subjects in the high-choice conditions of induced compliance experiments who are provided with a misattribution cue experience dissonance arousal, but not dissonance motivation.

Misattribution and Other Attitude-Change Processes

The misattribution approach clearly has proven fruitful in terms of providing evidence that dissonance arousal exists. In addition, it has proven useful in terms of fulfilling the goal mentioned earlier of determining whether a given attitude-change finding is the culmination of a dissonance process or of some other process. Fazio et al. (1977) employed a misattribution approach in an attempt to differentiate dissonance and self-perception processes. They proposed that dissonance and self-perception theories be regarded not as competing formulations, but as complementary ones, each applicable to its own particular domain. They argued that dissonance theory is relevant to the context of attitude-discrepant behavior (for in such a case the action produces an aversive consequence, i.e., a state of affairs that one finds objectionable) and self-perception theory to attitude-congruent behavior (for in such a case the consequences of the action are acceptable). As an operationalization of attitude-discrepant versus attitude-congruent behavior, Fazio et al. suggested use of the construct of latitudes of acceptance and rejection (Sherif & Hovland, 1961). The latitude of acceptance refers to statements that are found acceptable in a continuum of extreme pro- to extreme antiattitudinal positions. The latitude of rejection includes the entire range of positions that are found objectionable. It was proposed that a dissonance process follows the endorsement of a position within one's latitude of rejection and a self-perception process the endorsement of a position within the latitude of acceptance.

Under the rubric of a political survey, subjects first completed a latitudes measure regarding conservatism–liberalism. Half the subjects then committed themselves to endorsing a position within their latitudes of acceptance; the remaining subjects endorsed a position within their latitudes of rejection. In order to establish that the manipulations and procedure were sufficiently effective to produce attitude change, some subjects were committed under conditions of high choice and others under conditions of low choice. As is to be expected, if all relevant variables were properly operationalized, high-choice subjects displayed more extreme final attitudes than did low-choice subjects in both the accept and reject conditions (see Table 5-2).

In order to determine whether these attitude-change effects were due to dissonance or to self-perception processes, another set of high-choice conditions was included. Like the other high-choice subjects, these subjects freely committed themselves to endorsing either an acceptable or an objectionable position. However, they were also provided with a potential misattribution cue. Immediately after committing themselves, these subjects completed a "Departmental Equipment Inquiry," intended to make salient to the subject the possibility that any arousal he or she might be experiencing was possibly due to the small, soundproof booth in which the subject was seated. It was predicted that subjects in the reject condition, since they are hypothesized to undergo a dissonance process, would experience dissonance arousal and misattribute it to the booth. Hence, they would not experience dissonance motivation and would not display attitude change. Subjects in the accept condition, on the other hand, are hypothesized to be engaged in a passive self-perception process. Since they are not experiencing any arousal, they should remain unaffected by the misattribution cue and should display attitude change, just as their counterparts in the no-misattribution condition did. These predictions were confirmed (see Table 5-2). Within the reject conditions, final attitudes in the high-choice–misattribution condition and the low-choice conditions were equivalent and were less extreme than in the high-choice–no-misattribution condition. Within the accept conditions, the two high-choice conditions

TABLE 5-2. Adjusted Means

LATITUDE	LOW CHOICE	HIGH CHOICE–NO BOOTH	HIGH CHOICE–BOOTH
Accept	20.33$_{ab}$	22.70$_c$	22.39$_c$
Reject	18.77$_a$	21.14$_{bc}$	18.89$_a$

Note. The higher the mean, the more liberal subjects perceived themselves to be. Cell means not sharing a common subscript differ beyond the 5% significance level (except the low-choice–accept vs. high-choice–booth–accept comparison, which is at $p = .06$). From "Dissonance and self-perception: An integrative view of each theory's proper domain of application" by R. H. Fazio, M. P. Zanna, & J. Cooper, *Journal of Experimental Social Psychology,* 1977, *13,* 464–479. Copyright 1977 by Academic Press. Reprinted by permission.

displayed equivalent attitudes, significantly more extreme than final attitude scores in the low-choice condition.

On the Necessity of Arousal

The research discussed above demonstrates the necessity of a proper attribution for one's arousal if one is to experience dissonance motivation. Completing the analogy of dissonance to the Schachter and Singer model of emotions, Cooper, Zanna, and Taves (1978) have demonstrated that arousal itself is necessary. After agreeing to ingest any of three drugs (an amphetamine, a tranquilizer, and a placebo) for an experiment ostensibly concerned with short-term memory, all subjects in this experiment were told that they had been assigned to the placebo condition and ingested a capsule. For one-third of the subjects, the capsule did consist only of milk powder. The remaining subjects, although led to believe that they were taking a placebo, actually ingested either the amphetamine or the tranquilizer. During a "break" in the memory experiment, all subjects participated in a standard induced compliance experiment. Half the subjects were asked to write a counterattitudinal essay in support of the pardon of Richard Nixon and half were required to do so. Subjects' final attitudes toward the pardon are displayed in Table 5-3. Within the placebo conditions, the typical effect was apparent; high-choice subjects reported more extreme attitudes than low-choice subjects. Most relevant to the present concern are the findings in the tranquilizer conditions, wherein the high- and low-choice subjects did not differ. Thus, when the occurrence of arousal was prevented by a drug, high-choice subjects, apparently failing to experience dissonance arousal, felt no need to change their attitudes.

TABLE 5-3. Mean Scores of Attitudes toward the Pardoning of Richard Nixon

DECISION FREEDOM	DRUG CONDITION		
	TRANQUILIZER	PLACEBO	AMPHETAMINE
High choice	8.6$_a$	14.7$_b$	20.2$_c$
Low choice	8.0$_a$	8.3$_a$	13.9$_b$

Note. $n = 10$ subjects per cell. Higher means on the 31-point scale indicate greater agreement with the attitude-discrepant essay. Cell means with different subscripts are different from each other at the .05 level by the Newman–Keuls procedure. The mean in the survey control condition is 7.9$_a$. From "Arousal as a necessary condition for attitude change following induced compliance" by J. Cooper, M. P. Zanna, & P. A. Taves, *Journal of Personality and Social Psychology,* 1978, *36,* 1101–1106. Copyright 1978 by the American Psychological Association. Reprinted by permission.

Interpretation of External Arousal as Dissonance Motivation

The amphetamine conditions of the Cooper *et al.* (1978) experiment also revealed an interesting effect. In both the low-choice and high-choice conditions, attitude change was evident (see Table 5-3). Apparently, the arousal resulting from the amphetamine was misattributed to the essay writing. Believing that they had ingested a nonarousing placebo, the subjects appear to have interpreted their arousal as dissonance motivation and, consequently, changed their attitudes.

The result suggests that dissonance motivation can be created or enhanced by the individual's misinterpretation of arousal that is actually due to some external source. A similar implication is provided by an earlier study conducted by Worchel and Arnold (1974). These investigations also considered the effect of combined arousal states on attitude change. Dissonance arousal in conjunction with the perceived arousal created by task interruption was examined. Zeigarnik (1927) hypothesized that task interruption aroused tension within the individual aimed at task completion. It is presumably this arousal that results in the "Zeigarnik effect" of increased recall of the task material (cf. Mandler, 1964). In the Worchel and Arnold experiment, subjects chose, or were required, to listen to an objectionable, counterattitudinal tape-recorded speech. In order to manipulate task interruption, the tape "broke" during the conclusion for half the subjects. Final attitude scores indicated that high-choice subjects who had been interrupted displayed significantly greater attitude change than did the uninterrupted, high-choice subjects. This finding is consistent with the notion that any arousal resulting from task interruption was misinterpreted as, and contributed to, dissonance motivation. Unlike the findings of Cooper *et al.*, however, this effect was not observed in the low-choice conditions. Neither interrupted nor uninterrupted low-choice subjects revealed significant attitude change.

Thus, the findings of Cooper *et al.* and Worchel and Arnold are consistent in suggesting that misattribution of arousal due to an external source to dissonance motivation can accentuate the already existing dissonance arousal experienced by subjects given decision freedom. Yet the findings are discrepant with respect to the possibility that misinterpretation of external arousal can produce dissonance motivation even when dissonance arousal normally does not exist because of the lack of decision freedom. This discrepancy, and the general problem of drawing inferences from experiments such as Cooper *et al.*'s that involve the use of actual drugs that may produce multiple and unknown effects (cf. Higgins *et al.*, 1979), motivated Fazio and Martin to attempt a conceptual replication of the amphetamine conditions in the Cooper *et al.* experiment. These researchers employed the excitation transfer paradigm developed by Zillmann (1971, 1978; see also Chapter 8, this volume). Zillmann has suggested that after an arousing activity, residues of the arousal tend to linger and affect subsequent experiential states. Since the Fazio and Martin experiment was modeled after a study by Cantor, Zillmann, and Bryant (1975) that tested this transfer hypothesis, it will be useful to review this experiment. Cantor *et al.* identified three distinct phases of recovery from exercise. During phase 1, shortly after the exercise, physiological measures of systolic blood pressure and heart rate revealed arousal and, furthermore, subjects accurately reported that they were aroused. During phase 2, the unperceived, residual arousal stage, measured arousal remained elevated above baseline, but subjects reported no longer being aroused. Phase 3 involved a return of measured arousal to baseline. Cantor *et al.* had subjects ride an exercise bicycle and then exposed the subjects to an erotic film during one of the three recovery phases. Subjects then evaluated the erotic film and reported their degree of sexual arousal. Both sets of ratings revealed a significant transfer effect for the subjects in phase 2. These subjects apparently misattributed residual arousal from the exercise to the film and, consequently, reported feeling more sexually aroused and found the film more exciting than subjects in phase 3. It was expected that in phase 1 (perceived residual excitation) subjects' perceptions of residual arousal might lead them to misattribute arousal due to the erotic film to the residual arousal from exercise. Thereby, these subjects might underestimate their true response to the film. This was not the case, however. Subjects' ratings were equivalent to those of subjects in phase 3, suggesting that the subjects were able to apportion their arousal to the two arousal-inducing agents, exercise and erotica.

Fazio and Martin applied this same logic and procedure to dissonance, substituting dissonance arousal for erotica. Excitation transfer, resulting in accentuated attitude change, was expected for subjects who committed the dissonant action during phase 2. No prediction was made for phase 1 subjects. Misattribution of dissonance arousal to just having exercised, and a resulting attenuation of attitude change, appears theoretically possible. Yet the lack of a similar effect in the Cantor *et al.* experiment casts some doubt on this possibility.

In a pretest experiment, Fazio and Martin had subjects ride an exercise bicycle and then measured their systolic blood pressure at regular intervals during the 10 minutes following exercise. Subjects also reported their perception of their arousal levels. From these data the three critical phases of arousal recovery was identified. Subjects' reports of arousal level revealed a perceived return to baseline within approximately 5 minutes after exercise. On the other hand, actual systolic blood pressure did not return to baseline until approximately 8 minutes after exercise. On the basis of these data, subjects in the main experiment committed themselves to the dissonant action either 2 minutes (phase 1, perceived residual excitation; in this case, the experimenter began the description of the essay task almost immediately after the exercise and the actual request occurred within roughly 2 minutes), 5 minutes (phase 2, unperceived residual excitation), or 10 minutes (no residual excitation) after riding the exercise bicycle.

After the timing manipulation was accomplished, the experimenter informed the subject of another study that he was conducting and that the subject could participate in during this "break" in the experiment. The experimenter explained that he needed subjects to write essays in favor of federally financed abortions (a position that was extremely counterattitudinal for this subject population). The essays were presumably to be employed in future persuasion studies. Half the subjects were explicitly asked to volunteer to participate in this other study. The remaining subjects were not. Immediately after the subjects were committed to writing the essay, the subjects indicated their attitudes toward federally financed abortions. An additional group of subjects from the same student population also completed this attitude measure as part of an "attitude survey" and, hence, served as a survey control condition.

Table 5-4 presents mean attitude scores in each condition, following a reciprocal transformation of the data (necessitated by its skewness). Among those subjects who committed themselves to write the essay during the third phase of recovery, the typical induced compliance effect is observed. High-choice subjects reported greater agreement with the position they were to support than did low-choice subjects, indicating that decision freedom was properly manipulated. Predictions were also confirmed with regard to phase 2 (unperceived residual excitation) subjects. Both high- and low-choice subjects displayed more extreme attitudes than their

TABLE 5-4. Mean Transformed Attitude Scores toward Federally Financed Abortion

DECISION FREEDOM	RECOVERY PHASE		
	1	2	3
High choice	.290$_a$	.189$_a$	.299$_a$
Low choice	.209$_a$	.310$_a$	.671$_b$

Note. $n = 11$ subjects per cell. Means are based on a reciprocal transformation of the attitude data. Lower means indicate greater agreement with the attitude-discrepant position that the subject was committed to support. Cell means with different subscripts are significantly different at the 5% level. The mean in the survey control condition is .642$_b$.

counterparts in phase 3, although the comparison was statistically significant only for the low-choice subjects. The latter finding provides a conceptual replication of the Cooper *et al.* result and suggests that arousal from an external source can be misinterpreted as dissonance motivation, even when subjects are not provided with any actual decision freedom.

The data in the phase 1 conditions were somewhat surprising. As in Cantor *et al.*, there was no indication of misattribution of dissonance arousal to exercise. Just why misattribution of dissonance arousal did not occur is not clear. However, it is interesting to note that in most of the experiments concerned with the misattribution of dissonance arousal, the ostensible alternate source of arousal (i.e., the misattribution cue) was not itself actually arousing. Conceivably, when the "alternate" source of arousal actually produces an arousal state prior to the induction of dissonance (as with exercise in the present case), individuals attempt to apportion the arousal between the two sources. In Cantor *et al.*'s experiment subjects appeared to apportion arousal between exercise and erotica fairly accurately; phase 1 and phase 3 subjects displayed equivalence. This was not so in the present case. Means in the low-choice/phase 1 and low-choice/phase 3 conditions were not equivalent. Instead, the phase 1 subjects displayed significant attitude change. Subjects seem to have apportioned "too much" of the arousal due to exercise to dissonance motivation.

Despite the perplexity of the findings regarding phase 1, the data are quite clear in suggesting that misinterpretation of arousal from an external source can produce or enhance dissonance motivation. Along with the amphetamine condition in Cooper *et al.*, the present data strongly suggest that excitation transfer can prompt attitude change even when decision freedom does not exist. Hence, they imply that arousal, and misinterpretation of that arousal to one's having produced a potentially aversive consequence, are sufficient to prompt dissonance motivation and attitude change, even when one cannot be held personally responsible for the consequence. In general, the findings provide further evidence of the critical role that arousal exerts in the dissonance process of attitude change.

PHYSIOLOGICAL MEASUREMENT

The analogy proposed by Zanna and Cooper (1974) between dissonance arousal and the Schachter–Singer model of emotions has proven exceedingly fruitful. It has succeeded in generating much research—the findings of which imply that arousal is involved in the dissonance process. It has also provided a technique by which attitude change as a result of dissonance can be distinguished from attitude change occurring via other processes. Finally, it has served to elucidate the critical attribution process by which dissonance arousal (or arousal due to some external source) becomes dissonance motivation, the state of tension and pressure to change one's attitudes that Festinger alluded to in his original proposal.

The approach does raise some questions about misattribution processes in general, however. Does misattribution occur at a sufficient level of awareness that individuals can accurately report on the process (see Nisbett & Wilson, 1977)? Need the arousal itself be perceived at a level that the individuals can report its existence for a misattribution process to begin? Although not specific to the area of dissonance, these are questions that future research on misattribution needs to address.

More relevant to the present concerns are the many questions specific to dissonance arousal itself that the misattribution approach leaves unanswered (see Ronis & Greenwald, 1979; Fazio, Zanna, & Cooper, 1979). For, despite its success, the misattribution approach remains an indirect, inferential technique by which the presence of dissonance arousal can be detected. What is the time course of dissonance arousal in the induced compliance procedure? Just when after one has performed an objectionable behavior does the conditioned emotional state we referred to earlier occur? Does the labeling of the general, undifferentiated state of dissonance arousal as dissonance motivation or as arousal due to some external agent affect the level of arousal experienced? What variables do determine the level of arousal that is experienced?

It is difficult to see how data relevant to questions such as the above can be garnered readily from investigations employing the misattribution approach. It would seem that direct physiological measurement of the state would be necessary. Unfortunately, there exists a paucity of experiments employing such direct measurement in the literature. The prevalent notion that seems to be held by most dissonance researchers is that measurement of dissonance arousal has been attempted, but has proven fruitless. For that reason, presumably, very few reports of such experiments can be found in the literature.

In the sections that follow, we will review the available literature. We will then present the results of a new experiment that does succeed in obtaining reliable physiological measurements during a dissonance-inducing task. Taken together, the research will lead us to have greater confidence in the notion that cognitive dissonance is a state of arousal that has direct physiological ramifications.

Earlier Research

Physiological Correlates of Dissonance Reduction

At least four reports in the literature have concerned the use of physiological measures in order to examine physiological changes occurring as a consequence of dissonance reduction. These experiments serve to indicate that dissonance reduction can be accompanied by more quiescent physiological activity. Brehm, Back, and Bogdonoff (1964) have provided some suggestive evidence concerning perceptions of hunger and concentrations of free fatty acids in the blood. Essentially, the data suggest that food-deprived individuals who commit themselves to further fasting under conditions of minimal external justification not only report being less hungry but also display a lower concentration of free fatty acids (indicating less hunger physiologically) than do individuals provided with external justification for continued fasting. Similarly, three studies have employed physiological measurement to examine whether individuals who voluntarily commit themselves to undergoing a stressful event subsequently experience less stress. Zimbardo, Cohen, Weisenberg, Dworkin, and Firestone (1969) provided subjects with either high or low justification for accepting painful electric shocks and found that the latter subjects displayed less stress while enduring the shocks than the former subjects, as measured by galvanic skin responses (GSRs). In an attempt to replicate this experiment conceptually, Glass and Mayhew (1969) examined skin conductance responses while subjects observed a stressful film. Subjects who voluntarily agreed to watch the film displayed more quiescent autonomic reactivity to the film than did subjects who had been required to watch. Unfortunately, this relatively lower physiological activity was true for subjects who volunteered to watch the film regardless of whether they had or had not been provided with strong justification for complying. Since dissonance theory would not predict any effects given high justification, the findings could be interpreted to suggest that the lack of choice increased electrodermal activity, rather than dissonance reduction decreasing electrodermal activity.

Yet another conceptual replication of the Zimbardo *et al.* experiment did find a justification manipulation to have a physiological impact. Totman (1975) exposed subjects' inner forearms to painful radiant heat stimuli. Subjects were then asked or required to receive an experimental injection that ostensibly was a drug that "may temporarily alter your perception of thermal stimuli around the injected area," but actually was a placebo. Some of the choice subjects were promised a monetary payment; the others were not. Those subjects who chose to receive the injection for no payment rated a second series of heat stimuli as less painful than the first set and displayed lower GSR amplitude while undergoing the second series than the first. The reductions observed among these subjects were significantly greater than among subjects who were required to receive the injection. Furthermore, and most supportive of the proposition that dissonance reduction was responsible for the decreased arousal, these reductions were significantly greater than among subjects who chose to receive the injection, but did so for monetary payment.

These findings imply that the cognitive changes that occur as a result of dissonance reduction can be mirrored by physiological changes. Con-

sequently, these experiments serve more to reveal the power of dissonance processes than to provide information about dissonance arousal.

Physiological Measurement of Dissonance Arousal

An extensive search of the literature brought to our attention only four
reports of experiments in which physiological assessment of dissonance
arousal was attempted. Of these, the most prominent and most frequently
cited is an experiment by Gerard (1967) that employed the "free-choice"
paradigm. This particular dissonance paradigm involves subjects' selection
of which of a pair of alternatives among a set of earlier rank-ordered
possibilities they desire to have as their own. The magnitude of dissonance
is typically manipulated by having some subjects choose between alternatives very disparate in their desirability and others between nearly equally
desirable alternatives. Dissonance is more likely to be aroused in the latter
case because of the greater negative consequences associated with "giving
up" all the positive qualities of the nonchosen alternative. Typically, this
dissonance is reduced by "spreading apart the alternatives." That is, attitudes toward the chosen alternative become more positive and/or attitudes
toward the nonchosen more negative.

In the Gerard experiment, subjects first evaluated a set of paintings.
Subjects were then offered a choice between two paintings. In the high-
dissonance condition, the two were the third- and fourth-ranked; in the
low-dissonance condition, the third- and eighth-ranked. During this decision sequence, measures of changes in finger pulse amplitude were recorded by a plethysmograph. Stress is revealed by a decrease in pulse
amplitude as a result of constriction of blood vessels. Gerard predicted that
such a decrease would be evident immediately after the committing decision, at least for subjects in the high-dissonance condition. Amplitude
measures recorded immediately before and immediately after the decision
were compared and confirmed the prediction. Ten of the 12 subjects in the
high-dissonance condition displayed constriction, whereas only four of
the 11 in the low-dissonance condition did so.

The finding is certainly supportive of the proposition that dissonance
involves an arousal state. Unfortunately, there are at least two problems
that need to be kept in mind when considering the extent of this support.
First, attitudinal evidence of a dissonance process was somewhat weak.
When asked to rerank the entire set of paintings, subjects in the high-
dissonance condition displayed only marginally significantly greater
spreading apart of the alternatives than did subjects in the low-dissonance
condition (one-tailed $p < .10$). Second, as is frequently the problem with
the free-choice paradigm, seven subjects displayed choice inversions; that
is, they chose the lower ranked of the two alternatives. These subjects, six
of whom were in the high-dissonance condition, were apparently replaced
by other subjects. As Gerard notes, this potentially introduces a problem

of self-selection bias. Nevertheless, Gerard's findings are, at minimum, encouraging in suggesting that dissonance arousal can be measured physiologically.

Two unpublished experiments have employed heart rate and skin conductance measures in order to attempt to assess dissonance arousal. An unpublished dissertation by Buck (1970) reports an experiment in which heart rate and skin conductance were monitored in a situation that was theoretically dissonance arousing. During the first phase of the experiment, these measures were recorded while the subject was presented with a series of auditory tones. In the second phase, subjects were induced, under conditions of high choice, to deliver a series of intense shocks (high dissonance), mild shocks (low dissonance), or harmless tones (no dissonance) to an innocent victim. Delivery of the shock (or tone) activated the same tone the subject had heard in the first phase. Thus, the stimulation received was identical in the two phases, but the second series of measurements potentially included dissonance arousal. Differences in heart rate and in skin conductance between the two phases provided a physiological index of dissonance arousal. Although the heart rate index revealed no effects, a significant linear trend in response to the three levels of dissonance was apparent on the skin conductance index. High-dissonance subjects displayed the greatest increase in skin conductance, just as predicted.

Unfortunately, such mixed results are difficult to interpret. As Lacey and his colleagues have pointed out (Lacey, 1967; Lacey, Kagan, Lacey, & Moss, 1963), it is not uncommon for two distinct measures of physiological responding to fail to covary substantially and, hence, to lead to different conclusions about the level of physiological excitation. In this case the heart rate data revealed no reliable effects, whereas the skin conductance data displayed the predicted pattern. Thus, the findings provide, at best, only minimal evidence consistent with the notion that dissonance involves a state of physiological arousal. Again, however, satisfaction about even such partial corroboration must be tempered by lack of independent evidence that dissonance was properly manipulated. A variety of attitudinal measures failed to reveal the expected dissonance effect of attitude change. Evaluation of the "victim," estimates of the painfulness of the shock, judgments of the importance of the study, reported enjoyment of the experiment, and reported concern that the other person might be suffering were collected, together with some other potential measures of dissonance reduction. None displayed a linear trend corresponding to the effect on skin conductance.

In contrast to the Buck experiment, Gleason and Katkin (1978) observed effects on both heart rate and skin conductance measures in an investigation of dissonance arousal. Unfortunately, there is some question as to whether the procedure incorporated all the elements known to be necessary to produce dissonance. Two groups were created. In the dissonant condition, subjects were instructed to spend 5 minutes (in preparation for delivering a speech) thinking about arguments in support of reducing average grades at the university. This position was known to be counter-attitudinal for the subjects from their completion of a premeasure several weeks earlier. This group was compared to subjects in a consonant condition who had been instructed to consider arguments against reducing average grades. During the 5-minute "thinking" period, significantly greater elevations in heart rate and in the frequency of spontaneous skin conductance responses were displayed by subjects in the dissonant condition than by subjects in the consonant condition. In addition, a subsequent attitude measure revealed significant change from pre- to postassessment for the dissonant but not for the consonant subjects. The data, then, appear quite supportive. Nevertheless, the findings can only be regarded as suggestive, for it is conceivable that some process other than dissonance was responsible for both the physiological and attitudinal effects. The problem is that it is unclear that the subjects experienced perceived freedom or anticipated aversive consequences as a result of their speeches—two necessary conditions for a dissonance process. Had decision freedom been manipulated and the observed effects been apparent in a high-choice but not in a low-choice condition, we could be far more confident that the results reflected a dissonance process.

Yet another promising, although again inconclusive, approach to the measurement of dissonance arousal has been provided by McMillen and Geiselman (1974) and McMillen, Geiselman, and Jones (1975).[3] These investigators argued that since dissonance centers around cognitive events, it may be more appropriate to employ measures of central nervous system activity than such autonomic measures as GSR and pulse rate. Their experiment involved the use of electroencephalographic (EEG) recordings of alpha waves. They cited a number of investigations that demonstrated that high alpha frequency activity is associated with relaxation and tranquility (e.g., Brown, 1974; Kamiya, 1969) and, consequently, predicted that dissonance arousal would suppress alpha output.

Subjects were recruited for an experiment ostensibly concerned with the effects of sensory deprivation upon reaction time to an auditory stimulus and the relations between reaction time and physiological measurements. During the initial 10 minutes, subjects sat motionless and blindfolded while baseline alpha activity was recorded. (Two EEG electrodes were placed "approximately 2 cm above and lateral to the occipital protuberance,

---

3. McMillen and Gieselman (1974) is a published summary of a paper presented at the 1974 American Psychological Association Convention. McMillen, Geiselman, and Jones (1975) present a lengthier and more detailed description of this same experiment, together with a report of a second experiment. We do not describe the second experiment above because the procedures employed are of dubious relevance to a dissonance process.

one on the right and one on the left side of the scalp.") Then the experimenter instructed the subject that the auditory stimuli would be presented during the next part of the experiment and that upon hearing each tone, the subject was to press a button. The subject was informed that this procedure would last for 20 minutes. At this point, the manipulation took place. Two conditions relevant to the present concerns were created. In one, termed the high-justification condition, the subjects were told that their participation in the study was extremely useful. In the low-justification condition, subjects were told that all necessary data had already been collected, that the data they provided would be essentially useless, and that the experimenter had arranged for them to participate only because they had already been scheduled. Although we will comment further on this in a moment, the apparent intent of the manipulation was to create differential justification (and hence differential dissonance) for subjects' participation in the tedious and boring reaction-time task. The authors reasoned that the low-justification subjects would experience dissonance and display suppressed alpha activity during the 20-minute task. The predicted difference between the two conditions was observed. Low-justification subjects displayed a continued decrease in alpha activity from baseline through the 20-minute period, whereas high-justification subjects showed an increase.

The alpha findings are certainly of interest, but their relevance to dissonance processes is unclear because of the unusual manner by which the experimenters attempted to create dissonance. Their justification manipulation and instructions were modeled after an experiment by Freedman (1963), who had subjects write random numbers and provided the same high or low justification for their doing so. After finishing, subjects in the low-justification condition reported having enjoyed the task more than did subjects in the high-justification condition. In the present case, no such data (enjoyment of the reaction time task) were collected. Once again, then, there is a lack of attitudinal evidence that the dissonance process occurred. Furthermore, the attitudinal effect observed by Freedman is to be expected only to the extent that subjects voluntarily engaged in the boring task. In the present case, it is not at all clear that subjects perceived decision freedom. Apparently, no explicit statements about choice were made and, furthermore, all the subjects were introductory psychology students who were participating in order to fulfill a course requirement. They might have felt that they would not receive their experimental credit unless they participated. In sum, we cannot be very confident that the experimental procedure invoked a dissonance process. Yet we feel that McMillen and Geiselman have raised an intriguing possibility and demonstrated the workability of alpha measurement for use in social psychological experiments in general, and as a potential indicant of dissonance arousal, in particular.

Arousal and Dissonance: New Findings

To this point, the studies linking dissonance and physiological arousal lead us to make two observations. First, the findings are encouraging but have not provided conclusive evidence that dissonance has arousal properties. Second, a pervasive finding that renders ambiguous many of the results of previous research is the failure to employ standard dissonance paradigms and/or to find independent evidence of dissonance reduction with attitudinal measurements. In both Gleason and Katkin's and McMillen and Geiselman's studies, it is not evident that the procedure incorporated all the elements necessary to produce cognitive dissonance. In both Gerard's and Buck's studies, the usual attitudinal consequences of dissonance were not found even though some evidence was presented on the physiological measures.

Perhaps more convincing evidence can be presented if we do not construe the absence of attitudinal effects as the absence of dissonance but rather as the misattribution of dissonance arousal to the electronic gadgetry. Previous research has shown that subjects will misattribute arousal to fluorescent lights, small rooms, or pills. It should not be surprising, then, that subjects would misattribute their arousal to transducers strapped to their fingers, heart, or head. Such misattribution would not eliminate the arousal that is detected via the physiological measures employed, yet it would attenuate attitude change. To present an adequate test of the arousal state of dissonance, an experiment should be conducted that (1) replicates a paradigm that has shown the effects of dissonance in the past, (2) produces attitudinal results in a set of subject's who participate in the dissonance-arousing procedure but who are not strapped to the physiological recorders, and (3) finds evidence of physiological arousal for subjects in the dissonance arousing procedure.

An experiment conducted by Cooper and Croyle (1981) attempted to accomplish just that. The experiment used a standard induced compliance design with subjects' writing counterattitudinal essays on a controversial topic. Some subjects participated in a high-choice condition, others in a low-choice condition. Still a third set of subjects wrote attitude-consistent essays under high-choice conditions.

The research was conducted as two experiments. In the first study, subjects volunteered to participate in a study of attitudes. They were recruited from campus dormitories and had, earlier in the semester, completed an attitude survey which included the item, "Alcohol use should be totally banned from the university campus and eating clubs." Only subjects who disagreed with this statement were recruited for the study.

When subjects entered the laboratory, they were informed that the municipal government and the university were jointly studying an issue which had become a problem in the community. They were told that because of difficulty enforcing the minimum drinking age for alcoholic beverages, the Committee on Campus–Borough Relations was entertaining a proposal to ban totally all alcoholic beverages on the campus.

Subjects in the two counterattitudinal essay conditions were informed that the committee wanted to obtain arguments on both sides of this important issue, and that one of the best ways to understand the arguments on both sides was to have a person write a strong and forceful essay favoring just one side. What he wanted the subject to do was to write an essay taking the position that college students should not be allowed to drink on campus. In the proattitudinal condition, the subject was informed that his task was to write his essay opposed to the proposed ban.

In the two high-choice conditions, subjects were reassured that their participation was completely voluntary. The experimenter asked for a verbal statement as to whether the subject wished to continue. In addition, the subject was given a "consent form" to sign which once again made clear that subject's decision to continue was completely his own. In the low-choice condition, no mention of the voluntary nature of the task was presented and subjects were merely given pencil and paper with which to write their counterattitudinal essay.

At the conclusion of the essay, the experimenter obtained each subject's attitude with a one-item question identical to the question asked on the pretest several weeks before. Their responses to the attitude questionnaire are displayed in the first column of Table 5-5. The entries represent change scores between the two testing periods. The one-way analysis of variance reveals a significant effect, $F(2,26) = 7.92$, $p < .01$. The high-choice–counterattitudinal essay condition showed more change than either of the other two conditions.[4]

The second phase of the research was the attempt to measure physiological arousal in this paradigm. Following the lead of recent research in psychophysiology (e.g., Masling, Price, Goldband, & Katkin, 1981), the physiological arousal was measured by the frequency of spontaneous electrodermal activity. Specifically, the frequency of spontaneous skin conductance responses (SCRs) was measured with a Grass Model 7 polygraph and preamplifier. Electrodes were attached to masked areas on the

4. It should be noted that the attitude change results are not inconsistent with the findings of Fazio, Zanna, and Cooper (1977). In that experiment, high-choice subjects who wrote an "attitude-consistent" essay displayed significant attitude change. However, these subjects endorsed a statement that represented the most extreme position within their latitudes of acceptance. In the present case, subjects in the attitude-consistent condition were not induced to support a specific extreme, although acceptable, position. Instead, they were free to support their own view (their most acceptable position, in the terminology employed by Fazio *et al.*) in their essays, an endorsement that did not produce attitude change.

TABLE 5-5. Mean of Subjects' Attitudes and Electrodermal Responses

CONDITION	MEAN ATTITUDE-CHANGE SCORES (EXPERIMENT 1)	MEAN ADJUSTED FREQUENCY OF SKIN CONDUCTANCE RESPONSE (EXPERIMENT 2)
High-choice–dissonance	7.4	8.1
High-choice–consonance	2.4	4.6
Low-choice–dissonance	2.5	5.5

Note. From *Cognitive dissonance: Evidence for physiological arousal* by J. Cooper & R. Croyle. Unpublished manuscript, Princeton University, 1981. Reprinted by permission.

medial phalanx of the index and second fingers of the subject's nonpreferred hand.

Subjects were recruited in a manner similar to that described above. The purpose of the study, they were told, was to "examine the impact of simple mental and physical tasks on electrical activity of the skin." Subjects were recruited from the same dormitories and with regard to the same issue as those in the first study. In order to have subjects habituate to the machines, two filler tasks (i.e., memory and anagram solution) and three 1-minute rest periods were presented.

The next task that the experimenter described to the participants was identical to the essay-writing task of the first study. Subjects were randomly assigned to high-choice–counterattitudinal, low-choice–counterattitudinal, and high-choice–proattitudinal conditions. The latter condition served as a check on the degree of arousal that might obtain by simply giving individuals a free decision to make within the experimental session. Following the essay writing, the subjects were given a 3-minute rest period. It was expected that differences in arousal would be manifested during the 3-minute resting period. Subjects in all conditions were expected to become aroused during the essay-writing phase. However, subjects in the high-dissonance condition (i.e., high-choice–counterattitudinal essay) were expected to maintain that arousal rather than to habituate rapidly to their base rate. The second column of Table 5-5 shows the mean of the electrodermal response adjusted for the subjects' pre-essay resting measure. An analysis of covariance conducted on this measure revealed a significant effect of experimental condition, $F(2,23) = 4.34$, $p < .03$. The means in the high-choice–consonant and low-choice–dissonant conditions indicate a typical habituation by subjects to the experimental environment. Participants in the high-choice–counterattitudinal essay condition, however, maintained their high level of arousal in the final rest period.

Following the final rest period, subjects were asked to express their opinions on the one-item attitude scale that had been used in the first experiment. This time, however, there were no reliable differences among experimental conditions. The lack of attitudinal evidence for dissonance reduction is consistent with Gerard's and Buck's failure to find similar supporting evidence. However, in the present study, independent evidence from subjects drawn from the same population and assigned to identical conditions without having the misattributional electronic stimuli attached did show attitudinal support consistent with dissonance theory predictions.

In sum, these two experiments provide the strongest support of any physiological recording research to date that dissonance involves an arousal state. The second experiment revealed that a standard induced compliance manipulation clearly produced arousal. The first experiment demonstrated that the procedure employed was indeed successful in replicating the typical attitudinal effects observed following induced compliance. Considered in the context of these significant attitude-change effects, the lack of attitude change in the physiological recording experiment suggests that these subjects misattributed the arousal to the electronic gadgetry and, hence, did not experience dissonance motivation. Although the arousal was misinterpreted by the subjects, the physiological data make it quite clear that the arousal existed. Furthermore, the design of the experiment makes it evident that this arousal emanated from subjects' freely choosing to write a counterattitudinal essay.

CONCLUSION

Taken together, the evidence for dissonance having physiological arousal properties is impressive. Starting with studies whose goal was to show that dissonance interfered with learning in the same way as do other arousing drives, and examining evidence that implicates arousal through misattribution, we now have direct measurement of physiological activity when dissonance is aroused. The electrodermal recording opens the door for the answers to many heretofore unanswered questions. Researchers may be able to identify the time sequence of dissonance arousal and may also be able to differentiate in a clear way those changes of attitudes due to dissonance from those that are due to other nonarousing processes such as impression management or self-perception. Rather than merely answering a question that has been left unanswered since Festinger proposed dissonance theory in 1957, the physiological data raise significant questions that we may now be at the threshold of being able to answer.

REFERENCES

Aronson, E., & Mills, J.   The effects of severity of initiation on liking for a group. *Journal of Abnormal and Social Psychology*, 1959, 59, 177–181.

Axsom, D., & Cooper, J. Reducing weight by reducing dissonance: The role of effort justification in inducing weight loss. In E. Aronson (Ed.), *Readings about the social animal* (3rd ed.). San Francisco: W. H. Freeman, 1981.

Bem, D. J. Self-perception: An alternative interpretation of cognitive dissonance phenomena. *Psychological Review*, 1967, 74, 183–200.

Brehm, J. W. Postdecision changes in the desirability of alternatives. *Journal of Abnormal and Social Psychology*, 1956, 52, 384–389.

Brehm, J. W., & Cohen, A. R. *Explorations in cognitive dissonance.* New York: Wiley, 1962.

Brehm, M. L., Back, K. W., & Bodgonoff, M. D. A physiological effect of cognitive dissonance under stress and deprivation. *Journal of Abnormal and Social Psychology*, 1964, 69, 303–310.

Brown, B. B. *New mind, new body.* New York: Harper & Row, 1974.

Buck, R. W., Jr. *Relationships between dissonance-reducing behavior and tension measures following aggression.* Unpublished doctoral dissertation, University of Pittsburgh, 1970.

Cantor, J. R., Zillmann, D., & Bryant, J. Enhancement of experienced sexual arousal in response to erotic stimuli through misattribution of unrelated residual excitation. *Journal of Personality and Social Psychology*, 1975, 32, 69–75.

Cooper, J. Personal responsibility and dissonance: The role of foreseen consequences. *Journal of Personality and Social Psychology*, 1971, 18, 354–363.

Cooper, J. Reducing fears and increasing assertiveness: The role of dissonance reduction. *Journal of Experimental Social Psychology*, 1980, 16, 199–213.

Cooper, J., & Croyle, R. *Cognitive dissonance: Evidence for physiological arousal.* Unpublished manuscript, Princeton University, 1981.

Cooper, J., & Fazio, R. H. The formation and persistence of attitudes that support intergroup conflict. In W. G. Austin & S. Worchel (Eds.), *The social psychology of intergroup relations.* Monterey, Calif.: Brooks/Cole, 1979.

Cooper, J., Fazio, R. H., & Rhodewalt, F. Dissonance and humor: Evidence for the undifferentiated nature of dissonance arousal. *Journal of Personality and Social Psychology*, 1978, 36, 280–285.

Cooper, J., & Worchel, S. Role of undesired consequences in arousing cognitive dissonance. *Journal of Personality and Social Psychology*, 1970, 16, 199–206.

Cooper, J., Zanna, M. P., & Goethals, G. R. Mistreatment of an esteemed other as a consequence affecting dissonance reduction. *Journal of Experimental Social Psychology*, 1974, 10, 224–233.

Cooper, J., Zanna, M. P., & Taves, P. A. Arousal as a necessary condition for attitude change following induced compliance. *Journal of Personality and Social Psychology*, 1978, 36, 1101–1106.

Cottrell, N. B., Rittle, R. H., & Wack, D. L. The presence of an audience and list type (competitional or noncompetitional) as joint determinants of performance in paired-associates learning. *Journal of Personality*, 1967, 35, 425–434.

Davis, K. E., & Jones, E. E. Changes in interpersonal perception as a means of reducing cognitive dissonance. *Journal of Abnormal and Social Psychology*, 1960, 61, 402–410.

Doob, A. N., Carlsmith, J. M., Freedman, J. L., Landauer, T. K., & Tom, S. Effect of initial selling price on subsequent sales. *Journal of Personality and Social Psychology*, 1969, 11, 345–350.

Fazio, R. H., Zanna, M. P., & Cooper, J. Dissonance and self-perception: An integrative view of each theory's proper domain of application. *Journal of Experimental Social Psychology*, 1977, 13, 464–479.

Fazio, R. H., Zanna, M. P., & Cooper, J. On the relationship of data to theory: A reply to Ronis and Greenwald. *Journal of Experimental Social Psychology*, 1979, 15, 70–76.

Festinger, L. *A theory of cognitive dissonance.* Stanford, Calif.: Stanford University Press, 1957.

Festinger, L., & Carlsmith, J. M. Cognitive consequences of forced compliance. *Journal of Abnormal and Social Psychology*, 1959, 58, 203–211.

Freedman, J. L.   Attitudinal effects of inadequate justification. *Journal of Personality*, 1963, *31*, 371–385.

Gerard, H. B.   Choice difficulty, dissonance, and the decision sequence. *Journal of Personality*, 1967, *35*, 91–108.

Gerard, H. B., & Mathewson, G. C.   The effects of severity of initiation on liking for a group: A replication. *Journal of Experimental Social Psychology*, 1966, *2*, 278–287.

Glass, D. C., & Mayhew, P.   The effects of cognitive processes on skin conductance reactivity to an aversive film. *Psychonomic Science*, 1969, *16*, 72–74.

Gleason, J. M., & Katkin, E. S.   *The effects of cognitive dissonance on heart rate and electrodermal response.* Paper presented at the Society for Psychophysiological Research, Madison, Wis., 1978.

Goethals, G. R., Cooper, J., & Naficy, A.   Role of foreseen, foreseeable, and unforeseeable behavioral consequences in the arousal of cognitive dissonance. *Journal of Personality and Social Psychology*, 1979, *37*, 1179–1185.

Gonzalez, A. E. J., & Cooper, J.   What to do with leftover dissonance: Blame it on the lights. (Data reported in Zanna & Cooper, 1976.)

Greenwald, A. G., & Ronis, D. L.   Twenty years of cognitive dissonance: Case study of the evolution of a theory. *Psychological Review*, 1978, *85*, 53–57.

Higgins, E. T., Rhodewalt, F., & Zanna, M. P.   Dissonance motivation: Its nature, persistence, and reinstatement. *Journal of Experimental Social Psychology*, 1979, *15*, 16–34.

Jones, R. A., & Brehm, J. W.   Attitudinal effects of communicator attractiveness when one chooses to listen. *Journal of Personality and Social Psychology*, 1967, *6*, 64–70.

Kamin, L. J.   Predictability, surprise, attention, and conditioning. In B. A. Campbell & R. M. Church (Eds.), *Punishment and aversive behavior.* New York: Appleton-Century-Crofts, 1969.

Kamiya, J.   Operant control of the EEG alpha rhythm and some of its reported effects on consciousness. In C. Tart (Ed.), *Altered states of consciousness.* New York: Wiley, 1969.

Kiesler, C. A., & Pallak, M. S.   Arousal properties of dissonance manipulations. *Psychological Bulletin*, 1976, *83*, 1014–1025.

Knox, R. E., & Inkster, J. A.   Postdecision dissonance at post time. *Journal of Personality and Social Psychology*, 1968, *8*, 319–323.

Lacey, J. I.   Somatic response patterning and stress: Some revisions of activation theory. In M. H. Appley & R. Trumbull (Eds.), *Psychological stress: Issues in research.* New York: Appleton-Century-Crofts, 1967.

Lacey, J. I., Kagan, J., Lacey, B. C., & Moss, H. A.   The visceral level: Situational determinants and behavioral correlates of autonomic response. In P. H. Knapp (Ed.), *Expression of the emotions in man.* New York: International Universities Press, 1963.

Linder, D. E., Cooper, J., & Jones, E. E.   Decision freedom as a determinant of the role of incentive magnitude in attitude change. *Journal of Personality and Social Psychology*, 1967, *6*, 245–254.

Mandler, G.   The interruption of behavior. In *Nebraska Symposium on Motivation* (Vol. 12). Lincoln: University of Nebraska Press, 1964.

Masling, J., Price, J., Goldband, S., & Katkin, E. S.   Oral imagery and autonomic arousal in social isolation. *Journal of Personality and Social Psychology*, 1981, *40*, 395–400.

McMillen, D. L., & Geiselman, J. H.   Effect of cognitive dissonance on alpha frequency activity: The search for dissonance. *Personality and Social Psychology Bulletin*, 1974, *1*, 150–151.

McMillen, D. L., Geiselman, J. H., & Jones, W. B.   *Effects of dissonance manipulations on occipital cortex alpha output.* Unpublished manuscript, Mississippi State University, 1975.

Mowrer, O. H.   On the dual nature of learning: A reinterpretation of "conditioning" and "problem-solving." *Harvard Educational Review*, 1947, *17*, 102–148.

Mowrer, O. H.   *Learning theory and behavior.* New York: Wiley, 1960.

Nel, E., Helmreich, R., & Aronson, E.   Opinion change in the advocate as a function of the persuasibility of his audience: A clarification of the meaning of dissonance. *Journal of Personality and Social Psychology*, 1969, *12*, 117–124.

Nisbett, R. E., & Schachter, S.   Cognitive manipulation of pain. *Journal of Experimental Social Psychology*, 1966, *2*, 227–236.

Nisbett, R. E., & Wilson, T. D.   Telling more than we can know: Verbal reports on mental processes. *Psychological Review*, 1977, *84*, 231–259.

Pallak, M. S., & Pittman, T. S.   General motivation effects of dissonance arousal. *Journal of Personality and Social Psychology*, 1972, *21*, 349–358.

Pallak, M. S., Pittman, T. S., Heller, J. F., & Munson, P.   The effect of arousal on Stroop Color-World Task performance. *Bulletin of the Psychonomic Society*, 1975, *6*, 248–250.

Pittman, T. S.   Attribution of arousal as a mediator in dissonance reduction. *Journal of Experimental Social Psychology*, 1975, *11*, 53–63.

Ronis, D. L., & Greenwald, A. G.   Dissonance theory revised again: Comment on the paper by Fazio, Zanna, and Cooper. *Journal of Experimental Social Psychology*, 1979, *15*, 62–69.

Rosenberg, M. J.   When dissonance fails: On eliminating evaluation apprehension from attitude measurement. *Journal of Personality and Social Psychology*, 1965, *1*, 28–42.

Ross, L., Rodin, J., & Zimbardo, P. G.   Toward an attribution therapy: The reduction of fear through induced cognitive–emotional misattribution. *Journal of Personality and Social Psychology*, 1969, *4*, 279–288.

Schachter, S., & Singer, J. E.   Cognitive, social, and physiological determinants of emotional state. *Psychological Review*, 1962, *69*, 379–399.

Sherif, M., & Hovland, C. I.   *Social judgment: Assimilation and contrast effects in communication and attitude change.* New Haven, Conn.: Yale University Press, 1961.

Spence, K. W.   *Behavior theory and conditioning.* New Haven, Conn.: Yale University Press, 1956.

Spence, K. W., Farber, I. E., & McFann, H. H.   The relation of anxiety (drive) level to performance in competitional paired-associates learning. *Journal of Experimental Psychology*, 1956, *52*, 296–305.

Storms, M. D., & Nisbett, R. E.   Insomnia and the attribution process. *Journal of Personality and Social Psychology*, 1970, *2*, 319–328.

Tedeschi, J. T., Schlenker, B. R., & Bonoma, T. V.   Cognitive dissonance: Private ratiocination or public spectacle? *American Psychologist*, 1971, *26*, 685–695.

Tiller, M.   *A model for goal setting in a participative budgeting context: An empirical investigation of the effects of cognitive dissonance on budget commitment and performance.* Unpublished doctoral dissertation, Indiana University, 1980.

Totman, R.   Cognitive dissonance and the placebo response: The effect of differential justification for undergoing dummy injections. *European Journal of Social Psychology*, 1975, *5*, 441–456.

Wicklund, R. A., & Brehm, J. W.   *Perspectives on cognitive dissonance.* Hillsdale, N. J.: Erlbaum, 1976.

Worchel, S., & Arnold, S. E.   The effect of combined arousal states on attitude change. *Journal of Experimental Social Psychology*, 1974, *10*, 549–560.

Worchel, S., & Cooper, J.   *Understanding social psychology.* Homewood, Ill.: Dorsey, 1979.

Zanna, M. P.   *The effect of distraction on resolving cognition dilemmas.* Paper presented at the American Psychological Association Convention, Chicago, 1975.

Zanna, M. P., & Cooper, J.   Dissonance and the pill: An attribution approach to studying the arousal properties of dissonance. *Journal of Personality and Social Psychology*, 1974, *29*, 703–709.

Zanna, M. P., & Cooper, J.   Dissonance and the attribution process. In J. H. Harvey, W. J. Ickes, & R. F. Kidd (Eds.), *New directions in attribution research.* Hillsdale, N.J.: Erlbaum, 1976.

Zanna, M. P. Higgins, E. T., & Taves, P. A.   Is dissonance phenomenologically aversive? *Journal of Experimental Social Psychology*, 1976, *12*, 530–538.

Zeigarnik, B.   Uber das Behalten von erledigten und unerledigten Handlungen. *Psychologische Forschung*, 1927, *9*, 1–35.

Zillmann, D.   Excitation transfer in communication-mediated aggressive behavior. *Journal of Experimental Social Psychology*, 1971, *7*, 419–434.

Zillmann, D.   Attribution and misattribution of excitatory reaction. In J. H. Harvey, W. J.

Ickes, & R. F. Kidd (Eds.), *New directions in attribution research* (Vol. 2). Hillsdale, N.J.: Erlbaum, 1978.

Zimbardo, P. G., Cohen, A. R., Weisenberg, M., Dworkin, L., & Firestone, I. The control of experimental pain. In P. G. Zimbardo (Ed.), *The cognitive control of motivation.* Glenview, Ill.: Scott, Foresman, 1969.

CHAPTER 6

Cognitive and Physiological Processes in Fear Appeals and Attitude Change: A Revised Theory of Protection Motivation

Ronald W. Rogers
University of Alabama

INTRODUCTION

If you have forgotten what a fear appeal is, a passage from Jonathan Edwards's "Sinners in the Hands of an Angry God" may refresh your memory.

> O Sinner! Consider the fearful danger you are in. It is a great furnace of wrath, a wide and bottomless pit, full of the fire of wrath. . . . The use of this awful sermon may be for awakening unconverted persons in the congregation. This that you have heard is the case of every one of you. . . . And now you have an extraordinary opportunity, a day wherein Christ has thrown the door of mercy wide open . . . a day wherein many are flocking to him, and pressing into the kingdom of God.

This passage contains all of the crucial ingredients of a fear appeal. The preacher is telling you that (1) the threatened event is severe, (2) that, oh yes, it *can* happen to you, (3) but that there is an effective way to avoid the danger, (4) if you will only abandon your wicked, wicked ways, and accept his recommendation.

Fear appeals are ubiquitous. Preachers still use them. So do politicians, parents, advertisers, and public health organizations. Communications that attempt to change our attitudes by appealing to that unpleasant emotion of fear have been the object of a great deal of research. We review some of that research in this chapter.

Overview of the Chapter

This chapter has three purposes. First, it provides an opportunity to evaluate critically the empirical data on fear and persuasion in order to determine what conclusions may be drawn. The second purpose is to identify some of the critical issues requiring additional study. Finally, we integrate the data and concepts into a coherent theoretical framework: an expanded and revised theory of protection motivation.

The review of the literature on fear appeals and attitude change is divided into five major sections. First, we examine the relationship between fear and attitude change. Second, the three major theories of fear and persuasion that have evolved to guide research and explain results are reviewed. The third section examines those studies of attitude change directly manipulating physiological arousal, focusing on the implications for theories of emotion as well as attitude change. The fourth section reviews the data bearing on the role of physiological processes in mediating or producing attitude change. The third and fourth sections focus primarily on my program of research. The chapter concludes with a revised theory of protection motivation that incorporates the empirical and conceptual advances reviewed in the chapter.

The Relation of Fear to Attitude Change

The interrelationship among environmental stimuli, physiological arousal, emotion, and attitudes has been a topic of enduring interest. Although social psychological approaches to the study of emotion have employed a wide range of perspectives (cf. Harris & Katkin, 1975), our approach has focused on cognitive evaluations of autonomic nervous system activity. The research reported in the third and fourth sections attempts to integrate the social and psychophysiological approaches, applying them to the investigation of fear and persuasion. A fuller understanding of fear appeals and attitude change may require knowledge of physiological, as well as phenomenological, processes.

In the research paradigm designed to investigate the effects of fear appeals on attitude change, an individual typically is exposed to persuasive communications that depict the noxious consequences accruing to a specified course of action. The message usually portends bodily harm to the individual. Recommendations are presented that can avert the danger if the individual adopts the appropriate attitudes and acts on them. Fear-arousing stimuli seek to eliminate response patterns that produce aversive consequences (e.g., cigarette smoking) or establish response patterns that might prevent the occurrence of noxious events (e.g., taking prescribed inoculations).

Historically, fear has been conceptualized as a motivational state protecting one against danger (e.g., Cannon, 1915; Freud, 1936). A "motivational theory of emotion," especially the emotion of fear, is perhaps the most typical conceptualization of the emotions (cf. Izard, 1977; Leeper, 1965; Spence, 1956). A close relationship between emotion and muscular activity has been postulated in a long and rich tradition (e.g., Cannon, 1915; Darwin, 1872/1965; Sherrington, 1906). According to this tradition, the emotional disturbance of the viscera facilitates the muscular activity that protects the organism from the dangerous environmental stimulus: hence the etiology of the word "emotion" itself from the Latin *emovere*, *e* meaning out, and *movere* to move.

The emotion of fear has been of interest because of its role in mediating attitude and behavior change. According to the fear-as-acquired-drive model, fear is acquired through the classical conditioning of a noxious unconditioned stimulus to autonomic and skeletal responses. Fear is the conditioned form of the pain reaction. These conditioned intereoceptive responses act as an acquired drive to evoke instrumental avoidance behavior. The instrumental avoidance response is reinforced by drive reduction. Fear is referred to as an acquired drive because it is learned as a response to previously neutral cues. Fear is called a drive because it can produce the learning of new responses. In the initial theoretical formulation of the effects of fear on attitude change, Hovland, Janis, and Kelley (1953) adopted the fear-as-acquired-drive model.

THEORIES OF FEAR AND PERSUASION

The effects of fear on persuasion have been interpreted from three theoretical perspectives. Each theory has been presented in detail by the original author and thus will be reviewed only briefly here. The interested reader should refer to Beck and Frankel's (1981) excellent critical evaluation of all three theories.

Janis's Extension of the Drive Model

One of the first systematic theories of fear and persuasion was provided by Janis (1967), who adopted and extended the fear-as-acquired-drive model. According to this model, if a persuasive communication arouses fear, people are motivated to reduce this unpleasant drive state. Attitudes are changed when they reduce this state of arousal. The amount of attitude change depends on the amount of drive reduction contiguous with rehearsal of the communicator's recommendations. Janis also proposed that fear arousal has both facilitating and interfering effects. Because of these two contrasting effects, persuasion is an inverted-U-shaped function of the level of fear aroused. Thus, at a low level of arousal, any interfering effects will be outweighed by the facilitating effects of heightened vigilance and the need to seek reassurance. As fear arousal increases, the interfering effects will come to match the facilitating effects. This point is the optimal level of arousal. Beyond this point, facilitating effects are outweighed by interfering effects. Unfortunately, perhaps, the vast majority of tests of this interesting relationship have rejected it. A review of some of the formal inadequacies of this position may be found in Beck and Frankel (1981), Leventhal (1970), and Rogers (1975).

The empirical data have overwhelmingly rejected the drive model of fear appeals and attitude change. The model had to be abandoned for a variety of reasons. First, many variables that should interact with fear arousal (e.g., efficacy of recommendations, specificity of recommendations) did not interact in the manner predicted by drive theory (see the reviews by Beck & Frankel, 1981; Leventhal, 1970). Second, studies manipulating false physiological feedback of fear arousal revealed that arousal per se, not arousal reduction as required by drive theory, produced attitude change (Giesen & Hendrick, 1974; Hendrick, Giesen, & Borden, 1975). These data were interpreted in terms of a cognitive analysis: People use physiological feedback as a cognitive source of information from which to infer their attitudes. Finally, Leventhal's and Rogers's experiments never found a direct relationship between emotional responses (drive) and attitude change. Although the drive model must be rejected, we should remember that this theory not only initiated research in this area, but started the research in a theoretically elegant fashion by applying sophisticated learning theory principles to the study of fear appeals and attitude change.

Leventhal's Parallel Response Model

Leventhal's extensive research program led him to reject the fear-as-acquired-drive model. In its place, Leventhal (1970) proposed a parallel response model that distinguishes between emotional reactions to a threat and attempts to cope with the threat. According to Leventhal, a fear appeal may initiate a danger control process, which attempts to avoid the threatened danger, and/or a fear control process, which functions to reduce fear. These two processes are parallel or independent. Attempts to control fear are not necessary to produce adaptive behavior. Adaptive behavior results primarily from the danger control process. Thus, fear appeals may arouse the emotion of fear, but protective action results from the attempt to control the danger, not to control the fear. Research guided by the parallel response model has focused on how people respond to health threats and noxious medical examinations rather than fear and persuasion. Nevertheless, this research has demonstrated convincingly that emotional responses (i.e., fear control) are independent of and do not directly facilitate the danger control process of coping (Leventhal, Meyer, & Gutmann, 1980). The parallel response model performed the invaluable service of differentiating emotional from cognitive responses to fear-arousing communications.

Rogers's Original Protection Motivation Theory

I attempted to take the next logical steps of (1) specifying the components of a fear appeal initiating the coping process (i.e., the danger control process), and (2) analyzing this coping process in more detail. In one of the earliest theoretical analyses of fear arousal and persuasion (Hovland *et al.*, 1953), fear appeals were characterized as communications describing the unfavorable consequences that might result from failure to adopt the communicator's recommendations. This definition was sufficiently sweeping to allow fear-arousing communications to be operationalized in a variety of ways. And they were. For example, different levels of fear have been aroused by varying (1) the amount of information in the communications (e.g., the number of references to physical danger; Powell, 1965), (2) the type of information (e.g., use of personalized "It can happen to you" statements; Janis & Feshbach, 1953), (3) presence or absence of films (e.g., Leventhal & Watts, 1966), and (4) what information is emphasized (e.g., the degree of emphasis on negative consequences; Janis & Feshbach, 1953). Furthermore, high versus low fear has been manipulated in some studies by presenting information on the amount of bodily injury *and* the likelihood of exposure in both high- and low-fear conditions (e.g., Chu, 1966) by omitting the latter information only in the low-fear condition (e.g., Janis & Feshbach, 1952) and by omitting the latter information entirely (e.g., Rogers & Thistlethwaite, 1970). Because fear-arousing communications are multifaceted stimuli, their persuasive impact may be due to any one or more of the components. Thus, the effective content stimuli that produce attitude change may not have been firmly established.

If studies have varied types of communication content, it would be difficult to compare experiments and determine the communication variables producing the theoretically relevant changes in attitudes. I believed that conceptualizations of fear appeals had been too global and that they had to be refined if more precise and unequivocal relations were to be generated. An important conceptual and empirical task was to identify the effective content variables and their associated mediational processes.

I proposed that an expectancy–value model, which includes all the factors of concern to investigators on fear communication and to workers with the health belief model (e.g., Becker, Haefner, Kasl, Kirscht, Maiman, & Rosenstock, 1977), be applied to the fear communication problem in a more systematic manner (Rogers, 1975). The three most crucial variables in a fear appeal are (1) the magnitude of noxiousness of a depicted event (the value component), (2) the conditional probability that the event will occur provided that no adaptive activity is performed (an expectancy), and (3) the effectiveness of a coping response that might avert the noxious event (another expectancy). These three constructs are similar to those in the general category of expectancy–value theories. According to this class of theory, the tendency to perform a particular act is a function of the expectancy that the act will be followed by certain consequences and the value of those consequences. Hopefully, progress in understanding the fear communication problem will be facilitated by a theoretically based classification schema that is linked to more general psychological theories.

It was assumed that each of the three components of a fear appeal initiates a corresponding cognitive mediating process. Each of these processes appraises communication information about (1) noxiousness, (2) probability, or (3) efficacy by placing each stimulus on dimensions of (1) appraised severity of the depicted event, (2) expectancy of exposure to the event, or (3) belief in the efficacy of the recommended coping response, respectively. It has been demonstrated that these cognitive processes are independent (Rogers & Mewborn, 1976). Each of these appraisal processes will be roughly proportional to the strength of the associated message variable. The representation will not be exact, since individuals have different styles of appraising threatening events (cf. Lazarus & Launier, 1978).

It is also assumed that these three cognitive processes mediate the effects of the components of fear appeals on attitudes by arousing what has been termed "protection motivation." The intent to adopt the communicator's recommendation is a function of the amount of protection motivation aroused. Protection motivation is an intervening variable that has the typical characteristics of a motive: It arouses, sustains, and directs activity. The basic postulate is that protection motivation arises from the cognitive appraisal of a depicted event as noxious and likely to occur, together with the belief that a recommended coping response can effectively prevent the threatened event from occurring.

The model asserts that attitude change is not mediated by or a result of an emotional state of fear, but rather is a function of the amount of protective motivation aroused by the cognitive appraisal processes. The emphasis is thus on cognitive processes and protection motivation, rather than on fear as an emotion.

The basic assumption of the original statement of protection motivation theory, that the three crucial components of a fear appeal are noxiousness, probability, and response efficacy, has been confirmed in numerous studies. It was originally assumed that these three components would combine multiplicatively. That is, when persuasion is plotted against any one of the components, the other two components should form a fan of diverging curves. The original multiplicative combinatorial rule has been rejected. We shall now briefly review the evidence bearing on these three components of a fear appeal.

The noxiousness component has been operationalized, for example, by essays arguing that excessive drinking produces either severe injury or minor irritation to the internal organs (Stainback & Rogers, in press). The magnitude of noxiousness of the depicted threat exerts a main effect on intentions (1) to stop smoking (Rogers & Deckner, 1975; Rogers & Thistlethwaite, 1970), (2) to conserve energy (Hass, Bagley, & Rogers, 1975), (3) to abstain from drinking alcohol (Stainback & Rogers, in press), and (4) to help an endangered animal species (Shelton & Rogers, 1981). With respect to overt behavior, noxiousness increases the percentage of smokers who are able to stop smoking (Rogers, Deckner, & Mewborn, 1978) and reduces driver education students' error rates on their driving simulators (Griffeth & Rogers, 1976).

Response efficacy has a main effect on intentions to protect oneself (Rogers & Mewborn, 1976; Rogers & Thistlethwaite, 1970), on intentions to protect others (Shelton & Rogers, 1981), and on overt behavior (Chu, 1966). Response efficacy has been operationalized, for example, by essays arguing that there is no effective method to treat venereal disease or that simple medical treatment cures it (Rogers & Mewborn, 1976). Also, response efficacy is effective if combined with another original component of protection motivation theory: The probability of the threat's occurrence. This combination is referred to as "reassurance." Reassurance that the recommended coping response can reduce one's chances of exposure to a threat enhances intentions to adopt that response (Mewborn & Rogers, 1979).

When the probability of the threat's occurrence is manipulated independently of response efficacy, there is some evidence of a simple main effect on intentions (Janis & Mann, 1965; Leventhal & Watts, 1966; Stainback & Rogers, in press). The probability of occurrence component has been operationalized, for example, by persuasive essays arguing that a smoker has a very high chance of contracting lung cancer or that, although smoking can cause cancer, the chances of any particular smoker developing cancer are actually quite small (Rogers & Mewborn, 1976). Rogers and Mewborn (1976) and Kleinot and Rogers (1982) found an interaction between probability of occurrence and response efficacy. Figure 6-1 shows that if the recommended coping response is a highly effective preventive practice, increasing the probability of exposure to the danger increases intentions to adopt that practice; if the response is ineffective, increasing probability decreases intentions to adopt the response (i.e., smokers intend to increase their cigarette consumption, Rogers & Mewborn, 1976; and social drinkers intend to increase their alcohol consumption, Kleinot &

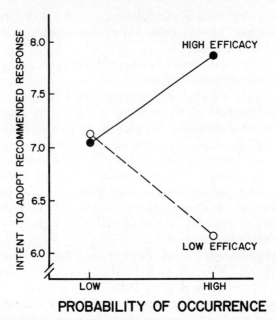

FIGURE 6-1. Intentions as a function of the probability of the threat's occurrence (vulnerability) and response efficacy. From "Fear appeals and attitude change: Effects of a threat's noxiousness, probability of occurrence, and the efficacy of coping responses" by R. W. Rogers & C. R. Mewborn, *Journal of Personality and Social Psychology*, 1976, **34**, 54–61. Copyright 1976 by the American Psychological Association. Reprinted by permission.

Rogers, 1982). It is small wonder that psychologists (e.g., Corah, Koch, & Eisenberg, 1977) frequently conclude that fear tactics should be abandoned because they can backfire!

In sum, most of the empirical evidence supports the original theory of protection motivation. There are (at least) three components of a fear appeal that, independently and in combination, affect attitude change. Furthermore, the effects of these communication variables are *mediated* by the cognitive appraisal processes originally proposed. In the section dealing with a revised theory of protection motivation, we shall retain these features of protection motivation theory and build a slightly more elaborate model around them. But first we need to review the research investigating the role of physiological arousal in mediating the effects of fear appeals on attitude change.

MANIPULATIONS OF PHYSIOLOGICAL AROUSAL

According to Schachter and Singer's (1962) well-known theory of emotion, emotion is determined by physiological arousal and situational cues. There is also evidence that the affective component of an attitude is influenced similarly (cf. Rogers & Deckner, 1975). Rogers and Deckner (1975) investigated the possibility of extending Schachter's theory to determine if physiological arousal and situational cues interact to affect, not only the emotional state of fear, but attitude and behaviors hypothesized to be mediated by the emotion of fear. In a series of experiments, physiological arousal was manipulated directly by injections of epinephrine. Epinephrine was the drug of choice because it is classified as an autonomic arousal agent that closely approximates the discharge of the sympathetic nervous system (Levy & Ahlquist, 1971). Epinephrine enhances vascular, muscular, and metabolic activity in response to stress. A total of 279 cigarette smokers were administered either epinephrine or a placebo and then exposed to situation cues suggestive of disparate emotional states (Experiment 1) or different intensities of the same emotion—fear (Experiment 2). In Experiment 1, disparate emotional states were aroused by exposing subjects to either a low-fear-arousing film or emotionally neutral material. In Experiment 2, the low-fear film, which was the same film used in Experiment 1, portayed a smoker's discovery that he has lung cancer. The high-fear film consisted of the same scenes plus a 5-minute operation removing the smoker's cancerous lung.

Self-reports of fear, shown in Table 6-1, did not simply fail to replicate Schachter and Singer's classic study; they suggested two modifications of the theory. First, the data from the no-film condition of the first experiment indicated that when there are no compelling situational cues to which to attribute a state of unexplained physiological arousal, epinephrine-induced arousal is interpreted as a state of fear. Marshall and Zimbardo (1979) and Maslach (1979) attempted to replicate Schachter and Singer's

TABLE 6-1. Mean Scores on Self-Report of Fear

	EPINEPHRINE	PLACEBO
Experiment I		
No film*	5.3$_a$	2.8$_b$
Low-fear film†	6.0$_a$	5.1$_a$
Experiment II		
High-fear film†	6.2$_a$	6.0$_a$
Low-fear film†	4.9$_b$	4.4$_b$

Note. Range = 1 to 9. Means that do not share a common subscript differ significantly; $p < .05$. From Rogers and Deckner (1975).

*Epinephrine-induced arousal may be interpreted as fear.

†Cognitive cues may be more important than physiological activity in labeling emotional states.

study, but they too found a negative bias in the interpretation of un-explained arousal.

The second modification of the original theory is derived from the equivalence of the emotional response in the epinephrine and placebo groups in the low- and high-fear film condition. When situational cues clearly suggest an emotion, the emotional response may be attributed to the situational cues and not to the manipulated arousal. Marshall and Zimbardo reached a similar conclusion. A great deal of evidence has been amassed by Lazarus and his colleagues (see reviews by Lazarus, Averill, & Opton, 1970; Lazarus & Launier, 1978) demonstrating that the manipula-tion of cognitive cues can enhance or inhibit emotional states. Therefore, the available data strongly suggest that the cognitive appraisal of environ-mental events is more important than peripheral, physiological activity in labeling emotional states.

The major research question posed by Rogers and Deckner was: Would the manipulation of physiological arousal affect attitudes and be-havior change? The answer was no. Since fear was not affected by the experimental manipulations as Schachter's theory predicted, the extension of the theory to attitude change mediated by the emotional state was also rejected. Neither the analyses of variance nor the correlational analyses revealed any relationship between physiological arousal and persuasion. However, the high-fear appeal significantly increased intentions to stop smoking, and a 3-month follow-up revealed that, compared to the low-fear condition, a significantly higher percentage of smokers in the high-fear condition had been able to stop smoking completely. Also, the response–efficacy communication reduced cigarette consumption. In sum, the mes-sages containing information changed cognitive appraisals, which in turn changed attitudes and behavior; the physiological arousal did not.

THE MEDIATIONAL ROLE OF PHYSIOLOGICAL AROUSAL

Empirical Studies of Physiological Arousal and Fear Appeals

We shall now review attitude-change studies that, although not manipu-lating physiological arousal directly, manipulated fear and employed con-tinuous monitoring of multiple autonomic functions.

Many conceptualizations of emotion maintain that emotion has several component subsystems, including cognitive and physiological components (e.g., Lazarus et al., 1970; Schachter & Singer, 1962). If emotions are defined as syndromes, no single response system may be adequate to infer an emotion. Therefore, it behooves us to measure physiological arousal in studies of fear and persuasion. Studies of other negative affective states, especially stress and anxiety, typically measure self-reports and autonomic activity. For example, Shapiro and Crider (1968) reported that "activation of the autonomic nervous system is used by psychologists as a measure of choice in the study of stress" (p. 34).

In addition to considering emotion in general as having component subsystems, many definitions of the emotion of fear consider it to have cognitive and physiological subsystems (e.g., Lang, 1971; Lazarus *et al.*, 1970). Yet despite the fact that a physiological component is an integral part of many definitions of emotion and the emotion of fear in particular, few studies of fear and persuasion have simultaneously measured self-report and autonomic measures of fear.

In a rare exception, Corah *et al.* (1977) investigated high- versus low-fear-arousing communications on the topic of dental hygiene. The manipulation of fear had no effects on galvanic skin responses, heart rate, or self-reports of fear. The manipulations simply were not successful. Hendrick *et al.* (1975) investigated false physiological feedback of fear arousal. They found that the false feedback of arousal changed attitudes, but did not affect measures of heart rate or galvanic skin responses. Beck (1979) found that false physiological feedback of negative arousal was related to changes in attitudes and beliefs and that false physiological feedback of positive arousal was related to changes in intentions. However, the manipulations of arousal had no effect on heart rate. Thus, studies of false feedback of emotional arousal indicate that persuasion is independent of physiological activity.

Mewborn and Rogers (1979) showed research participants either a high- or low-fear film on the topic of venereal disease. The low-fear film blandly depicted laboratory procedures for serum detection of syphilis. The high-fear film demonstrated surgical procedures for removing tissue damaged by venereal disease. These two films were of equal length and had been used successfully by Rogers and Mewborn (1976). Half of the subjects were given high reassurance about the effectiveness of the recommended coping response, while half were given low reassurance. In addition to postexperiment measures of emotion and intentions, heart rate and skin conductance were monitored continuously. The results shown in Table 6-2 indicate that an identical pattern of findings emerged on the

TABLE 6-2. Mean Scores on Measures of Fear

	SELF-REPORT	HEART RATE (BEATS PER MINUTE)	SKIN CONDUCTANCE (μmhos)
High-fear condition	5.8	86.6	9.9
Low-fear condition	3.7	83.6	8.7

Note. From Mewborn and Rogers (1979).

cardiovascular, electrodermal, and self-report measures: The high-fear film produced significantly stronger arousal than the low-fear film.

The fear-arousing film was chosen for study because it is typical of the films used in studies of fear and persuasion (e.g., Leventhal & Watts, 1966; Rogers & Mewborn, 1976). Since the fear manipulation had a main effect on self-reports and autonomic indices of arousal, we can be confident that prior studies employing similar manipulations have also aroused "fear."

The construct validity and generality of paper-and-pencil measures of fear has been enhanced. The significant relationship between these different response measures should be comforting to users of either one. Furthermore, these data tend to weaken two criticisms of self-report measures: (1) People do not possess the appropriate language to report bodily states, and (2) people may be unwilling to report truthfully. The similar pattern of data yielded by the dependent measures of fear indicate that self-report data may be sufficient to check on the adequacy of manipulations. Furthermore, time of measurement interacted with the fear and the reassurance variables on the self-report measure (these interactions were not significant on the heart rate and the skin conductance measures), which suggested that the verbal measure may be more sensitive than the physiological measures.

The intragroup correlation between heart rate and skin conductance was a substantial .70. Thus, although each of these measures may be sensitive to different kinds of events (e.g., skin conductance to novelty, heart rate to action-instigating properties of stimuli), when there is an attempt to arouse fear, there is a great deal of convergence and commonality. However, the self-report measure correlated only .36 with heart rate and .39 with skin conductance. These low correlations are not surprising because each response system serves multiple functions, militating against high correlations (e.g., autonomic activity is responsive to reflexive and homeostatic processes). In addition, whereas the autonomic measures were continuous, the verbal measure required a retrospective report over the preceding 6 to 7 minutes. Students had to select a single value to represent the fluctuating levels of their affective reactions. The multiple correlation among self-report, heart rate, and skin conductance was .44 during the film, but diminished to a negligible .15 during the communication, suggesting that verbal and autonomic measures converge only momentarily after a rather dramatic event. This suggests that the measures will correspond only when their controlling conditions covary. These data support the position of Lang (1971), Lazarus et al. (1970), and Leventhal (1970) that these response systems are only loosely integrated—that they are interactive but largely independent except after a dramatic event.

With respect to the role of fear arousal in mediating attitude change, these results disclosed that fear was successfully aroused but did not mediate attitude change. Evidence reviewed in the preceding section led us to conclude that cognitive appraisal of environmental events is more important than peripheral, physiological activity in *labeling* emotional states (i.e., the films used in the Rogers and Deckner studies affected the labeling of emotion, but the manipulation of physiological arousal did not affect labeling). Taken together, these experiments indicate that the autonomic components of fear are of secondary importance in both the labeling of the emotional state and changing the attitudes hypothesized to be mediated by the emotion of fear. These data are consistent with our path analytic findings that fear arousal does not facilitate attitude change unless this arousal directly affects the cognitive appraisal of the severity of that threat (Rogers & Mewborn, 1976; Shelton & Rogers, 1981).

A Conceptual Review of Physiological Arousal and Cognitive Processes

We have reviewed several studies in which manipulations of fear have changed attitudes or behavioral intentions, but there was no evidence for a mediational role of physiological processes. Let us review the reasons for these negative findings. First, direct manipulations of physiological arousal by injections of the sympathomimetic agent epinephrine did not facilitate attitude change (Rogers & Deckner, 1975). Second, studies monitoring physiological arousal indicated that the arousal was not associated with attitude change (Beck, 1979; Giesen & Hendrick, 1974; Hendrick et al., 1975; Mewborn & Rogers, 1979). Third, fear arousal has been found to have no direct effect on attitude change, but only an indirect effect via the cognitive appraisal of the severity of the threat. Fourth, rejection of the drive model casts doubt on the mediational role of physiological processes, although rejecting the former does not require rejecting the latter. Finally, Cacioppo's (1979) research on his biosocial model of attitude change (other than fear appeals) has demonstrated that a manipulation of heart rate facilitated cognitive elaboration, but had no direct effect on attitude change. Cacioppo concluded "recent evidence casts doubt on a *direct* link between affective and heart rate responses" (p. 496). In sum, the available evidence reveals no direct relationship between physiological arousal and attitude change with (1) perceived but nonveridical changes in autonomic nervous system (ANS) functioning (Beck, 1979; Hendrick et al., 1975), (2) actual but unperceived changes in ANS functioning (Cacioppo, 1979), and (3) actual and perceived changes in ANS functioning (Mewborn & Rogers, 1979; Rogers & Deckner, 1975).

Despite these data, it may be premature to deny physiological processes a mediational role in changing attitudes. Social psychologists need more sophisticated conceptualizations of the physiological processes underlying social phenomena (e.g., the role of negative feedback between the reticular activating system and the baroreceptors of the aortic arch and carotid sinus). We also need more sophisticated measures (e.g., the transit time of the blood pulse wave to index catecholamine excretion). In a nutshell, we need more collaboration with psychophysiological researchers, which should be mutually beneficial.

How can the data denying physiological processes a mediational role in attitude change be reconciled with the knowledge that in response to a threat, our autonomic nervous system reacts with vascular, muscular, and metabolic activity that serve an adaptive function? These bodily changes mobilize us for flight or fight. The answer may be that these bodily responses play a crucial role *if an immediate bodily response is required to cope with the threat.* No such immediate action is required in studies of attitude change. Therefore, threats requiring immediate action are facilitated by physiological activity. On the other hand, the vast majority of psychological and education interventions designed to change attitudes and behavior are directed toward a very different class of responses. These responses typically do not have to be made immediately and usually must be made repeatedly over a long period of time (e.g., drive safely, take medication). These protective responses must be made after an emotional state and accompanying physiological arousal have vanished. The theory of protection motivation assumes that protection from danger frequently requires long-sustained processes, cognitive representations, rather than reflexive responsivity to physiological events.

There are numerous other advantages to the emphasis on cognitive constructs. With respect to investigations of animal instrumental avoidance learning (an area where peripheral explanations might be expected to be preferred to cognitive ones), Rescorla and Solomon (1967) concluded from their review of the literature that "we have not yet identified any peripheral CRs [conditioned responses] which are necessary to mediate avoidance behavior" (p. 169). They further suggest that physiological activity is merely an index of a central state that mediates the avoidance learning. Mineka (1979) concluded: "There is often a marked dissociation between fear and avoidance responding that had led a number of theorists to question whether fear plays any role at all in mediating avoidance responding" (p. 985). Our conclusion is also consistent with the position of Obrist and his colleagues (e.g., Obrist, Gaebelein, Shanks, Langer, & Botticelli, 1976) that changes in heart rate and somatic activity are both mediated by a common central nervous system integrating mechanism. Although bodily responses do not control emotion, however, they can be used as indices of emotional states (cf. Grings & Dawson, 1978). Thus, the deemphasis on the mediational role of physiological processes is consistent with empirical data and emerging conceptualizations. Both emotional responses and coping responses are products of cognitive appraisal. The cognitive appraisal processes are the crucial mediating processes. We shall now attempt to extend the theory of protection motivation reviewed earlier, focusing on these cognitive mediational processes.

A REVISED THEORY OF PROTECTION MOTIVATION

One of the major purposes of this chapter is to revise and extend protection motivation theory. The revised theory includes (1) a broader statement about the sources of information initiating the coping process, (2) additional cognitive mediating processes, and (3) a fuller exposition of the modes of coping. The components of the original model remain intact in the revision. The components of a fear appeal are part of the "verbal persuasion" source of information. The associated cognitive mediational processes are now part of a more comprehensive model. A schema of protection motivation theory is shown in Figure 6-2.

Sources

The sources of information initiating the cognitive mediating processes can be environmental or intrapersonal. The environmental sources include verbal persuasion (especially fear appeals) and observational learning (seeing what happens to others). The intrapersonal sources include personality variables and prior experiences with similar threats (including feedback from coping activity). Any source of information can lead to any of the mediating processes. The focus of protection motivation theory is on the cognitive mediational processes, regardless of the source.

Cognitive Mediating Processes

The sources of information initiate two appraisal processes: threat appraisal and coping appraisal (which are similar to Lazarus's primary and secondary appraisals, respectively).[1] The components of these appraisal processes may be viewed as the 4 cells of a 2×2 table. These cognitive processes appraise (1) either the maladaptive or adaptive response(s), and (2) the variables increasing or decreasing the probability of the occurrence of the response.

We shall consider threat appraisal first. The maladaptive response can be a behavior currently engaged in (e.g., drinking excessively) or one that

1. A principal distinction between Lazarus's position and the protection motivation position is that the latter organizes the cognitive mediating processes around (1) the maladaptive versus the adaptive response, and (2) the factors increasing versus decreasing response probability (see Figure 6-2). Thus, protection motivation theory is more specific about the component cognitions of threat appraisal (e.g., beliefs in severity and vulnerability) and of coping appraisal (e.g., beliefs in self-efficacy).

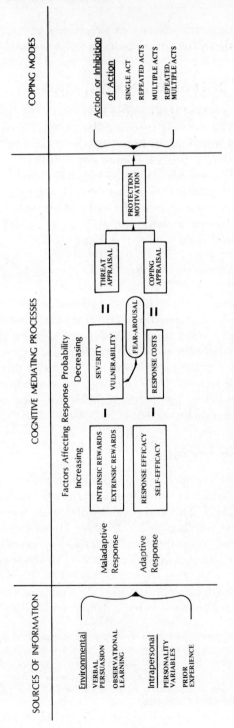

FIGURE 6-2. Schema of protection motivation theory.

168

could be adopted (e.g., starting to smoke). The factors increasing the probability of the maladaptive response (i.e., positive reinforcers) include both intrinsic rewards (e.g., bodily pleasure, satisfaction) and extrinsic rewards (e.g., social approval). The factors decreasing the probability of the occurrence of the maladaptive response (i.e., punishers) are the severity of the threat and the expectancy of being exposed to the threat (i.e., one's vulnerability). Although severity usually refers to bodily harm, it can also involve intrapersonal threats (e.g., self-esteem) and interpersonal threats (e.g., family and work relationships). It is assumed that the appraisal of these factors increasing and decreasing the probability of the maladaptive response will summate algebraically to produce the final appraisal of threat.

We have seen that fear arousal was originally thought to be the crucial mediator of the effects of fear appeals on attitude and behavior change (cf. Hovland *et al.*, 1953). The preceding sections of this chapter have shown that physiological activity is cognitively appraised and these central nervous system events mediate protective activity. Our emphasis on "protection motivation" rather than "fear" is designed to emphasize the importance of cognitive processes rather than visceral ones. According to protection motivation theory (Rogers & Mewborn, 1976), the emotional state of fear influences attitude and behavior change, not directly, but only indirectly through the appraisal of the severity of the danger. Note in Figure 6-2 that arousal has no direct link to protection motivation or coping.

The coping appraisal process evaluates one's ability to cope with and avert the threatened danger. As seen in Figure 6-2, the beliefs that increase the probability of the adaptive response are the beliefs that the recommended coping response is effective (e.g., "stopping smoking is an effective way to avoid the dangers associated with smoking") and that one can successfully perform the coping response (e.g., "I can stop smoking"). Coping appraisal is a summation of these appraisals of response efficacy, self-efficacy, and any "costs" of adopting the recommended preventive response: inconvenience, expense, unpleasantness, difficulty, complexity, side effects, disruption of daily life, and overcoming habit strength.

Self-efficacy is the major new component of the theory. According to Bandura (1977), a self-efficacy expectancy is the belief that one is or is not capable of performing a behavior. Self-efficacy is so important that Bandura proposed that *all* processes of psychological change are mediated by changes in an individual's sense of self-efficacy or mastery. According to Bandura, the cognitive appraisal of self-efficacy determines if coping behavior will be initiated, which behavior(s) will be chosen, how much effort will be expended, and how long it will persist.

Virtually every expectancy-value theory has omitted the self-efficacy concept. Research on fear and attitude change, however, has referred to it. Leventhal (1970) noted that not only must a coping response be effective, but one must possess the ability to make that coping response. Leventhal operationalized this concept in terms of "specific action instructions," which consistently has been found to facilitate coping. Recently, he included self-efficacy as a component of his self-regulatory model of dealing with health threats (Leventhal *et al.*, 1980). He also noted that early research in the fear and persuasion area investigating the personality variable of self-esteem was concerned with a similar issue; however, research with a new scale to measure dispositional self-efficacy has found it is relatively independent of self-esteem (Sherer, Maddux, Mercadante, Prentice-Dunn, Jacobs, & Rogers, 1982). The most thorough analysis of the role of self-efficacy for fear appeals has been offered by Beck and his colleagues (Beck & Frankel, 1981; Beck & Lund, 1981). Beck argued that self-efficacy (he prefers to label it personal efficacy) is not only an important construct but that it is critical to each of the three existing theories of how people cope with threats to their health. The only experiment I am aware of that manipulated self-efficacy in the context of an attitude-change study found that self-efficacy tended to increase intentions to adopt the communicator's recommendation (Maddux, Sherer, & Rogers, 1982). Our ability to understand and predict the effects of fear appeals on persuasion is greatly advanced by including the concept of self-efficacy.

Figure 6-2 shows that the amount of protection motivation elicited is a function of the threat appraisal and coping appraisal processes. Protection motivation, like any intervening variable, can be measured several ways, but it is assumed that protection motivation is best measured by behavioral intentions. The major assumptions of protection motivation theory are that the motivation to protect oneself from danger is a positive linear function of four beliefs: (1) the threat is severe, (2) one is personally vulnerable to the threat, (3) one has the ability to perform the coping response, and (4) the coping response is effective in averting the threat. Furthermore, the motivation is a negative linear function of (1) the reinforcements associated with the maladaptive response, and (2) the response costs.

The additive model holds *within* each appraisal process. When combining components *between* the two processes, second-order interaction effects occur (see Figure 6-1). It is assumed that if response efficacy (or self-efficacy) is high, severity and/or vulnerability will have a simple main effect on intentions; if response efficacy (or self-efficacy) is low, increments in severity and/or vulnerability will either have no effect or a boomerang effect, actually reducing intentions to comply with the recommendations. Thus, the model predicts outcomes that violate a completely rational decision-making process. There are at least two conditions in which individuals feel incapable of protecting themselves: (1) if the only available coping response is ineffective (i.e., low response efficacy), and (2) if they cannot perform the necessary coping response (i.e., low self-efficacy). We have obtained no evidence indicating that the boomerang effect shown in

Figure 6-1 is a product of defensive avoidance, denial, or reactance (Kleinot & Rogers, 1982; Rogers & Mewborn, 1976). It is assumed that the inability to protect oneself induces feelings of helplessness and loss of control. These feelings may motivate attempts to restore *perceived* control of one's fate, which can be accomplished by consciously and vigorously choosing to perform the behavior that will lead to the inescapable danger.

These assumptions yield six sufficient conditions that are prerequisite to eliciting protection motivation and coping behavior: An individual must believe that (1) the threat is severe, (2) he or she is vulnerable, (3) he or she can perform the coping response, (4) the coping response is effective, (5) the rewards associated with the maladaptive response are outweighed by the factors decreasing the probability of making the maladaptive response, and (6) the costs of the adaptive response are outweighed by the factors increasing the probability of making the adaptive response.

This model does not assume that the decision maker is rational. Each of the appraisal processes will be biased by heuristic judgments (Tversky & Kahneman, 1981) and the vividness of the sources of information (Nisbett & Ross, 1980). For example, in a recent study of vividness, we discovered that manipulations of the concreteness of information in a fear appeal affected the threat appraisal process (Sherer & Rogers, submitted for publication). That is, although information about the magnitude of bodily damage was held constant, the more detailed and specific the information, the more severe the threat was believed to be. Another aspect of vividness is how emotionally interesting information is. If the people depicted in the fear appeal messages were upset by the health threat (problem drinking in the Sherer and Rogers experiment) and were similar to the subjects, the subjects' intentions to protect themselves (i.e., moderate alcohol use) were stronger than if the people depicted in the messages were not upset and were dissimilar to the subjects. Thus, at least two components of vividness affect the threat appraisal process and intentions to protect onself. In addition to these cognitive biases, there are dynamic tendencies of defensively avoid threats (cf. Janis & Mann, 1977). Detailed consideration of these cognitive and motivational sources of bias is beyond the scope of this chapter. These biasing processes will prevent a one-to-one mapping of the objective information, but the final appraisals will reflect them. Thus, protection motivation should correspond closely with final threat and coping appraisals.

Coping Modes

Protection motivation eventuates in a single act, repeated acts (e.g., return to clinic for follow-up visits), multiple acts, or repeated multiple acts. Furthermore, the acts can either involve direct action or the inhibition of action. That is, coping with a threat may require that one actively do something (e.g., stop smoking, take medication) or *not* start something (e.g., do not start smoking). Attempts to persuade people to take direct action is usually the goal of remedial programs (i.e., illness and sick role behaviors); attempts to persuade people to refrain from an act is the goal of prevention programs.

Having hypothesized that protection motivation is best measured by behavioral intentions, a comment on the relation between intentions and behavior is in order. This relationship has been the subject of extensive and intensive research, guided by Fishbein's model. This research (e.g., Fishbein & Ajzen, 1975) has demonstrated that intentions accurately predict behavior if (1) the behavior, object, situation, and time are measured at the same level of specificity, and (2) the measure of intention reflects intention at the time the behavior is measured.

Three final observations are important. First, what about the factors, which are not included in protection motivation theory, known to affect coping with threats? These factors are assumed to be "external" or "distal" determinants of protection motivation. That is, those conditions not explicitly included in the model influence protection motivation and coping behavior *indirectly* by affecting threat appraisal and/or coping appraisal. Second, we should note that the theory has moved beyond fear appeals and persuasion. The theory is now sufficiently broad to apply to any situation involving threat (e.g., health behavior, coping with stress, compliance). Finally, protection motivation theory is one of a class of theories that differ from each other only in detail. It is similar to the health belief model (Becker *et al.*, 1977) and the models of Lazarus (Lazarus & Launier, 1978) and Leventhal (Leventhal *et al.*, 1980). These theories deal with essentially the same beliefs, but organize them differently and assume slightly different mediational processes.[2] It would be comforting to believe

2. There are several differences between the health belief model (HBM) and the protection motivation model. (Some distinctions between our position and Lazarus's and Leventhal's positions have been noted previously.) First, the components of the HBM are organized like predictors in a multiple regression equation; the components of protection motivation theory are organized and differentiated according to (1) the maladaptive versus the adaptive response, and (2) the factors increasing versus decreasing response probability (see Figure 6-2). A related distinction is that the models assume different mediating processes. Threat appraisal and coping appraisal (especially the component of self-efficacy) are unique to protection motivation. Third, the HBM has difficulty accounting for the frequently observed lack of effects of severity or vulnerability, but our model can account for them. Fourth, the HBM does not deal explicitly with emotional arousal, which has been shown to have an indirect effect in our model. Fifth, the concepts of the HBM have not been connected to antecedent conditions (especially components of persuasive communication) as precisely as those of the protection motivation model. Finally, the HBM assumes that the presence of the appropriate components will lead to changes in health behavior, whereas our model assumes that the appropriate components will lead to changes in motivation to protect oneself, which is best indexed by behavioral intentions. We assume that intentions are related to behavior according to Fishbein's well-known theory of reasoned action.

that these similarities mean that our theories are as advanced as unified theories of particle interaction, which also differ from each other only in detail. (It would also be delusional.) Nevertheless, I interpret this convergence in theory construction to be a strength.

CONCLUSION

Fear added wings to his feet.—Vergil (*The Aeneid*)

Social psychologists realized long ago that fear might do for attitudes what it did for feet. The original theoretical formulation borrowed heavily from the reinforcement theories of the time. Several different theories have evolved, each attempting to rectify the inadequacies of the previous positions. In this sense, theory construction has advanced in a systematic, cumulative fashion. One of the major goals of this chapter was to describe a revision of one of those theories.

We discovered several different types of experiments designed to investigate the role of physiological processes in attitude change. Some studies actually manipulated physiological arousal, others led people to believe they were aroused, and others measured physiological activity. All roads led to the same conclusion: There is very little, if any, evidence supporting the proposition that physiological processes mediate fear-based attitude change. We learned that fear arousal (which includes a physiological component) can affect attitude change only by first altering the cognitive appraisal of the severity of the threatening event. This relationship was incorporated into the revised theory of protection motivation. Furthermore, as the evidence unfolded, it became increasingly apparent that cognitive processes were much more important than physiological ones in changing attitudes and behavior. Protection motivation theory incorporated these new findings into an organized and sequential framework. Basically, any source of information about a threat, especially a fear appeal, initiates a threat appraisal process and a coping appraisal process. The former evaluates the consequences of acting maladaptively, and the latter evaluates the consequences of coping adaptively. Furthermore, the components of the two cognitive appraisal processes were organized according to whether they increased or decreased the probability of the adaptive and maladaptive responses.

According to protection motivation theory, the sinners in Jonathan Edwards's congregation would weigh the rewards associated with their wicked ways against their beliefs that they might be consigned to an everlasting Hell. The congregation also would quickly assess the effectiveness of the preacher's recommendation and their ability to follow his instructions despite the "costs" involved. The outcome of these two appraisal processes would determine the flock's motivation to take protective action. Fear may add wings to the sinners' feet so they can run faster, but protection motivation adds the wings that will enable them to soar over the bottomless pit.

REFERENCES

Bandura, A. Self-efficacy: Toward a unifying theory of behavioral change. *Psychological Review*, 1977, *84*, 191–215.

Beck, K. H. The effects of positive and negative arousal upon attitudes, belief acceptance, behavioral intention, and behavior. *Journal of Social Psychology*, 1979, *107*, 239–251.

Beck, K. H., & Frankel, A. A conceptualization of threat communications and preventive health behavior. *Social Psychology Quarterly*, 1981, *44*, 204–217.

Beck, K. H., & Lund, A. K. The effects of health threat seriousness and personal efficacy upon intentions and behavior. *Journal of Applied Social Psychology*, 1981, *11*, 401–415.

Becker, M. H., Haefner, D. P., Kasl, S. V., Kirscht, J. P., Maiman, L. A., & Rosenstock, I. M. Selected psychosocial models and correlates of individual health-related behaviors. *Medical Care*, 1977, *15*, 27–46.

Cacioppo, J. T. Effects of exogenous changes in heart rate on facilitation of thought and resistance of persuasion. *Journal of Personality and Social Psychology*, 1979, *37*, 489–498.

Cannon, W. B. *Bodily changes in pain, hunger, fear, and rage.* New York: Appleton, 1915.

Chu, C. C. Fear arousal, efficacy, and imminency. *Journal of Personality and Social Psychology*, 1966, *4*, 517–524.

Corah, N. L., Koch, B. E., & Eisenberg, L. S. *Use of fear appeals to change oral hygiene behavior.* Paper presented at the meeting of the International Association for Dental Research, Copenhagen, 1977.

Darwin, C. *The expression of the emotions in man and animals.* Chicago: University of Chicago Press, 1965. (Originally published, 1872.)

Fishbein, M., & Ajzen, I. *Belief, attitude, intention, and behavior.* Reading, Mass.: Addison-Wesley, 1975.

Freud, S. *The problem of anxiety.* New York: W. W. Norton, 1936.

Giesen, M., & Hendrick, C. Effects of false positive and negative arousal feedback on persuasion. *Journal of Personality and Social Psychology*, 1974, *30*, 449–457.

Griffeth, R., & Rogers, R. Effects of fear-arousing components of driver education on students' attitudes and simulator performance. *Journal of Educational Psychology*, 1976, *69*, 501–506.

Grings, W. W., & Dawson, M. E. *Emotions and bodily responses: A psychophysiological approach.* New York: Academic, 1978.

Harris, V. A., & Katkin, E. S. Primary and secondary emotional behavior: An analysis of the role of autonomic feedback on affect, arousal, and attribution. *Psychological Bulletin*, 1975, *82*, 904–916.

Hass, J., Bagley, G., & Rogers, R. Coping with the energy crisis: Effects of fear appeals upon attitudes toward energy consumption. *Journal of Applied Psychology*, 1975, *60*, 754–756.

Hendrick, C., Giesen, M., & Borden, R. False physiological feedback and persuasion: Effect of fear arousal vs. fear reduction on attitude change. *Journal of Personality*, 1975, *43*, 196–214.

Hovland, C., Janis, I., & Kelley, H. *Communication and persuasion.* New Haven, Conn.: Yale University Press, 1953.

Izard, C. *Human emotions.* New York: Plenum, 1977.

Janis, I. L. Effects of fear arousal on attitude change: Recent developments in theory and experimental research. In L. Berkowitz (Ed.), *Advances in experimental social psychology* (Vol. 3). New York: Academic, 1967.

Janis, I. L., & Feshbach, S. Effects of fear-arousing communications. *Journal of Abnormal and Social Psychology*, 1953, *48*, 78–92.

Janis, I. L., & Mann, L. Effectiveness of emotional role-playing in modifying smoking habits and attitudes. *Journal of Experimental Research in Personality*, 1965, *1*, 84–90.

Janis, I. L., & Mann, L. *Decision making*. New York: Free Press, 1977.

Kleinot, M. C., & Rogers, R. W. Identifying effective components of alcohol misuse prevention programs. *Journal of Studies on Alcohol*, 1982, *43*, 802–811.

Lang, P. J. The application of psychophysiological methods to the study of psychotherapy and behavior modification. In A. E. Bergin & S. L. Garfield (Eds.), *Handbook of psychotherapy and behavior change: An empirical analysis*. New York: Wiley, 1971.

Lazarus, R. S., Averill, J. R., & Opton, E. M. Toward a cognitive theory of emotion. In M. Arnold (Ed.), *Feelings and emotion*. New York: Academic, 1970.

Lazarus, R. S., & Launier, R. Stress-related transactions between person and environment. In L. Pervin & M. Lewis (Eds.), *Perspectives in interactional psychology*. New York: Plenum, 1978.

Leeper, R. Some needed developments in the motivational theory of emotions. In D. Levine (Ed.), *Nebraska Symposium on Motivation*. Lincoln: University of Nebraska Press, 1965.

Leventhal, H. Findings and theory in the study of fear communications. In L. Berkowitz (Ed.), *Advances in experimental social psychology* (Vol. 5). New York: Academic, 1970.

Leventhal, H., Meyer, D., & Gutmann, M. The role of theory in the study of compliance to high blood pressure regimens. In R. Haynes & M. Mattson (Eds.), *Patient compliance to prescribed antihypertensive medication regimens: A report to the National Heart, Lung, and Blood Institute* (NIH Publ. No. 81-2102). Bethesda, Md.: U.S. Department of Health and Human Services, 1980.

Leventhal, H., & Watts, J. Sources of resistance to fear-arousing communications on smoking and lung cancer. *Journal of Personality*, 1966, *34*, 155–175.

Levy, B., & Ahlquist, R. Adrenergic drugs. In J. R. Dipalma (Ed.), *Drill's pharmacology in medicine* (4th ed.). New York: McGraw-Hill, 1971.

Maddux, J. E., Sherer, M., & Rogers, R. W. Self-efficacy expectancy and outcome expectancy: Their relationship and their effects on behavioral intentions. *Cognitive Therapy and Research*, 1982, *6*, 207–211.

Marshall, G. D., & Zimbardo, P. G. Affective consequences of inadequately explained physiological arousal. *Journal of Personality and Social Psychology*, 1979, *37*, 970–988.

Maslach, C. Negative emotional biasing of unexplained arousal. *Journal of Personality and Social Psychology*, 1979, *37*, 953–969.

Mewborn, C. R., & Rogers, R. W. Effects of threatening and reassuring components of fear appeals on physiological and verbal measures of emotion and attitudes. *Journal of Experimental Social Psychology*, 1979, *15*, 242–253.

Mineka, S. The role of fear in theories of avoidance learning, flooding, and extinction. *Psychological Bulletin*, 1979, *86*, 985–1010.

Nisbett, R., & Ross, L. *Human inference: Strategies and shortcomings of social judgment*. Englewood Cliffs, N.J.: Prentice-Hall, 1980.

Obrist, P. A., Gaebelein, C. J., Shanks, E. M., Langer, A. W., & Botticelli, L. J. Cardiovascular behavioral interactions. In D. Mostofsky (Ed.), *Behavior control and modification of physiological activity*. Englewood Cliffs, N.J.: Prentice-Hall, 1976.

Powell, F. The effect of anxiety-arousing messages when related to personal, familial, and impersonal referents. *Speech Monographs*, 1965, *32*, 102–106.

Rescorla, R., & Solomon, R. L. Two-process learning theory: Relationships between Pavlovian conditioning and instrumental learning. *Psychological Review*, 1967, *14*, 151–182.

Rogers, R. W. A protection motivation theory of fear appeals and attitude change. *Journal of Psychology*, 1975, *91*, 93–114.

Rogers, R. W., & Deckner, C. W. Effects of fear appeals and physiological arousal upon emotion, attitudes, and cigarette smoking. *Journal of Personality and Social Psychology*, 1975, *32*, 222–230.

Rogers, R. W., Deckner, C. W., & Mewborn, C. R.   An expectancy-value theory approach to the long-term modification of smoking behavior. *Journal of Clinical Psychology*, 1978, *34*, 562–566.

Rogers, R. W., & Mewborn, C. R.   Fear appeals and attitude change: Effects of a threat's noxiousness, probability of occurrence, and the efficacy of coping responses. *Journal of Personality and Social Psychology*, 1976, *34*, 54–61.

Rogers, R. W., & Thistlethwaite, D. L.   Effects of fear arousal and reassurance upon attitude change. *Journal of Personality and Social Psychology*, 1970, *15*, 227–233.

Schachter, S., & Singer, J. E.   Cognitive, social, and physiological determinants of emotional state. *Psychological Review*, 1962, *69*, 379–399.

Shapiro, D., & Crider, A.   Psychophysiological approaches in social psychology. In G. Lindzey & E. Aronson (Eds.), *The handbook of social psychology* (Vol. 3). Reading, Mass.: Addison-Wesley, 1968.

Shelton, M. L., & Rogers, R. W.   Fear-arousing and empathy-arousing appeals to help: The pathos of persuasion. *Journal of Applied Social Psychology*, 1981, *11*, 366–378.

Sherer, M., Maddux, J. E., Mercadante, B., Prentice-Dunn, S., Jacobs, B., & Rogers, R.   The self-efficacy scale: Construction and validation. *Psychological Reports*, 1982, *51*, 663–671.

Sherer, M., & Rogers, R. W.   *Impact of vividness of information on persuasiveness of fear appeals.* Manuscript submitted for publication.

Sherrington, C. S.   *The integrative action of the nervous system.* London: Constable, 1906.

Spence, K. W.   *Behavior therapy and conditioning.* New Haven, Conn.: Yale University Press, 1956.

Stainback, R. D., & Rogers, R. W.   Identifying effective components of alcohol abuse prevention programs: Effects of fear appeals, message style, and source expertise. *International Journal of the Addictions*, in press.

Tversky, A., & Kahneman, D.   The framing of decisions and the psychology of choice. *Science*, 1981, *211*, 453–458.

CHAPTER 7

Bogus Physiological Feedback

Richard Hirschman
Kent State University
Michael Clark
VA Medical Center
Chillicothe, Ohio

INTRODUCTION

The technique of bogus physiological feedback is closely akin to biofeedback, in which a digital or analog representation of an individual's physiological activity is "fed back" to the individual for the purpose of self-control. However, with bogus physiological feedback, the information is non-veridical. That is, the information is either unrelated to the individual's ongoing physiological activity or it is directly related but disguised or altered prior to its presentation. In both cases the individual presumably believes that the information represents his or her physiological activity. The technique requires the presentation of the physiological information and a belief manipulation that the information parallels the functioning of one or more existing physiological response systems. This latter aspect is an important one which we examine later in the chapter.

Initially, bogus physiological feedback was used to study the relationship between the perception of physiological activity and the generation or modification of emotions or the attribution of emotions (Valins, 1966, 1967). Subsequently, it was used to study the efficacy of biofeedback treatments (Gatchel, Hatch, Watson, Smith, & Gaas, 1977; Klinge, 1972; Rupert & Holmes, 1978), the attribution of intrinsic and extrinsic motivation (Pittman, Cooper, & Smith, 1977), the mechanisms of attitude change and persuasion (Giesen & Hendrick, 1974; Harris & Jellison, 1971; Hendrick, Giesen, & Borden, 1975; S. E. Taylor, 1975), and the reduction of fear (Gaupp, Stern, & Galbraith, 1972; Valins & Ray, 1967) and other symptoms (e.g., depressive cognitions: G. S. Stern, Berrenberg, Winn, & Dubois,

1978; physical distress: G. S. Stern, Miller, Ewy, & Grant, 1980). All of these areas of application pertain directly to the broader area of emotion. For instance, the fear reduction and biofeedback applications were attempts to control or modify emotions; the attitude and persuasion applications were attempts to induce or vary an emotion in order to examine its impact on attitude formation and persuasion. Thus, the general framework that is adopted in this chapter is to examine the impact and mechanisms of the technique on emotion.

In the following sections we examine briefly contemporary views of bogus feedback. We also examine the attempts to apply the technique. Our primary emphasis throughout this chapter is on the relative importance of cognitive and physiological explanatory factors. The complex way in which these factors interact during emotional experience is perhaps the most important contribution to emerge from the bogus feedback area.

CONTEMPORARY VIEWS

As noted elsewhere in this book, there has been much discussion about the relative importance of the physiological component of emotional experience. Suffice it to say that neither the felt experience of actual physiological activity (e.g., feeling more aroused with a concomitant increase in heart rate) nor the exteroceptive appraisal of actual physiological activity (e.g., noticing that one's palms are sweaty) can fully account for the range and variability of emotional experience. In response to this, some theorists have expanded James's (1890) original notion of a preemotional stimulus appraisal process into cognitively based theories of emotion. Most relevant to this chapter is the theory proposed by Schachter and Singer (1962; see also Lazarus, 1966). Schachter and Singer proposed that given a state of general physiological arousal for which no ready explanation exists, the emotional label attached to the experience is determined by one's cognitions concerning the situation. Thus, a state of unexplained arousal creates a need for cognitions that account for the experience. When one's arousal can be explained by relating it to some causative situation, no alternative cognitions are necessary. In fact, an emotion may not occur unless it is justified by the situation. Although physiological arousal is necessary in order to experience emotions, situationally dependent cognitions are the means by which emotional labels are differentiated.

The gradual historical process of emphasizing the causal role of cognitive factors was given an empirical boost with Valins's (1966, 1967) studies, which were based on the premise that sympathetic activity may be incidental to the experience of emotion. He reasoned that if epinephrine-induced, interoceptive cues create a need to rely on situationally relevant cognitions in labeling an experience as emotional, then exteroceptive cues of one's internal state should result in a similar process. Valins (1966) tested this idea by presenting male subjects with slides of seminude females while they were listening to prerecorded auditory beeps. One group was told that the beeps were their actual ongoing heart rate; another group was told that the beeps were extraneous sounds. Subjects were exposed to increasing beep frequency, decreasing beep frequency, or no change in beep frequency during the presentation of the slides. When subjects were later asked to rate the attractiveness of the slides, Valins found that those subjects who were exposed to changing bogus heart rate feedback (increase and decrease) rated the accompanying slides as more attractive than the slides accompanied by nonchanging bogus heart rate feedback. (This is often referred to as the "Valins effect.") No such difference occurred for subjects exposed to the same sounds labeled as extraneous noise. In addition, slides accompanied by heart rate increases were rated as more attractive than slides accompanied by heart rate decreases. Valins concluded that the perceptions of internal changes, regardless of actual internal changes, influenced the slide attractiveness ratings. In a later study, Valins (1967) utilized a similar paradigm to examine the role of individual differences. In addition to replicating his earlier results, he found that the effect of changing bogus heart rate feedback on subjective ratings was more pronounced on emotional subjects than on unemotional subjects.[1]

Following these encouraging results, Valins and Ray (1967) examined bogus heart rate feedback in a practical context. The prevailing view at that time was that successful fear reduction first required concomitant changes in physiological activation. However, Valins and Ray proposed that perhaps the belief of being physiologically aroused was more critical for the determination and maintenance of fear than actually being physiologically aroused. To examine this possibility, they presented volunteers with slides of snakes, as well as with slides of the word "shock," followed by actual finger shock. During the presentation, one-half of the subjects heard sounds identified as their heart beats, while the remaining subjects heard the same sounds identified as noise. For all subjects the sounds increased in frequency for the "shock" slides but remained stable for the snake slides. When the data were analyzed without including those subjects who had previously handled snakes, the "heart rate" subjects showed significantly more snake-approach behavior than the "noise" subjects. Similar findings were reported in a second experiment in which only snake-fearful subjects were used. Based on these findings, Valins and Ray concluded that fear reduction may be accomplished in the absence of actual physiological changes (e.g., a reduction in heart rate) if subjects' beliefs about their physiological responses to fear stimuli are appropriately altered.

The reaction to this research was both intense and prolific because Valins was challenging not only Schachter and Singer's well-formulated

1. See Lykken (1967) for a critique of Valins's method for measuring emotionality.

theory, but also traditional psychophysiological assumptions that relegated a major causal role to physiological arousal in the generation of affective state.[2] Since that time, Valins's original findings have been replicated within a variety of emotional contexts. Increases and reductions of the intensity of emotional attributions have been found with various combinations of bogus feedback and (1) aversive stimuli (Bloemkolk, Defares, Van Enckevort, & Van Gelderen, 1971; Hirschman, 1975), (2) ambiguous stimuli (Reisman, Insko, & Valins, 1970; White & Wilkins, 1973), and (3) actual life stressors (Borkovec, Wall, & Stone, 1974; Lick, 1975). More specific information concerning these studies as well as the others mentioned throughout this chapter may be seen in Table 7-1. (The reader is encouraged to refer to this table to understand more fully those studies that are mentioned briefly in the text.)

Liebhart (1980) proposed a comprehensive cognitively oriented model to account for these and other successful demonstrations of the Valins effect. According to Liebhart, the Valins effect is mediated by three cognitive processes: explanation search, attribution, and attention to the perceived causes of the bogus physiological changes. The concomitant presentation of bogus feedback (e.g., accelerating heart rate) and another stimulus (e.g., a slide of a nude) presumably is experienced as incongruous; that is, there is a failure to appreciate a causal link between the two. To resolve this discrepancy, an *explanation search* is initiated; the stimulus in question (e.g., the nude) is *attended* to until an *attribute* is found (e.g., attractiveness of the nude) that can account for the bogus physiological changes. It is only then that the attribution might influence actual physiological responses and other behaviors.

Although Liebhart (1980) offered much empirical support for his cognitive model, there is also the possibility that actual physiological cues may be a part of the mediation process, depending on the context and the characteristics of the subject population (Detweiler & Zanna, 1976; Goldstein, Fink, & Mettee, 1972; Hirschman, 1975). To put it another way, there may be two qualitatively different experiences associated with the Valins effect, depending on the parameters of the individual and the social context—a *physiologically based experience* (significant physiological activity and its perception) or a *cognitively based experience* (no significant physiological activity). With respect to emotions, Harris and Katkin (1975) labeled these experiences primary emotion and secondary emotion, respectively. For example, Hirschman (1975) noted that with bogus feedback, actual physiological cues (appraised exteroceptively or interoceptively) may be more salient for high-anxious subjects and high autonomic perceivers than for low-anxious subjects and low autonomic perceivers, respectively. If actual

---

2. See Kleinke (1977) for additional evidence concerning the importance of the cognitive labeling of bodily reactions.

TABLE 7-1. Summary of Bogus Feedback Studies

Study	Task or Stimulus	Type of Bogus Feedback	Direction of Bogus Feedback	Impact of Bogus Feedback*			Remarks
				Verbal	Behavioral	Physiological	
Barefoot & Straub (1971)	Slides of female nudes	(1) Bogus heart rate	(1) Feedback of presence of heart rate reaction to some slides	Yes (attractiveness)	—	—	Stimulus exposure times affected impact of bogus feedback
Bloemkolk & Defares (1971)	Slides of pleasant, neutral, sexual, or aversive content	(1) Bogus heart rate	(1a) Increasing and no-change feedback (1b) No-change feedback only	Yes (attractiveness)	—	Yes (heart rate)	Bogus feedback altered perceptions of both pleasant and unpleasant stimuli
Borkovec (1973)	Live snake	(1) Bogus heart rate	(1a) Increasing (1b) Decreasing	—	Yes (approach)	Yes (heart rate)	Failed to replicate Valins & Ray (1967) study
Borkovec & Glasgow (1973)	Live snake	(1) Bogus heart rate (2) Extraneous sounds	(1) Decrease (2) Decrease	—	Yes (snake handling)	Yes (heart rate)	Preexposure to feared stimulus attenuated effects of bogus feedback
Borkovec, Wall, & Stone (1974)	Present speech	(1) Bogus heart rate (2) Extraneous sounds (3) No feedback	(1a) Increasing (1b) Decreasing (1c) No change (2) Increasing	Yes (anxiety)	Yes (speech disfluencies and overt anxiety)	No (heart rate)	No anxiety-reduction effects of bogus feedback relative to controls; significant effects were for feedback conditions
Botto, Galbraith, & Stern (1974)	Slides of seminude females	(1) Bogus heart rate	(1) Increasing, decreasing, and no change	Yes (attractiveness)	—		Replicated Valins (1966) effect without evidence

(continued)

TABLE 7-1. (Continued)

Study	Task or Stimulus	Type of Bogus Feedback	Direction of Bogus Feedback	Impact of Bogus Feedback*			Remarks
				Verbal	Behavioral	Physiological	
		(2) Extraneous sounds (3) Extraneous sounds—task attention	(2) Same as (1) (3) Same as (1)				for an attentional factor
Carver & Blaney (1977a)							
Experiment 1	Live snake	(1) Bogus heart rate	(1a) Increasing (1b) No change	No (fear)	Yes (approach)	—	
Experiment 2	Live snake	(1) Bogus heart rate (2) No feedback	(1a) Increasing (1b) No change	Yes (fear)	Yes (approach)	—	No-change bogus feedback facilitated approach of phobic subjects
Experiment 3	Live snake	(1) Bogus heart rate (2) No feedback	(1a) Increasing (1b) No change	No (fear)	Yes (approach)	—	Bogus feedback affected approach of high-aversion subjects only
Carver & Blaney (1977b)	Live snake	(1) Bogus heart rate	(1a) Increase (1b) No change	Yes (attention to behavior)	Yes (approach)	—	Confidence level for task interacted with bogus feedback
Conger, Conger, & Brehm (1976)	Live snake Slides of the word "shock" Slides of snakes	(1) Bogus heart rate (2) Extraneous sounds	(1) Increase to slides of the word "shock"; no change to slides of snakes (2) Same as (1)	No (anxiety)	Yes (approach)	—	Bogus heart rate feedback enhanced the approach behavior of low-fear subjects

Study	Task	Feedback conditions	Direction	Self-report	Behavioral	Physiological	Results
Decaria, Proctor, & Malloy (1974)	Slides of geometric shapes	(1) Bogus heart rate	(1) Increasing, decreasing, and no change	Yes (anxiety)	—	No (heart rate)	
DeGood, Elkin, Lessin, & Valle (1977)	Enhance or suppress alpha levels	(1) Veridical alpha (2) Bogus alpha	(2) Increasing or decreasing alpha which was the reverse of actual alpha activity	No (alpha experiences)	—	No (alpha levels)	
Detweiler & Zanna (1976)	Characteristics of nations	(1) Bogus electrodermal and heart rate	(1) Increasing, no change, decreasing, and no feedback	No (attitudes)	—	Yes (heart rate)	No effect of bogus feedback on attitudes; some evidence for relationship between actual heart rate and attitudes
Gatchel, Hatch, Maynard, Turns, & Taunton-Blackwood (1979)	Present speech	(1) Veridical heart rate (2) Bogus heart rate (3) No feedback (systematic desensitization)	(2) Decreasing	Yes (anxiety)	Yes (overt anxiety)	No (heart rate)	Bogus feedback resulted in equivalent improvements in anxiety reports and behaviors relative to veridical feedback
Gatchel, Hatch, Watson, Smith, & Gaas (1977)	Present speech	(1) Veridical heart rate (2) Veridical heart rate (with relaxation) (3) Bogus heart rate (4) No feedback (relaxation only)	(3) Decreasing	Yes (anxiety)	Yes (overt anxiety)	No (skin conductance and heart rate)	Equal reductions in self-report and behavioral measures of anxiety despite physiological differences

(continued)

183

TABLE 7-1. (*Continued*)

Study	Task or Stimulus	Type of Bogus Feedback	Direction of Bogus Feedback	Impact of Bogus Feedback*			Remarks
				Verbal	Behavioral	Physiological	
Gaupp, Stern, & Galbraith (1972)	Live snake Slides of the word "shock" Slides of snakes	(1) Bogus heart rate	(1) Increasing to slides of the word "shock"; no change to snake slides	Yes (fear)	Yes (approach)	Yes (heart rate)	Bogus feedback failed to facilitate approach relative to other experimental groups; significant difference between groups (1) and (4)
		(2) Extraneous sounds	(2) Same as (1)				
		(3) Veridical heart rate					
		(4) No feedback					
Giesen & Hendrick (1974)							
Experiment 1	Listen to a communication	(1) Bogus "arousal"	(1a) High arousal (1b) low arousal	Yes (arousal)	—	—	
		(2) No feedback					
Experiment 2	Listen to a communication	(1) Bogus "arousal"	(1a) Low arousal during baseline; low during communication	Yes (arousal)	—	—	
			(1b) High to high arousal				
			(1c) Low to high arousal				
		(2) No feedback					
Goldstein, Fink, & Mettee (1972)							
Part 1	Slides of nude females	(1) Bogus heart rate	(1) Increasing and no change	Yes (attractiveness)	—	Yes (heart rate)	

Study	Task	Manipulation	Levels				
Part 2	Slides of nude females and nude males	(1) Bogus heart rate (2) No feedback	(1a) Increasing (1b) No change	No (attractiveness of nude males)	—	No (heart rate)	
Hanna, Wilfling, & McNeill (1975)	Present speech	(1) Veridical and bogus muscle feedback and periods of no feedback	—	—	Yes (stuttering)	Unclear	Credibility of bogus muscle feedback was questioned
Harris & Jellison (1971) Experiment 1	Listen to communication	(1) Bogus "fear" arousal	(1a) Low arousal throughout communication (1b) Low to high to low arousal (1c) Low to high arousal (1d) Variable	Yes (arousal)	—	—	
Experiment 2	Same as above with change in feedback instructions	Same as above	Same as above	Yes (arousal)	—	—	
Hendrick, Giesen, & Borden (1975) Experiment 1	Listen to communication	(1) Bogus arousal	(1a) High arousal (1b) Medium arousal (1c) High to low arousal (1d) Medium to low arousal	Yes (persuasion)	—	—	

(continued)

TABLE 7-1. (Continued)

Study	Task or Stimulus	Type of Bogus Feedback	Direction of Bogus Feedback	Impact of Bogus Feedback* Verbal	Behavioral	Physiological	Remarks
Experiment 2	Listen to communication	Same as above	(1a) Low arousal (1b) High arousal (1c) High to low arousal	Yes (persuasion)	—	—	
Hirschman (1975)	Slides of violent deaths	(1) Bogus heart rate (2) Extraneous sound	(1a) Increase (1b) No change (2a) Increase (2b) No change	Yes (discomfort)	—	Yes (skin conductance and galvanic skin responses)	
Hirschman, Clark, & Hawk (1977)	Slides of nude females	(1) Bogus heart rate (2) Extraneous sound	(1) Increase and no change (2) Same as (1)	Yes (attractiveness)	—	No (galvanic skin responses)	Effects of heart and sound on ratings were equivalent
Hirschman & Hawk (1978)	Slides of violent deaths	(1) Bogus heart rate	(1a) Increasing (1b) No change	Yes (unpleasantness)	—	Yes (skin conductance)	
Hirschman & Revland (in preparation, 1983)	Videotape of a dental procedure	(1) Veridical heart rate (2) Inverted heart rate	(1a) Task-increase (1b) Task-decrease (2a) Task-increase (2b) Task-decrease	Yes (unpleasantness)	—	Yes (heart rate)	Perception of physiological change was more important than actual change in altering the ratings
Holmes & Frost (1976)	Shocks	(1) Bogus heart rate	(1a) Increase (1b) Decrease	Yes (anxiety and shock intensity)	—	No (heart rate)	
Kent, Wilson, & Nelson (1972)	Live snake Slides of the word "shock" Slides of snakes	(1) Bogus heart rate (2) Extraneous sounds	(1) Increasing to "shock" slides; no change to snake slides (2) Same as (1)	Yes (fear)	No (approach)	—	

Study	Task	Feedback conditions	Feedback direction	Self-report measure	Behavioral measure	Physiological measure	Comments
Kerber & Coles (1978)	Slides of nude females	(1) Bogus heart rate	(1) Increasing and no change	Yes (attractiveness)	—	Yes (skin conductance and heart rate)	
Klinge (1972)	Relax or think	(1) Veridical electrodermal (2) Bogus electrodermal (3) Extraneous meter activity	(2a) Positive (in compliance with instructions) (2b) Negative (not in compliance)	—	—	Yes (galvanic skin response)	Accurate feedback most conducive to electrodermal control
Koenig (1973)	Solve math problem	(1) Bogus electrodermal	(1a) High and no feedback (1b) Average and no feedback	Yes (anxiety)	Yes (response latency)	—	
Koenig & Del Castillo (1969)							
Experiment 1	Shock presentation in conditioned emotional response study	(1) Bogus electrodermal (2) Extraneous meter activity with attention (3) Extraneous meter activity (4) No feedback	(1) High meter activity (2) High meter activity (3) High meter activity	—	—	Yes (skin conductance)	
Experiment 2	Same as above with extended trials	(1) Bogus electrodermal (2) No feedback	(1) High meter activity	—	—	Yes (skin conductance)	
Kondo & Canter (1977)	Record headache activity	(1) Veridical muscle feedback (2) Bogus muscle feedback	(2) Decreasing	No (number of headaches)	—	No (muscle tension)	

(continued)

TABLE 7-1. (Continued)

Study	Task or Stimulus	Type of Bogus Feedback	Direction of Bogus Feedback	Impact of Bogus Feedback*			Remarks
				Verbal	Behavioral	Physiological	
Lick (1975)	Live snake or spider	(1) Bogus electrodermal and placebo (2) No feedback—desensitization (3) No feedback—placebo (4) No feedback—no treatment	(1) Decreasing	Yes (fear)	Yes (approach)	Yes (heart rate)	
Misovich & Charis (1974)	Slides of nude females or of accident victims	(1) Bogus heart rate	(1) Verbal feedback of slides which incurred "most" and "least" change	Yes (attractiveness)	No (time looking at slides)	No (heart rate)	
Parkinson & Manstead (1981)	Slides of skin diseases	(1) Bogus heart rate (2) Extraneous sounds	(1) Increasing and no change (2) Same as (1)	No (unpleasantness)	No (recall of slides)	—	Failed to replicate the Valins effect
Pittman, Cooper, & Smith (1977)	Reward manipulation game	(1) Bogus electrodermal	(1a) Verbal feedback of arousal pattern indicative of interest in the game (1b) Verbal feedback of arousal pattern indicative of interest in reward	Yes (arousal)	Yes (playing time)	—	

Study	Instructions	Conditions	Manipulation			
Plotkin (1980)	Learn alpha control	(1) Veridical alpha (2) Bogus alpha (3) Extraneous sounds—concentration exercise (4) Extraneous sounds—brain-wave stimulation (5) Combination of 3 and 4 (6) Extraneous sounds—self-induction	(2) Feedback of successful alpha enhancement Sounds for groups (3), (4), (5), and (6) same as those for (2)	Yes (alpha experiences)	—	Yes (alpha level)
Pressner & Savitsky (1977)	Learn alpha control	(1) Veridical alpha (2) Bogus alpha	(2) Feedback of successful alpha enhancement	No (mood)	–	No (alpha level)
Reisman, Insko, & Valins (1970)	Rorschach stimuli	(1) Bogus heart rate	(1) Increasing and no change	Yes (positive-negative)	—	—
Rosen, Rosen, & Reid (1972)	Slides of the word "shock" Slides of snakes	(1) Bogus heart rate (2) Extraneous sounds (3) No feedback (no treatment)	(1a) Increase to "shock" slides; no change to snake slides (1b) Reverse of (1a) (2) Same as (1a)	Yes (anxiety)	No (approach)	No (heart rate)

(continued)

TABLE 7-1. (*Continued*)

Study	Task or Stimulus	Type of Bogus Feedback	Direction of Bogus Feedback	Impact of Bogus Feedback*			Remarks
				Verbal	Behavioral	Physiological	
Rupert & Holmes (1978)	Learn heart rate control	(1) Veridical heart rate (2) Bogus heart rate (3) No feedback (4) No feedback (no treatment)	(2a) Increasing (2b) Decreasing	No (anxiety)	—	No (heart rate)	
G. S. Stern, Berrenberg, Winn, & Dubois (1978)	Learn heart rate control	(1) Veridical heart rate (2) Bogus heart rate (3) No feedback	(2a) Increasing (2b) Decreasing	Yes (depression)	—	No (heart rate)	
G. S. Stern, Miller, Ewy, & Grant (1980)	Learn heart rate control	(1) Bogus heart rate (2) No feedback	(1a) Decreasing (ascending success) (1b) Decreasing (equally distributed success)	Yes (life stress symptoms)	—	—	
R. M. Stern, Botto, & Herrick (1972) Experiment 1	Slides of female nudes; ignore feedback stimuli	(1) Bogus heart rate (2) Extraneous sound	(1a) Increase and no change (1b) Decrease and no change (2) Increase, no change, and decrease	Yes (attractiveness)	—	No (heart rate) No (skin resistance)	

Study	Stimuli	Treatments	Results				
Experiment 2	Same as above except attend to feedback stimuli	(1) Extraneous sound	(1) Increase and no change	No (attractiveness)	—	—	—
Experiment 3	Rate slides of injured people	(1) Bogus heart rate (2) Extraneous sound (3) Extraneous sound; attend to the feedback stimuli	(1) Increase, decrease, and no change (2) Same as (1) (3) Same as (1)	Yes (unpleasantness)	—	Yes (heart rate) No (skin resistance)	Effects of bogus feedback similar to those of sound-attention group
Sushinsky & Bootzin (1970)	Live rat or snake Slides of snakes or rats	(1) Bogus heart rate (2) Extraneous sound (3) No feedback (no treatment)	(1) Increase to snake slides; no change to rat slides (2) Same as (1)	No (discomfort)	No (approach)	—	—
S. E. Taylor (1975)	Slides of clothed males	(1) Bogus electrodermal (2) No feedback	(1a) Feedback of presence of electrodermal response to preferred slide (1b) Feedback of presence of electrodermal response to nonpreferred slide	Difference in attractiveness ratings between preferred and nonpreferred slides greater for group (1a) than (1b), but only when no future consequences of ratings were foreseen	Yes (viewing time)	—	—

(continued)

TABLE 7-1. (Continued)

| Study | Task or Stimulus | Type of Bogus Feedback | Direction of Bogus Feedback | Impact of Bogus Feedback* | | | Remarks |
				Verbal	Behavioral	Physiological	
Thornton & Hagan (1976)	Slides of skin diseases	(1) Bogus heart rate (2) No feedback	(1a) Increasing and no change (1b) No change	Yes (un-pleasantness)	—	No (heart rate)	
Valins (1966)	Slides of female nudes	(1) Bogus heart rate (2) Extraneous sound	(1a) Increase and no change (1b) Decrease and no change (2a) Same as (1a) (2b) Same as (1b)	Yes (attractiveness)	Yes (choice of slides)	—	
Valins (1967)	Same as above with addition of emotionality measure	Same as above	Same as above	Yes (attractiveness)	Yes (choice of slides)	—	Bogus feedback differentially affected slide choice and ratings of high-emotional subjects relative to low-emotional subjects
Valins & Ray (1967)							
Experiment 1	Live snake Slides of the word "shock" Slides of snakes	(1) Bogus heart rate (2) Extraneous sound	(1) Increase to "shock" slides; no change to snake slides (2) Same as (1)	—	Yes (approach)	—	
Experiment 2	Live snake	Same as above	Same as above	No (fear)	Yes (incentive to approach)	—	

192

Valle & Levine (1975)	Enhance or suppress alpha	(1) Veridical alpha (2) Bogus alpha	(2) Increasing or decreasing alpha, which was the reverse of actual alpha activity	—	—	Yes (alpha levels)	—
White & Wilkins (1973)	Presentations of Thematic Apperception cards	(1) Bogus electrodermal (2) Extraneous meter activity	(1) High and no change in meter activity (2) Same as (1)	—	Yes (response thresholds)	—	Perception of emotional state differentially affected response threshold of sensitizers and repressors
Wilson (1973)	Live snake	(1) Bogus arousal feedback (2) No feedback—slide exposure (3) No feedback—no treatment	(1) Feedback of presence of arousal to selected slides	Yes (fear)	No (approach)	—	
Woll & McFall (1979)	Slides of nude males	(1) Bogus heart rate	(1) Increasing and no change	Yes (attractiveness)	—	Yes (heart rate) No (skin resistance)	No effect for degree of autonomic awareness
Young, Hirschman, & Clark (1982)	Videotape of a dental procedure	(1) Bogus heart rate	(1a) Increasing (1b) Decreasing	Yes (unpleasantness)	—	Yes (heart rate)	

Note. Only main effects of bogus feedback are presented. Interactions are not presented because of their complexity. Our purpose is to highlight the paradigms and the impact of bogus feedback on three components of emotional experience (verbal, behavior, and physiological).

* A "yes" in these columns indicates a significant effect for bogus feedback; a "no" indicates the absence of a significant effect; a dash indicates the absence of a measure.

physiological cues are salient (i.e., a physiologically based experience), then, in Liebhart's terms, these cues would require an explanation instead of, or in addition to, an explanation for the bogus feedback cues. Presumably, a subject would then initiate a "search" of the stimulus in question (e.g., a slide of a nude) for explanatory factors; that is, a *cyclic physiological–cognitive* feedback loop would occur. Obviously, this loop would not occur if actual physiological cues are minimal or are undetected exteroceptively or interoceptively (i.e., a cognitively based experience).

We regard the issue of cognitive versus physiological mediation of the Valins effect to be most important. It has an important bearing on the validity of physiologically based theories of emotion and on the usefulness of therapeutic techniques (e.g., biofeedback) that rely on a causal link between physiological and emotional change. It is for these reasons that we will continue to explore this issue in the subsequent sections of this chapter.

PHYSIOLOGICAL MEDIATION

Unfortunately, Valins's original conclusions regarding the primacy of cognitive factors were not completely justified because he failed to report in detail the ongoing physiological responses of his subjects. The lack of supporting physiological data failed to exclude the possibility that changes in the self-reports that he found were due to one of the following: (1) the exteroceptive perception of actual physiological changes (e.g., noticing sweaty palms), (2) the interoceptive sensation (felt sensation) of actual physiological changes (e.g., feeling more aroused), and (3) undetected actual physiological changes which nevertheless may modulate experience by acting on the central nervous system (see Cacioppo & Petty, 1982). A first step to rule out these possibilities would be to show that actual physiological changes do not occur in response to bogus feedback and/or that they do not covary with other changes of emotionality (e.g., self-reports) that are elicited by bogus feedback. These possibilities resulted in numerous studies of the *physiological mediation* issue. Many of these studies yielded data consistent with Valins's position. For instance, although Rosen, Rosen, and Reid (1972), found that, for some subjects, increasing bogus heart rate feedback resulted in self-reports of anxiety to slides of snakes and slides of the word "shock," no comparable effect was found on actual heart rate. Similarly, bogus feedback had no effect on heart rate with speech-anxious subjects (Borkovec et al., 1974), under nonarousing conditions (Decaria, Proctor, & Malloy, 1974), with aversive stimuli (Holmes & Frost, 1976; Thornton & Hagan, 1976), and with positively and negatively affective stimuli (Misovich & Charis, 1974).

However, the failure to find bogus feedback effects on physiological responses has not been consistent. For example, Koenig and Del Castillo

(1969) found that bogus electrodermal feedback, indicative of increased activity, retarded the extinction of conditioned galvanic skin responses. In a study of emotional attributions, R. M. Stern, Botto, and Herrick (1972) found that male subjects who heard increasing or decreasing bogus heart rate feedback with slides of seminude females showed biphasic heart rate responses, including an initial heart rate acceleration. Subjects who heard extraneous sounds with the slides showed uniphasic heart rate deceleration.[3] In a more comprehensive study, Goldstein *et al.* (1972) also found that the *rate* of bogus heart rate feedback influenced actual heart rate responses to slides of seminude females. Male subjects reacted with larger heart rate changes to a bogus heart rate increase–slide condition than to a bogus heart rate no change–slide condition. This "mimic" effect was not found when presumably more offensive male nude slides were used. In addition, there was a positive correlation between actual heart rates and ratings of emotional potency for the male nudes but not for the female nudes. Goldstein *et al.* concluded that during exposure to the presumably offensive male nudes, contradictions between actual heart rate changes and bogus feedback were resolved by a reliance on actual heart rate changes, in a manner which they did not specify; in the minimally provocative situation (slides of seminude females), bogus heart rate cues were more critical than actual heart rate changes.

Unfortunately, the acceptance of Goldstein *et al.*'s conclusions is tempered, to some extent, by the following. Clear documentation of the importance of the meaning of bogus feedback requires careful control for the differential effects of the stimuli themselves regardless of their meaning. However, Goldstein *et al.* (1972) did not use appropriate noise control conditions. The importance of this was shown in a study by Hirschman, Clark, and Hawk (1977). They found that accelerating bogus heart rate feedback and the same stimuli labeled as extraneous noise both increased the self-ratings of pleasantness to slides of female nudes. Thus, it is difficult to determine whether the attributional effects of bogus feedback in the Goldstein *et al.* study were due to the meaning of the feedback (sounds identified as heart rate) or to the pattern of impinging auditory stimuli.

A more important objection that can be raised with the Goldstein *et al.* study is their use of *any* change in heart rate to define a "mimicking" effect. Collapsing the data in this way may have shrouded the *in vivo* effects of specific directional heart rate changes. The notion of directional fractionation (J. I. Lacey, Kagan, Lacey, & Moss, 1963) may help to clarify this point. J. I. Lacey *et al.* found that the intake of nonnoxious environmental stimuli is associated with heart rate decreases, while the rejection of noxious environmental stimuli is associated with heart rate increases. In fact, when

---

3. See Harris and Katkin (1975) for a critique of the analyses in this study.

Goldstein *et al.* analyzed just for differential heart rate increases, the effect of the rate of bogus feedback washed out. Given that there are apparently two unique heart rate responses which are indicative of two *qualitatively* different arousal states, it might be appropriate to look, in detail, at a unidirectional indicant of arousal (e.g., the electrodermal response), in order to delineate *quantitative* changes in physiological arousal.

This was examined more closely in a study by Hirschman (1975). Subjects were exposed to 10 successive slides of people who died violently. One group also heard continuous auditory tones, purported to be their own heart rate, increase 20 seconds before each slide onset and remain at an increased level throughout each slide presentation. A second group heard tones, labeled as heart rate, which did not vary in frequency. Two other groups heard the same tones, respectively, but were led to believe that they were extraneous sounds. Separate electrodermal analyses were obtained for anticipatory periods, slide stimulus periods, and intertrial intervals. During all three data collection periods, the concomitant presentation of bogus feedback and noxious slides resulted in more electrodermal activity when compared to the sound–slide combinations. As expected, differences were found between the heart and sound conditions in both amplitude and frequency of electrodermal responses during the anticipatory period. Furthermore, amplitude during slide anticipation was significantly greater for the heart–increase group than for the other three groups. Although not significant, a similar trend was found for the frequency measure. Subjects were also asked to respond on a self-discomfort continuum subsequent to each slide presentation. Typically in previous studies, self-reports of emotion were defined operationally by an attribution of stimulus quality, such as unpleasantness. Intuitively, a report of self-discomfort would be more akin to an assessment of emotional experience. Again, as expected, subjects in the heart–increase group reported significantly more discomfort than subjects in the heart–no-change, sound–increase, and sound–no-change groups.

To infer that the changes in electrodermal activity (i.e., sympathetic arousal) mediated the changes in the self-reports of discomfort in the Hirschman (1975) study, it would have been necessary to demonstrate a relationship between these indicators. However, the Pearson product-moment correlations were, at best, moderate. (The highest correlation was .37.) This discrepancy between subjective ratings and actual physiological activity is not an atypical finding (Hirschman, Young, & Nelson, 1979; Kerber & Coles, 1978; Woll & McFall, 1979). In one such study (Young, Hirschman, & Clark, 1982) dentally anxious subjects were presented with either increasing or decreasing bogus heart rate feedback while they were viewing a videotape of a "first-person" dental procedure. Dentally anxious males in the decrease condition responded to the dental procedure with less discomfort than did dentally anxious males in the increase condition. No comparable effect was found for females. Male and female subjects in the decrease condition demonstrated a significant decrease in actual heart rate across dental segments, whereas male and female subjects in the increase condition demonstrated a significant increase in actual heart rate across dental segments. Although male and female subjects showed this physiological "mimic" effect, differential discomfort ratings were elicited only for male subjects. This suggests that the observed heart rate changes were unrelated to the discomfort ratings.

The failure to consistently link bogus feedback-induced changes in physiological activity (e.g., electrodermal responses) and cognitive appraisals (e.g., ratings of autopsy slides) remains a crucial obstacle for attributing the changes in cognitive appraisals to changes in physiological activity. In fact, in only two studies has there been a concordance between physiological activity and self-report cognitive appraisals, if the problematic experiment of Goldstein *et al.* is excluded. In the first study, Detweiler and Zanna (1976) exposed subjects to bogus heart rate feedback and galvanic skin response feedback that increased, decreased, or did not change, while the subjects indicated attitudes toward various nations. Subjects in the three feedback conditions showed significantly larger heart rate decreases than did subjects in a control condition. In addition, there was a significant relationship between attitudes and heart rate changes such that greater heart deceleration was predictive of more positive attitudes. In the second study, Gaupp *et al.* (1972) utilized Valins and Ray's (1967) bogus feedback desensitization design to examine the effects of bogus feedback on snake-approach behaviors and subjective fear ratings. They found that subjects exposed to snake slides and no change bogus heart rate feedback showed a greater decline in their heart rate responses to the slides than subjects exposed to the slides and the same bogus stimuli labeled as noise. However, these groups did not show differential GSR responses. Subsequently, the bogus feedback subjects also demonstrated less subjective fear and more snake-approach behavior than did subjects in a no-treatment condition. When the snake-approach behavior of subjects who showed a decrease in heart rate was compared to those demonstrating either no change or an increase in heart rate, the "decrease" subjects showed more approach behavior than did subjects in the latter groups.

Although Detweiler and Zanna's (1976) study and Gaupp *et al.*'s (1972) study offer some support for the idea that bogus feedback may be mediated by physiological change, this possibility needs to be considered in the context of their methodologies. As with Goldstein *et al.*'s (1972) study, Detweiler and Zanna failed to compare the autonomic and subjective responses of subjects exposed to bogus feedback with the responses of subjects exposed to the same sounds labeled as extraneous noise. In addition, their data provide little support for the idea that the exteroceptive perception of physiological change was a critical antecedent. Possibly any stimuli (e.g., feedback stimuli not labeled as such) that varied on a "degree of stimulation" dimension might have had a similar effect on heart rate. What they did show was a relationship between actual heart rate and attitude rather than a relationship among directional bogus feedback, heart rate, and attitude.

With respect to the Gaupp *et al.* study, the bogus feedback group did show greater heart rate reductions in response to the snake slides relative to the noise group. However, there were no significant differences in subjective fear levels or change in approach behavior between the two groups. Only the no-feedback control group (i.e., no exposure to either the slides or to the bogus feedback) responded with greater fear and less change in approach behavior than the feedback group, a finding that again highlights the importance of including appropriate noise control groups. Furthermore, the greater change in approach for individuals showing heart rate reductions relative to those demonstrating steady or increasing heart rates were based on breakdowns independent of treatment group assignment and therefore provides no information as to the potential links between physiological levels and the cognitive effects of bogus feedback.

In summary, although bogus feedback apparently affects physiological activity in some situations, the effect is not consistent. Even in those situations in which physiological changes have occurred, the changes have not necessarily been related to the self-reports of emotionality or to the characteristics of the stimuli in question. However, it may be that actual physiological changes are more pronounced in response to bogus feedback only for certain individuals. It is to this issue that we now turn our attention.

INDIVIDUAL DIFFERENCES AND BOGUS FEEDBACK

The bases for our belief that individual differences may be important are the following:

> 1. Physiological responsivity to emotional stimuli, in part, may be a function of individual differences (Harvey & Hirschman, 1980; Hirschman & Katkin, 1971).
> 2. The ability to voluntarily control physiological activity, in part, may be a function of individual differences (Hirschman & Favaro, 1980).
> 3. The effects of voluntary physiological control on perceived affect during stress, in part, may be a function of individual differences (Clark & Hirschman, 1980; Hirschman & Revland, 1979).

That individuals may differentially perceive and utilize their actual physiological activity has been examined with bogus feedback in several ways. The first approach presupposes that if actual physiological activity affects emotional appraisals, subjects more exteroceptively or interoceptively aware of this activity should show greater correspondence between the perception of this activity and measures of emotionality. The effects of bogus feedback should be stronger for those subjects who are less aware of their actual physiological activity and for those who are less physiologically reactive. These possibilities were examined in two studies (Borkovec, 1973; Woll & McFall, 1979) in which portions of the Autonomic Perception Questionnaire (APQ—Mandler, Mandler, & Uviller, 1958) were used. This questionnaire consists of 30 items that measure awareness of autonomic changes in various circumstances. Borkovec (1973), using a modification of this questionnaire, exposed snake-fearful subjects to either increasing or decreasing bogus heart rate feedback during the second of two snake-approach tasks. The relevant findings are as follows. Autonomically aware subjects showed a greater increase in approach behavior than did unaware subjects but only under a suggestion-for-improvement condition. In addition, autonomically aware subjects who exhibited a strong pretest autonomic reaction (as measured by heart rate) and who were exposed to increasing bogus feedback showed greater change in approach behavior than did the other subjects. Subjects exposed to increasing bogus feedback and who were in the suggestion for improvement condition also showed significant reductions in actual heart rate over the two snake-approach tasks. Most important, Borkovec failed to replicate the bogus feedback effect found by Valins and Ray (1967).

Woll and McFall (1979) examined these same issues by exposing autonomically aware and autonomically unaware female subjects to slides of partially clad males while they heard increasing or constant bogus heart rate feedback. Subjects rated the slides accompanied by increasing feedback as more attractive than the slides accompanied by constant feedback. There was a similar feedback effect on self-ratings of arousal. Although there was an initial heart rate acceleration in both conditions, a subsequent decelerative response was more pronounced in response to the bogus heart rate increase–slide combination. Furthermore, high autonomic perceivers (defined by scores on the APQ) did not show a significant relationship between subjective ratings and heart rate and they were not differentially affected by the feedback manipulation.

The second approach to the issue of the differential utilization of actual physiological cues presupposes that individuals who are more physiologically active might have more cues available for exteroceptive or interoceptive appraisal and therefore might demonstrate greater physiological, self-report correspondence than less physiologically active individuals. In these studies, classification of preexperimental physiological activity was based on indirect self-report assessments or on measures of actual physiological activity. The former method is illustrated by a previously mentioned study (Valins, 1967) in which male subjects were classified on an emotional activity dimension by their scores on Lykken's emotionality questionnaire

(Lykken, 1957). Valins found that the ratings of slides of female nudes made by emotional male subjects were more affected by bogus feedback than the ratings made by unemotional male subjects (i.e., emotional male subjects responded with higher attractiveness ratings than did unemotional male subjects). However, as with his earlier study (Valins, 1966), Valins did not monitor actual autonomic activity, which again precluded the attribution of this effect to cognitive or physiological factors.

In an attempt to rectify this, physiological activity was monitored in a study by Hirschman and Hawk (1978) in which subjects were exposed to slides of people who died violently and concomitant increasing or constant bogus heart rate feedback. Two measures of preexperimental activity were used: Taylor Manifest Anxiety Scale scores (J. A. Taylor, 1953) and resting nonspecific electrodermal activity. Analyses using both breakdowns yielded significant feedback effects; that is, there were higher unpleasantness ratings to slides accompanied by increasing feedback. However, only the analysis based on resting electrodermal activity revealed an effect for individual differences. Here, as expected, the high-autonomic-activity subjects reported more unpleasantness and showed higher skin conductance responses to the slide–heart rate feedback combination than did the low-autonomic-activity subjects. This was particularly evident in the heart-increase condition. Although bogus feedback affected visceral activity and subjective ratings, in part as a function of preexperimental autonomic activity, the changes in both response modalities were not necessarily coincident. For example, the high-autonomic-activity subjects were electrodermally responsive to the bogus feedback, regardless of rate. Yet the most extreme unpleasantness ratings were elicited in the heart-rate-increase condition.

In summary, the failure to find concordance between physiological responses (e.g., heart rate) and verbal reports (e.g., attractiveness of nudes) in these studies again argues against the physiological mediation hypothesis. Possibly the importance of actual physiological responses is more consistently apparent only in emotionally volatile situations in which high levels of physiological activity typically are elicited. This possibility will now be explored.

EMOTIONALLY VOLATILE SITUATIONS AND BOGUS FEEDBACK

Several contemporary techniques (e.g., biofeedback) that are used for the reduction of anxiety are based on the assumption that anxiety and physiological quiescence are incompatible and that by promoting the latter, the former will be reduced. If bogus feedback can also be shown to reduce anxiety or fear in emotionally volatile situations, particularly in the absence of physiological change, this would indeed be damaging to the physiological mediation hypothesis.

Interest in the more direct application of bogus feedback to emotionally volatile situations was catalyzed by a study mentioned previously (Valins & Ray, 1967) in which snake phobics showed approach improvement after being exposed to bogus heart rate feedback and slides of snakes. This finding was replicated by Borkovec and Glasgow (1973) but only with subjects who were not exposed to a live snake prior to the feedback–slide presentations. However, Borkovec and Glasgow did not find concomitant group differences in heart rate; unfortunately, in the Valins and Ray study, as well as in several other studies in which bogus feedback affected self-reports or behavioral indexes of fear (e.g., Conger, Conger, & Brehm, 1976; Wilson, 1973), physiological activity was not monitored.

Three attempts to replicate the findings from the Valins and Ray study were unsuccessful (Gaupp *et al.*, 1972; Kent, Wilson, & Nelson, 1972; Sushinsky & Bootzin, 1970). However, Borkovec and Glasgow (1973) noted some important methodological problems in these studies: for example (1) the use of behavioral pretest that may have increased fear, and (2) the use of a low-demand (nontherapeutic) instructional set. Of even greater importance, the feedback presentation in these studies occurred only during a slide presentation task which intervened between pretest and posttest exposures to the actual phobic stimulus. Apropos of this, Borkovec *et al.* (1974) exposed speech-anxious subjects to bogus heart rate feedback while they engaged in an actual speech presentation task. There were no striking effects of the feedback manipulation on behavioral indicants of anxiety during the speech presentation. However, during a subsequent speech presentation not paired with feedback, subjects who previously had heard either heart-rate-decrease feedback or heart-rate-no-change feedback reported significantly less anxiety and showed fewer overt anxiety signs and speech disfluencies than did subjects who had heard heart-rate-increase feedback. Perhaps, as Borkovec *et al.* suggested, the decrease and no-change conditions may have had a minimal effect beyond that which would have been expected from repetitive speech presentations. From another perspective, Borkovec *et al.* reported that all subjects demonstrated relatively high prespeech physiological arousal. As such, the fear behavior of the heart-increase group may have been enhanced by the interactive effect of high visceral activity and congruent exteroceptive cues. Against the backdrop of relatively short speech durations (3 minutes), the high visceral activity may have tempered the fear-attenuation effects of the heart-no-change and the heart-decrease manipulations. Thus, a longer task exposure might permit a more precise charting of temporal changes in emotionality as a function of continuous feedback.

There is yet another explanation for the failures to replicate the findings of Valins and Ray (1967). Subjects in the replication studies were more fearful than subjects in the Valins and Ray study (Borkovec & Glasgow, 1973). Presumbly, the high-fear subjects had more salient internal physiological cues than low-fear subjects in the presence of the feared stimulus. The less noticeable internal state of the low-fear subjects might have increased their susceptibility to the bogus feedback. In support, snake-approach behavior was enhanced with decreasing bogus heart rate feedback to a greater degree in low-fear subjects than in high-fear subjects (Conger *et al.*, 1976). However, in another study constant bogus heart rate feedback facilitated approach behavior and accelerating bogus heart rate feedback inhibited approach behavior in high-fear subjects but not in low-fear subjects (Carver & Blaney, 1977a). The latter finding may have been due to a heterogeneous group of low-fear subjects who may have differed in their confidence to approach and handle the feared stimulus (Carver & Blaney, 1977a, 1977b). In fact, subjects with moderate fear who reported that they could handle a snake responded to bogus feedback like subjects with low fear. Subjects with moderate fear who reported that they were uncertain that they could handle a snake responded to bogus feedback like subjects with high fear (Carver & Blaney, 1977a).

Information obtained from studies such as these could have an important bearing on the understanding of the mechanisms by which anxiety may be reduced. For example, if cognitive mediators are of prime importance in anxiety reduction and subsequent behavior change, it may be less critical to elicit physiological responses incompatible with anxiety as posited in the reciprocal inhibition-counterconditioning model (Wolpe, 1958, 1971) or to lower arousal as posited in the habituation model (Mathews, 1971). Diminution of physiological responding would be a critical component of the anxiety-reduction process if one were to adhere to these latter models. To the extent that *cognitive* appraisals of arousal are more critical, their direct alteration may provide an alternative, possibly a more efficient base for anxiety-reduction techniques. However, support for the latter possibility is still tenuous considering the inconsistent behavioral and self-report data and the absence of physiological data in some of the studies that we have reviewed.

Another approach that has been used to examine the importance of actual physiological activity on negatively emotional states has been to compare the effectiveness of veridical feedback and bogus feedback on altering subjective reports of distress. If it is assumed that actual physiological change is a critical mediator of emotionality, then bogus feedback should not be as effective in altering emotionality as the amplified signals of actual physiological change (i.e., veridical heart rate feedback).[4] Following earlier observations regarding the effectiveness of heart rate biofeedback

4. See the following for examples with (1) electroencephalographic alpha-wave veridical feedback—DeGood, Elkin, Lessin, and Valle (1977), Plotkin (1980), Pressner and Savitsky (1977), Valle and Levine (1975)—and (2) electromyographic veridical feedback—Kondo and Canter (1977).

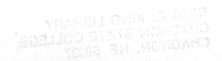

(Gatchel & Proctor, 1976), Gatchel *et al.* (1977) compared the effects of heart rate feedback, muscular relaxation, combined heart rate feedback/ muscular relaxation, and bogus heart rate feedback on speech anxiety. They found that only the veridical feedback procedures led to significant reductions in heart rate and skin conductance levels. However, all groups demonstrated significant and equivalent reductions in the self-report component of public-speaking anxiety. In a similar experiment, Gatchel, Hatch, Maynard, Turns, and Taunton-Blackwood (1979) compared the effects of heart rate feedback, systematic desensitization, and bogus heart rate feedback on speech anxiety. They found that although the veridical feedback group showed less of an increase in heart rate than did the other groups, all three groups showed similar reductions in public-speaking anxiety. Interestingly, the improvement in self-report was maintained in all groups at a one-month follow-up session during which subjects gave another speech. Clearly, the bogus feedback (placebo) condition used in Gatchel's studies had a "therapeutic impact" on the self-reports of public-speaking anxiety. In summarizing these studies, Gatchel (1979) concluded that the perception of having control over an anxiety-competing response (e.g., heart rate) can reduce anxiety even if the perception of control is inaccurate.

Bogus heart rate feedback was also used as a placebo condition in a study with patients who were hospitalized with anxiety-related problems (Rupert & Holmes, 1978). In this study bogus heart rate feedback did not induce heart rate changes, whereas veridical feedback induced heart rate increases. Neither veridical feedback nor bogus feedback had an effect on subjective feelings of anxiety; thus, it would be difficult to extrapolate the findings from this study to our more general concern—the relative importance of physiological mediation.

Hirschman and Revland (in preparation, 1983), utilizing a different approach to the mediation issue, preselected 32 dentally anxious subjects and had them view and rate their discomfort and anxiety to a stressful videotape of a dental procedure. During the tape presentation, eight subjects were instructed to increase their heart rate and eight subjects were instructed to decrease their heart rate by monitoring their heart rate on a digital voltmeter positioned within their field of vision. Heart rate accelerations relative to resting levels were accompanied by positive beats-per-minute values on the feedback meter (increase-accurate condition), while heart rate decelerations were accompanied by negative beats-per-minute values on the meter (decrease-accurate condition). There were two additional conditions (eight subjects per condition) in which subjects received directionally inaccurate feedback; that is, the sign on the feedback meter was reversed, resulting in negative beats-per-minute values for heart rate accelerations (increase-inaccurate group) and positive beats-per-minute values for heart rate decelerations (decrease-inaccurate group).

Subjects were unaware of this reversal. Subsequent comparisons among the groups revealed that the increase-inaccurate group demonstrated heart rate decreases indistinguishable from the decrease-accurate group, while the decrease-inaccurate group demonstrated heart rate increases indistinguishable from the increase-accurate group. The unpleasantness ratings and the state anxiety responses to the dental presentation were consistent with subjects' beliefs about the feedback task rather than with their actual heart rate changes. There were no significant differences in unpleasantness ratings and state anxiety ratings between the increase-accurate group and the increase-inaccurate group or between the decrease-accurate group and the decrease-inaccurate group. Relative to the increase groups, the decrease groups rated the dental presentation as being significantly less unpleasant. It should be noted that all subjects in the two inaccurate groups believed that the feedback was veridical.

In summary, the results of these studies do not generally support the physiological mediation hypothesis. Physiological changes at times occurred in response to bogus feedback, owing perhaps to reactions to the feedback stimuli or to the situational context. Yet these changes did not consistently parallel changes in other response systems that are presumably indicative of emotionality (e.g., self-reports). In addition, Gatchel and his coworkers showed that veridical heart rate feedback, which presumably induces a consistent heart rate change, was no more effective than bogus feedback in altering self-report and behavioral indicants of emotionality.

We have argued throughout this chapter that the *cognitive appraisal* of physiological activity, regardless of veridicality, is the primary modus operandi of bogus feedback on emotional experience. In fact, it would be difficult to view emotional experience in general as not being dependent on cognitive mediation (Lazarus, 1981). We are not arguing that physiological activity is, by definition, vestigial vis-à-vis emotional experience. Rather, theories of emotion that require the demonstration of observable physiological changes and which presume consistent correspondence between cognitions and actual physiological arousal may not be as generalizable as was once thought.

METHODOLOGICAL ISSUES

Although there has been little, if any, concern about the replicability of the Valins effect (Parkinson & Manstead, 1981), the effect may not be solely dependent on the perception and the exteroceptive utilization of bogus feedback cues. The following variables have been considered most often as alternative explanations for the effect or as components of the procedure that are essential for the effect to occur: attention, expectancy, information search, and cue credibility.

Attention

Bogus feedback is a salient exteroceptive cue; as such it may alter the focus of attention, which in turn may alter self-reports and physiological responses to emotionally provocative stimuli. This explanation is plausible if one considers that attentional processes (e.g., orienting) influence physiological activity (e.g., electrodermal responses) and other behaviors. However, when the importance of attention was explored by Botto, Galbraith, and Stern (1974), they were able to replicate the typical Valins effect with bogus heart rate feedback and slides of seminude females, but they were unable to find a comparable effect with an attention manipulation. The latter finding contrasts with that of another study from Stern's laboratory (R. M. Stern *et al.*, 1972). In this earlier study, subjects *attending* to extraneous sounds and slides of injured or dead people showed heart rate responses and self-reports that were comparable to the responses elicited by bogus feedback. Parkinson and Manstead (1981) also found that instructing subjects to attend to increasing or no-change bogus heart rate feedback or comparable electronic "bleeps" produced differential ratings of slides of skin diseases, regardless of the meaning of the feedback stimuli. It should be noted that Parkinson and Manstead excluded particularly arousing slides. Thus, if the slides were only moderately arousing, subjects may have been primed to use any change in the quality of the feedback stimulus (e.g., increasing) in order to evaluate the slides. Thus, at present, the evidence for the importance of attentional factors is inconclusive. Perhaps the issue needs to be examined in greater detail. For example, changes in the rate of feedback may elicit more attention than no change in rate regardless of the meaning of the feedback; that is, a change in rate may be more salient than no change in rate, or perhaps the feedback itself is more salient than "extraneous noise," regardless of "attend" or "ignore" instructions.

Expectancy

In theory, the differential effects of bogus feedback relative to control procedures could be attributed to (1) the differences in expectations regarding the meaningfulness of the information, (2) the meaningfulness of the information, and (3) the beliefs regarding the demands of the experiment. Wilson (1973) examined the first possibility by exposing snake-fearful subjects to either pictures of snakes or to blank slides and either bogus feedback (general physiological arousal) or no feedback. Wilson found that although the bogus feedback selectively influenced fear ratings, expectations of success were equivalent in all four treatment groups. Lick (1975) manipulated expectancy levels directly in an examination of the impact of systematic desensitization, bogus electrodermal feedback with placebo instructions, and placebo instructions alone on the fear levels of snake- and spider-phobic subjects. Lick reported that all three manipulations were associated with significant improvement (less fear) relative to a no-treatment group on various behavioral, physiological, and self-report outcome measures. However, the responses of the feedback with placebo group were different from those of the placebo-only group on two self-report measures, suggesting that the processes underlying the feedback and placebo effects were not necessarily equivalent. Finally, we have already alluded to Borkovec's (1973) view concerning the importance of a suggestion for improvement (high-demand) instruction.

The available data suggest that expectancy factors play a role, to some degree, in the mediation of bogus feedback effects. The degree of their impact appears to vary with the experimental context. For example, the explicit improvement suggestions usually provided in applied bogus feedback studies probably have a greater effect than the ignore-the-tones instructions that are typical of attributional studies mentioned previously. Yet in neither case do these factors account for the entirety of bogus feedback effects.

Information Search

Another potentially important cognitive factor in bogus feedback paradigms is information search. Barefoot and Straub (1971) tested Valins's (1966) contention that increasing bogus heart rate feedback leads to a search for stimulus attributes that would account for the change in the sound frequency of the feedback. They compared the effects of short (5-second) and long (20-second) exposure times of slides of female nudes on attributions of attractiveness to the slides. It was expected that only subjects in the long exposure time would be affected by the feedback stimuli. Barefoot and Straub found that subjects who viewed the slides for 5 seconds were not affected by the bogus feedback, whereas the reverse was true for subjects who viewed the slides for 20 seconds. Although a 5-second slide exposure time may be too short for information search and attribution processes to occur, Hirschman's (1975) results suggest that stimulus factors may also be involved. Using aversive slides, Hirschman found significant bogus feedback effects using 5-second stimulus exposure times. That aversive stimuli may require less exposure time than less negative stimuli suggests that aversive stimuli may not demand the same degree of active information search.

Woll and McFall (1979) provided additional support for the importance of information search. They exposed female subjects to seminude male slides in a typical bogus feedback paradigm and collected attractiveness ratings in response to the slides and ratings for specific attitudes in response to the slides. They found that rate-related feedback effects occurred not only for overall slide ratings but also for three specific attributes of each slide, suggesting that complex cognitive search and evaluative processes were stimulated by the feedback.

Cue Credibility

There are two important aspects of cue credibility: credibility of the bogus feedback and consistency between the feedback and the experimental context. As mentioned before, bogus feedback paradigms require that subjects believe that the bogus feedback is veridical. Typically, this has been assessed during postexperimental subject debriefings. Generally, few subjects, including autonomically aware or highly reactive subjects, have questioned the authenticity of bogus *autonomic* feedback, except when the feedback has been extremely inconsistent with their past experiences. (See the clinical addendum in Kent *et al.*, 1972, for an example of a failure to accept bogus autonomic feedback.) However, it may be more difficult to establish the credibility of bogus *somatic* feedback because actual somatic cues may be more discernible. For example, Hanna, Wilfling, and McNeill (1975) found that when they exposed a single subject to bogus electromyographic feedback following veridical electromyographic feedback, the subject refused to accept the bogus feedback as veridical.

The importance of the experimental context is more apparent when considering the relatively limited impact of decreasing bogus heart rate feedback in studies of fear and emotional attribution. For example, decreasing bogus heart rate feedback was less effective than increasing bogus heart rate feedback on increasing the ratings of attractiveness to slides of female nudes (Valins, 1966). Also, in fear-reduction studies, the differential effects of decreasing bogus heart rate feedback, constant bogus heart rate feedback, and no feedback have been inconsistent (see Borkovec & Glasgow, 1973; Borkovec *et al.*, 1974). One explanation for this is that feedback cues which are indicative of less autonomic activity (e.g., decreasing bogus heart rate feedback) may not be credible in the presence of a feared stimulus. Thus, reliable demonstrations of the effects of bogus feedback may require the presentation of cues that are, to some extent, consistent with situational context.

CONCLUSIONS AND IMPLICATIONS

Much of the previously cited research has focused on the input aspects of perceived arousal. In operational terms, the primary aim has been to establish a bogus feedback procedure that will alter the processing of other stimulus-bound, emotionally laden information in a predictable fashion. However, the specific mechanisms by which such information is in fact internally processed are unclear. One speculative account is that arousal cognitions affect the flow of ongoing cognitive processes so as to select and direct the encoding and decoding mechanisms (Hendrick, 1968). Perhaps these mechanisms might also enhance or activate particular response tendencies available for a particular situation, that is, a kind of energizing or alteration of motivation effect. These are certainly areas ripe for examination by cognitively oriented psychologists.

With respect to the relationship between bogus feedback and the alteration of emotional experience, generally there appears to be a positive linear relationship between levels of bogus physiological arousal, perceived exteroceptively, and the heightening of emotional experience, at least within the bounds of arousal created by the stimuli that have been used. Under conditions in which there is a tendency to experience an already heightened positive emotion (e.g., males viewing nude females), increased bogus physiological arousal, perceived exteroceptively, apparently enhances this tendency. However, under conditions in which an already heightened negative emotion is attenuated (e.g., fear reduction), the effects of bogus feedback appear to be less straightforward. In this case bogus feedback does not necessarily elicit fear-attenuating cognitions; rather, the extent of the effect is dependent on the complex interaction of the intraindividual and experimental factors that were previously discussed.

We have emphasized that cognitive processes are important mediators of the effects of bogus feedback. Changes in actual physiological activity probably are less critical considering the failures to elicit consistent physiological responses to bogus feedback and the independence between self-reports of emotionality and physiological responses. Nor do the effects of bogus feedback appear to be artifactual, as neither expectancy nor attentional factors can fully account for its impact. That attention and expectancy at times may exert an interactive effect with bogus feedback indicates the complexity of the technique and the relative importance of individual differences in appraisal processes and response capabilities as compared to biologically based commonalities. A corollary of our cognitive view is that the appraisal of actual physiological activity may not be a necessary component of all emotional experiences, regardless of whether an individual is appraising his or her own state (e.g., feeling pleasant) or making an attribution to an external stimulus (e.g., the stimulus is attractive). We have even found that cognitive appraisals also may override the effects of actual physiological activity on attributions to innocuous external stimuli (Hirschman & Brumbaugh-Buehler, 1975). High-anxious subjects (defined by Taylor Manifest Anxiety Scale scores) perceived nonchanging moderate and low tones as increasing in intensity over trials, while their electrodermal responses to the tones were habituating. If the electrodermal responses mimicked or affected the cognitive appraisals of the tones (i.e., change in intensity), a dishabituation of the electrodermal response should have occurred. To the extent that cognitive factors generally are prepotent, it may be necessary to reassess some of the assumptions underlying physiologically based theories of emotion and physiologically based treatments for anxiety (e.g., biofeedback, systematic desensitization, and progressive relaxation). To an extent this reevaluation has already begun, as witnessed by the growing concern over the lack of a relationship between physiological activity and affective states (Tarler-Benlolo, 1978; Turk, Meichenbaum, & Berman, 1979) and the increasing use of cognitively oriented therapies (e.g., Meichenbaum, 1973, 1975).

Although changes in physiological activity have not necessarily covaried with changes in self-reports of emotional experience in the studies that we have reviewed, we are not trying to totally negate the importance of physiological activity as a component of phenomenological experience. First, emotion is a construct with multiple operational definitions, many of which include a physiological component (Borkovec, Weerts, & Bernstein, 1977; Lang, 1968; Liebhart, 1979). Second, physiological activity may influence a variety of experiences (e.g., attitudes) by being detected exteroceptively or interoceptively and may even have an effect without being detected (Cacioppo & Petty, 1982; see Cacioppo, 1979, and B.C. Lacey & Lacey, 1978, for examples of the effects of physiological activity that is undetected, and Reeves & Shapiro, 1982, for examples of the effects of physiological activity that is detected exteroceptively). Apropos of this review, the limited success of bogus feedback with highly fearful subjects may have been due to a greater production of veridical cues, which if experienced may have contradicted or may have minimized the acceptance of bogus cues. Finally, the intense physical sensations that frequently accompany emotional experiences such as embarrassment or acute panic or fear do not always remain independent of emotional appraisals. It may be that physiological activity that is experienced exteroceptively (e.g., noticing that one's palms are sweaty) or that is experienced interoceptively (e.g., a felt sensation) is most important for *reevaluating* initial cognitive appraisals; in Lazarus's (1966) terms, it may be most critical for secondary appraisals. Perhaps Lazarus's view could be amended in the following manner. For some individuals veridical or "imagined" physiological activity may be used exteroceptively to reevaluate an emotional experience.

Physiological activity may also be more or less important depending on the *intensity of an emotional experience*. Although cognitive factors may be more important during the experience of mild or moderately intense emotions, physiological factors may be more important as emotional intensity increases. To put it another way, if the emotion is dictated by cognitive factors (possibly during mild emotions), individual differences in cognitive appraisals, fear level, and cue credibility may exert a more critical influence on the experience. In contrast, if the emotion is dictated by physiological factors (possibly during intense emotions), actual physiological activity may exert a more critical influence on experience by being perceived exteroceptively, by being sensed interoceptively, or by exerting an undetected effect on the central nervous system. If it is true that only mild or moderately intense emotions have been typically elicited in bogus feedback studies, this might account for the greater potency of cognitive factors than physiological factors in these studies.

Another offshoot of this idea is that positive and negative emotions may not be comparable on an intensity dimension and therefore may be mediated by different processes. Perhaps strongly negative emotions (e.g., fear) are more intense and are easier to identify than strongly positive emotions (e.g., love). Intuitively, this is reasonable if one considers that the experience of negative emotions may be a warning that biological survival (or psychological survival) is at stake and that a strong "built-in" sympathetic response occurs, presumably to ensure survival. The need for positive emotions to be recognized is less critical from a survival perspective. If this view of *bipartite emotionality* on an intensity dimension is correct, it would not be surprising to discover that physiological factors are a more salient feature of negative emotions and that cognitive factors are a more salient feature of positive emotions. Bogus feedback could be used to clarify this possibility much as it has been used to clarify other issues concerning the mediation of emotion.

ACKNOWLEDGMENT

Preparation of this chapter was supported in part by NIDR Grant DE 06294 awarded to the first author.

REFERENCES

Barefoot, J. C., & Straub, R. B. Opportunity for information search and the effect of false heart-rate feedback. *Journal of Personality and Social Psychology*, 1971, *17*, 154–157.

Bloemkolk, D., Defares, P., Van Enckevort, G., & Van Gelderen, W. Cognitive processing of information on varied physiological arousal. *European Journal of Social Psychology*, 1971, *1*, 31–46.

Borkovec, T. D. The effects of instructional suggestion and physiological cues on analogue fear. *Behavior Therapy*, 1973, *4*, 185–192.

Borkovec, T. D., & Glasgow, R. E. Boundary conditions of false heart-rate feedback effects on avoidance behavior: A resolution of discrepant results. *Behaviour Research and Therapy*, 1973, *11*, 171–177.

Borkovec, T. D., Wall, R. L., & Stone, N. M. False physiological feedback and the maintenance of speech anxiety. *Journal of Abnormal Psychology*, 1974, *83*, 164–168.

Borkovec, T. D., Weerts, T. C., & Bernstein, D. A. Behavioral assessment of anxiety. In A. Ciminero, K. Calhoun, & H. E. Adams (Eds.), *Handbook of behavioral assessment*. New York: Wiley, 1977.

Botto, R. W., Galbraith, G. G., & Stern, R. M. Effects of false heart rate feedback and sex-guilt upon attitudes toward sexual stimuli. *Psychological Reports*, 1974, *35*, 267–274.

Cacioppo, J. T.   Effects of exogenous changes in heart rate on facilitation of thought and resistance to persuasion. *Journal of Personality and Social Psychology*, 1979, *37*, 489–498.

Cacioppo, J. T., & Petty, R. E.   A biosocial model of attitude change. In J. T. Cacioppo & R. E. Petty (Eds.), *Perspectives in cardiovascular psychophysiology*. New York: Guilford, 1982.

Carver, C. S., & Blaney, P. H.   Avoidance behavior and perceived arousal. *Motivation and Emotion*, 1977, *1*, 61–73. (a)

Carver, C. S., & Blaney, P. H.   Perceived arousal, focus of attention, and avoidance behavior. *Journal of Abnormal Psycholgoy*, 1977, *86*, 154–162. (b)

Clark, M., & Hirschman, R.   Effects of paced respiration on affective responses during dental stress. *Journal of Dental Research*, 1980, *59*, 1533.

Conger, J. C., Conger, A. J., & Brehm, S. S.   Fear level as a moderator of false feedback effects in snake phobics. *Journal of Consulting and Clinical Psychology*, 1976, *44*, 135–141.

Decaria, M. D., Proctor, S., & Malloy, T. E.   The effect of false heart rate feedback on self-reports of anxiety and on actual heart rate. *Behaviour Research and Therapy*, 1974, *12*, 251–253.

DeGood, D. E., Elkin, B., Lessin, S., & Valle, R. S.   Expectancy influence on self-reported experience during alpha feedback training. Subject and situational factors. *Biofeedback and Self-Regulation*, 1977, *2*, 183–194.

Detweiler, R. A., & Zanna, M. P.   Physiological mediation of attitudinal responses. *Journal of Personality and Social Psychology*, 1976, *33*, 107–116.

Gatchel, R. J.   Biofeedback and the treatment of fear and anxiety. In R. J. Gatchel & K. P. Price (Eds.), *Clinical applications of biofeedback: Appraisal and status*. Elmsford, N.Y.: Pergamon, 1979.

Gatchel, R. J., Hatch, J. P., Maynard, A., Turns, R., & Taunton-Blackwood, A.   Comparison of heart rate biofeedback, false biofeedback, and systematic desensitization in reducing speech anxiety: Short- and long-term effectiveness. *Journal of Consulting and Clinical Psychology*, 1979, *47*, 620–622.

Gatchel, R. J., Hatch, J. P., Watson, P. J., Smith, D., & Gaas, E.   Comparative effectiveness of voluntary heart rate control and muscular relaxation as active coping skills for reducing speech anxiety. *Journal of Consulting and Clinical Psychology*, 1977, *45*, 1093–1100.

Gatchel, R. J., & Proctor, J. D.   Effectiveness of voluntary heart rate control in reducing speech anxiety. *Journal of Consulting and Clinical Psychology*, 1976, *44*, 381–389.

Gaupp, L. A., Stern, R. M., & Galbraith, G. G.   False heart-rate feedback and reciprocal inhibition by aversion relief in the treatment of snake avoidance behavior. *Behavior Therapy*, 1972, *3*, 7–20.

Giesen, M., & Hendrick, C.   Effects of false positive and negative arousal feedback on persuasion. *Journal of Personality and Social Psychology*, 1974, *30*, 449–457.

Goldstein, D., Fink, D., & Mettee, D. R.   Cognition of arousal and actual arousal as determinants of emotion. *Journal of Personality and Social Psychology*, 1972, *21*, 41–51.

Hanna, R., Wilfling, F., & McNeill, B.   A biofeedback treatment for stuttering. *Journal of Speech and Hearing Disorders*, 1975, *40*, 270–273.

Harris, V. A., & Jellison, J. M.   Fear-arousing communications, false physiological feedback, and the acceptance of recommendations. *Journal of Experimental Social Psychology*, 1971, *7*, 269–279.

Harris, V. A., & Katkin, E. S.   Primary and secondary emotional behavior: An analysis of the role of autonomic feedback on affect, arousal, and attribution. *Psychological Bulletin*, 1975, *81*, 904–916.

Harvey, F., & Hirschman, R.   The influence of extraversion and neuroticism on heart rate responses to aversive visual stimuli. *Personality and Individual Differences*, 1980, *1*, 97–100.

Hendrick, C.   *Fear arousal and attitude change: A general hypothesis*. Unpublished manuscript, Kent State University, 1968.

Hendrick, C., Giesen, M., & Borden, R.   False physiological feedback and persuasion: Effect of fear arousal vs. fear reduction on attitude change. *Journal of Personality*, 1975, *43*, 196–214.

Hirschman, R.   Cross-modal effects of anticipatory bogus heart rate feedback in a negative emotional context. *Journal of Personality and Social Psychology*, 1975, *31*, 13–19.

Hirschman, R., & Brumbaugh-Buehler, R.   Electrodermal habituation and subjective responses: The effects of manifest anxiety and autonomic arousal. *Journal of Abnormal Psychology*, 1975, *84*, 46–50.

Hirschman, R., Clark, M., & Hawk, G.   Relative effects of bogus physiological feedback and control stimuli on autonomic and self-report indicants of emotional attribution. *Personality and Social Psychology Bulletin*, 1977, *3*, 270–275.

Hirschman, R., & Favaro, L.   Relationship between imagery vividness and voluntary heart rate control. *Personality and Individual Differences*, 1980, *1*, 129–133.

Hirschman, R., & Hawk, G.   Emotional responsivity to nonveridical heart rate feedback as a function of anxiety. *Journal of Research in Personality*, 1978, *12*, 235–242.

Hirschman, R., & Katkin, E. S.   Relationships among attention, GSR activity and perceived similarity of self and others. *Journal of Personality*, 1971, *39*, 277–289.

Hirschman, R., & Revland, P.   Effects of heart rate feedback on dental stress. *Journal of Dental Research*, 1979, *58*, 323. (Abstract)

Hirschman, R., & Revland, P.   *Effects of accurate and inverted heart rate feedback on response to stress: A cognitive mediation view.* Manuscript in preparation, 1983.

Hirschman, R., Young, D., & Nelson, C.   Physiologically based techniques for stress reduction. In B. D. Ingersoll & W. R. McCutcheon (Eds.), *Clinical research in behavioral dentistry.* Morgantown: West Virginia University Foundation, 1979.

Holmes, D. S., & Frost, R. D.   Effect of false autonomic feedback on self-reported anxiety, pain perception and pulse rate. *Behavior Therapy*, 1976, *7*, 330–334.

James, W.   *The principles of psychology* (Vol. 2). New York: Holt, 1890.

Kent, R. N., Wilson G. T., & Nelson, R.   Effects of false heart-rate feedback on avoidance behavior: An investigation of "cognitive desensitization." *Behavior Therapy*, 1972, *3*, 1–6.

Kerber, K. W., & Coles, M. G. H.   The role of perceived physiological activity in affective judgments. *Journal of Experimental Social Psychology*, 1978, *14*, 419–433.

Kleinke, C. L.   Self-labeling of bodily states. *Catalog of Selected Documents in Psychology*, 1977, *7*, 38–39. (MS. 1468)

Klinge, V.   Effects of exteroceptive feedback and instructions on control of spontaneous galvanic skin responses. *Psychophysiology*, 1972, *9*, 305–317.

Koenig, K. P.   False emotional feedback and the modification of anxiety. *Behavior Therapy*, 1973, *4*, 193–202.

Koenig, K. P., & Del Castillo, D.   False feedback and longevity of the conditioned GSR during extinction: Some implications of aversion therapy. *Journal of Abnormal Psychology*, 1969, *74*, 505–510.

Kondo, C., & Canter, A.   True and false electromyographic feedback: Effect on tension headache. *Journal of Abnormal Psychology*, 1977, *86*, 93–95.

Lacey, B. C., & Lacey, J. I.   Two way communication between the heart and the brain: Significance of time within the cardiac cycle. *American Psychologist*, 1978, *33*, 99–113.

Lacey, J. I., Kagan, J., Lacey, B. C., & Moss, H. A.   The visceral level: Situational determinants and behavioral correlates of autonomic response patterns. In P. Knapp (Ed.), *Expression of the emotions in man.* New York: International Universities, Press, 1963.

Lang, P. J.   Fear reduction and fear behavior: Problems in treating a construct. In J. M. Schlien (Ed.), *Research in psychotherapy* (Vol. 3). Washington, D.C.: American Psychological Association, 1968.

Lazarus, R. S.   *Psychological stress and the coping process.* New York: McGraw-Hill, 1966.

Lazarus, R. S.   A cognitivist's reply to Zajonc on emotion and cognition. *American Psychologist*, 1981, *36*, 222–223.

Lick, J.   Expectancy, false galvanic skin response feedback, and systematic desensitization in the modification of phobic behavior. *Journal of Consulting and Clinical Psychology*, 1975, *43*, 557–567.

Liebhart, E. H.   Information search and attribution: Cognitive processes mediating the effect of false autonomic feedback. *European Journal of Social Psychology*, 1979, *9*, 19–37.

Liebhart, E. H.   Perceived autonomic changes as determinants of emotional behavior. In

D. Görlitz (Ed.), *Perspectives on attribution research and theory: The Bielefeld Symposium.* Cambridge, Mass.: Ballinger, 1980.

Lykken, D. T.   A study of anxiety in the sociopathic personality. *Journal of Abnormal and Social Psychology,* 1957, *55,* 6–10.

Lykken, D. T.   Valins' "emotionality and autonomic reactivity": An appraisal. *Journal of Experimental Research in Personality,* 1967, *2,* 49–55.

Mandler, G., Mandler, J. M., & Uviller, E. T.   Autonomic feedback: The perception of autonomic activity. *Journal of Abnormal and Social Psychology,* 1958, *56,* 367–373.

Mathews, A. M.   Psychophysiological approaches to the instigation of desensitization and related procedures. *Psychological Bulletin,* 1971, *76,* 73–91.

Meichenbaum, D.   Cognitive factors in behavior modification: Modifying what clients say to themselves. In C. M. Franks & G. T. Wilson (Eds.), *Annual review of behavior therapy: Theory and practice.* New York: Brunner/Mazel, 1973.

Meichenbaum, D.   Toward a cognitive theory of self control. In G. Schwartz & D. Shapiro (Eds.), *Consciousness and self-regulation: Advances in research.* New York: Plenum, 1975.

Misovich, S., & Charis, P. C.   Information need, affect, and cognition of autonomic activity. *Journal of Experimental Social Psychology,* 1974, *10,* 274–283.

Parkinson, B., & Manstead, A. S. R.   An examination of the roles played by meaning of feedback and attention to feedback in the "Valins effect." *Journal of Personality and Social Psychology,* 1981, *40,* 239–245.

Pittman, T. S., Cooper, E. E., & Smith, T. W.   Attribution of causality and the overjustification effect. *Personality and Social Psychology Bulletin,* 1977, *3,* 280–283.

Plotkin, W. B.   The role of attributions of responsibility in the facilitation of unusual experiential states during alpha training: An analysis of the biofeedback placebo effect. *Journal of Abnormal Psychology,* 1980, *89,* 67–78.

Pressner, J. A., & Savitsky, J. C.   Effect of contingent and noncontingent feedback and subject expectancies on electroencephalogram biofeedback training. *Journal of Consulting and Clinical Psychology,* 1977, *45,* 713–814.

Reeves, J. L., & Shapiro, D.   Heart rate biofeedback and cold pressor pain. *Psychophysiology,* 1982, *19,* 393–403.

Reisman, S., Insko, C. A., & Valins, S.   Triadic consistency and false heart-rate feedback. *Journal of Personality,* 1970, *38,* 629–640.

Rosen, G. M., Rosen, E., & Reid, J. B.   Cognitive desensitization and avoidance behavior: A reevaluation. *Journal of Abnormal Psychology,* 1972, *80,* 176–182.

Rupert, P. A., & Holmes, D. S.   Effects of multiple sessions of true and placebo heart rate biofeedback training on the heart rates and anxiety levels of anxious patients during and following treatment. *Psychophysiology,* 1978, *15,* 582–590.

Schachter, S., & Singer, J. E.   Cognitive, social, and physiological determinants of emotional state. *Psychological Review,* 1962, *69,* 379–399.

Stern, G. S., Berrenberg, J. L., Winn, D., & Dubois, D. L.   Contingent and noncontingent feedback in pulse rate change and reduction in depressive cognitions. *Biofeedback and Self-Regulation,* 1978, *3,* 277–285.

Stern, G. S., Miller, C. R., Ewy, H. W., & Grant, P. S.   Bogus pulse rate feedback and reported symptom reduction for individuals with accumulated stressful life events. *Biofeedback and Self-Regulation,* 1980, *5,* 37–49.

Stern, R. M., Botto, R. W., & Herrick, C. D.   Behavioral and physiological effects of false heart rate feedback: A replication and extension. *Psychophysiology,* 1972, *9,* 21–29.

Sushinsky, L. W., & Bootzin, R. R.   Cognitive desensitization as a model of systematic desensitization. *Behaviour Research and Therapy,* 1970, *8,* 29–33.

Tarler-Benlolo, L.   The role of relaxation in biofeedback training: A critical review of the literature. *Psychological Bulletin,* 1978, *85,* 727–755.

Taylor, J. A.   A personality scale of manifest anxiety. *Journal of Abnormal and Social Psychology,* 1953, *48,* 285–290.

Taylor, S. E.   On inferring one's attitudes from one's behavior: Some delimiting conditions. *Journal of Personality and Social Psychology*, 1975, *31*, 126–131.

Thornton, E. W., & Hagan, P. J.   A failure to explain the effects of false heart-rate feedback on affect by induced changes in physiological response. *British Journal of Psychology*, 1976, *67*, 359–365.

Turk, D. C., Meichenbaum, D. H., & Berman, W. H.   Application of biofeedback for the regulation of pain: A critical review. *Psychological Bulletin*, 1979, *86*, 1322–1338.

Valins, S.   Cognitive effects of false heart-rate feedback. *Journal of Personality and Social Psychology*, 1966, *4*, 400–408.

Valins, S.   Emotionality and information concerning internal reactions. *Journal of Personality and Social Psychology*, 1967, *6*, 458–463.

Valins, S., & Ray, A. A.   Effects of cognitive desensitization on avoidance behavior. *Journal of Personality and Social Psychology*, 1967, *7*, 345–350.

Valle, R. S., & Levine, J. M.   Expectation effects in alpha wave control. *Psychophysiology*, 1975, *12*, 306–309.

White, M. D., & Wilkins, W.   Bogus physiological feedback and response thresholds of repressers and sensitizers. *Journal of Research in Personality*, 1973, *7*, 78–87.

Wilson, G. T.   Effects of false feedback on avoidance behavior: "Cognitive" desensitization revisited. *Journal of Personality and Social Psychology*, 1973, *28*, 115–122.

Woll, S. B., & McFall, M. E.   The effects of false feedback on attributed arousal and rated attractiveness in female subjects. *Journal of Personality*, 1979, *47*, 214–229.

Wolpe, J.   *Psychotherapy by reciprocal inhibition.* Stanford, Calif.: Stanford University Press, 1958.

Wolpe, J.   The behavioristic conception of neurosis: A reply to two critics. *Psychological Review*, 1971, *78*, 341–343.

Young, D., Hirschman, R., & Clark, M.   Nonveridical heart rate feedback and emotional attribution. *Bulletin of the Psychonomic Society*, 1982, *20*, 301–304.

CHAPTER 8

Transfer
of Excitation
in Emotional Behavior

Dolf Zillmann
Indiana University

In this chapter the theory of excitation transfer (Zillmann, 1978, 1979) is presented in paradigm form, the assumptions on which this theory is based are elaborated, and the propositions of the theory are developed. The conditions under which excitation transfer occurs or does not occur are specified and discussed in the light of the available research evidence. Individual differences in the propensity for transfer are considered. Phases are distinguished in the dissipation of excitation, and the phase for transfer is delineated. The mediation of delayed behavior that is instigated by emotional experiences is analyzed. Finally, differences in the mechanics of transfer in humans and subhuman species are discussed, and a unified theory of excitation transfer, applicable to higher and lower vertebrates as well as to humans, is outlined.

EXCITATION-TRANSFER THEORY

The paradigm of excitation transfer addresses the influence of emotional reactions on subsequent, potentially unrelated emotional behaviors and emotional experiences. More specifically, it pertains to contiguous sequences of emotional responses, and it deals with the conditions under which a preceding emotional reaction will or will not intensify a subsequent one. Excitation-transfer theory is the application of the three-factor theory of emotion (Zillmann, 1978, 1979) to such behavior sequences. It projects the intensification of subsequent emotional behaviors and emotional experiences as a function of residual sympathetic excitation from preceding emotional reactions. Figure 8-1 presents a transfer model in which residues of excitation from prior stimulation combine additively with excitation in response to subsequent stimulation, with the combined sympathetic ac-

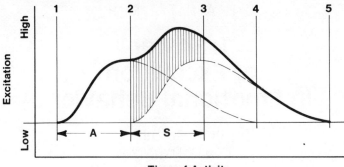

FIGURE 8-1. Model of excitation transfer in which residual excitation from a preceding excitatory reaction combines additively with the excitatory reaction to current stimulation. An antecedent stimulus condition (A), persisting from time 1 to time 2, is assumed to produce excitatory activity that has entirely decayed only at time 4. Similarly, a subsequent stimulus condition (S), persisting from time 2 to time 3, is assumed to produce excitatory activity that has entirely decayed only at time 5. Residual excitation from condition A and excitation specific to condition S combine from time 2 to time 4. The extent to which the transfer of residues from condition A increases the excitatory activity associated with condition S is shown in the shaded area. From **Hostility and aggression** by D. Zillmann, Hillsdale, N.J.: Erlbaum, 1979, p. 337. Copyright 1979 by Lawrence Erlbaum Associates. Reprinted by permission.

tivity expected to intensify the emotional experience and emotional behaviors during the subsequent stimulation.

In brief, three-factor theory distinguishes among the dispositional, excitatory, and experiential components of emotional behavior.

The *dispositional* component is conceived of as a response-guiding mechanism, with motoric reactions largely under stimulus and reinforcement control. The initial skeletal–motor behavior associated with emotions is thus seen as a direct response to emotion-inducing stimuli that can be made without the considerable latency characteristic of complex cognitive mediation.

The *excitatory* component is conceived of as a response-energizing mechanism. Excitatory reactions, analogous to skeletal–motor reactions, are also assumed to be under stimulus and reinforcement control, again without the necessary involvement of complex cognitive mediation. In accordance with Cannon's (1929) proposal of the "emergency" nature of emotional behavior, the excitatory reaction associated with emotional states is viewed as heightened activity in the sympathetic nervous system, primarily, that prepares the organism for the temporary engagement in vigorous action such as that needed for fight or flight. The provision of energy for vigorous skeletal–motor behavior can be seen as motivating the organism to perform such behavior. It is not assumed, however, that any impulsion to act has specific appetitive properties. This is to say that, unlike in deprivation-based behaviors such as hunger and thirst, the excitatory emergency reaction in emotion is impartial to specific emotions (e.g., fear vs. anger) and depends on independent response-guiding mechanisms.

The *experiential* component of emotional behavior, finally, is conceptualized as the conscious experience of either the skeletal–motor or the excitatory reaction or of both these aspects of the response to a stimulus condition. It is thus assumed that exteroceptive and/or interoceptive information about any facet of an immediate emotional reaction may reach the awareness level, enabling the individual to appraise the precipitating and experiential circumstances, and fostering a continual monitoring of his or her behavior. Such monitoring allows the individual to assess the utility and appropriateness of emotional reactions and actions, and—within limits —to modify and correct behavioral efforts. In principle, then, the experiential component of emotions is viewed as a corrective that can substantially alter unfolding emotional behavior. It can be construed as a cognitive means of influence capable of modifying and, potentially, of overriding the more archaic, basic mechanics of stimulus and reinforcement control.

Figure 8-2 further explicates the three-factor theory of emotion.

Applied to emotional reactions in sequence, three-factor theory projects excitatory reactions that are unlearned (e.g., startle) or learned (e.g., acquired phobias). However, although the initial reactions, especially their magnitude, are assumed to elude voluntary control, the dissipation of excitation—or the maintenance of high levels of excitation, respectively— may be greatly influenced by appraisal and monitoring. Analogously, initial skeletal–motor reactions, including reactions in the facial muscles, are unlearned or learned. As such reactions are being monitored, however, they are likely to be modified or inhibited. Since skeletal–motor activities are largely under voluntary control, the inhibition of incipient responses may be complete and comparatively fast. Taken together, the organism seems capable of rapid adjustment to stimulus changes only with regard to skeletal–motor behavior. Excitatory adjustment is inefficient, and it tends to be incomplete for extended periods of time. It is this imperfection in the excitatory adjustment, of course, that is the basis of transfer theory: Residues of excitation from a preceding emotional reaction enter into and intensify (i.e., they are being *transferred* into) a subsequent state which is the result of appropriate dispositional and experiential assimilation of a change in the stimulus condition.

Assumptions

Transfer theory is based on the following assumptions (cf. Zillmann, 1978).

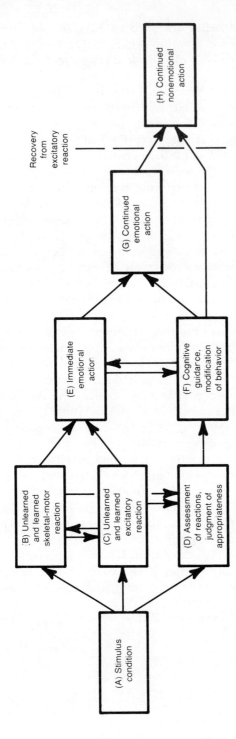

FIGURE 8-2. Essentials of three-factor theory. A stimulus (A) elicits skeletal-motor (B) and excitatory (C) reactions. Both B and C (the dispositional and excitatory component, respectively) are under stimulus and reinforcement control and combine to produce immediate emotional action (E). B includes reactions in the facial muscles and overt and covert verbal reactions. All reactions under B and C, through afferent impulses and perception of external effects, are monitored under D (the experiential component). Reactions deemed inappropriate are corrected (i.e., partially or completely inhibited, strengthened, altered); reactions deemed appropriate maintained (F). Incipient reactions (E) may thus be stopped and redirected by processes under D and F. Continued emotional action (G) derives from E, but is modified by D and F. Action under G can be continued or delayed beyond the dissipation of excitation. Processes under F can motivate action under H. See the text for further explanation.

218

1. The excitatory activity of emotions that are characterized by sympathetic dominance in the autonomic nervous system is largely nonspecific.
Across such emotions, there is considerable redundancy in the pattern of
excitatory reactions.

The assumed excitatory redundancy in these so-called "active emotions" (cf. Leventhal, 1979) is viewed as the result of the organism's
preparedness for energy expenditure. This preparedness is often due to
the behavioral emergency—Cannon's (1929) fight-or-flight reaction—that
many active emotions entail. In states of anger or fear, for instance, the
preparedness for energy expenditure potentially serves the termination or
reduction of aversion through attack of or escape from the aversive condition. However, this preparedness may also serve energy-consuming behaviors that appear to be devoid of aversive elements. Reproductive behavior is a case in point.

It is generally held that the action component of acute emotional
states constitutes an evolutionary remnant. The preparedness for vigorous
motor activity and for endurance, accomplished mainly through the dilation of the blood vessels in the muscles by discharge from the posterior
hypothalamus through the sympathetic cholinergic nerves (cf. Gellhorn,
1967; Grossman, 1967), had great survival value in earlier times. For life in
modern society, much of this value has been lost. In fact, the impulsion
toward motor discharge during acute emotions has become potentially
maladaptive. It is certainly the exception that emotional problems can be
resolved through immediate, vigorous responses. Notwithstanding the
loss of adaptive value and the potentiality for maladaption, the preparedness for energy expenditure has persisted in humans as a most salient
component of emotional reactions (cf. Gellhorn, 1968; MacLean, 1964;
Malmo, 1975; Zillmann, 1979).

The assumption of excitatory redundancy accommodates the research
evidence on the specificity versus nonspecificity of excitatory reactions in
emotional states (cf. Shapiro & Crider, 1969). Nonspecificity has been
observed both in peripheral manifestations of sympathetic excitation, such
as heart rate acceleration, blood pressure elevation, and increased vasoconstriction (e.g., Adamson, Romano, Burdick, Corman, & Chebib, 1972;
Averill, 1969; Craig & Wood, 1971), and in excitatory endocrine processes,
such as increased circulation of catecholamines (e.g., Levi, 1965, 1967;
Pátkai, 1971). On the other hand, emotion-specific excitatory response
patterns have also been recorded in both peripheral manifestations (e.g.,
Ax, 1953; Engel, 1960; J. Schachter, 1957; Wenger & Cullen, 1958) and
endocrine processes (e.g., Barclay & Little, 1972; Elmadjian, Hope, &
Lamson, 1957, 1958; Funkenstein, 1956). Many of the apparent inconsistencies may be due to differences in the research procedures employed
(cf. Wenger, Clemens, Coleman, Cullen, & Engel, 1961), to differences in

the specific excitatory responses sampled (cf. Zillmann, 1983), and to the enormous difficulties in creating genuine emotional reactions in laboratory subjects (cf. Chessick, Bassan, & Shattan, 1966). Regardless of the particular source of the discrepant findings, however, the evidence at hand supports neither an assumption of pure nonspecificity nor one of pure specificity. This assessment, it should be noted, does not detract from the fact that all vital emotions have strong sympathetic discharge as a common element (cf. Grossman, 1967, 1968; Kety, 1970; Oken, 1967). Surely, there are excitatory differences among emotions. In a state of sexual arousal, for instance, tumescence should be more pronounced than in a state of anger or fear. But strong sympathetic discharge should be common to all these states.

The assumed excitatory redundancy, then, is projected primarily in terms of sympathetic activity, and it might be characterized as "sympathetic nonspecificity" or, perhaps more appropriately, as "sympathetic commonality."

The projection of sympathetic commonality is independent of hedonic considerations. Counter to earlier contentions in which negative emotions such as grief were thought to be accompanied by a general decrease in physiological functioning (e.g., Wenger, Jones, & Jones, 1956), positive and negative emotions have been shown to hold comparable sympathetic charges. Mirth and sadness (e.g., Averill, 1969) and pleasure and distress (e.g., Levi, 1965; Pátkai, 1971) have been found to be sympathetically comparable.

Furthermore, the projection of sympathetic commonality is most compatible with the proposal of individual excitatory response stereotypy (Lacey, 1967; Lacey & Lacey, 1958). The plasticity of the autonomic nervous system is not in doubt (cf. DiCara, 1970), and considerable individual differences in the pattern of autonomic responses to emotion-evoking stimuli must be expected on the basis of different conditioning histories (cf. Kimmel, 1974). Individual response stereotypy—that is, the individual's tendency to display somewhat similar autonomic reaction patterns in different emotions—may result from a selective utilization and sensitization of particular autonomic structures. Regardless of the possible mechanics of stereotypy formation, individual autonomic response stereotypy has been recorded (e.g., Lacey, 1950; Lacey, Bateman, & VanLehn, 1953). It has been found to be comparatively weak, however (e.g., Goldstein, Grinker, Heath, Oken, & Shipman, 1964; Wenger, Clemens, Coleman, Cullen, & Engel, 1961). Thus, although it seems possible to create unique, highly personalized excitatory response patterns through the arbitrary and deliberate management of reinforcement contingencies, it must be considered very unlikely that under common environmental and social conditions the formation of stereotypy could fundamentally alter characteristic excitatory response patterns. In terms of both theory (cf. Grossman, 1968; Tarpy, 1977) and research (cf. Frankenhaeuser, 1978; Grings & Dawson, 1978), the sympathetic reaction component of emotions, in particular, appears to be highly persistent and robust. It is to be expected, then, that individual autonomic response stereotypy will modify the excitatory response to emotion-evoking stimuli; it will do so, however, without critically altering the basic, sympathetic response tendencies—even without disturbing the high degree of redundancy that is to be expected among the various sympathetic activities (e.g., Schnore, 1959).

If, as is suggested, individual autonomic response stereotypy is limited in scope and does not entirely control sympathetic activity, it may be considered most conducive to excitation transfer. Obviously, the greater the degree of structural similarity in the patterned response to different emotions, the easier it should be for residues from one particular emotion to merge with the excitatory pattern of another.

As will be recalled, the assumption of substantial autonomic nonspecificity was limited to emotions characterized by sympathetic dominance. Transfer predictions are based primarily on residues of sympathetic excitation. These residues are expected to combine with sympathetic activity evoked by subsequent stimulation. It follows that states that fail to provide such residues cannot produce transfer, and that states that are characterized by subnormal levels of sympathetic activity cannot be meaningfully enhanced by residual sympathetic excitation from preceding experiences. It has been observed, for instance, that depressed persons tend to be hypoactive sympathetically (e.g., Frankenhaeuser & Pátkai, 1965; Schildkraut, 1973; Schildkraut & Kety, 1967). To the extent that depression is regarded an emotion, it thus should not be expected to enhance subsequent emotions through excitation transfer, or to be enhanced by excitation transfer from other emotions. Similarly, the transfer paradigm does not apply directly to depression-related states such as apathy; nor does it apply directly to other experiential states that are potentially hyposympathetic, such as feelings of acceptance and trust (Plutchik, 1980).

> 2. Interoception of activity in the autonomic nervous system is highly nonspecific to emotion. Exteroceptive feedback is similarly nonspecific.[1]

Interoceptive and exteroceptive nonspecificity is due largely to the high degree of nonspecificity of the autonomic activity itself. In addition, however, both interoception and exteroception appear to be poorly developed and fail to provide accurate representations of prevailing patterned states of excitation. In fact, even feedback of elementary autonomic

---

1. Interoception refers to symptoms of an arousal state that originate inside the body (e.g., palpitation, sensation of increased tenseness). Exteroception refers to the perception of external concomitants and manifestations of an arousal state (e.g., perspiration, tremble of hands).

changes, such as heart rate acceleration or blood pressure elevation, seems ambiguous and usually yields rather unreliable accounts. Research into the accuracy of autonomic perception (e.g., Mandler & Kahn, 1960; Mandler & Kremen, 1958; Mandler, Mandler, Kremen, & Sholiton, 1961; Thayer, 1967, 1970) indeed shows such perception to be quite imprecise. On the other hand, it appears that the mammalian organism is endowed with the capacity for considerable interoceptive sensitivity (cf. Adám, 1967; Chernigovskiy, 1967), and that humans, if properly trained, are capable of discriminating comparatively minute autonomic changes (cf. Brener, 1974, 1977; Schwartz, 1976, 1977). The commonly observed imprecision of autonomic perception, then, seems not to be a consequence of insufficient faculties, but rather the result of the lack of utilization of an existing capacity. Presumably, interoceptive feedback of autonomic activity has less adaptive utility than feedback from potentially more sensitive structures, such as the facial muscles (e.g., Izard, 1977; Leventhal, 1979; Tomkins, 1962, 1963). It probably also has less utility than information from the immediate environment (e.g., Mandler, 1962; S. Schachter, 1964). The relative neglect of this feedback, especially the limitation of awareness of specific autonomic changes, may thus have served adaptation by minimizing interference with the attentional control of the environment and with the preparation and execution of appropriate actions (cf. Shapiro, 1974).

> 3. Individuals can determine the intensity of their excitatory reactions through interoception and/or exteroception. However, only comparatively gross excitatory changes will draw attention and produce awareness of the state of excitation.

This assumption is in accordance with the demonstrated imprecision of the perception of specific autonomic changes. As Mandler (1975) suggested, the *functional* autonomic feedback in emotion is probably "general autonomic arousal" that varies "in degree but not in discriminable pattern" (p. 128).

Additionally, the assumption accords with considerations of feedback from general somatic activity, especially from activity in the muscles. Gellhorn (e.g., 1964) has stressed the close correspondence between autonomic and somatic processes. Apparently, sympathetic excitation and muscle tone undergo parallel changes. "Upward" discharges from the posterior hypothalamus to the cerebral cortex are associated with sympathetic–somatic "downward" discharges of proportional intensity. Proprioceptive impulses from the muscles reach the cerebellum and the motor cortex, and collaterals from the specific afferent systems feed into the reticular formation and the hypothalamus. The involvement of these structures fosters diffuse excitation, and proprioception is likely to reflect this diffuseness. Somatic feedback, then, appears to parallel autonomic feedback in that it represents a variation in intensity, not in patterned specificity. The systems thus seem highly redundant functionally. However, with interoception of autonomic processes having received considerable attention (e.g., Mandler, 1975; Valins, 1970) and proprioception of somatic processes having been largely neglected (e.g., Shields & Stern, 1979), the relative contribution of these feedback systems to the formation of emotional experiences and to the energization of emotional behaviors remains to be determined.

> 4. Individuals tend to link excitatory reactions of which they become aware to conditions that apparently induced these reactions. The linkages and their constituents may be recalled at later times, probably in the form of emotional experiences (i.e., feeling states) of which they are an integral part.

Clearly, the linkages can be construed as causal attributions (e.g., Jones & Davis, 1965; Kelley, 1967, 1971). Individuals appear to ascribe an effect (i.e., the excitatory reaction) to a particular cause (i.e., the inducing condition). The specifics of this presumed ascription are quite unclear and controversial, however. At issue is the extent to which such attributions are motivated by epistemic pressures (i.e., a need to comprehend the cause-and-effect relationship) and the degree to which they are formally executed (i.e., thought out explicitly or recognized in fragments).

Many investigators (e.g., Konečni, 1975; Rule, Ferguson, & Nesdale, 1979) have followed S. Schachter (1964) in assuming that the perception of increased autonomic arousal occasions a search for an explanation that eventually, via the causal attribution of the arousal reaction, produces an emotion-defining label for the experience. The universality of this process in the genesis of emotional reactions appears highly questionable, however (cf. Zillmann, 1978). Schachter's approach to emotion is at variance with the fact that emotional reactions tend to be executed before the organism can attain feedback from autonomic changes. Behavioral responses to emotion-inducing stimuli can be quasi-instantaneous; the peripheral manifestations of autonomic responses, in contrast, have a characteristic latency of 3 to 15 seconds (e.g., Grossman, 1967; Newman, Perkins, & Wheeler, 1930). Quite obviously, emotional behavior would have had little adaptive value if individuals would have had to await feedback from excitation in peripheral structures in order to comprehend their reaction and decide on an appropriate course of action. Regardless of such evolutionary considerations, however, epistemic searches that would serve the explanation of perceived autonomic activity seem mostly superfluous because individuals are provided with emotion-determining feedback from potentially more sensitive structures prior to the unfolding of autonomic reactions. Any overt behavioral reaction, according to long-standing theory on emotion (e.g., Henle, 1876; James, 1884), virtually forces upon individuals the recognition of their emotions. In the absence of skeletal-muscular action, reactions in the facial muscles—even only incipient motion—furnish the proprioception capable of instantly determining emotional reactions in kind (e.g., Gellhorn, 1964; Izard, 1977; Leventhal, 1979). It would seem quite misleading, then, to implicate cognitive efforts toward resolving emerging autonomic ambiguities with a critical emotion-determining function.

Whereas autonomic feedback is probably of little, if any, consequence in the determination of specific emotional reactions, it is likely to be significantly involved in the determination of emotional *experiences*. In concert with other sources of information about excitatory activity (e.g., somatic feedback), it provides individuals with information about the existence and strength of excitatory reactions. In other words, it aids in the subjective assessment of emotional states, especially in the assessment of their intensity. This assessment has, of course, significant implications both for the emotional states themselves and for subsequent behaviors (cf. Zillmann, 1978, 1979).

The assessment is likely to involve some form of attribution of the excitatory reaction to an inducer. Even if these attributions are not considered to be motivated by a need to explain an otherwise incomprehensible reaction, but are regarded instead as acquired verbal habits, the question about their specific manifestations remains to be answered. Some investigators (e.g., Barefoot & Straub, 1971; Nisbett & Valins, 1971) have projected a time-consuming reasoning process, presumably executed in covert linguistic operations at the awareness level. Others (e.g., Rule *et al.*, 1979) have suggested that attributions can be made without the individuals' awareness and that—although the attributions are supposed to satisfy a search for the cause of a reaction—they can occur simultaneously with the onset of a physiological reaction. Attributions, in short, have been conceived of both as inferences drawn in some sort of inner monologue and as entirely hypothetical entities that are without specified manifestations and whose performance does not consume an appreciable amount of time.

Alternatively, it has been suggested (Zillmann, 1978, 1979) that attributions are implicit in covert verbal responses to situational stimuli and/or to the overt and covert bodily reactions elicited by these stimuli. A person might respond to provocation, for example, with "You stupid idiot!," "This isn't fair!," or "Boy, I'll get you for this!" The verbal responses will thus make obtrusive the kind of emotion experienced, namely annoyance and anger, as well as the inducing condition. Similarly, a person who responds with "My God, this gives me the creeps!" will experience little need to infer more formally the specifics of the emotional experience. It is suggested, then, that the flow of covert (and occasionally overt) verbal responses to a situation, highly idiosyncratic as it may be, constitutes the cognitive side of emotional experiences and determines, through implicit attribution, the subjective typology of such experiences. Upon reflection, and especially upon querying in a research situation, individuals should, of course, be able to convert implicit causal linkages into more formal causal attributions. The response "You stupid idiot!," for example, may readily be transformed into "His behavior annoyed me," or "He made me very angry."

The flow of covert verbal responses may be greatly influenced by autonomic and somatic feedback. Strong sensations of tenseness in response to provocation, for example, may prompt strong verbiage. Similarly, the perception of intense palpitation in response to acute danger may foster extreme verbal responses. These "labels" may be considered part and parcel of emotional experiences. As responses, they signal the intensity of affect; and this signaling function makes them stimuli, in turn, for emotional actions to follow. Covert verbal responses are an essential part of the experiential component of emotion and probably influence the course of events to a large measure. It is likely, for instance, that they greatly facilitate the recall of emotional experiences, especially the recall of the intensity of these experiences (cf. Maltzman, 1968; Osgood, 1953; Staats & Staats, 1963). In addition, they probably aid the reinstatement of components of emotional reactions, and they may serve in the perpetuation of behavioral intentions that were expressed at times of intense excitation. Responses such as "I will get you for this . . . and if it's the last thing I do!" not only index the intensity of anger during acute emotion and in retrospect, but—because of the traces they leave behind—may instigate retaliatory action long after the dissipation of the emotional experience proper (cf. Zillmann, 1983).

> 5. Individuals do not partition excitation compounded from reactions to different inducing conditions. Autonomic and/or somatic feedback permits neither the isolation of all factors that contribute to a state of excitation, nor the apportionment of excitation to the various contributing factors. As a result, individuals tend to ascribe their excitatory reaction in toto to one specific, though potentially complex inducing condition.

This assumption implies that, in general, individuals fail to engage continually in a careful accounting of their excitatory activity. Moreover, it implies that individuals are incapable of monitoring the independent time courses of concurrent excitatory reactions with any degree of precision. Individuals seem unable, hence, to link specific reactions to specific inducers in a complex stimulus–response situation. Even if a person were instructed to focus attention on these relationships, it is unlikely that they could be delineated by procedures better than guessing. It must be expected, as a result, that individuals will misconstrue the induction of their excitatory activity to some extent.

Misperceptions concern both simultaneously induced reactions and reactions elicited in succession. A person who is provoked while exposed to loud tones, for example, is likely to be ignorant of the fact that the noise contributes to his excitatory state; he is bound to construe it (by implication!) as provocation-induced, to experience inappropriately intense anger, and eventually to aggress more strongly against his annoyer (e.g., Konečni, 1975). Similarly, a person who has seen an exciting motion picture and is provoked while still aroused from the film is apt not to recognize this circumstance and misconstrue his arousal in toto as anger and aggressiveness (e.g., Donnerstein, Donnerstein, & Barrett, 1976).

It appears that, in these misperceptions, individuals favor the strongest or most noticeable of a number of excitatory reactions. The dominant response is likely to draw attention and suggest an inducer in the immediately preceding conditions. The choice of the particular inducer seems to be determined mainly by beliefs, valid or erroneous as they may be, about stimulus–response linkages concerning arousal. It may be expected, for example, that a youngster who— based on past experience—believes rock music to be arousing and girls unexciting, and who listens to such music in the presence of his girlfriend, will erroneously attribute his entire excitatory state to the music. Analogously, a youngster who believes girls to be arousing and rock music to be unexciting will erroneously attribute prevailing excitation to the girl's presence. If both the music and the girl are deemed arousing, the linkage should be determined by the stimulus condition that was the immediate antecedent of a noticed excitatory reaction (i.e., that occurred when the reaction fostered awareness). The *preceding* stimulus is likely to be construed as the *precipitating* stimulus. If it was a particular segment of the music, the music will be implicated; if it was a long look at the girl, the girlfriend becomes the inducer. This is not to say, however, that attentional focus quasi-mechanically controls attribution (Rule *et al.*, 1979). In the absence of the belief that, for example, mental arithmetic is arousing, any excitatory reaction produced by it is likely to be ascribed to events other than the performance of arithmetical operations, regardless of the extent to which such operations are made "salient" attentionally. The suggested dependence on attentional focus relies, instead, on the plausibility of an apparent connection. Excitatory reactions will be attributed to particular inducing conditions only if such linkages strike individuals as "obvious." Attributions concerning emotional experiences, then, are viewed as being greatly influenced by established belief systems. They may, in fact, be viewed as being culturally confined, because they are—in part, at least—subject to consensual validation (cf. Barden, Zelko, Duncan, & Masters, 1980; Zillmann, 1978).

> 6. Excitatory activity, especially autonomic activity, does not terminate abruptly. Because of humoral processes involved, sympathetic excitation— in particular—dissipates comparatively slowly. Residues of this slowly decaying sympathetic excitation may thus enter into subsequent, potentially independent emotional reactions and emotional experiences.

In terms of endocrine manifestations, sympathetic excitation is activity in the sympathetic–adrenomedullary system. The release of the catechol-amines epinephrine and norepinephrine produces the emergency reaction discussed earlier (cf. Smith, 1973; Turner & Bagnara, 1971). The circulating amines mediate excitation, of course, until they are chemically converted to a nonsympathomimetic agent (cf. Axelrod, 1959, 1971). The peripheral concomitant of this conversion is the characteristic, slow decay of heart rate and blood pressure reactions, among others. Emotional behavior is also associated with increased activity in the pituitary–adrenal cortical system, where the release of corticosteroids is likely to produce elevated levels of excitation that extend far beyond the time course of emergency reactions (cf. Conner, 1972; Hennessy & Levine, 1979). There can be no doubt, then, that increased excitatory activity does not terminate with the discontinuation of emotional instigation, and that it persists to a degree that should significantly affect subsequent behavior.

Propositions

Based on these assumptions, the implications of residual excitation for emotional behavior and emotional experience can be specified as follows (cf. Zillmann, 1978).

> 1. Given a situation in which (a) individuals respond to emotion-inducing stimuli and assess their responses, (b) levels of sympathetic excitation are still elevated from prior, potentially unrelated stimulation, and (c) individuals are not provided with obtrusive intero- and/or exteroceptive cues that link their excitatory state to prior stimulation, residues of excitation from prior stimulation will inseparably combine with the excitatory reaction to the present stimuli and thereby intensify both emotional behavior and emotional experience.
> 2. Emotional behavior and/or emotional experience will be enhanced in proportion to the magnitude of transferred residual excitation.
> 3. Both the period of time during which transfer can occur and the magnitude of residues for transfer are a function of (a) the magnitude of the preceding excitatory reaction and/or (b) the rate of recovery from the associated excitatory state.
> 4. Individuals' potential for transfer is (a) proportional to their excitatory responsiveness and (b) inversely proportional to their proficiency to recover from excitatory states.

It is assumed that, in general, residual excitation and excitation generated by the emotion into which the residues transfer combine in a summative fashion (see Figure 8-1). Such an assumption is parsimonious and has proved useful in that it satisfactorily accommodates pertinent research findings (cf. Zillmann, 1979). It should be clear, however, that predictions of transfer effects cannot be based on the additive combination of two or more excitatory reactions that are assessed against basal levels. This procedure would, of course, violate the law of initial values (cf. Sternbach, 1966; Wilder, 1957). It must be assumed that the magnitude of excitatory reactions is a function of prevailing levels of excitation (i.e., prestimulus levels). Specifically, excitatory reactions are likely to be inversely proportional to prestimulus levels of excitation. Such a qualification, which is necessary mainly to prevent the prediction of excitatory intensity above maximally possible levels, gives extreme residues little power to influence extreme emotional reactions. In contrast, it projects comparatively strong transfer effects for moderate residues that enter into moderate emotional reactions.

The qualification can be readily expressed as a correction to be applied to the prediction of the intensity of the subsequent excitatory response. A linear correction, for example, would take the form

$$\alpha = 1 - \frac{p - b}{m - b}$$

where p is the prestimulus, b the basal, and m the maximal level of excitation. The factor α would modify the "normal" intensity of the subsequent excitatory response (i.e., its intensity assessed against basal levels). This intensity, clearly, would not be affected if $p = b$. If $p = m$, in contrast, it is reduced to zero. Nonlinear corrections may prove to be more appropriate, but are certainly not demanded by the scarce data at hand.

The implications of the proposition concerning individual differences in the propensity for transfer (No. 4), expressed in terms of differences in cardiovascular fitness, are visualized in Figure 8-3.

RESEARCH EVIDENCE

Transfer theory has been validated by research dealing with a wide range of emotional phenomena. It has been demonstrated, for example, that residues of excitation from physical exertion can intensify feelings of anger and aggressive behavior (Zillmann & Bryant, 1974; Zillmann, Katcher, & Milavsky, 1972) or the experience of sexual excitement (Cantor, Zillmann, & Bryant, 1975). Similarly, it has been shown that residues of sexual arousal can potentiate aggression (e.g., Donnerstein & Hallam, 1978; Meyer, 1972; Zillmann, 1971; Zillmann, Bryant, Comisky, & Medoff, 1981), that residual excitation from exposure to music can have similar effects (Bryant & Zillmann, 1979; Day, 1980), that residual sexual arousal can promote prosocial behavior (Jaffe, 1981; Mueller & Donnerstein, 1981), and that residues from either sexual arousal or disgust reactions can facilitate such diverse experiences as the enjoyment of music

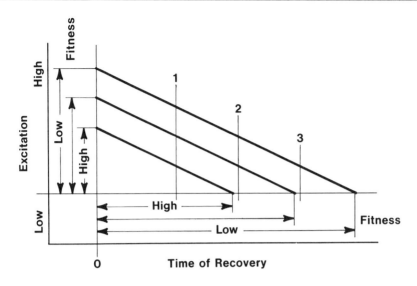

FIGURE 8-3. Illustration of the inverse relationship between cardiovascular fitness and the propensity for transfer. As shown in the simplified decay gradients, the excitatory reaction to a particular stimulus (time 0) and the time of recovery from that reaction decrease as cardiovascular fitness increases. At time 1, residual excitation for transfer exists in all fitness conditions in differing amounts. At time 2, recovery to basal levels of excitation is complete for high fitness, but the propensity for transfer is maintained, to different degrees, for intermediate and low fitness. At time 3, the propensity for transfer is maintained only for low fitness. From **Hostility and aggression** by D. Zillmann, Hillsdale, N.J.: Erlbaum, 1979, p. 345. Copyright 1979 by Lawrence Erlbaum Associates. Reprinted by permission.

(Cantor & Zillmann, 1973), appreciation of humor (Cantor, Bryant, & Zillmann, 1974), and dysphoric empathy (Zillmann, Mody, & Cantor, 1974). Residues from dysphoric empathy, in turn, can facilitate the enjoyment of drama (Zillmann, 1980). It has also been observed that humor is capable of generating arousal (Levi, 1965) that can enhance motivated aggressive behavior (Mueller & Donnerstein, 1977; Tannenbaum, 1972). Additionally, there is evidence in support of the predictions regarding individual differences in the propensity for transfer (Cantor, Zillmann, & Day, 1978; Cox, Evans, & Jamieson, 1979; Zillmann, Johnson, & Day, 1974).

These and other demonstrations of transfer effects, which have been fully reviewed elsewhere (e.g., Zillmann, 1978, 1979, 1983), will not be discussed further here. Rather, the discussion will concentrate on selected studies whose findings clarify some of the assumptions underlying transfer theory.

Critical Periods in the Dissipation of Excitation

The assumptions concerning awareness of strong excitatory reactions (No. 3) and the linkage of these reactions to inducers (No. 4) project characteristic phases in the decay of transferable excitation. In a first phase, pronounced excitatory activity should foster awareness; and this awareness, in turn, should foster the linkage of this activity to a particular inducing condition. The linkage should be "undeniable" as long as obtrusive feedback from the excitatory activity prevails (i.e., sensations of tenseness, trembling hands, heavy breathing, heart pounding, etc.). As obtrusive feedback vanishes, due primarily to the partial decay of excitation, awareness of excitatory residues and their linkage should fade as well. The dissociation of residues and inducer, together with the likely lack of recognition of the residues, defines the onset of a second phase. This second phase, then, is characterized by the persistence of excitatory residues that are no longer linked to the inducing condition. Finally, a third phase comes into being with the complete dissipation of the excitatory residues (i.e., recovery to basal levels). Figure 8-4 presents the described relationship between perceived and actual residual excitation in hypothetical gradients.

In accordance with the first proposition of transfer theory, transfer effects should occur only during phase 2. The strength of transfer effects during this phase should, of course, be proportional to the magnitude of residues transferred (see proposition 2). The strength of effects, then,

FIGURE 8-4. Phases of perceived and actual excitation during recovery. In phase 1 (point 1 to point 2), excitatory activity is still elevated and is recognized as being still elevated. In phase 2 (point 2 to point 4), excitatory activity is still elevated to different degrees, but complete recovery is perceived. In phase 3 (beyond point 4), recovery is achieved and properly perceived. Excitation transfer is expected to occur in phase 2 only, the strength of effects being proportional to the magnitude of residual excitation prevailing (i.e., strongest at point 2; successively weaker toward point 4).

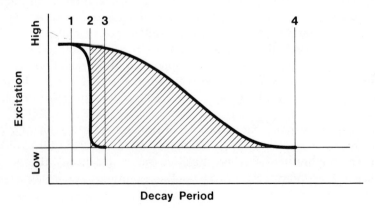

favors the initial period of the transfer phase (i.e., phase 2). In further accordance with the first proposition, transfer effects should not occur in phase 3 (see stipulation b) or in phase 1 (see stipulation c).

The validity of these conceptions has been demonstrated most clearly in an investigation by Cantor *et al.* (1975). This investigation explored transfer from exertion into sexual excitement. In a pretest, male subjects performed strenuous physical exercise. Their excitatory reactions, measured in peripheral manifestations, were assessed immediately after exertion and intermittently during recovery. The subjects' perception of the extent to which they were still aroused from exertion was assessed concurrently. The findings revealed that subjects indeed perceived recovery long before they actually had recovered. The discrepancy between perceived and actual residual excitation, which Figure 8-4 expresses in simplified gradients, was observed despite the focus of attention on arousal. To the extent that this "sensitization" may have fostered artificially long periods during which excitatory residues were reported, the discrepancy may actually be stronger. Possible bias, then, would be conservative.

The discrepant gradients were used to construct the three pertinent decay phases for the main experiment. In that experiment, male subjects were exposed to erotica and their reactions of sexual excitement were assessed. Exposure took place during the first, the second, or the third phase. Exactly as expected, sexual excitement was intensified by residual excitation in the second phase only. Subjects who were exposed to erotica during the first phase exhibited levels of sexual excitement comparable to those of subjects whose exposure to erotica occurred during the third phase. Presumably, this was because they were still short of breath, and so on, from exertion—the recognition of which prevented them from perceiving their excitedness as resulting from exposure to the erotica.

The failure of excitatory residues of great magnitude to produce transfer effects during phase 1 has also been observed in research on aggression. In an investigation by Zillmann *et al.* (1974), male subjects were provoked, performed strenuous physical exercise, and were then either immediately (phase 1) or after a delay (phase 2) provided with an opportunity to retaliate. Phases were cross-varied with levels of cardiovascular fitness. It was found that subjects behaved quite nonaggressively during phase 1, regardless of level of fitness. During phase 2, although residual excitation was of lesser magnitude, subjects' aggressive behavior was greatly intensified by prevailing residues. Superbly fit subjects, however, had fully recovered at this later time and their aggressive behavior—in accordance with transfer theory—was not intensified.

Additionally, an investigation by Younger and Doob (1978) showed that merely suggesting a causal linkage between an inducing condition and an excitatory reaction can remove much of the intensity of an emotional experience. Subjects ingested a placebo tablet and were led to expect either an arousal or a relaxation reaction. This manipulation was cross-varied with the presence or absence of subsequent provocation. It was observed that, when an opportunity for retaliation was provided, the provoked subjects who believed that the placebo was a sympathomimetic aggressed significantly less against their tormentor than their counterparts who believed it to be a sedative. In fact, the level of aggressiveness in the former condition was not appreciably different from that in the no-provocation conditions. The subjects' erroneous presumption that their excitatory reaction to the provocation treatment was due to the sympathomimetic thus seems to have deprived the aggression-mediating experience of anger of its excitatory concomitant.

Taken together, these investigations attest to both the proposed great imprecision in the intero- and/or exteroceptive assessment of residual excitation and the proposed transfer-preventing recognition of arousal-inducer linkages.

Mediation of Delayed Emotional Behavior

The assumption concerning the recall of emotional experiences that are linked to specific inducers (No. 4) has interesting consequences for delayed emotional behavior. Contingencies of reinforcement that govern human conduct frequently demand the inhibition of the overt components of motivated emotional reactions (cf. Zillmann, 1979). Also, regardless of inhibitory forces, the conditions for effective action on the emotion-inducing events are often unfavorable; consequently, immediate action is inadvisable or simply not possible. Behavior may thus be motivated by emergency reactions, but cannot be executed. Individuals are thus confined to potentially very intense emotional experiences. During these experiences, they may become cognizant of their behavioral inclinations. These intentions, in turn, may be reinstated (or reactivated, if individuals did not become cognizant of them) as the experience is recalled at later times, usually due to the encounter of experience-related stimuli. Actions that had been intended during the initial emotional experience may then be taken—possibly independent of the extent of excitatory activity produced by the recall of the experience.

The outlined relationship between emotional experience and emotional behavior frequently exists in emotional hostility and aggression. Severely provoked individuals may experience acute annoyance without being able to do anything about it at the time. However, as favorable conditions for retaliation arise at later times, they may take punitive actions whose intensity reflects that of their earlier emotional experience rather than that of the prevailing excitatory state.

These possibilities have been explored within transfer research. In an investigation by Zillmann and Bryant (1974), excitatory residues from exertion were transferred into provocation, and retaliation was delayed to a time when transferable residues had dissipated. Residual excitation was found to intensify both immediate annoyance and delayed aggressive behavior.

In this investigation, excitatory activity was traced in peripheral manifestations (blood pressure, heart rate). It could hence be argued that, although it has been shown that excitation had dissipated peripherally, it might still have lingered on in other manifestations. At the time of retaliation, then, excitation may still have been differentiated as the result of exertion. In order to rule out such an account, Bryant and Zillmann (1979) conducted a follow-up investigation in which the opportunity to retaliate was delayed by an entire week. Residual excitation from exposure to communication was transferred into provocation, intensifying the experience of annoyance. As expected, the differences created in the experienced intensity of this annoyance produced corresponding differences in delayed retaliatory behavior.

In more general terms, these investigations suggest that intense emotional experiences can profoundly influence substantially delayed emotional (or pseudoemotional) behaviors. The mechanics of this influence remain rather unclear, however. Specifically, it is unclear to what extent the effect is mediated by the recall of the circumstances that precipitated and followed the emotional experience and to what extent it depends on the recall of the bodily and cognitive manifestations of the experience itself. The extent to which processes other than recall are involved is equally unclear. It is conceivable, for instance, that the seemingly deliberate recall of emotional experiences revives, to some degree, their original excitatory accompaniment. Alternatively, however, it is conceivable that such revival is under stimulus control in learning-theoretical terms, and that the vivid recall of the various facets of emotional experiences is initiated and greatly facilitated by the activation of stimulus–response connections that were formed during the initial experiences. The likely partial recreation of the excitatory activity associated with the original emotional experiences, in turn, may be critically involved in the mediation of delayed emotional behaviors. Research has simply failed to explore the possible mechanics, despite their potential significance for emotional behavior.

TOWARD A UNIFIED THEORY

Excitation transfer appears to be a phenomenon that occurs in many species, potentially in all species in which comparatively time-consuming humoral processes are critically involved in the mediation of behavior-

energizing, excitatory reactions.[2] Such likely generality of excitation transfer raises the question as to what, in transfer, is common to both humans
and subhuman species, and what, if any, differences exist. In terms of
theory building, the issue becomes the construction of a set of propositions
that apply to all species considered, and the addition of propositions to
account for the presumably more complex behavior of humans. Since
excitation-transfer theory was initially conceived to explain human behavior, the reverse procedure suggests itself: Is it possible to isolate those
propositions that address uniquely human aspects of behavior and eliminate
them so as to construct the broader paradigm by reduction?

Such a reduction is readily accomplished. It is the experiential component with its behavior-modifying implications, as identified in the three-
factor theory of emotion (Zillmann, 1978, 1979), that needs to be eliminated. In subhuman species, transfer effects are the result of the interaction
of only two factors: the dispositional and the excitatory component. This
interaction projects that environmental cues *direct* the animals' behavior in
both the antecedent and the subsequent situation (see Figure 8-1), and
that residual excitation *intensifies* the directed behavior in the subsequent
situation.

2. Ethologists have noted that the discontinuation of excited behaviors tends to produce
seemingly artificially intense subsequent behaviors in numerous species (cf. Eibl-Fibesfeldt,
1970; Hinde, 1970). This phenomenon has been discussed under the headings "displacement
activity," "substitute activity," and "redirection activity." All these labels refer to such
matters as birds turning to vigorous preening or beak wiping after social encounters in
aggressive or sexual situations, fish engaging in extensive fanning after conflict, and rodents
grooming excessively after vacillating between withdrawal and approach in exploratory
endeavors. Tinbergen (1940, 1952) suggested that such displacement activities result from
the "sparking over" of surplus nervous energy that the ceased preceding activity left behind.
Bindra (1959) analyzed these activities in behavior-theoretical terms. He proposed that, as
the animal is prevented from engaging in vital behaviors instigated by prevailing stimuli,
levels of arousal are likely to be heightened, and that the heightened arousal persists "for
some time after the obstruction in the original activity" (p. 253). Bindra noted that "activities
that are categorized as displacement phenomena typically occur when the animal is highly
excited" (p. 253). But he went on to propose, on the basis of heightened arousal, a selective
bias toward activities associated with high habit strength. The focus on high-habit responses
is also apparent in Hull's (1943, 1952) theorizing, where diffuse drive is considered to activate
behavior that is prepotent in the habit structure. However, Hull's proposals are commonly
interpreted as suggesting that such drive also intensifies ("energizes") behavior (cf. McFarland,
1966; Zillmann, 1978, 1979). In contrast to the behavior-theoretical approach, transfer
theory concentrates on the prediction of the *intensity* of subsequent behaviors. Displacement
activities are explained as stimulus-bound reactions whose intensity (i.e., vigor, persistence)
is determined by residual sympathetic excitation from the preceding, arousing activities that
were interrupted. Strong, acquired habits and potentially innate responses of the fixed-
action-pattern variety should, of course, influence the selection of subsequent behaviors. It
should be added that excitation transfer in subhuman species has not only been recorded in
ethological research, but has also been experimentally demonstrated in laboratory research
(e.g., Barfield & Sachs, 1968; Crowley, Popolow, & Ward, 1973).

The changes required in the propositions are minimal. In proposition 1, the section under stipulation a that concerns the subjective assessment of emotional reactions, and stipulation b are to be deleted. The reference to emotional experience in propositions 1 and 2 should also be removed. Propositions 3 and 4 remain unchanged.

For subhuman species, then, the transfer paradigm is greatly simplified. The behavior-monitoring function that characterizes emotional experience in humans is inoperative for these species, and the consequences of this function—mainly the prevention of emotional reactions that are deemed inappropriate and the extension of emotional behavior through the rehearsal and recall of emotional experiences—cannot manifest themselves.

REFERENCES

Adám, G. *Interoception and behavior: An experimental study.* Budapest: Publishing House of the Hungarian Academy of Sciences, 1967.

Adamson, J. D., Romano, K. R., Burdick, J. A., Corman, C. L., & Chebib, F. S. Physiological responses to sexual and unpleasant film stimuli. *Journal of Psychosomatic Research*, 1972, 16, 153–162.

Averill, J. R. Autonomic response patterns during sadness and mirth. *Psychophysiology*, 1969, 5, 399–414.

Ax, A. F. The physiological differentiation of fear and anger in humans. *Psychosomatic Medicine*, 1953, 15, 433–442.

Axelrod, J. Metabolism of epinephrine and other sympathomimetic amines. *Physiological Reviews*, 1959, 39, 751–776.

Axelrod, J. Noradrenaline: Fate and control of its biosynthesis. *Science*, 1971, 173, 598–606.

Barclay, A. M., & Little, D. M. Urinary acid phosphatase secretion under different arousal conditions. *Psychophysiology*, 1972, 9, 69–77.

Barden, R. C., Zelko, F. A., Duncan, S. W., & Masters, J. C. Children's consensual knowledge about the experiential determinants of emotion. *Journal of Personality and Social Psychology*, 1980, 39, 968–976.

Barefoot, J. C., & Straub, R. B. Opportunity for information search and the effect of false heart-rate feedback. *Journal of Personality and Social Psychology*, 1971, 17, 154–157.

Barfield, R. J., & Sachs, B. D. Sexual behavior: Stimulation by painful electric shock to skin in male rats. *Science*, 1968, 161, 392–393.

Bindra, D. *Motivation: A systematic reinterpretation.* New York: Ronald, 1959.

Brener, J. Learned control of cardiovascular processes: Feedback mechanisms and therapeutic applications. In K. S. Calhoun, H. E. Adams, & K. M. Mitchel (Eds.), *Innovative treatment methods in psychophysiology.* New York: Wiley, 1974.

Brener, J. Sensory and perceptual determinants of voluntary visceral control. In G. E. Schwartz & J. Beatty (Eds.), *Biofeedback: Theory and research.* New York: Academic, 1977.

Bryant, J., & Zillmann, D. Effect of intensification of annoyance through unrelated residual excitation on substantially delayed hostile behavior. *Journal of Experimental Social Psychology*, 1979, 15, 470–480.

Cannon, W. B. *Bodily changes in pain, hunger, fear and rage: An account of researches into the function of emotional excitement* (2nd ed.). New York: Appleton-Century, 1929.

Cantor, J. R., Bryant, J., & Zillmann, D.   Enhancement of humor appreciation by transferred excitation. *Journal of Personality and Social Psychology*, 1974, *30*, 812–821.

Cantor, J. R., & Zillmann, D.   The effect of affective state and emotional arousal on music appreciation. *Journal of General Psychology*, 1973, *89*, 97–108.

Cantor, J. R., Zillmann, D., & Bryant, J.   Enhancement of experienced sexual arousal in response to erotic stimuli through misattribution of unrelated residual excitation. *Journal of Personality and Social Psychology*, 1975, *32*, 69–75.

Cantor, J. R., Zillmann, D., & Day, K. D.   Relationship between cardiorespiratory fitness and physiological responses to films. *Perceptual and Motor Skills*, 1978, *46*, 1123–1130.

Chernigovskiy, V. N.   *Interoceptors*. Washington, D.C.: American Psychological Association, 1967.

Chessick, R. D., Bassan, M., & Shattan, S.   A comparison of the effect of infused catecholamines and certain affect states. *American Journal of Psychiatry*, 1966, *123*, 156–165.

Conner, R. L.   Hormones, biogenic amines, and aggression. In S. Levine (Ed.), *Hormones and behavior*. New York: Academic, 1972.

Cox, J. P., Evans, J. F., & Jamieson, J. L.   Aerobic power and tonic heart rate responses to psychosocial stressors. *Personality and Social Psychology Bulletin*, 1979, *5*, 160–163.

Craig, K. D., & Wood, K.   Autonomic components of observers' responses to pictures of homicide victims and nude females. *Journal of Experimental Research in Personality*, 1971, *5*, 304–309.

Crowley, W. R., Popolow, H. B., & Ward, O. B., Jr.   From dud to stud: Copulatory behavior elicited through conditioned arousal in sexually inactive male rats. *Physiology and Behavior*, 1973, *10*, 391–394.

Day, K. D.   *The effect of music differing in excitatory potential and hedonic valence on provoked aggression.* Unpublished doctoral dissertation, Indiana University, 1980.

DiCara, L. V.   Plasticity in the autonomic nervous system: Instrumental learning of visceral and glandular responses. In F. O. Schmitt (Ed.), *The neurosciences: Second study program*. New York: Rockefeller University Press, 1970.

Donnerstein, E., Donnerstein, M., & Barrett, G.   Where is the facilitation of media violence: The effects of nonexposure and placement of anger arousal. *Journal of Research in Personality*, 1976, *10*, 386–398.

Donnerstein, E., & Hallam, J.   Facilitating effects of erotica on aggression against women. *Journal of Personality and Social Psychology*, 1978, *36*, 1270–1277.

Eibl-Eibesfeldt, I.   *Ethology: The biology of behavior*. New York: Holt, Rinehart & Winston, 1970.

Elmadjian, F., Hope, J. M., & Lamson, E. T.   Excretion of epinephrine and norepinephrine in various emotional states. *Journal of Clinical Endocrinology and Metabolism*, 1957, *17*, 608–620.

Elmadjian, F., Hope, J. M., & Lamson, E. T.   Excretion of epinephrine and norepinephrine under stress. In G. Pincus (Ed.), *Recent progress in hormone research* (Vol. 14). New York: Academic, 1958.

Engel, B. T.   Stimulus-response and individual-response specificity. *AMA Archives of General Psychiatry*, 1960, *2*, 305–313.

Frankenhaeuser, M.   Psychoneuroendocrine approaches to the study of emotion as related to stress and coping. In H. E. Howe, Jr., & R. A. Dienstbier (Eds.), *Nebraska Symposium on Motivation, 1978*. Lincoln: University of Nebraska Press, 1978.

Frankenhaeuser, M., & Pátkai, P.   Interindividual differences in catecholamine excretion during stress. *Scandinavian Journal of Psychology*, 1965, *6*, 117–123.

Funkenstein, D. H.   Nor-epinephrine-like and epinephrine-like substances in relation to human behavior. *Journal of Mental Diseases*, 1956, *124*, 58–68.

Gellhorn, E.   Motion and emotion: The role of proprioception in the physiology and pathology of the emotions. *Psychological Review*, 1964, *71*, 457–472.

Gellhorn, E.   *Principles of autonomic–somatic integrations: Physiological basis and psychological and clinical implications*. Minneapolis: University of Minnesota Press, 1967.

Gellhorn, E.   Attempt at a synthesis: Contribution to a theory of emotion. In E. Gellhorn

(Ed.), *Biological foundations of emotion: Research and commentary.* Glenview, Ill.: Scott, Foresman, 1968.

Goldstein, I. B., Grinker, R. R., Sr., Heath, H. A., Oken, D., & Shipman, W. G.   Study in psychophysiology of muscle tension: I. Response specificity. *AMA Archives of General Psychiatry*, 1964, *11*, 322–330.

Grings, W. W., & Dawson, M. E.   *Emotions and bodily responses: A psychophysiological approach.* New York: Academic, 1978.

Grossman, S. P.   *A textbook of physiological psychology.* New York: Wiley, 1967.

Grossman, S. P.   The physiological basis of specific and nonspecific motivational processes. In W. J. Arnold (Ed.), *Nebraska Symposium on Motivation, 1968.* Lincoln: University of Nebraska Press, 1968.

Henle, J.   *Anthropologische Vorträge.* Braunschweig: Vieweg, 1876.

Hennessy, J. W., & Levine, S.   Stress, arousal, and the pituitary–adrenal system: A psychoendocrine hypothesis. In J. M. Sprague & A. N. Epstein (Eds.), *Progress in psychobiology and physiological psychology.* New York: Academic, 1979.

Hinde, R. A.   *Animal behavior: A synthesis of ethology and comparative psychology* (2nd ed.). New York: McGraw-Hill, 1970.

Hull, C. L.   *Principles of behavior: An introduction to behavior theory.* New York: Appleton-Century-Crofts, 1943.

Hull, C. L.   *A behavior system: An introduction to behavior theory concerning the individual organism.* New York: Wiley, 1952.

Izard, C. E.   *Human emotions.* New York: Plenum, 1977.

Jaffe, Y.   Sexual stimulation: Effects on prosocial behavior. *Psychological Reports*, 1981, *48*, 75–81.

James, W.   What is emotion? *Mind*, 1884, *9*, 188–204.

Jones, E. E., & Davis, K. W.   From acts to dispositions: The attribution process in person perception. In L. Berkowitz (Ed.), *Advances in experimental social psychology* (Vol. 2). New York: Academic, 1965.

Kelley, H. H.   Attribution theory in social psychology. In D. Levine (Ed.), *Nebraska Symposium on Motivation, 1967.* Lincoln: University of Nebraska Press, 1967.

Kelley, H. H.   Causal schemata and the attribution process. In E. E. Jones, D. E. Kanouse, H. H. Kelley, R. E. Nisbett, S. Valins, & B. Weiner (Eds.), *Attribution: Perceiving the causes of behavior.* Morristown, N.J.: General Learning Press, 1971.

Kety, S. S.   Neurochemical aspects of emotional behavior. In P. Black (Ed.), *Physiological correlates of emotion.* New York: Academic, 1970.

Kimmel, H. D.   Instrumental conditioning of autonomically mediated responses in human beings. *American Psychologist*, 1974, *29*, 325–335.

Konečni, V. J.   The mediation of aggressive behavior: Arousal level versus anger and cognitive labeling. *Journal of Personality and Social Psychology*, 1975, *32*, 706–712.

Lacey, J. I.   Individual differences in somatic response patterns. *Journal of Comparative and Physiological Psychology*, 1950, *43*, 338–350.

Lacey, J. I.   Somatic response patterning and stress: Some revisions of activation theory. In M. H. Appley & R. Trumbull (Eds.), *Psychological stress: Issues in research.* New York: Appleton-Century-Crofts, 1967.

Lacey, J. I., Bateman, D. E., & VanLehn, R.   Autonomic response specificity: An experimental study. *Psychosomatic Medicine*, 1953, *15*, 8–21.

Lacey, J. I., & Lacey, B. C.   Verification and extension of the principle of autonomic response stereotypy. *American Journal of Psychology*, 1958, *71*, 50–73.

Leventhal, H.   A perceptual-motor processing model of emotion. In P. Pliner, K. R. Blankstein, & I. M. Spigel (Eds.), *Advances in the study of communication and affect* (Vol. 5). *Perception of emotion in self and others.* New York: Plenum, 1979.

Levi, L.   The urinary output of adrenalin and noradrenalin during pleasant and unpleasant emotional states. *Psychosomatic Medicine*, 1965, *27*, 80–85.

Levi, L.   Stressors, stress tolerance, emotions and performance in relation to catecholamine excretion. In L. Levi (Ed.), *Emotional stress: Physiological and psychological reactions; medical, industrial and military implications.* New York: American Elsevier, 1967.

MacLean, P. D.   Man and his animal brains. *Modern Medicine,* 1964, *32,* 95–106.

Malmo, R. B.   *On emotions, needs, and our archaic brain.* New York: Holt, Rinehart & Winston, 1975.

Maltzman, I.   Theoretical conceptions of semantic conditioning and generalization. In T. R. Dixon & D. L. Horton (Eds.), *Verbal behavior and general behavior theory.* Englewood Cliffs, N.J.: Prentice-Hall, 1968.

Mandler, G.   Emotion. In R. Brown, E. Galanter, E. H. Hess, & E. Mandler, *New directions in psychology.* New York: Holt, Rinehart & Winston, 1962.

Mandler, G.   *Mind and emotion.* New York: Wiley, 1975.

Mandler, G., & Kahn, M.   Discrimination of changes in heart rate: Two unsuccessful attempts. *Journal of the Experimental Analysis of Behavior,* 1960, *3,* 21–25.

Mandler, G., & Kremen, I.   Autonomic feedback: A correlational study. *Journal of Personality,* 1958, *26,* 388–399.

Mandler, G., Mandler, J. M., Kremen, I., & Sholiton, R. D.   The response to threat: Relations among verbal and physiological indices. *Psychological Monographs,* 1961, *75* (9, Whole No. 513).

McFarland, D. J.   On the causal and functional significance of displacement activities. *Zeitschrift fuer Tierpsychologie,* 1966, *23,* 217–235.

Meyer, T. P.   The effects of sexually arousing and violent films on aggressive behavior. *Journal of Sex Research,* 1972, *8,* 324–331.

Mueller, C. W., & Donnerstein, E.   The effects of humor-induced arousal upon aggressive behavior. *Journal of Research in Personality,* 1977, *11,* 73–82.

Mueller, C. W., & Donnerstein, E.   Film-facilitated arousal and prosocial behavior. *Journal of Experimental Social Psychology,* 1981, *17,* 31–41.

Newman, E. B., Perkins, F. T., & Wheeler, R. H.   Cannon's theory of emotion: A critique. *Psychological Review,* 1930, *37,* 305–326.

Nisbett, R. E., & Valins, S.   Perceiving the causes of one's own behavior: In E. E. Jones, D. E. Kanouse, H. H. Kelley, R. E. Nisbett, S. Valins, & B. Weiner (Eds.), *Attribution: Perceiving the causes of behavior.* Morristown, N.J.: General Learning Press, 1971.

Oken, D.   The psychophysiology and psychoendocrinology of stress and emotion. In M. H. Appley & R. Trumbull (Eds.), *Psychological stress: Issues in research.* New York: Appleton-Century-Crofts, 1967.

Osgood, C. E.   *Method and theory in experimental psychology.* New York: Oxford University Press, 1953.

Pátkai, P.   Catecholamine excretion in pleasant and unpleasant situations. *Acta Psychologica,* 1971, *35,* 352–363.

Plutchik, R.   A general psychoevolutionary theory of emotion. In R. Plutchik & H. Kellerman (Eds.), *Emotion: Theory, research, and experience* (Vol. 1). *Theories of emotion.* New York: Academic, 1980.

Rule, B. G., Ferguson, T. J., & Nesdale, A. R.   Emotional arousal, anger, and aggression: The misattribution issue. In P. Pliner, K. R. Blankstein, & I. M. Spigel (Eds.), *Advances in the study of communication and affect* (Vol. 5). *Perception of emotion in self and others.* New York: Plenum, 1979.

Schachter, J.   Pain, fear, and anger in hypertensives and normotensives. *Psychosomatic Medicine,* 1957, *19,* 17–29.

Schachter, S.   The interaction of cognitive and physiological determinants of emotional state. In L. Berkowitz (Ed.), *Advances in experimental social psychology* (Vol. 1). New York: Academic, 1964.

Schildkraut, J. J.   Neuropharmacology of the affective disorders. *Annual Review of Pharmacology,* 1973, *13,* 427–454.

Schildkraut, J. J., & Kety, S. S.   Biogenic amines and emotion. *Science,* 1967, *156,* 21–30.

Schnore, M. M.   Individual patterns of physiological activity as a function of task differences and degree of arousal. *Journal of Experimental Psychology,* 1959, *58,* 117–128.

Schwartz, G. E.   Self-regulation of response patterning: Implications for psychophysiological research and therapy. *Biofeedback and Self-Regulation*, 1976, *1*, 7–30.

Schwartz, G. E.   Biofeedback and patterning of autonomic and central processes: CNS-cardiovascular interactions. In G. E. Schwartz & J. Beatty (Eds.), *Biofeedback: Theory and research*. New York: Academic, 1977.

Shapiro, D.   Operant-feedback control of human blood pressure: Some clinical issues. In P. A. Obrist, A. H. Black, J. Brener, & L. V. DiCara (Eds.), *Cardiovascular psychophysiology: Current issues in response mechanisms, biofeedback, and methodology*. Chicago: Aldine, 1974.

Shapiro, D., & Crider, A.   Psychophysiological approaches in social psychology. In G. Lindzey & E. Aronson (Eds.), *The handbook of social psychology* (2nd ed., Vol. 3). Reading, Mass.: Addison-Wesley, 1969.

Shields, S. A., & Stern, R. M.   Emotion: The perception of bodily change. In P. Pliner, K. R. Blankstein, & I. M. Spigel (Eds.), *Advances in the study of communciation and affect* (Vol. 5). *Perception of emotion in self and others*. New York: Plenum, 1979.

Smith, G. P.   Adrenal hormones and emotional behavior. In E. Stellar & J. M. Sprague (Eds.), *Progress in physiological psychology*. New York: Academic, 1973.

Staats, A. W., & Staats, C. K.   *Complex human behavior: A systematic extension of learning principles*. New York: Holt, Rinehart & Winston, 1963.

Sternbach, R.   *Principles of psychophysiology*. New York: Academic, 1966.

Tannenbaum, P. H.   Studies in film- and television-mediated arousal and aggression: A progress report. In G. A. Comstock, E. A. Rubinstein, & J. P. Murray (Eds.), *Television and social behavior* (Vol. 5). *Television's effects: Further explorations*. Washington, D.C.: U.S. Government Printing Office, 1972.

Tarpy, R. M.   The nervous system and emotion. In D. K. Candland, J. P. Fell, E. Keen, A. I. Leshner, R. M. Tarpy, & R. Plutchik, *Emotion*. Monterey, Calif.: Brooks/Cole, 1977.

Thayer, R. E.   Measurement of activation through self-report. *Psychological Reports*, 1967, *20*, 663–678.

Thayer, R. E.   Activation states as assessed by verbal report and four psychophysiological variables. *Psychophysiology*, 1970, *7*, 86–94.

Tinbergen, N.   Die Übersprungbewegung. *Zeitschrift fuer Tierpsychologie*, 1940, *4*, 1–40.

Tinbergen, N.   "Derived" activities: Their causation, biological significance, origin, and emancipation during evolution. *Quarterly Review of Biology*, 1952, *27*, 1–32.

Tomkins, S. S.   *Affect, imagery, consciousness* (Vol. 1). *The positive affects*. New York: Springer, 1962.

Tomkins, S. S.   *Affect, imagery, consciousness* (Vol. 2). *The negative affects*. New York: Springer, 1963.

Turner, C. D., & Bagnara, J. T.   *General endocrinology* (5th ed.). Philadelphia: Saunders, 1971.

Valins, S.   The perception and labeling of bodily changes as determinants of emotional behavior. In P. Black (Ed.), *Physiological correlates of emotion*. New York: Academic, 1970.

Wenger, M. A., Clemens, T. L., Coleman, D. R., Cullen, T. D., & Engel, B. T.   Autonomic response specificity. *Psychosomatic Medicine*, 1961, *23*, 185–193.

Wenger, M. A., & Cullen, T. D.   ANS response patterns to fourteen stimuli. *American Psychologist*, 1958, *13*, 423. (Abstract)

Wenger, M. A., Jones, F. N., & Jones, M. H.   *Physiological psychology*. New York: Holt, 1956.

Wilder, J.   The law of initial values in neurology and psychiatry: Facts and problems. *Journal of Nervous and Mental Disease*, 1957, *125*, 73–86.

Younger, J. C., & Doob, A. N.   Attribution and aggression: The misattribution of anger. *Journal of Research in Personality*, 1978, *12*, 164–171.

Zillmann, D.   Excitation transfer in communication-mediated aggressive behavior. *Journal of Experimental Social Psychology*, 1971, *7*, 419–434.

Zillmann, D.   Attribution and misattribution of excitatory reactions. In J. H. Harvey, W. J. Ickes, & R. F. Kidd (Eds.), *New directions in attribution research* (Vol. 2). Hillsdale, N.J.: Erlbaum, 1978.

Zillmann, D.   *Hostility and aggression*. Hillsdale, N.J.: Erlbaum, 1979.

Zillmann, D.   Anatomy of suspense. In P. H. Tannenbaum (Ed.), *The entertainment functions of television.* Hillsdale, N.J.: Erlbaum, 1980.

Zillmann, D.   Arousal and aggression. In R. G. Geen & E. Donnerstein (Eds.), *Aggression: Theoretical and empirical reviews* (Vol. 1). New York: Academic, 1983.

Zillmann, D., & Bryant, J.   Effect of residual excitation on the emotional response to provocation and delayed aggressive behavior. *Journal of Personality and Social Psychology,* 1974, *30*, 782-791.

Zillmann, D., Bryant, J., Comisky, P. W., & Medoff, N.J.   Excitation and hedonic valence in the effect of erotica on motivated intermale aggression. *European Journal of Social Psychology,* 1981, *11*, 233-252.

Zillmann, D., Johnson, R. C., & Day, K. D.   Attribution of apparent arousal and proficiency of recovery from sympathetic activation affecting excitation transfer to aggressive behavior. *Journal of Experimental Social Psychology,* 1974, *10*, 503-515.

Zillmann, D., Katcher, A. H., & Milavsky, B.   Excitation transfer from physical exercise to subsequent aggressive behavior. *Journal of Experimental Social Psychology,* 1972, *8*, 247-259.

Zillmann, D., Mody, B., & Cantor, J. R.   Empathetic perception of emotional displays in films as a function of hedonic and excitatory state prior to exposure. *Journal of Research in Personality,* 1974, *8*, 335-349.

B · AFFECT AND EMOTIONS

CHAPTER 9

Electromyographic Studies of Facial Expressions of Emotions and Patterns of Emotions

Alan J. Fridlund
Martinez VA Medical Center
and CSPP–Berkeley

Carroll E. Izard
University of Delaware

INTRODUCTION

Although nearly 30 years have elapsed since Ax's pioneering experiment (Ax, 1953) concerning visceral response patterning in fear and anger, the investigation of the physiological correlates of human emotion remains largely unelaborated. While earlier investigators focused on neural and visceroautonomic correlates of emotion (see Leshner, 1977, and Tarpy, 1977, for recent reviews), current work has explored the electromyographic (EMG) measurement of the striate musculature of the face as a promising quantitative index both of overt expressive behavior and of subjective emotional state. That the emotions might be fully detectable and discriminable through the use of facial EMG has significance for theories of human emotion, for the formulation of criterion-valid methods of exploring emotional changes in psychophysiological research and therapies, for psychodiagnosis of affective disorder, and for studies of social interaction.[1]

This chapter is intended to survey current thinking and research related to the use of facial EMG techniques in the assessment of human emotions. First, an attempt is made to place these research efforts in a theoretical and historical context. Second, difficulties in formulating, implementing, and

1. The present chapter was written from an implicit differential emotions perspective (Darwin, 1872/1965; Izard, 1971, 1972, 1977, 1979; Tomkins, 1962, 1963), which assumes a reduced typology of fundamental emotions from which the complete range of emotion displays and experiences is constructed. Implicit also is the monistic stance that since emotions are phenomenologically discriminable, they are *eo ipso* physiologically discriminable as well.

interpreting facial EMG–emotion studies (as well as studies of emotion in general) are discussed. Third, a critical synopsis of the extant research is undertaken in light of these difficulties. Fourth, some new theoretical and methodological approaches are described which may allow for more rigorous and meaningful research in the physiology of emotion.

FACIAL ACTION, EMOTION, AND ELECTROMYOGRAPHY

The exquisite capability of the facial musculature to express emotional states was first systematically investigated in the mid-nineteenth century by the French anatomist Duchenne, who employed electrical stimulation of facial muscle tissue to assess the role of specific muscles in the generation of facial expressions (Duchenne, 1867/1959). However, it was Charles Darwin (1872/1965) who emphasized the social, communicative, and survival value of facial expressions. For Darwin, instances of interspecies isomorphism in emotional behavior constituted evidence of a phyletic basis for the motor patterning seen in emotional displays. For example, the sagging head and shrugged shoulders of a demoralized human may be presumed homologous to the lowered head and tail and crouching posture of a punished dog. Similarly, the human expression of anger (or in nonhumans, the elicited "rage" reaction) almost universally involves an erect head and posture, and bared teeth. The idea that the facial actions involved in emotional display might have an innate component led to early studies designed to distill the "basic" human emotions, and to ascertain the extent of their cross-cultural generality (e.g., Feleky, 1914; Frois-Wittman, 1930; Landis, 1929; Levy & Schlosberg, 1960), efforts which continue to the present day (Ekman, 1982; Izard, 1971; and see the updated review by Fridlund, Ekman, & Oster, in press). Recent investigations employing systems for coding facial response in terms of individual muscle actions (Ekman & Friesen, 1978) or correlated muscle groupings (Izard, 1979; see Ekman, 1981, for a review of methods for coding facial behavior), have shown support for cross-culturally recognized basic human emotions, such as joy, sadness, anger, fear, contempt, and disgust (Izard, 1977, 1979).

Facial muscle action in emotional behavior has not only been regarded as a feedforward process serving a display function; patterned afferent feedback from contracting facial musculature has also been postulated to be a component of emotion experience (Izard, 1971; Tomkins, 1962, 1963). Such theorizing proceeds directly from William James's theory of emotion (James, 1884), which holds that patterns of contraction of facial and somatic musculature (as well as the less differentiated visceroautonomic responses) are, in great part, responsible for the experience of emotion. Although there are demonstrable neurological substrates (Starr, McKeon, Skuse, & Burke, 1981), the status of facial-feedback theories of emotion experience is controversial (Buck, 1980). Recent data unsupportive of a primary role of facial feedback in mediating emotion experience (Tourangeau & Ellsworth, 1979) have encountered severe criticism (Hager & Ekman, 1981; Izard, 1981; Tomkins, 1981; and see the spirited rebuttal by Ellsworth & Tourangeau, 1981). However, one important deduction from James's peripheralist theory of emotion is that patterned striate-muscle responses would be detectable at any level of emotional responsiveness, from expansive overt displays of emotion (e.g., grief or rage reactions), to low levels of felt emotion without discernible overt behavior (e.g., during affectively tainted imagery). This hypothesis formed the basis for many of the early facial EMG–emotion studies (e.g., Schwartz, Fair, Salt, Mandel, & Klerman, 1976a, 1976b).

The use of facial EMG in studies of emotion is a recent development, with the body of previous facial EMG research having been done in the context of rehabilitation medicine (see Basmajian, 1978). Facial EMG techniques employ implanted wire electrodes or surface recording disks to detect the electrical discharges (the "muscle action potentials," or MAPs) of contracting muscle fibers. The discrete microvolt-level MAPs which aggregate during motor-unit recruitment (Basmajian, 1978) are amplified, filtered to maximize signal-to-noise ratio, rectified, and then integrated to provide a varying dc voltage that is roughly proportional to the level of isometric contraction of the muscle(s) detected at the recording site (Moritani & DeVries, 1978). Fridlund and Fowler (1978) and Fridlund, Price, and Fowler (1982) offer a technical description of the signal-processing stages necessary for securing the EMG signal.

The use of facial electromyography present three advantages over visual facial coding techniques for the detection of facial muscular action. First, the EMG signal is instantaneously detectable and thereby lends itself to immediate recording, whereas coding systems presently require large amounts of time for observer judgments and manual recording of the facial actions. Second, the EMG signal is a very precise index of the degree of a muscle contraction, offering a more fine-grained measure of muscle activity than that provided by raters. Third, the use of EMG techniques allows the detection of muscle contractions which are too small to be observable, as in the affective-imagery studies to be reported subsequently. Facial EMG techniques are not without their liabilities, and these are examined in the next section.

PROBLEMS WITH FACIAL EMG–EMOTION RESEARCH

Before delving into the experimental literature using facial EMG in the assessment of emotion states and emotion expressions, it will be necessary to acquaint the reader with several of the constraints that plague studies of emotion in general, and facial EMG–emotion studies in particular. These

are issues that debatably vitiate to some extent the validity and inter-
pretability of any experimental findings, on both theoretical and methodological grounds. Chief among these are intrusion of the measurement
apparatus, experimental demand characteristics, methodological problems
with EMG measurement techniques, and arousal confounds.

Intrusion of Measurement Apparatus

Unlike facial coding systems, which typically rely on ratings of videotaped
facial behavior, EMG techniques require direct contact with the subject's
face. In the case of implanted wire electrodes (e.g., Sumitsuji, Matsumoto, &
Kaneko, 1965), the electrodes are inserted through the skin (often with
some pain or irritation), and may terminate on a collar which surrounds
the face and prevents the accidental removal of the electrodes. In surface
EMG recording (e.g., Fridlund, Schwartz, & Fowler, 1983), 1-cm-diameter
paired differential recording disks are taped to the skin using adhesive collars
(Strong, 1970). In both cases, the subject is manifestly aware of the electrode placements. With surface recording in particular, the electrodes may
obstruct facial action to some degree, and thus the subject may be able to
sense making small facial movements that would otherwise be impercep-
tible.

Experimental Demand Characteristics

Because the subject is exposed to a lengthy electrode-application procedure
and remains more or less aware of the electrode placements throughout a
facial EMG experiment, he or she can typically be expected to discern that
the experiment has something to do with the face, if not necessarily facial
expression. The effects of this inference may be accentuated when the
subject is presented (and possibly asked to rate) emotion stimuli that elicit
facial actions or facial expressions. The influence of experimental demand
characteristics in facial EMG–emotion experiments is likely to be dependent
on the subject's set as he or she enters the experiment (Rosenthal, 1976).
Subjects may want to please the experimenter and "make good faces";
others may wish to sabotage the experiment and inhibit facial behavior;
still others may feel embarrassed at the monitoring of their facial expressions and generate attenuated or distorted expressions (Kleck, Vaughan,
Cartwright-Smith, Vaughan, Colby, & Lanzetta, 1976).

The generation of facial expressions in an attempt to please the
experimenter (or to "contribute to science") is especially problematic for
those experiments that purport to measure covert facial EMG correlates of
affective imagery (e.g., Fridlund et al., 1983; Schwartz et al., 1976a, 1976b).
In these studies, it is never clear how much the EMG patterning associated with the imagery items reflects experimental demand (i.e., simulated

emotion) or "real" emotion elicited by the items.[2] This distinction may bear not only on the intensity, but also the morphology, of imagery-related EMG activity (Ekman, Hager, & Friesen, 1981; Hager & Ekman, Chapter 10, this volume). Although it may be objected that emotional behavior is *always* embedded within a context of social demand (thus making the question moot—see the sociological account of emotion by Kemper, 1978), it is nonetheless proper to ask whether, under the contrived conditions of the laboratory, subjects are generating verisimilar data. In this regard, recent studies have seriously questioned whether brief verbal affective-imagery items (representative of those used in many facial EMG–emotion studies) are indeed valid elicitors of emotion (Buchwald, Strack, & Coyne, 1981; Polivy & Doyle, 1980). Polivy and Doyle (1980) state that self-referent mood statements are quite susceptible to experimental demand, and that "demand characteristics both contribute to [affective change] and falsely inflate measurements of it" (p. 290).

Strategies that can be employed to attenuate the effects of experimental demand include the use of dummy nonfacial electrode placements (Cacioppo & Petty, 1979; Carney, Hong, O'Connell, & Amado, 1981; Schwartz *et al.*, 1976a); cover stories to the effect that brain waves (or the like) are being measured (e.g., Fridlund *et al.*, 1983; Vaughan & Lanzetta, 1980); and explicit counterdemand instructions to subjects (Orne, 1962). Subjects may also be offered money (or otherwise motivated) to guess the purposes of the experiment at its conclusion—those who do are paid and excluded from, or separately grouped within, the study. To date, no facial EMG–emotion studies have been performed to assess the effects of experimental demand on facial EMG patterning.

Methodological Problems in EMG Measurement Techniques

The EMG data in facial EMG–emotion studies are often difficult to interpret because of the uniqueness of the EMG methodology employed in each experiment, and because of some constraints intrinsic to the EMG techniques themselves. First, the choice of electrode type determines the specificity of pickup site. Implanted wire electrodes provide a selectivity restricted to the muscle fibers in which they are inserted. Surface electrodes show broad pickup areas not confined to the muscle group(s) underlying the electrodes. Consequently, researchers employing surface electrodes in their studies must carefully interpret any data as reflecting "muscle

---

2. The similarity of affective-imagery procedures to many hypnotic inductions should be fully appreciated. As an aside, our arguments regarding demand characteristics may also pertain to the kinesthetic imagery–EMG studies of Jacobson and others (e.g., Jacobson, 1973). These studies, although enshrined in cognitive psychophysiology as suggesting a peripheralist conception of thinking, have never, to our knowledge, been replicated with appropriate counterdemand procedures.

regions" (Schwartz, Ahern, & Brown, 1979) or "tensional zones" (Fridlund, Fowler, & Pritchard, 1980). Low pickup-site selectivity may be especially troublesome in the investigation of overt expressions, wherein large muscle responses may result in the dislocation of the surface electrodes from their positions overlying the targeted muscle group. This dislocation may cause changes in signal amplitude, or complete loss of electrical contact with the skin. Additionally, the large-amplitude facial actions occurring during overt expression may produce considerable intermuscle-site crosstalk, with consequent spurious signal correlations between proximal EMG sites. For example, a strongly contracted masseter may produce myopotentials which easily override those from any other facial muscle, thereby inducing intolerable crosstalk even in lateral frontalis or corrugator sites.

Lack of measurement conventions for the processing of the EMG signals yields only limited comparability among EMG data in facial EMG–emotion studies. Whereas some studies present only the raw EMG signals in oscillographic form (Sumitsuji et al., 1965), others have employed integrated EMG levels over imagery periods from 20 seconds (Fridlund et al., 1983) to 3 minutes (Schwartz et al., 1976a). Analyses based on mean EMG-site levels over extended trial lengths always obscure temporal EMG response patterning and neglect dynamic properties of the EMG signals which may contain important information (Fridlund, Cottam, & Fowler, 1982). Differences in EMG detection passband also complicate attempts to compare EMG levels across studies, with detection bandwidth affecting the amplitude of detected signal (Hayes, 1960), degree of inter-site crosstalk (DeBacher & Basmajian, 1977), and system signal-to-noise ratio (see Fridlund & Fowler, 1978, for an extended discussion of these issues).

Davidson (cited in Ekman, 1981) has raised yet another difficulty common to facial EMG studies of emotion: the lack of a standardized atlas of facial electrode placements (such as the one developed by Davis, 1952, for trunk and limb muscle sites). Use of standard electrode placements based on facial anatomical landmarks could only result in improved measurement validity and reliability. Finally, an important caution in designing facial EMG–emotion studies is the dictum that EMG levels from one muscle site are never comparable with those from another muscle site (Grossman & Weiner, 1966). Differences in muscle size, α-motoneuron innervation ratios, muscle locations relative to bone (a current sink), and differing substrates of neural control (see Fridlund et al., in press) render such attempted comparisons invalid. Failures to heed this principle (even from contralateral, homologous muscle sites, as in the "laterality" studies to be reviewed subsequently) may lead to spurious results. What can be compared are changes within specific EMG sites across experimental conditions (within subjects), or across randomized groups of subjects.

Arousal Confounds

Psychophysiological studies of emotion in general have been subjected to the criticism that any differences in physiological response which may be observed among induced emotion states are not in fact due to emotion, but rather to differences in generalized arousal produced by the emotion stimuli. A complete understanding of this criticism requires placement in theoretical context.

The James–Lange theory of emotion (James's theory was modified by Lange, 1885, to emphasize perception of visceral, as opposed to striate-muscle responses, as mediators of emotion experiences) was subjected to serious criticism by Cannon (1927). Cannon described the action of physiological systems in emotion as the formation of an undifferentiated background state (arousal state), "a kind of bubbling physiological soup" (Lang, 1979), against which the emotional behavior occurred. This centralist conception of emotion (see M. L. Goldstein, 1968, for a review of physiological theories of emotion), together with the behavioristic zeitgeist, resulted in the relegation of the concept of emotion to the status of an intervening variable affecting response strength (Skinner, 1953), a Hullian drive variable (Brown & Farber, 1951), or an "energizer" (Duffy, 1962, 1972; Malmo, 1959). One line of experimentation seemed to substantiate an arousal-plus-cognition theory of emotion (e.g., Cantril & Hunt, 1932; Schachter & Singer, 1962), but failures to replicate the basic experiments in this series suggest otherwise—that undifferentiated arousal cannot be considered a neutral state modulated or channeled by a cognitive appraisal or evaluation process (Marshall & Zimbardo, 1979; Maslach, 1979).[3]

Alternative evidence supports the existence of physiological response patterning in states of arousal or emotion (Lacey, 1967; Schwartz, 1980); that is, it has been found that physiological systems in emotion do not always act in unifactorial fashion. Schwartz (1975, 1977, 1980) embraces the neogestaltist viewpoint that the dissociations among response systems may encode information pertaining to emotion state, whereas behavior of a single system may be relatively uninformative. Certainly, the use of facial striate-muscle response as an index of overtly expressed emotion would seem to disarm criticism from the arousal standpoint, since the configurative nature of *overt* facial expression is part of everyday experience (Chernoff, 1971; Ekman & Friesen, 1975; Izard & Dougherty, 1980). However, EMG studies of *covert* facial behavior (in which the facial responses may, or may not, be configurative) may still be vulnerable to

---

3. It is not widely appreciated that the centralist–peripheralist controversy applies strictly to the question of the determinants of the subjective-experience, or feeling, component of emotion. It does not apply to the issue of the viability of the notion of feedforward physiological patterning in states of emotion.

arousal confounds which may render results ambiguous and not strictly interpretable as representing "emotion." In the following review of the facial EMG–emotion literature we present instances in which arousal confounds may contravene unambiguous interpretations of findings. Following that, we offer some new research with methodological refinements which may allow more definitive interpretation of facial EMG data as reflecting distinctly emotional processes.

REVIEW OF THE LITERATURE

The present section attempts to provide a critical synopsis of the facial EMG–emotion literature to date. This review focuses on those studies that have employed facial EMG techniques to investigate differential emotions (see Table 9-1 for outline of key studies in the facial EMG–emotion literature). Studies that used facial EMG placements to assess "stress" or "arousal" (e.g., the common use of the forehead lateral frontalis placement arguably to measure "tension"; see Fridlund *et al.*, 1980) will not be included, nor will psychophysiological studies that employed non-EMG measures of facial behavior (e.g., Öhman & Dimberg, 1978). The developing literature on the use of multiple-site facial EMG in rehabilitation medicine (e.g., Balliet, Shinn, & Bach-y-Rita, 1982) will be excluded, as will research that utilized facial EMG placements as indicants of cognitive, nonaffective responding (but see Cacioppo & Petty, 1981a, for recent review).

This review first presents studies of facial EMG correlates of affective imagery and affective disorder. Second, studies of overt facial expression are reviewed. Third, recent work using facial EMG in studies of social interaction and communication is considered.

Facial EMG Studies of Affective Imagery and Affective Disorder

Among the earliest reported studies using electromyography to investigate facial response in changing mood states was a pilot study reported by Izard (1971). In this experiment, a single female subject was presented a graded anxiety-desensitization imagery protocol. EMG activity was recorded from a mixed frontalis–corrugator surface placement. (See Figure 9-1 for some of the major expressive muscles of the face and their function in overt expression.) The amplitude of the electromyogram was reported to increase as the subject moved up the stimulus hierarchy (p. 391). Izard (1971) proposed the use of facial EMG as a sensitive indicator of subjective emotion states, thus echoing the early sentiments of Malmo and Shagass (1949), who stated: "It would appear that the study of striate muscle function in emotion should receive far more attention" (p. 23).

TABLE 9-1. Key Facial EMG–Emotion Studies

STUDY	NUMBER AND TYPE OF SUBJECTS	EMG DETECTION METHOD: ELECTRODE SITES	EXPERIMENTAL MANIPULATION	MAJOR REPORTED FINDINGS
		AFFECTIVE IMAGERY/AFFECTIVE DISORDER		
Carney, Hong, O'Connell, & Amado (1981)	21 clinically depressed female inpatients	Differential surface integrated (DSI) EMG—left corrugator, zygomatic, and splenius-capitis regions	Tricyclic antidepressant medication	Initial corrugator and zygomatic levels predictive of treatment outcome
Fridlund, Schwartz, & Fowler (1983)	12 normal college females	DSI EMG—left lateral frontalis, corrugator, orbicularis oculi, and orbicularis oris regions	Affective-imagery instructions for happiness, sadness, anger, and fear; posed expressions	Reliable multivariate classification of emotion-specific EMG patterns for imagery and posed expressions
Oliveau & Willmuth (1979)	40 clinically depressed and nondepressed inpatients (21 women, 19 men)	DSI EMG—right corrugator region	Self-constructed affective imagery for happiness, sadness, and "a typical day"	Failed to differentiate depressed vs. nondepressed patients
Schwartz, Ahern, & Brown (1979)	10 male and 10 female college students	DSI EMG—left and right corrugator and zygomatic regions	Reflective questions involving happiness, sadness, excitement, and fear; posed expressions	Lateralization of zygomatic-region activity for positive- vs. negative-emotion questions
Schwartz, Brown, & Ahern (1980)	30 male and 30 female college students	DSI EMG—left lateral frontalis, corrugator, zygomatic, and masseter regions	Affective-imagery instructions for happiness, sadness, anger, and fear; posed expressions	Higher EMG amplitudes in females for both imagery and posed-expression conditions
Schwartz, Fair, Mandel, Salt, Mieske, & Klerman (1978)	14 female and 5 male clinically depressed outpatients (in original sample)	DSI EMG—right corrugator region	Tricyclic antidepressant medication ($n = 7$) vs. placebo ($n = 5$)	Initial corrugator level predictive of treatment outcome
Schwartz, Fair, Salt, Mandel, & Klerman (1976a)	12 self-reported depressed clinic outpatients, 12 non-depressed controls (mixed sexes)	DSI EMG—right corrugator, zygomatic, mentalis, and depressor regions	Instructions to "think about" vs. "feel" self-constructed affective imagery	Higher EMG amplitudes in "feel" condition; differentiation of depressed vs. control subjects

(continued)

TABLE 9-1. (*Continued*)

STUDY	NUMBER AND TYPE OF SUBJECTS	EMG DETECTION METHOD: ELECTRODE SITES	EXPERIMENTAL MANIPULATION	MAJOR REPORTED FINDINGS
Schwartz, Fair, Salt, Mandel, & Klerman (1976b)	24 females: 6 clinically depressed outpatients, 6 self-reported depressed volunteers, 12 nondepressed controls	DSI EMG—right lateral frontalis, corrugator, masseter, and depressor regions	Self-constructed affective imagery for happiness, sadness, anger, and "a typical day"	Differentiation of emotion types, and of depressed from nondepressed controls
Teasdale & Bancroft (1977)	5 female outpatients with mixed dysphoric and depressive symptoms	DSI EMG—left corrugator and masseter regions	Self-constructed "happy and unhappy thoughts"	Corrugator EMG activity tracked self-reported mood ratings within subjects
Teasdale & Rezin (1978)	5 female and 4 male clinically depressed outpatients	DSI EMG—left corrugator region	Thought-stopping for "depressive thinking"	Corrugator EMG activity correlated with negative-thought frequency but not depressed mood

POSED EXPRESSIONS

Rusalova, Izard, & Simonov (1975)	23 Stanislavski actors and 12 nonactor controls (mixed sexes)	DSI EMG—lateral frontalis, corrugator, masseter, and depressor regions	Instructions to reproduce emotion displays using imagery; effects of motor inhibition and emotion mimicry	Differentiation of emotion types; superiority of actors in both display-suppression and mimicry conditions

Sumitsuji, Matsumoto, Tanaka, Kashiwagi, & Kaneko (1967)	14 male and 14 female volunteer hospital staff	Implanted wire electrodes—10 sites including all sites in Figure 9-1	Instructions to rest, supinate, and perform discrete facial expressive actions	Determination of EMG patterns characteristic of each facial movement
Sumitsuji, Matsumoto, Tanaka, Kashiwagi, & Kaneko (1977)	10 subjects: 1 actor, 1 actress, and 8 psychotics	Implanted wire electrodes—7 sites including all sites in Figure 9-1	Unspecified elicitors for emotion expressions	EMG-pattern factor scores related to Schlosberg's dimensional emotion typology
SOCIAL INTERACTION/COMMUNICATION				
Cacioppo & Petty (1979)	60 male college students	DSI EMG—left corrugator, zygomatic, depressor, and mentalis regions	Proattitudinal vs. counterattitudinal advocacy messages	Facial EMG activity differentiated affective valence of anticipation and reception of messages
Dimberg (1981)	9 male and 7 female college students	DSI EMG—left corrugator and zygomatic regions	Exposure to posed-expression photographs for anger and happiness	EMG responses differentiated type of photographic stimulus
Englis, Vaughan, & Lanzetta (1982)	11 female and 24 male college students	DSI EMG—left corrugator, orbicularis oculi, and masseter regions	Vicarious conditioning of observers under congruent vs. conflicting model/observer outcomes in gaming situation	EMG patterns differentiated empathetic from counterempathetic responses
Vaughan & Lanzetta (1980)	10 female and 6 male college students	DSI EMG—left medial frontalis, orbicularis oculi, and masseter regions	Vicarious conditioning to a model's pain display	EMG patterns in observers characteristic of anticipation and experience of pain
Vaughan & Lanzetta (1981)	34 male and 26 female college students	DSI EMG—left medial frontalis, orbicularis oculi, and masseter regions	Observers instructed to inhibit or amplify facial responses to model's pain display in vicarious-conditioning procedure	Modulation instructions affected instigated, but not conditioned, empathic responses

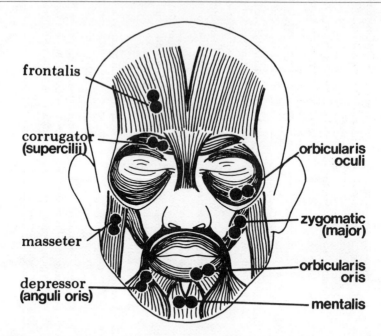

FIGURE 9-1. Diagram showing the chief expressive muscles of the face. Superimposed on each muscle region is typical placement for surface differential EMG recording disks. The muscular anatomy is simplified; there are usually individualized degrees of structural asymmetry, and irregularity and interleaving of muscle tissue. The functions of each muscle in overt expression follow: **frontalis** (lateral and medial portions): raises the (outer and inner) eyebrows, increasing the width between eyebrows and eyes; **corrugator** (supercilii): moves the eyebrows downward and inward, creating vertical furrows between the brows which extend down to the nasal root; **orbicularis oculi**: narrows or closes the eye fissure, and compresses the soft tissue in the eye region inward toward the fissure; **zygomatic** (major): draws the angle of the mouth backward and upward, tapering the end of the upper lip; **masseter**: clenches the teeth; **orbicularis oculi**: contracts the lips and moves them together and forward; **depressor** (anguli oris): lowers the upper lip outside the commissure, produces a downward concavity of the mouth, and deepens the depression at the mouth angle; **mentalis**: raises the tissue of the chin and pushes the lower lip upward. Muscle actions are abstracted from the more complete descriptions given by Izard (1979); diagram adapted from Schwartz (1977), original provided through the courtesy of Gary E. Schwartz.

Imagery and Depression

The first systematic studies of facial EMG response in differential emotion states were performed by Schwartz, Fair, and colleagues (Schwartz *et al.*, 1976a, 1976b). Schwartz *et al.* (1976b) sampled surface EMG activity from the lateral frontalis, corrugator, masseter, and depressor regions of the face in six depressed and six nondepressed female subjects (with "depression" determined from scores on the Zung Self-Rating Depression Scale).

Subjects were exposed to four 3-minute imagery trials in which they were asked to evoke their own specific images for "happiness," "sadness," "anger," and "a typical day." Results were difficult to interpret since univariate statistics were employed throughout (see the next section for an extended criticism of the use of univariate statistics in emotion studies). Taken together, the findings seemed to indicate some differentiation of the happy condition from the remaining three conditions, for both depressed and nondepressed subjects. This effect was largely due to decreased corrugator-region activity in the happy condition. Sadness was not well differentiated from anger. Depressed subjects were interpreted as generating attenuated happy patterns, and typical-day patterns that were high in corrugator-region activity and so were taken by Schwartz *et al.* to resemble sad patterns (the response of the nondepressed subgroup to the typical-day instruction was taken to resemble the happy pattern).

Problematic in this study is that EMG activity was expressed in terms of deviations from pretrial baselines. This procedure is based on the incorrect assumption that the striate musculature evinces a certain resting level of "tonus" which must then be subtracted from imagery-period levels. In fact, the facial musculature, like the rest of the striate musculature, can show complete electrical silence at rest (Basmajian, 1978; DeVries, 1965; Ralston & Libet, 1953; Vitti & Basmajian, 1976). Any EMG activity in facial sites during "rest" periods (with the possible exception of weight-bearing muscles such as the temporalis, which supports the lower jaw) is, at some level, instigated, and may properly be taken to reflect ongoing affective processes (Basmajian, 1978, p. 394). Therefore, baseline-corrected scores are of dubious discriminative efficiency in comparing nondepressed with depressed subjects, whose "resting" EMG activity may be of primary interest.

Schwartz *et al.* (1976a) explored the role of specific imagery instructions in eliciting facial EMG activity in 12 nondepressed and 12 depressed subjects (with "depression" again determined using Zung Scale ratings). Subjects were given happy and sad imagery items, first with the instruction to "think" about the imagery, then to "reexperience the feelings" associated with the imagery. Surface EMG activity was obtained from the corrugator, zygomatic, depressor, and mentalis regions. The results established the corrugator and zygomatic placements as the most responsive to the differentiation of happiness versus sadness in nondepressed subjects, with the instruction to "reexperience the feelings" producing the most differentiable patterns. For the depressed subjects, the "think" condition produced happy–sad differentiations only in the corrugator site, whereas the "feel" condition again produced differentiations in both EMG sites. These data suggest that the "feel" instruction may be a relatively more potent induction. These findings, as well as those of Schwartz *et al.* (1976b), are interesting in the light of the usual functional roles of the corrugator and zygomatic muscles in overt facial display (Figure 9-1): The corrugator is involved in the expression of sadness, anger, disgust, and fear; the zygomatic retracts the corners of the mouth to form a smile.

Designation of subjects as "depressed" in the two Schwartz *et al.* (1976a, 1976b) studies was based solely on self-report, not on clinical (e.g., behavioral and/or vegetative) indices of depression. As such, the differences in EMG patterns obtained between depressed and nondepressed subjects may well not have been related to any clinically significant depressive process, but rather to generalized anxiety or simple dysphoria. Oliveau and Willmuth (1979) attempted a partial replication of the findings of Schwartz *et al.* (1976b), using subjects selected for depression according to more stringent diagnostic criteria. Subjects were instructed to formulate and imagine happy and sad events, and events of a typical day. Integrated surface EMG activity was obtained from the corrugator region. The results supported the finding by Schwartz *et al.* (1976b) that significant EMG-level differences were obtained between happy and sad conditions for both depressed and nondepressed subjects. However, contrary to the findings of Schwartz *et al.*, the depressed and nondepressed groups were not distinguishable in any of the three imagery conditions.

In a largely within-subjects study which extended the procedures of Schwartz *et al.* (1976b), Teasdale and Bancroft (1977) instructed five clinically depressed subjects to formulate their own happy and unhappy thoughts for repeated 30-second periods, during which integrated EMG recordings were obtained from the corrugator and masseter regions. The instructions to think of the happy and unhappy thoughts were found, on the basis of a self-report mood scale, to produce significant changes in mood ratings. Corrugator-region EMG activity was found to correlate with mood rating (average correlation for the five subjects was approximately .70). Masseter-region activity was largely uncorrelated with mood ratings in four of the five subjects. The results of this study were important in that they established correlations between self-report ratings and facial EMG response within subjects, whereas the earlier studies employed only between-groups tests of significance.

Teasdale and Rezin (1978) furthered the within-subjects study of corrugator-region EMG activity in depressed moods in an investigation of the widely practiced behavior therapy technique of "thought stopping" (e.g., Wolpe, 1958). Nine depressed psychiatric day patients were trained in thought stopping for "negative" thoughts; a control procedure of "letting the mind wander" was also employed in the sessions. After training, surface corrugator-region EMG activity was measured during two experimental sessions. The thought-stopping technique was found to be only marginally effective in reducing negative-thought frequency (assessed using a button-pushing task), compared to the control periods. Effects of thought stopping on overall depressed mood (assessed using a self-report inventory) were not significant. Despite the ineffectiveness of the thought-stopping manipulation, corrugator-region EMG activity was found to correlate with frequency of negative thoughts ($r = .81$). However, the corrugator-region activity failed to show significant correlations with either "instantaneous mood" (obtained several times during the sessions) or overall depressed mood, although the latter effect had been obtained by Teasdale and Bancroft (1977). The authors stated that this failure to replicate the depressed-mood–corrugator correlation may have been due to the small sample size or to differences in experimental manipulations. Equally likely are problems of restricted range (Carroll, 1961) in both depression ratings and corrugator-region EMG levels (see Table 3, p. 100, in Teasdale & Rezin, 1978).

Facial EMG as a Prognostic Sign in Depression

Because corrugator-region EMG activity seemed to differentiate negative and positive emotion states, and perhaps depressed from nondepressed subjects (Schwartz *et al.*, 1976a, 1976b), Schwartz and colleagues (Schwartz, Fair, Mandel, Salt, Mieske, & Klerman, 1978) attempted to use it to assess improvement in depressive symptomatology with and without tricyclic antidepressant therapy. Twelve clinically depressed subjects were administered the Zung Scale and Taylor Manifest Anxiety Scale, were interviewed using the Hamilton Psychiatric Rating Scale for Depression, and measurement was made of their "resting" corrugator-region EMG levels before and after a 2-week period. Approximately half the subjects began tricyclic (amitriptyline) therapy at the beginning of the 2-week period. Results showed that when the subjects were divided using a median split on initial corrugator-region EMG levels, the Hamilton ratings of the "low"-EMG-level subgroup did not indicate as much clinical improvement as did the "high"-EMG-level subgroup. Zung and Taylor scores did not differentiate the subgroups. The amount of change in EMG levels was a function of initial EMG levels.

The authors interpret these findings as demonstrating that "changes in resting levels of corrugator EMG not only covary with observed clinical improvement, but also forecast subsequent change" (p. 359). However, there are alternative interpretations of the data. That the amount of EMG-level change was dependent on initial levels may simply reflect a confound involving the "Law of Initial Values" (Lykken, Rose, Luther, & Maley, 1966; Wilder, 1957; and see Cacioppo and Petty, Chapter 1, this volume), as the authors concede (p. 357). Second, the subgroups created by the median split on initial corrugator-region EMG levels were not balanced for subjects receiving tricyclics. In the "high"-EMG-level subgroup, four of six subjects received tricyclics; in the "low"-EMG-level subgroup, only three received tricyclics. This imbalance resulted in an inevitable confound of drug effect with EMG-level effect. A reanalysis of the Hamilton Scale data with balanced subgroups reveals that the Hamilton Scale differences are no longer significant when grouped according to corrugator-region EMG-level change.[4] Third, the pre–post changes for EMG levels and depression scale ratings were assessed over a 2-week period. Since antidepressant effects with tricyclics may not begin until at least 2 weeks have elapsed (Berger, 1977; Byck, 1975), the EMG "improvement" effects, in addition to regression artifact and effects of the Law of Initial Values, may also be attributable to sedation (as opposed to lifting of depression) occurring in the early phase of amitriptyline therapy.

More convincing data relating to the use of corrugator-site EMG activity as a prognostic indicant in depression are provided by Carney *et al.* (1981). Integrated EMG activity from left corrugator, zygomatic, and splenius capitis (occipital neck musculature) sites was obtained from 21 clinically diagnosed depressed female inpatients. The recordings were repeated 2 weeks after hospital admission. The Beck Depression Inventory (BDI; Beck, 1967) was administered to each patient before each recording session. The EMG records were obtained over an 8-minute period during which the patient was reclining and instructed to close her eyes and move as little as possible. All patients were medicated at admission (or just prior to admission) with tricyclic antidepressants. The authors failed to replicate the reported findings of Schwartz *et al.* (1978) that corrugator-site EMG-level changes were significantly related to changes in depressive symptoms (measured by Carney *et al.* in terms of BDI scores). Their data did corroborate a second finding by Schwartz *et al.*, that patients with higher *initial* corrugator-site EMG levels showed greater changes in BDI scores. Carney (1981) and his colleagues reported replication of these findings on 14 additional inpatients.

A critical challenge to the inference that depressed subjects may be making covert "sad" faces (e.g., Schwartz *et al.*, 1976a, 1976b, 1978) is the striking finding by Carney *et al.* (1981) that BDI change scores were also significantly positively correlated with initial zygomatic EMG levels! The coexistence of high corrugator- and zygomatic-site EMG levels in patients with lower subsequent BDI scores is problematic from a differential-emotions standpoint, unless many of the depressed patients were evincing covert "negative-affect smiles" (see Ekman, Friesen, & Ancoli, 1980) in addition to heightened corrugator-site activity. Carney (1981) and co-workers tentatively attribute this finding to a "hyperarousal" phenomenon, a putative depressive sign which was suggested by earlier investigators (e.g., Goldstein, 1965; Martin & Davies, 1965; Rimon, Stenback, & Hahmar,

4. Further reanalysis reveals that the statistics used to assess the Hamilton Scale group differences were erroneously computed (assuming the accuracy of the Table 1 data, p. 358, of Schwartz, Fair, Mandel, Salt, Mieske, & Klerman, 1978). Even given the nonorthogonal design (drug $\times$ corrugator levels are confounded), the Hamilton Scale differences are non-significant for $\alpha = .05$.

1966; cf. the "hyperponesis" hypothesis of Whatmore & Ellis, 1959, 1962; and see the review of these early studies by Goldstein, 1972). Carney, Hong, Kulkarni, and Kapila (1982) have recently confirmed that corrugator-site EMG levels are higher in depressed patients than in normal controls, when recordings were obtained from subjects who were merely asked to sit still.

More research is needed to determine whether the elevated EMG levels found in depressed subjects in these studies reflect an arousal process pronounced in depressions which are optimally responsive to tricyclic pharmacotherapy. Some clue is provided by Whatmore and Ellis (1959), who found that retarded depressives showed *higher* EMG levels than agitated depressives, and that these levels decline during successful treatment (Whatmore & Ellis, 1962). Since it is known that tricyclic anti-depressants produce maximal benefits in retarded forms of depression (Byck, 1975; Kuhn, 1958), those subjects in Schwartz *et al.* (1978) and Carney *et al.* (1981) who showed higher EMG levels (hence, by the preceding rationale, more retarded depressions) might be expected to respond prefer-entially to tricyclics. This relationship may underlie the seeming prognostic value of corrugator- and zygomatic-site EMG activity in tricyclic-treated patients.

Investigation of the arousal (vs. a "sad-face") explanation for the elevated EMG levels in depression will likely require inspection of the second-by-second EMG time-series data from individual subjects (see the discussion of the use of P-factored principal-component analysis for EMG data by Fridlund *et al.*, 1980, and Fridlund, Cottam, & Fowler, 1982). A find-ing of positive temporal covariance would favor an arousal process. Sizable negative covariance would suggest a differential-emotions (sad-face) proc-ess (see also recent findings regarding agitative processes in trait-anxious subjects by Fridlund, Hatfield, Cottam, & Fowler, 1981, for feasible analytic methods). If some "hyperponetic" mechanism can account for any prog-nostic value of facial EMG, it may be correlated with that subset of depres-sives that exhibits inhibited pituitary–adrenocortical response to dexa-methasone challenge; thus, facial EMG could provide a noninvasive alternative to the dexamethasone suppression test (Nelson, Orr, Stevenson, & Shane, 1982).

Facial EMG Lateralization for Emotion

In an extension of the growing body of research which suggests hemi-spheric specialization for emotion (Galin, 1974; Sackeim, Greenberg, Weiman, Gur, Hungerbuhler, & Geschwind, 1982), Schwartz *et al.* (1979) found evidence supportive of lateralization of facial EMG response to "emotion" stimuli (but see the criticism by Ekman *et al.*, 1981, p. 102). Surface EMG activity was recorded from both left and right corrugator and zygomatic regions in 10 male and 10 female subjects. Subjects were exposed to imagery instructions in the form of reflective questions designed to evoke happiness, sadness, excitement, and fear, and were also asked to produce overt expressions corresponding to the four affective categories. In the reflective-question condition (but not for posed expressions), positive-emotion items elicited relatively greater right- than left-zygomatic-region activity. Negative-emotion items produced relative left-zygomatic-site predominance. The corrugator-region placements showed no evidence for lateralization in either the reflective-question or the posed-expression condition. Some data were obtained which suggested greater lateralization in female than in male subjects. Similar lateralization effects were also reported for self-referent mood statements (e.g., Velten, 1968) by Sirota and Schwartz (1982).

Interpretation of these results as reflecting cerebral specialization for positive versus negative emotions must remain tentative. Several caveats engendered by such an interpretation should be stated. First, the EMG placements tap only peripheral, effector processes, whose neural substrates are, as stated by Schwartz et al. (1979), obscure. Additionally, the "laterality" effects may have been due to differential regression slopes in the right- and left-musculature EMG transforms to different intensities of emotion stimuli. In other words, the right and left musculature may not show parallel increases in EMG levels at increasing levels of emotion activation. The resulting "crossover" interaction in homologous lateral EMG sites may have produced the laterality effects (see Figure 9-2). This possible difference in right- and left-musculature regression slopes amounts to a complex arousal confound which could only be ruled out through the careful parametric study of self-reported emotion intensities and their regression on EMG-level amplitudes in the left and right musculature. Differences in slope could readily be postulated from evidence of asymmetry in facial bone structure, muscle size, and fatty deposits (see Hager, 1982, and Sackeim & Gur, Chapter 11, this volume). The noncollinearity of left and right zygomatic sites during bilateral activation was recently confirmed by Fridlund and Blood (1983; and see Fridlund, 1982).

Sex Differences in Facial EMG Response

Schwartz, Brown, and Ahern (1980) further investigated the sex differences which were obtained by Schwartz et al. (1979). Surface facial EMG activity was recorded from lateral frontalis, corrugator, zygomatic, and masseter regions (left side of face) in 30 males and 30 females. Subjects were presented imagery items engineered to evoke happiness, sadness, anger, and fear. Results indicated that females generated larger EMG amplitudes than males during the affective imagery. Females reported imagining the items more vividly than males (assessed using a self-report scale), showed greater correlations between imagery ratings and zygomatic- and corrugator-region EMG activity during imagery, and generated larger EMG amplitudes than males during a postimagery, posed-expression con-

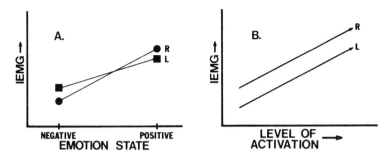

FIGURE 9-2. Possible "arousal" confound in facial EMG lateralization research. (A) Lateralization effect for left–right **zygomatic-major**-region integrated EMG activity (IEMG) as reported by Schwartz, Ahern, and Brown (1979); similar data were also reported by Sirota and Schwartz (1982). Left-zygomatic-site EMG activity was greater than that of the right zygomatic site in a negative-affect reflective-question condition; for positive-affect reflective questions, right-zygomatic-site EMG activity was observed to predominate. However, reporting this finding as demonstrating "lateralization for emotion" implicitly assumes (B), the collinearity of left–right EMG increments for differing degrees of zygomatic response. The crossover interaction observed in (A) may reflect noncollinearities of left–right zygomatic response due to asymmetries in muscle size, skin fatty deposits, α-motoneuron innervation ratios, or more central motor-control substrates, **as apart from** emotion processes per se. Lateralization effects for emotion may only be claimed by showing: (1) that a crossover interaction, as in (A), occurs with equality of EMG levels across the emotion conditions (i.e., there should be no overall EMG gradients from negative- to positive-affect conditions), and/or (2) that collinearity assumptions hold for left–right zygomatic-site EMG responses (or other muscle-site EMG responses for which crossovers are observed) across wide ranges of voluntary, non-emotion-related muscle contraction. Noncollinearity of left–right zygomatic-region EMG sites during bilateral activation was recently confirmed by Fridlund and Blood (1983). (Although we would not push the point, similar collinearity assumptions may underlie cortical EEG–laterality-for-emotion findings!)

dition. It is possible that these findings may have been especially affected by experimental demand. A number of studies have suggested that females may be more influenceable in the experimental context than males (see the review of Rosenthal, 1976, pp. 226–233). Differences in experimental demand might have produced higher vividness ratings, EMG activity, and greater EMG–self-report correlations (because of the expansion of range in both measures). This study is suggestive, and should be replicated with appropriate counterdemand procedures.

Facial EMG Studies of Overt Expressions

There have been relatively few EMG studies of overt facial expression. This is probably due to the relative ease of visual observation of overt expression, in contrast with the barely discernible facial actions which occur during affective imagery and which necessitate the use of facial electromyography. Several studies have nonetheless demonstrated that the use of facial EMG techniques may be valuable for the study of overt expression.

Schwartz *et al.* (1976b; see above) employed a posed-expression condition following the affective-imagery trials, but these data were not presented. However, in an abstract of an earlier unpublished study (Schwartz, Fair, Greenberg, Foran, & Klerman, 1975), results indicated that the facial EMG patterns accompanying affective imagery "were miniature representations of those occurring during overt facial expression" (p. 234). Although the data from the affective imagery experiments are generally suggestive that imagery-related EMG patterning is isomorphic with that occurring during overt expression (e.g., increased corrugator-region activity in negative-emotion imagery, and increased zygomatic-region activity in positive-emotion imagery), this important hypothesis has not yet been systematically tested. Voluntary-expression findings relating to questions of lateralization of facial response and to sex differences were presented previously (Schwartz *et al.*, 1979, 1980).

In an interesting study employing Stanislavski "method" actors, Rusalova, Izard, and Simonov (1975) exposed the actors and an untrained group of control subjects to three emotion conditions. First, the subjects were asked to imagine situations evoking the emotions of joy, fear, anger, and sadness. They were asked to react to the experienced situations with facial expressions. In the second experimental phase, the subjects were asked to reproduce the same emotion states while inhibiting facial expression. In the third phase, the subjects were asked to reproduce the facial expressions for the four emotion states without experiencing the corresponding emotions. Surface EMG activity was sampled from lateral frontalis, corrugator, masseter, and depressor regions, and heart rate and respiration measures were obtained. Results showed that the actors produced patterns of facial EMG activity which differentiated all four emotion states, whereas the untrained controls showed clear differentiation only between the "joy" situation and the negative emotions as a whole. Heart rate declined monotonically from the first experimental phase to the third. The authors interpret the results as emphasizing the role of facial expression in the differentiation of emotion states, and that of heart rate as a measure of generalized "emotional stress." Unfortunately, the lack of counterbalancing of the three experimental conditions makes the heart rate data confounded by habituation to the experimental situation. Nevertheless, the relationship between facial EMG activity and autonomic response systems across various modes of emotion expression and inhibition is an exciting area that merits further inquiry.

A most ambitious effort to systematize the EMG study of overt facial expression is that of Sumitsuji and his colleagues at the University of Osaka. Sumitsuji *et al.* (1965) detailed the methodology employed in their investigations. Sumitsuji *et al.* use a light plastic circular frame surrounding the face of the subject. This frame acts as a harness and terminus for up to

11 differential pair of stainless-steel wire EMG electrodes which are implanted in selected expressive muscles of the face. Sumitsuji *et al.* report excellent recording-site selectivity, sensitive low-noise recording, minimal discomfort to subjects, and little obtrusiveness to the formation of overt expressions.

Using these methods, Sumitsuji, Matsumoto, Tanaka, Kashiwagi, and Kaneko (1967) recorded the EMG activity from 10 muscles in 28 subjects who were each asked to perform a number of motor tasks: elevate the eyebrows, frown, close the eyes, open the mouth, whistle, and supinate with eyes closed. Although the complexity of their data precludes discussion here, both chart records and integrated EMG levels showed distinctive patterns for each of these conditions, many of which are components of facial action in emotion expressions (Izard, 1979). Although this patterning is to be expected for the overt facial actions employed, the confirmation of the sensitivity and practicality of the methodology described by Sumitsuji *et al.* (1965) should not be overlooked.

Sumitsuji, Matsumoto, Tanaka, Kashiwagi, and Kaneko (1977) expanded their inquiry to the direct study of overt facial expressions of emotion. In their brief report, they describe their effort to systematize facial expression according to Schlosberg's "three dimensions of emotion" (pleasant–unpleasant, tension–sleep, and attention–rejection; see Schlosberg, 1952, and a compendium of the dimensional framework of emotion discussed in Izard, 1971). EMG activity was sampled from seven sites in 10 subjects. Photographs were taken of the subjects' faces during moments of overt expression (the experimental manipulation was unspecified), and these photographs were matched with the concurrent electromyograms. A set of judges was employed to classify the photographed expressions according to the following emotion categories: laugh, relaxation, neutral, fear, anger, sadness, attention, surprise, or unclassified. These classifications were combined with ratings of the expressions along Schlosberg's three dimensions. These data, together with the EMG patterns for each expression, were subjected to a set of factor analyses. As before, the results are too complex to detail here, but they suggest that spatial plots of the EMG-pattern factor scores do show some concordance with the Schlosberg dimensional model. Knowles (1978) provided anecdotal data describing the use of similar methods to classify overt facial expressions. These studies are important in that they exploit the power of multivariate techniques for the systematic study of emotion expressions, as we emphasize later in this chapter.

Facial EMG Studies of Social Interaction

A variety of studies have used facial EMG techniques to assess the affectivity of social interaction processes. Specifically, facial EMG has been used in attempt to determine the emotion processes engendered in the presentation of social stimuli, in the delivery of attitudinal communications, and in vicarious (empathic) conditioning.

Dimberg (1981) found that mere presentation of still photographs of posed facial expressions was sufficient to elicit facial EMG responses in subjects. Sixteen subjects were each administered randomized presentations of eight happy faces and eight angry faces. Integrated EMG activity was obtained from left corrugator and zygomatic regions. Results indicated that corrugator-region EMG levels were elevated for the anger stimuli, and that zygomatic-region levels were higher for the happy stimuli. Heart rate and skin conductance responses were also monitored, and these failed to discriminate the two stimulus types. This finding underscores the augmented discriminability that may follow from facial EMG detection in emotion research.

As part of their extensive research program concerning the psychophysiology of attitudes and cognitions (Cacioppo & Petty, 1981a), Cacioppo and Petty (1979) examined multiple-site facial EMG responses in subjects exposed to audiotaped advocacy messages. Forty-eight males received a forewarning, then a presentation, of either a proattitudinal or counterattitudinal communication. Twelve males received a neutral communication. Facial EMG activity was monitored from left corrugator, zygomatic, depressor, and mentalis regions, preceding, and during, the 2-minute message period. Complete results from the multiple-site comparisons are too complex to detail here, but they generally showed discrimination of the affective nature of the subjects' responses. Corrugator-region activity increased significantly during forewarning periods for all groups, corroborating Darwin's notion (Darwin, 1872/1965) that the corrugator region was an indicant of generalized "disturbance" (cognitive *or* affective), not solely of negative affects. Zygomatic-region activity was higher during reception of the proattitudinal message than during either the neutral or counterattitudinal advocacies. Depressor-region activity was also elevated during the proattitudinal message, an interesting and puzzling finding considering the typical role of the depressor muscle in the expression of many negative affects (see Figure 9-1). Assessment of possible crosstalk from other muscles in depressor-region sites is indicated for future research. Mentalis-region activity showed increments during message presentation, regardless of the attitudinal valence of the message. These particular data are consistent with the frequent use of mentalis (as well as orbicularis oris) sites as indicants of general cognitive responding (Cacioppo, 1982; Cacioppo & Petty, 1981b).

Lanzetta and colleagues at Dartmouth College have evolved an ongoing research effort focusing on the empathic eliciting of affective responses using a "vicarious classical conditioning" procedure. In this procedure, a subject observes a model undergoing classical conditioning trials. Under the assumption that the model's emotional responses act as unconditional stimuli (USs) for the subject, the subject is assessed for conditioning effects toward the previously neutral conditional stimuli (CSs) to which the model was exposed.

Vaughan and Lanzetta (1980) studied the involvement of the observer's spontaneous facial responses in vicarious conditioning. They described two experiments designed "to explore the extent to which the facial expressive responses of a model instigate expressive as well as autonomic responses in an observer, and to determine from the expressive measures the extent to which the elicited emotional reaction is congruent with that displayed by the model" (p. 910). Sixteen subjects were shown a videotape of a confederate who displayed facial pain responses to CS+ (conditional stimuli for simulated shock delivery) presentations in a paired-associate word task. EMG responses from surface electrodes over medial frontalis, orbicularis oculi, and masseter regions were monitored. These sites were selected because of their hypothesized involvement in the facial expression of pain. Skin conductance activity was recorded adjunctively. Subjects' verbal responses were scored for their awareness of the specific class of word pairs serving as CS+s, and those serving as nonshock (CS−) stimuli. The physiological response data for the observers were analyzed with respect to both instigation effects (occurring during the model's pain display), and conditioning effects (occurring at CS+ offset, before the model reacted). Instigation effects were demonstrated for both electrodermal and facial EMG activity. During instigation periods, subjects showed greater skin conductance and heightened EMG activity in orbicularis oculi and masseter sites. Conditioning effects were shown to be highly dependent on the observers' awareness of the CS+/US contingency. During conditioning periods, observers showed increased skin conductance and *lower* activity in the three EMG sites. Results were interpreted as suggesting that observers responded as though they were anticipating pain during conditioning periods, and experiencing pain during instigation periods. The authors proposed a social-mimetic process to account for the vicarious responding.

In a correlational analysis of their vicarious-conditioning data, Vaughan and Lanzetta (1980) found that subjects who showed greater facial EMG response amplitudes during instigation periods also tended to show greater electrodermal conditioning. Realizing the possible implications of these data for a facial-feedback theory of emotional experience (Izard, 1971; Tomkins, 1962, 1963), Vaughan and Lanzetta (1981) systematically explored the effects of modulation of observers' expressivity of facial responding to a model's display of pain. Experimental procedures were as in Vaughan and Lanzetta (1980), except that observers were given instructions to inhibit their facial responses or to amplify them by posing pain expressions. A third group of observers was supplied no instructions. Heart rate was added to electrodermal response as a measure of autonomic functioning. The data showed that the "amplify" group of observers generated higher electrodermal conductance and heart rate (and, of course, facial EMG activity) during instigation than did the other two groups; the "inhibit" and uninstructed groups did not differ in autonomic or EMG response instigation. However, the "amplify" group did not show greater conditioning of autonomic or facial EMG measures. These data suggest that *posing* of expressions may have little effect on the modulation of conditioned emotion experienes, although such posed expressions may have facilitating effects on momentarily instigated affects. As the authors acknowledge (Vaughan & Lanzetta, 1981, pp. 28–29), the use of simple posing or modulation instructions as a test of the facial-feedback hypothesis of emotional experience assumes only the most facile interpretation of the hypothesis (see discussion of the facial-feedback hypothesis in the first section of this chapter).

Englis, Vaughan, and Lanzetta (1982) found the extent of vicarious responding to be strongly dependent on the congruence of a model's expressive behavior with the subsequent outcomes for the *observer*. Thirty-five observers were exposed to a gaming situation involving "stock market conditions," in which they were required to guess, in supposed participation with another subject, which market indices were rising or declining. "Correct" guesses (as determined by the experimenters) were monetarily rewarded; "wrong" guesses were punished by mild finger shock. During each session, observers were shown ostensible televised pictures of the other subject undergoing the game. However, the televised image was of a videotaped confederate. The game was not identified as being either promotive or contrient. For the "symmetric" group of subjects, successful market predictions by the models (accompanied by happy expressions) were followed by successful predictions for the observers, and wrong model predictions (accompanied by pain displays) yielded wrong observer predictions. For the "asymmetric" group, the observers were exposed to contingencies opposite of those of the models. A "vicarious" phase, following the gaming phase of the experiment, involved the monitoring of the observers' responses while merely watching the videotaped model, and not playing the game. The observers' skin conductance, heart rate, and integrated EMG activity from orbicularis oculi, masseter, and corrugator sites were recorded throughout the gaming and vicarious experimental phases. The extensive and thoughtful data analyses showed that symmetric model-observer outcomes resulted in greater "empathetic" responding in both phases; asymmetric outcomes resulted in weakened or even counter-empathetic responses. These responses were marked by heightened orbicularis oculi, masseter, corrugator, and skin conductance activity for empathetic responding to modeled pain displays; modeled happiness displays produced relative decrements in these responses. The observer heart rate data did not show differences for modeled pain versus happiness displays. The findings from this experiment were taken to support conditioning perspectives on empathetic responding which emphasize the predictive significance of modeled cues.

The facial EMG studies of vicarious conditioning are important in that they elucidate the role of emotion processes in the mediation of social learning. A minor encumbrance is the somewhat strained usage of Pavlovian terminology to describe the facial EMG responses engendered in the "vicarious classical conditioning" procedure. That this procedure (and the corollary facial EMG responses) is suitable for a classical-conditioning analysis is questionable because of both the extremely long CS-CR intervals (approximately 3 to 10 seconds; Vaughan & Lanzetta, 1980, p. 912), and the slow, nonreflexive temporal dynamics of the EMG responses in these experiments (e.g., Vaughan & Lanzetta, 1980, pp. 914, 918). Unless compelling evidence dictates otherwise, the facial EMG responses are perhaps best interpreted within learning theory as discriminated operants with as-yet-unclear (but theoretically interesting) functions.

Summary

The studies reviewed above strongly suggest that facial electromyography may be well suited for the detection and quantification of overt expression and subjective emotional and mood states. Taken together, these studies support several conclusions:

1. Facial EMG techniques reveal highly differentiated EMG patterns during overt emotion expressions; these are in accord with the specific facial actions that occur during overt expression (see Figure 9-1, and Izard, 1979).
2. The EMG patterning associated with affective imagery instructions is much less differentiated, but may be emotion specific nonetheless (the methodology necessary to investigate this is detailed in the next section of this chapter). The most robust effects are those of increased corrugator-region activity in imagery related to negative emotions, and of increased zygomatic-site activity in positive-emotion imagery.
3. The hypothesis of isomorphism of imagery-related and posed-expression EMG patterns is suggested, but has not yet been systematically investigated.
4. Facial EMG effects related to differentiation of depressed from non-depressed subjects have been tentatively confirmed. However, interpretation of the effects in terms of a differential-emotions perspective (i.e., depressed individuals show covert "sad" faces) was premature. More recent evidence lends credence to earlier notions of a generalized "hyperponetic" process, especially in retarded depressions.
5. Findings pertaining to sex differences and lateralization for emotion in facial EMG activity have not at present been convincingly demonstrated. These tantalizing findings await more definitive experimentation.

6. Facial EMG activity during affective imagery may reflect complex "blended" affect (i.e., patterns of emotions), as well as discrete fundamental emotions. Some unpublished data suggest that this hypothesis may hold true (Polonsky & Schwartz, cited in Schwartz, 1980). The hypothesis of blended EMG patterns was also confirmed by Fridlund *et al.* (1983; see the upcoming section of this chapter).

7. The social-interaction studies show that facial EMG presents a promising adjunctive measure in social psychological research, one that may afford specific information on the role of affective processes in social learning and human interaction.

A PATTERN-CLASSIFICATION APPROACH TO THE STUDY OF FACIAL EMG PATTERNING IN EMOTION

The purpose of this section is to elaborate a methodological approach that may allow more meaningful research in the psychophysiology of emotion. First, conventional paradigms for such research are presented. Second, theoretical considerations that develop from a multivariate perspective on the physiology of emotion are discussed. Third, the implementation of a pattern-classification system for the study of facial EMG response in emotion states is described.

Conventional Paradigms for the Psychophysiological Study of Emotion

Most of the extant experimentation in the psychophysiology of emotion has involved induction of affective states in subjects, and then entertained the question: Is emotion *A* distinguishable from emotion *B* on response *X*? Such experiments have, for the most part, been large-*n*, between-subjects designs summarized by univariate statistical analyses of variance.

Approaches of this type are not ideal for the psychophysiological study of emotion. This is true for several reasons. First, the groups design obscures individual differences in response patterns which are known to exist in states of arousal and emotion (Lacey, 1967). Second, we are in substantial agreement with Meehl (1978) when he asserts: "If you have enough cases and your measures are not totally unreliable, the null hypothesis will always be falsified, regardless of the truth of the substantive theory" (p. 822). Thus, the emphasis on tests of statistical significance in groups designs may not yield results that are interpretable or psychobiologically meaningful in terms of the emotion processes of the individual human being. Third, in the conventional univariate paradigm, any effects of emotion are hopelessly confounded with arousal or response intensity, since any variance in a psychophysiological response system may be due to either arousal or emotion processes. Fourth, it is impossible to discern coordinated multiple-system responses in emotion when the analytic methods are univariate.[5] Fifth, the conventional paradigm fails to address the issue of the *classifiability* of emotion states. Differential emotions theory posits that emotions can be characterized by identifiable neurophysiological signatures (e.g., Izard, 1977; Tomkins, 1962, 1963). The prospect of decoding and classifying emotion states would therefore seem to be a more stringent and meaningful test of discriminability of those states than are simple hypothesis tests of differences between means on single response variables.

Variables and Conformations of Variables

What is needed is an experimental approach that considers multiple response systems and their states and operations across emotion conditions. Numerous theorists have stressed the consideration of patterns of physiological response in the understanding of emotion (e.g., Izard, 1972, 1977; Schwartz, 1975, 1977, 1980). In operational terms, this emphasis may be seen as encompassing within the data analyses the conformation of response variables (their shapes and relative positions within a multivariable space of full rank) as well as the variables themselves.

The desirability of this enhanced approach may be demonstrated graphically (Figure 9-3). Figure 9-3A posits data samples from two organismic states in one subject, A and B (e.g., fear and anger), which are mapped on (measured using) physiological responses X and Y (e.g., EMG activity from two muscle regions). The dispersions of A and B are obviously discriminable (and completely nonoverlapping) in the 2-space formed by variables X and Y (variances in X and Y are shown here as orthogonal, although independence of response systems is not a necessary stipulation). It can readily be seen that attempts to discriminate A and B based on either X or Y alone would be difficult. In accordance with Meehl's (1978) aforementioned tenet, if the experiment contained enough samples of A and B,

---

5. An inductive error made all too commonly in facial EMG–emotion studies was pinpointed in another context by Bear (1979). The error arises as in the following example. A group of subjects is exposed to, say, "fear" and "anger" situations during which lateral frontalis- and corrugator-region EMG activity is monitored. Univariate group tests show that frontalis-site activity is significantly higher in fear than in anger, whereas corrugator-site activity is higher in anger than in fear. An erroneous interpretation of these data would state: "Results showed that subjects in fear situations evinced higher frontalis-site levels and lower corrugator-site levels. In anger situations, subjects showed higher corrugator-site levels and lower frontalis-site levels." The implication of such a statement would be that in fear versus anger, the frontalis and corrugator regions acted in reciprocal fashion (i.e., a patterned negative covariance of the two EMG sites is assumed). However, no such statement can be validly made given the group univariate analyses, since different *subgroups* of the subjects, showing nonhomogeneous responses to the emotion inductions, may have accounted for the significant differences in each case. Only appropriate multivariate tests allow valid pattern interpretations of data sets involving multiple dependent measures.

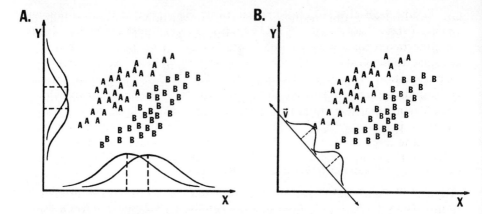

FIGURE 9-3. Scatterplots of two hypothetical emotion states, **A** and **B**, mapped on (measured using) two psychophysiological response measures, **X** and **Y**. (A) Superposition of marginal distributions of **A** and **B** on **X** and **Y** demonstrates considerable overlap despite clear separability of **A** and **B** in the 2-space formed by variables **X** and **Y**. (B) Superposition of vector **V** on which the dispersions of **A** and **B** are maximally separated. **V** is a linear composite of **X** and **Y** derived from linear discriminant analysis. Adapted from Nunnally (1978, p. 457).

the univariate tests for differences on either X or Y might reach significance. Yet little information would be gained in terms of classifying the affective state of the subject even if statistical significance is achieved easily. Moreover, such tests are, like those employed in much of previous emotion research, extremely vulnerable to arousal confounds. Figure 9-3A demonstrates that, although statistical tests based on either measure X or measure Y may be detecting genuine differences *between* A and B, they inexorably detect variation *within* both A and B which may be a function of the level of emotional response and which obscures emotion discriminations. In this way, information is lost and evidence is rendered ambiguous whenever a patterned organismic state is considered within a univariate analytical frame.

How, then, are A and B to be distinguished? Figure 9-3B shows one such method, that of linear discriminant analysis. A linear combination (discriminant function) of the form

$$\mathbf{V}(X, Y) = C(X) + D(Y)$$

where C and D are appropriate weighting coefficients, and X and Y represent values for psychophysiological response systems X and Y, is constructed on which separation of A and B is maximized. Figure 9-3B demonstrates that the distributions of A and B on the resultant vector solution (vector $\mathbf{V}$) could then be used to classify reliably the affective state of the subject.

Figure 9-3B also suggests that accurate classification of an unknown emotion state according to its score on linear discriminant function **V** may be undertaken for a wide range of conjoint values of X and Y. Thus, it is possible to separate the dimensions of emotion intensity and emotion discrimination. The vulnerability of this discriminant solution to arousal confounds is thereby reduced, since while the magnitudes of the individual variables may largely reflect arousal (i.e., arousal would be reflected by a sample's position within an emotion cluster), only the conjoint values within the multivariate space would target the particular emotion cluster to which the sample belonged. (In Figure 9-3B, the *intensity* of emotion of a sample would largely be reflected by its placement along the long axis of either A or B, as opposed to its position along discriminant vector **V**. The long axes of A and B are, in fact, linear functions of X and Y derived from principal-component analysis; see Cooley & Lohnes, 1971, pp. 36–38.)

The issue of variables versus conformations of variables may be interpreted as a mathematical distillation of the gestaltist axiom, "The whole is more than the sum of the parts," which in general systems theory is denoted as the *doctrine of emergence* (Fridlund, in preparation, 1983; Sunderland, 1973) and which has been applied by Schwartz (1977, 1980) to the question of physiological patterning in human emotion. That the conformations of response variables may offer more information than any univariate reductions in discriminating emotion states is shown in Figure 9-4. (The experiment from which the data in Figure 9-4 are taken will be described subsequently.)

Classification of Variable Conformations

Pattern-Classification Approach

Because of the considerations outlined above, recent research incorporates a pattern-classification approach to the study of the facial EMG correlates of affective imagery and posed expressions (Fridlund *et al.*, 1983). The pattern-classification paradigm is presented in Figure 9-5. Within this general paradigm, patterned input variables are transduced to a form suitable for quantification (*Transduction*). An iterative process ensues whereby features are derived from the input variables which maximally discriminate among sets of the variables (*Feature Extraction*), and show maximal hit rates on pre- or postdiction of those sets (*Classification*). In this approach, reliability of hit rate of classification indexes the success of the pattern-recognition procedure by demonstrating the degree of discriminability of input-variable conformations.

Experimental Implementation. For the present research, 12 right-handed females were administered 48 counterbalanced 20-second affective-imagery trials using verbal items preselected for relative purity along the dimen-

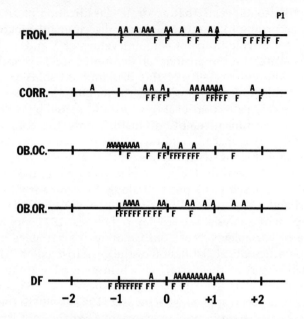

FIGURE 9-4. Plots of standard EMG scores for fear and anger affective-imagery responses of subject P1 mapped itemwise on each of four muscle regions, and on a linear composite of the four regions derived from linear discriminant analysis (see Figure 9-3). The superior discrimination of the anger and fear responses on the discriminant function demonstrates that consideration of variable conformations provides information which cannot be gleaned from any of the univariate reductions alone. Item codes: A, anger; F, fear. Abbreviations: FRON., lateral frontalis region; CORR., corrugator region; OB.OC., orbicularis oculi region; OB.OR., orbicularis oris region; DF, discriminant function.

sions of happiness, sadness, anger, and fear (Schwartz & Weinberger, 1980). After each trial, subjects rated the affective content of the image on all four of the emotion dimensions, using an abbreviated version of the Differential Emotions Scale (DES; Izard, 1972). The imagery trials were followed by 12 posed-expression trials, and by tests for maximal contraction of each of the muscle regions sampled.

EMG responses were recorded from left lateral frontalis, corrugator, orbicularis oculi, and orbicularis oris regions. Signals were detected with surface differential electrodes with detection passband of 90 to 250 Hz, processed through contour followers ($\tau = .025$ second; Fridlund, 1979), denoised in quadrature (geometric subtraction of average noise levels which recognizes the orthogonality of noise components; see DeVries, 1965), and sampled at 10 Hz throughout each trial using a 32-kRAM PDP-11/03 computer with requisite FORTRAN IV software. Signal amplitudes were resolved to .1 μV (avg.). A 4(muscle region) × 64 (trial) × 200 (samples/trial/muscle region) data file was created on floppy disk for each subject.

Preliminary Analyses. The collection and analysis of the data proceeded as shown in Figure 9-5B. All analyses were within-subject. Program FACE.FOR presented the affective imagery or posed expressions to be read to the subjects, performed data acquisition, and plotted the facial EMG amplitudes on a graphics terminal for monitoring by the experimenter (Figure 9-6).

Parameter extraction was performed by a FORTRAN routine which decounterbalanced the trials into the four a priori emotion categories, and extracted selected statistical parameters for each trial. Parameters included within-trial means, peaks, liabilities, baseline-corrected means and peaks, and range-corrected means and peaks.

Reduced subfiles were created for each parameter. The subfiles were edited in case the subject's DES ratings for any of the imagery items did not correspond to the a priori categorizations of the items. These subfiles

FIGURE 9-5. (A) Stylized pattern-classification system (after Duda & Hart, 1973). (B) Implementation of the pattern-classification approach showing successive stages of data analysis (after Fridlund, Schwartz, & Fowler, 1983).

A.

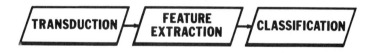

B.

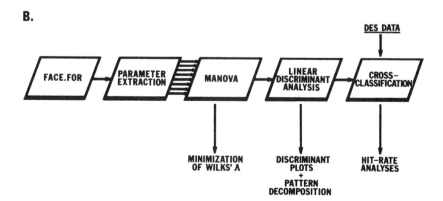

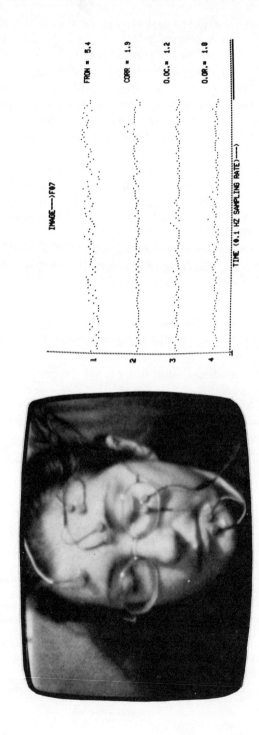

FIGURE 9-6. Left: Televised image of subject P2 showing electrode placements over lateral frontalis, corrugator, orbicularis oculi, and orbicularis oris regions. The subject was asked to imagine a "fear" item. Right: Cathode-ray-tube graphics plot of EMG activity in the four EMG sites throughout the 20-second imagery trial. (**Note:** Abscissa label is erroneous; sampling rate was 10 Hz.)

274

were sequentially input to one-way fixed-effects multivariate analyses of variance (MANOVAs; Cooley & Lohnes, 1971).[6] These MANOVAs formed the feature-extraction portion of the program sequence (Figure 9-6). Their results were evaluated for the parameter which minimized the value of the Wilks's Λ statistic (the ratio of the determinants of the within-groups to total-groups dispersion matrices). The minimal-Λ criterion was used as the measure of the parameter's ability to separate the emotion categories on the basis of the EMG sample vectors, and thus provided information about the signal properties that afforded maximal discrimination of the imagery-related facial EMG patterns. (For the posed-expression condition, in which subjects were instructed to maintain the expressions for 20 seconds, within-trial means were employed throughout the analyses.)

Tabulation of parameter-extraction results for the 12 subjects revealed that within-trial *means* satisfied the minimal-Λ criterion for 5 of the subjects, with the remainder evincing the minimal-Λ criterion for the following parameters: range-corrected means (3), peaks (2), and lability (2). These results suggest that subjects may produce different temporal patterns of striate-muscle activity during the imagery, and that these temporal characteristics may offer nonredundant sources of discriminability among emotion states.

The subfiles that fit the minimal-Λ criterion for each subject (thus showing maximal separations of muscle conformations) were input to a linear discriminant analysis routine. Output from the discriminant analysis consisted of a set of linear combinations (canonical variates or discriminant functions) of the four EMG sites. These allowed a spatial remapping of the conformational EMG-site responses to the imagery (or posed-expression) items such that they were maximally discriminated (as on vector **V** in Figure 9-2B). This remapping effected a projection of muscle-region conformations (which, for four muscle regions, are represented in 4-space)

---

6. Use of the fixed-effects model in the single-subject design, as presented here, proceeds directly from the cardinal assumption of differential emotions theory—that the imagery items constituted samples drawn from each of several independent emotion populations within the individual subject. Under this assumption, treatment-level (emotion) covariances were explicitly excluded from the MANOVAs. (Assumptions of independent emotion populations also underlay the use of standard χ^2 tests for independent data in the classification analyses.) The values of Wilks's Λ which resulted from the MANOVAs were not interpreted inferentially (as hypothesis tests), but rather as indices of relative success in parameter extraction. We would nevertheless argue the suitability of the single-subject use of MANOVA here, since autocorrelated errors in the MANOVAs were neutralized by the decounterbalancing procedure (see Gentile, Roden, & Klein, 1972). Our preference within the pattern-classification framework is to work at the single-subject level of analysis, and then to assess the congruence of the subjects' response patterns. Social psychologists, who may prefer to deal solely with group effects within a pattern-classification perspective, may employ an Emotions $\times$ Subjects repeated-measures MANOVA (e.g., Murphy, 1979), followed by standard classification analyses.

onto a reduced space. The resulting "emotive plot" provided a precise quantitative decomposition of the EMG patterns through the examination of the discriminant weights, and permitted the exact muscle-region conformations which characterized each emotion state to be ascertained (see Overall & Klett, 1972; Tatsuoka, 1971). Figure 9-7 shows the emotive plots for one subject, for both posed-expression and affective-imagery conditions.

The minimal-Λ subfiles for each subject were input to a multivariate classification routine (Anderson, 1958; Cooley & Lohnes, 1971; Overall & Klett, 1972). Output from this routine included a set of classification functions (see Anderson, 1958) which was used to classify the EMG vector from an "unknown" imagery (or posed-expression) trial in one of the four emotion categories. This procedure allowed either fitted, within-sample classifications, or given sufficient data, split-half cross-validation and assessment of true hit rates.

Preliminary analyses showed that within-sample cross-classifications of the EMG Conformations $\times$ Emotion Category during the affective-imagery condition were significant ($p < .05$, χ^2 test of contingency) in 11 of the 12 subjects. The use of 48 affective-imagery items provided sufficient data to allow split-half cross-validation on unknown items. These data are presented in Table 9-2. They revealed moderate success in classification, with hit rates of 51%, 49%, 49%, and 38% for happiness, sadness, anger, and fear, respectively.[7]

The wide range of differentiation in patterns seen across subjects (from 29% to 88% average hit rate) suggests that subject selection may be useful for particular facial EMG–emotion experimentation, and that hit rates may be improved considerably through the use of imagery training emphasizing the response properties of the imagery instructions (Lang, 1979). Measurement of more than four EMG sites will allow further discrimination of characteristic EMG patterns for each emotion category. The posed-expression data were not sufficient (three trials for each of four emotion categories) to permit χ^2 analysis or cross-validation, but within-sample classification revealed rates of 89%, 83%, 86%, and 86% for the four expression categories of happiness, sadness, anger, and fear, respectively.[8]

7. Performance of the classification analyses using the within-trial mean parameter (as opposed to the minimal-Λ parameter) for each subject showed little shrinkage in classification rates ($\approx 5\%$), indicating that the stated rates did not result from an appreciably overfit model.

8. In the present classification scheme, the analyses employed were variants of the general linear model. Higher-order nonlinear methods incorporating more complex decision surfaces may offer greater accuracy of classification. This hypothesis awaits further research. In addition, closer examination of the temporal clustering of multiple EMG-site responses may provide important classificatory information not revealed through covariance-structure analyses (see Colgan, 1978).

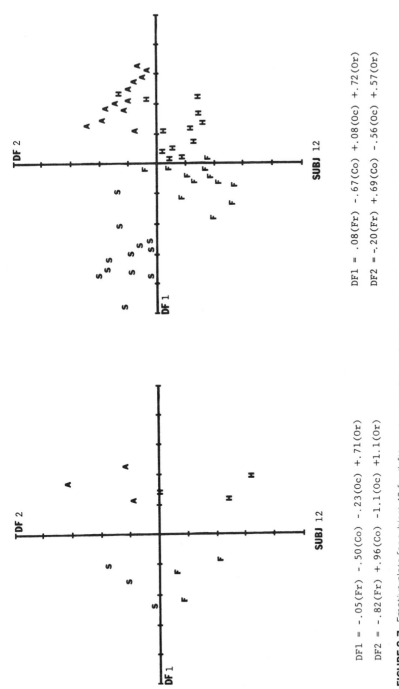

FIGURE 9-7. Emotive plots for subject 12 for (left) overt expression, and (right) imagery-related EMG activity. Each data point represents one trial. Pattern decompositions are provided by the discriminant functions for each plot. Subject 12 evinces a high degree of isomorphism of overt-expression and imagery-related EMG patterns. Item codes: H, happiness; S, sadness; A, anger; F, fear. Abbreviations: DF, discriminant function; Fr, lateral frontalis site; Co, corrugator site; Oc, obicularis oculi site; Or, orbicularis oris site.

DF1 = -.05(Fr) -.50(Co) -.23(Oc) +.71(Or)
DF2 = -.82(Fr) +.96(Co) -1.1(Oc) +1.1(Or)

DF1 = .08(Fr) -.67(Co) +.08(Oc) +.72(Or)
DF2 = -.20(Fr) +.69(Co) -.56(Oc) +.57(Or)

277

TABLE 9-2. Split-Half Cross-Validation on Imagery-Related EMG Vectors: Group Data

SUBJECT NO.	PERCENT									
	I_H	Ht_H	I_S	Ht_S	I_A	Ht_A	I_F	Ht_F	I_T	Ht_T
1	33	30	33	60	50	38	33	0	38	29
2	83	50	50	43	67	33	50	33	63	42
3	50	10	83	17	33	33	67	50	58	25
4	50	83	67	33	50	14	50	40	54	42
5	67	17	17	60	67	40	33	50	46	33
6	83	67	67	40	67	67	33	17	63	33
7	67	75	67	50	67	50	50	50	63	58
8	33	25	83	67	17	50	17	33	38	42
9	100	71	50	0	83	33	50	0	71	29
10	83	67	67	83	83	67	67	33	75	63
11	83	63	83	50	50	63	33	50	63	58
12	83	67	100	83	100	100	100	100	96	88
$\bar{x}$	68	51	64	49	61	49	49	38	61	45

Note. Abbreviations: I, percentage index of internal structure from derivation sample; Ht, hit rate on cross-validation sample; H, happy images; S, sad images; A, anger images; F, fear images; T, total; $\bar{x}$, group mean.

The pattern-classification results also suggested the following:

1. The MANOVA Wilks's Λ was a nearly ideal index of overall degree of emotion discrimination shown by individual subjects, producing significant ($p < .05$) correlations with both within-sample classification rates, and subsequent hit rates on cross-validation.

2. Subjects who generated highly differentiated imagery-related EMG patterns were not necessarily the ones who generated highly differentiated posed expressions; the correlation between the Wilks's Λ indices for the two conditions was .26 (not significant). This finding provided evidence against a simple demand interpretation of the EMG patterning seen in the affective-imagery condition.

3. The Wilks's Λ indices of emotion discrimination for the 12 subjects correlated significantly with both their ratings of imagery vividness, and of the reported average duration during each trial that the imagery was maintained.

4. Utilization of blended self-report scores from the DES (wherein each subject rated the content of each imagery item on all four emotion dimensions) decomposed significantly more of the EMG patterning seen in the imagery condition than did the use of only primary-emotion ratings (assessed using a paired-samples Hotelling T^2 test on normalized canonical

correlations of EMG patterns with blended vs. tetrachotomous self-report). The hypothesis that the facial musculature encoded complex, blended affect in the imagery condition was thus supported.

Implications for Emotion Research. The pattern-classification paradigm is offered as a valuable approach not only for the decoding and characterization of the emotions through facial EMG activity, but also for the quantitative substantiation of previous studies of facial expression and emotion, including cross-cultural research (Ekman, Friesen, & Ellsworth, 1972; Izard, 1971). Using this approach, the configurative emotion predictions adduced by facial coding systems such as MAX (Izard, 1979) and FACS (Ekman & Friesen, 1978) may be empirically validated. In a more general context, the perspective and procedures detailed here may enable the more sophisticated study of psychophysiological phenomena which have largely proven refractory to traditional univariate analyses, such as the autonomic concomitants of emotion,[9] and the physiological signatures which may correspond to specific psychophysiological disorders.

CONCLUSION

Electromyographic detection of facial striate-muscle activity offers the possibility of a dynamic psychophysiological measurement system which is highly sensitive to emotion states and displays. Facial EMG techniques present several advantages over observer coding schemes. They allow the capability of immediate quantification, the provision of high-resolution measurement of the magnitude of facial actions, and sensitivity to low-level facial actions which would otherwise be unobservable. Facial EMG techniques are not without their liabilities. These involve the intrusion of measurement apparatus and obstruction of facial vagility, experimental demand confounds due to subjects' ongoing awareness of the measure-

---

9. With regard to the use of autonomic responses for the decoding and classification of emotion states, we are encouraged by the frequent finding (often lamented by arousal theorists) that autonomic indices of "arousal" show either low or moderate intercorrelations (Lacey, 1967). Following from the standard psychometric approach, if one wished to construct a classification instrument with high discriminant validity, one would want to use a number of criterion-valid, yet minimally correlated, response variables. The fact that these criteria are met by traditional autonomic response measures seems advantageous from a multivariate perspective.

At this writing, a very innovative implementation of the pattern-classification approach is under way at Dartmouth under the direction of G. M. McHugo and J. T. Lanzetta. These researchers are using multivariate techniques to derive autonomic, facial EMG, and self-report response patterns to film segments standardized for affective valence according to multidimensional scaling procedures (McHugo, 1981). Clearly, this is quite a promising extension of facial EMG–emotion research.

ment procedure, methodological problems and lack of conventions in EMG-detection technology, and arousal confounds which may obscure observation of emotion-specific patterning.

Facial EMG–emotion research, although plagued by the foregoing limitations, has provided provocative findings relating both to covert facial-muscle patterning in affective imagery and in overt facial expressions. The affective-imagery studies suggest that low-level facial EMG may be a sensitive index of felt emotion states and, possibly, of depressive disorder. The overt-expression research indicates that facial EMG techniques may allow the rapid quantification, description, and categorization of the dimensionality of facial displays. They may also provide for the concurrent validation of emotion predictions of facial coding systems. Studies of facial EMG activity in social interaction and communication promise to reveal the power and extent of interpersonal emotion processes.

A multivariate pattern-classification approach to the psychophysiological study of emotion is offered for special application to facial EMG–emotion research. This approach recognizes the configurative nature of facial action in emotion, and permits the disentangling of arousal processes from those due to distinct emotions. Because of its emphasis on the *decoding* and *classification* of emotion states, the pattern-classification approach presents a superior analytic framework for the extension of psychophysiological studies of human emotions.

The findings that have emerged from the extant facial EMG–emotion research must be regarded as tentative. More rigorous and systematic investigation must proceed before facial EMG activity is adequately criterion-validated as a reliable and interpretable correlate of discrete emotions. But we are optimistic. The nascent facial EMG–emotion methodology has already produced the best evidence to date for the physiological discrimination of human emotion states. It may indeed offer considerable knowledge of the role of emotion processes in human behavior.

ACKNOWLEDGMENTS

The authors gratefully acknowledge the helpful and formative comments made by P. Ekman, S. C. Fowler, J. C. Hager, and G. J. McHugo on an earlier draft of the manuscript. The facial EMG pattern-classification research presented in this chapter was performed while the first author was a predoctoral research associate at the Psychophysiological Laboratory and Research Clinic, Yale University, under National Science Foundation Grant BNS76-81045 to G. E. Schwartz.

REFERENCES

Anderson, T. W. *Introduction to multivariate statistical analysis.* New York: Wiley, 1958.
Ax, A. F. The physiological differentiation between fear and anger in humans. *Psychosomatic Medicine*, 1953, 5, 433–442.

Balliet, R., Shinn, J. B., & Bach-y-Rita, P.   Facial muscle rehabilitation: Retraining selective muscle control. *International Rehabilitation Medicine*, 1982, *4*, 67–74.

Basmajian, J. V.   *Muscles alive: Their functions as revealed by electromyography* (4th ed.). Baltimore: Williams & Wilkins, 1978.

Bear, D. M.   The temporal lobes: An approach to the study of organic behavioral changes. In M. S. Gazzaniga (Ed.), *Handbook of behavioral neurobiology* (Vol. 2). *Neuropsychology*. New York: Plenum, 1979.

Beck, A. T.   *Depression*. New York: Harper & Row, 1967.

Berger, P. A.   Antidepressant medications and the treatment of depressions. In J. D. Barchas, P. A. Berger, R. D. Ciaranello, & G. R. Elliott (Eds.), *Psychopharmacology: From theory to practice*. New York: Oxford University Press, 1977.

Brown, J. S., & Farber, I. E.   Emotions conceptualized as intervening variables with suggestions toward a theory of frustration. *Psychological Bulletin*, 1951, *48*, 465–495.

Buchwald, A. M., Strack, S., & Coyne J. C.   Demand characteristics and the Velton mood induction procedure. *Journal of Consulting and Clinical Psychology*, 1981, *49*, 478–479.

Buck, R.   Nonverbal behavior and the theory of emotion: The facial feedback hypothesis. *Journal of Personality and Social Psychology*, 1980, *38*, 811–824.

Byck, R.   Drugs and the treatment of psychiatric disorders. In L. S. Goodman & A. Gilman (Eds.), *The pharmacological basis of therapeutics* (5th ed.), New York: Macmillan, 1975.

Cacioppo, J. T.   Social psychophysiology: A classic perspective and contemporary approach. *Psychophysiology*, 1982, *19*, 241–251.

Cacioppo, J. T., & Petty, R. E.   Attitudes and cognitive response: An electrophysiological approach. *Journal of Personality and Social Psychology*, 1979, *37*, 2181–2199.

Cacioppo, J. T., & Petty, R. E.   Electromyograms as measures of extent and affectivity of information-processing. *American Psychologist*, 1981, *36*, 441–456. (a)

Cacioppo, J. T., & Petty R. E.   Electromyographic specificity during covert information processing. *Psychophysiology*, 1981, *18*, 518–523. (b)

Cannon, W.B.   The James–Lange theory of emotions: A critical examination and an alternative theory. *American Journal of Psychology*, 1927, *39*, 106–124.

Cantril, H., & Hunt, W. H.   Emotional effects produced by the injection of adrenalin. *American Journal of Psychology*, 1932, 44, 300–307.

Carney, R. M.   Personal communication, June 1981.

Carney, R. M., Hong, B. A., Kulkarni, S., & Kapila, A.   A comparison of EMG and SCL in normal and depressed subjects. *Pavlovian Journal of Biological Science*, 1982, *16*, 212–216.

Carney, R. M., Hong, B. A., O'Connell, M. F., & Amado, H.   Facial electromyography as a predictor of treatment outcome in depression. *British Journal of Psychiatry*, 1981, *138*, 454–459.

Carroll, J. B.   The nature of the data, or how to choose a correlation coefficient. *Psychometrika*, 1961, *26*, 347–372.

Chernoff, H.   *The use of faces to represent points in n-dimensional space graphically* (Tech. Rep. No. 71). Stanford, Calif.: Stanford University, Department of Statistics, 1971.

Colgan, P. W. (Ed.).   *Quantitative ethology*. New York: Wiley, 1978.

Cooley, W. W., & Lohnes, P. R.   *Multivariate data analysis*. New York: Wiley, 1971.

Darwin, C.   *The expression of the emotions in man and animals*. Chicago: University of Chicago Press, 1965. (Originally published, 1872.)

Davis, J. F. *Manual of surface electromyography*. Montreal: Allan Memorial Institute of Psychiatry, Laboratory for Psychological Studies, 1952.

DeBacher, G., & Basmajian, J. V.   EMG feedback strategies in rehabilitation of neuromuscular disorders. In J. Beatty & H. Legewie (Eds.), *Biofeedback and behavior*. New York: Plenum, 1977.

DeVries, H. A.   Muscle tonus in postural muscles. *American Journal of Physical Medicine*, 1965, 44, 275–291.

Dimberg, U.   Facial reactions to facial expressions. *Uppsala Psychological Reports No. 303*, 1981.

Duchenne, G. B. A. [*Physiologie des mouvements*] (E. B. Kaplan trans.). Philadelphia: Saunders, 1959. (Originally published, 1867.)

Duda, R. O., & Hart, P. E. *Pattern analysis and scene classification.* New York: Wiley, 1973.

Duffy, E. *Activation and behavior.* New York: Wiley, 1962.

Duffy, E. Activation. In. N. S. Greenfield & R. A. Sternbach (Eds.), *Handbook of psychophysiology.* New York: Holt, Rinehart & Winston, 1972.

Ekman, P. Methods for measuring facial action. In K. Scherer & P. Ekman (Eds.), *Handbook on methods of nonverbal communications research.* New York: Cambridge University Press, 1981.

Ekman, P., & Friesen, W. V. *Unmasking the face.* Englewood Cliffs, N.J.: Prentice-Hall, 1975.

Ekman, P., & Friesen, W. V. *Facial action coding system.* Palo Alto, Calif.: Consulting Psychologists Press, 1978.

Ekman, P., Friesen, W. V., & Ancoli, S. Facial signs of emotional experience. *Journal of Personality and Social Psychology*, 1980, *39*, 1125–1134.

Ekman, P., Friesen, W. V., & Ellsworth, P. C. *Emotion in the human face.* Elmsford, N.Y.: Pergamon, 1972.

Ekman, P., Hager, J. C., & Friesen, W. V. The symmetry of emotional and deliberate facial actions. *Psychophysiology*, 1981, *18*, 101–106.

Ellsworth, P. C., & Tourangeau, R. On our failure to disconfirm what nobody ever said. *Journal of Personality and Social Psychology*, 1981, *40*, 363–369.

Englis, B. G. Vaughan, K. B., & Lanzetta, J. T. Conditioning of counterempathetic emotional responses. *Journal of Experimental Social Psychology*, 1982, *18*, 375–391.

Feleky, A. M. The expression of the emotions. *Psychological Review*, 1914, *21*, 33–34.

Fridlund, A. J. Contour-following integrator for dynamic tracking of electromyographic data. *Psychophysiology*, 1979, *16*, 491–493.

Fridlund, A. J. Artistry and artifact in facial EMG/emotion studies: Methodology, miscellany, and the multivariate imperative. *Psychophysiology*, 1982, *19*, 542–543. (Abstract)

Fridlund, A. J. *The doctrine of emergence and its application to psychophysiological research and therapy.* Manuscript in preparation, 1983.

Fridlund, A. J., & Blood, K. M. T. *Possible motor-control confounds in facial EMG "lateralization-for-emotion" research.* Manuscript submitted for publication, 1983.

Fridlund, A. J., Cottam, G. L., & Fowler, S. C. In search of the general tension factor: Tensional patterning during auditory stimulation. *Psychophysiology*, 1982, *19*, 136–145.

Fridlund, A. J., Ekman, P., & Oster, H. Facial expressions of emotion. In A. Siegman (Ed.), *Nonverbal communication: A functional perspective*, in press.

Fridlund, A. J., & Fowler, S. C. An eight-channel computer-controlled scanning electromyograph. *Behavior Research Methods and Instrumentation*, 1978, *10*, 652–662.

Fridlund, A. J., Fowler, S. C., & Pritchard, D. A. Striate muscle tension patterning in frontalis EMG biofeedback. *Psychophysiology*, 1980, *17*, 47–55.

Fridlund, A. J., Hatfield, M., Cottam, G. L., & Fowler, S. C. *The effects of trait anxiety on multiple-site EMG response amplitudes and covariance structures.* Paper presented at the 21st Annual Meeting of the Society for Psychophysiological Research, Washington, D.C., October 1981.

Fridlund, A. J., Price, A. W., & Fowler, S. C. Low-noise, optically isolated electromyographic preamplifier. *Psychophysiology*, 1982, *19*, 701–705.

Fridlund, A. J., Schwartz, G. E., & Fowler, S. C. *Facial EMG patterning and emotion: Implementation of multivariate pattern-classification strategies.* Manuscript submitted for publication, 1983.

Frois-Wittman, J. The judgment of facial expression. *Journal of Experimental Psychology*, 1930, *13*, 113–151.

Galin, D. Implications for psychiatry of left and right cerebral specialization. *Archives of General Psychiatry*, 1974, *31*, 572–583.

Gentile, J. R., Roden, A. H., & Klein, R. D. An analysis of variance model for the intra-subject replication design. *Journal of Applied Behavior Analysis*, 1972, *5*, 193–198.

Goldstein, I. B. The relationship of muscle tension and autonomic activity to psychiatric disorders. *Psychosomatic Medicine*, 1965, *27*, 39–52.

Goldstein, I. B. Electromyography. In N. S. Greenfield & R. A. Sternbach (Eds.), *Handbook of psychophysiology*. New York: Holt, Rinehart & Winston, 1972.

Goldstein, M. L. Physiological theories of emotion: A critical historical review from the standpoint of behavior theory. *Psychological Bulletin*, 1968, *69*, 23–40.

Grossman, W. I., & Weiner, H. Some factors affecting the reliability of surface electromyography. *Psychosomatic Medicine*, 1966, *28*, 78–83.

Hager, J. C. Asymmetries in facial expression. In P. Ekman (Ed.), *Emotion in the face: Guidelines for research and an integration of findings*. Cambridge: Cambridge University Press, 1982.

Hager, J. C., & Ekman, P. Methodological problems in Tourangeau and Ellsworth's study of facial expression and experience of emotion. *Journal of Personality and Social Psychology*, 1981, *40*, 358–362.

Hayes, K. J. Wave analyses of tissue noise and muscle action potentials. *Journal of Applied Physiology*, 1960, *15*, 749–752.

Izard, C. E. *The face of emotion*. New York: Appleton-Century-Crofts, 1971.

Izard, C. E. *Patterns of emotions*. New York: Academic, 1972.

Izard, C. E. *Human emotions*. New York: Plenum, 1977.

Izard, C. E. *The maximally discriminative facial movement coding system (MAX)*. Newark, Del.: University of Delaware, Instructional Resources Center, 1979.

Izard, C. E. Differential emotions theory and the facial feedback hypothesis of emotion activation: Comments on Tourangeau and Ellsworth's "The role of facial response in the experience of emotion." *Journal of Personality and Social Psychology*, 1981, *40*, 350–354.

Izard, C. E., & Dougherty, L. M. *System for identifying affect expressions by holistic judgment (AFFEX)*. Newark, Del.: University of Delaware, Instructional Resources Center, 1980.

Jacobson, E. Electrophysiology of mental activities and introduction to the psychological process of thinking. In F. J. McGuigan & R. A. Schoonover (Eds.), *The psychophysiology of thinking*. New York: Academic, 1973.

James, W. What is an emotion? *Mind*, 1884, *9*, 188–204.

Kemper, T. D. *A social interactional theory of emotions*. New York: Wiley, 1978.

Kleck, R. E., Vaughan, R. C., Cartwright-Smith, J., Vaughan, K. B., Colby, C. Z., & Lanzetta, J. T. Effects of being observed on expressive, subjective, and physiological responses to painful stimuli. *Journal of Personality and Social Psychology*, 1976, *34*, 1211–1218.

Knowles, P. L. A preliminary report on a technique for the classification of facial expressions. *Journal of General Psychology*, 1978, *98*, 155–156.

Kuhn, R. The treatment of depressive states with G22355 (imipramine hydrochloride). *American Journal of Psychiatry*, 1958, *115*, 459–464.

Lacey, J. I. Somatic response patterning and stress: Some revisions of activation theory. In M. H. Appley & R. Trumbull (Eds.), *Psychological stress*. New York: Appleton-Century-Crofts, 1967.

Landis, C. The interpretation of facial expression in emotion. *Journal of General Psychology*, 1929, *2*, 59–72.

Lang, P. J. A bio-informational theory of emotional imagery. *Psychophysiology*, 1979, *16*, 495–512.

Lange, C. G. *Om sindsbevaegelser. et psyko. fysiolog. studie*. Copenhagen: Krønar, 1885.

Leshner, A. I. Hormones and emotions. In D. K. Candland, J. P. Fell, E. Keen, A. I. Leshner, R. M. Tarpy, & R. Plutchik, *Emotion*. Monterey, Calif.: Brooks/Cole, 1977.

Levy, N., & Schlosberg, H. Woodworth scale of values of the Lightfoot pictures of facial expression. *Journal of Experimental Psychology*, 1960, *60*, 121–125.

Lykken, D. T., Rose, R., Luther, B., & Maley, M. Correcting psychophysiological measures for individual differences in range. *Psychological Bulletin*, 1966, *66*, 481–484.

Malmo, R. B. Activation: A neuropsychological dimension. *Psychological Review*, 1959, *66*, 367–383.

Malmo, R. B., & Shagass, C.   Physiologic studies of reaction to stress in anxiety and early schizophrenia. *Psychosomatic Medicine*, 1949, *11*, 9–24.

Marshall, G. D., & Zimbardo, P. G.   Affective consequences of inadequately explained physiological arousal. *Journal of Personality and Social Psychology*, 1979, *37*, 970–988.

Martin, I., & Davies, B. M.   The effect of sodium amytal in autonomic and muscular activity of patients with depressive illness. *British Journal of Psychiatry*, 1965, *111*, 168–175.

Maslach, C.   Negative emotional biasing of unexplained arousal. *Journal of Personality and Social Psychology*, 1979, *37*, 953–969.

McHugo, G. J.   Personal communication, June 1981.

Meehl, P. E.   Theoretical risks and tabular asterisks: Sir Karl, Sir Ronald, and the slow progress of soft psychology. *Journal of Consulting and Clinical Psychology*, 1978, *46*, 806–834.

Moritani, T., & DeVries, H. A.   Reexamination of the relationship between the surface integrated electromyogram (IEMG) and the force of isometric contraction. *American Journal of Physical Medicine*, 1978, *57*, 263–277.

Murphy, D. D.   *Program MRM: Multivariate repeated measures*. Unpublished manuscript, Florida International University, 1979.

Nelson, W. H., Orr, W. W., Stevenson, J. M., & Shane, S. R.   Hypothalamic–pituitary–adrenal axis activity and tricyclic response in major depression. *Archives of General Psychiatry*, 1982, *39*, 1033–1036.

Nunnally, J. C.   *Psychometric theory*. New York: McGraw-Hill, 1978.

Öhman, A., & Dimberg, U.   Facial expressions as conditioned stimuli for electrodermal responses: A case of "preparedness"? *Journal of Personality and Social Psychology*, 1978, *36*, 1251–1258.

Oliveau, D., & Willmuth, R.   Facial muscle electromyography in depressed and nondepressed hospitalized subjects: A partial replication. *American Journal of Psychiatry*, 1979, *136*, 548–550.

Orne, M. T.   On the social psychology of the psychological experiment: With particular reference to demand characteristics and their implication. *American Psychologist*, 1962, *17*, 776–783.

Overall, J. E., & Klett, C. J.   *Applied multivariate analysis*. New York: McGraw-Hill, 1972.

Polivy, J., & Doyle, C.   Laboratory induction of mood states through the reading of self-referent mood statements: Affective changes or demand characteristics? *Journal of Abnormal Psychology*, 1980, *89*, 286–290.

Ralston, H. J., & Libet, B.   The question of tonus in skeletal muscle. *American Journal of Physical Medicine*, 1953, *32*, 85–92.

Rimon, R., Stenback, A., & Hahmar, E.   Electromyographic findings in depressive patients. *Journal of Psychosomatic Research*, 1966, *10*, 159–170.

Rosenthal, R.   *Experimenter effects in behavioral research*. New York: Irvington, 1976.

Rusalova, M. N., Izard, C. E., & Simonov, P. V.   Comparative analysis of mimical and autonomic components of man's emotional state. *Aviation, Space, and Environmental Medicine*, 1975, *46*, 1132–1134.

Sackeim, H. A., Greenberg, M. C., Weiman, A. L., Gur, R. C., Hungerbuhler, J. P., & Geschwind, N.   Hemispheric asymmetry in the expression of positive and negative emotions: Neurological evidence. *Archives of Neurology*, 1982, *39*, 210–218.

Schachter, S., & Singer, J. E.   Cognitive, social, and physiological determinants of emotional state. *Psychological Review*, 1962, *69*, 379–399.

Schlosberg, H.   The description of facial expressions in terms of two dimensions. *Journal of Experimental Psychology*, 1952, *44*,229–237.

Schwartz, G. E.   Biofeedback, self-regulation, and the patterning of physiological processes. *American Scientist*, 1975, *63*, 314–324.

Schwartz, G. E.   Psychosomatic disorders and biofeedback: A psychobiological model of disregulation. In J. D. Maser & M. E. P. Seligman (Eds.), *Psychopathology: Experimental models*. San Francisco: W. H. Freeman, 1977.

Schwartz, G. E.   Psychophysiological patterning and emotion revisited: A systems perspective. In C. E. Izard (Ed.), *Measuring emotions in infants and children*. Cambridge: Cambridge University Press, 1980.

Schwartz, G. E., Ahern, G. L., & Brown, S. L.   Lateralized facial muscle response to positive and negative emotional stimuli. *Psychophysiology*, 1979, *16*, 561–571.

Schwartz, G. E., Brown, S. L., & Ahern, G. L.   Facial muscle patterning and subjective experience during affective imagery. *Psychophysiology*, 1980, *17*, 75–82.

Schwartz, G. E., Fair, P. L., Greenberg, P. S., Foran, J. M., & Klerman, G. L.   Self-generated affective imagery elicits discrete patterns of facial muscle activity. *Psychophysiology*, 1975, *12*, 234. (Abstract)

Schwartz, G. E., Fair, P. L., Mandel, M. R., Salt, P., Mieske, M., & Klerman, G. L.   Facial electromyography in the assessment of improvement in depression. *Psychosomatic Medicine*, 1978, *40*, 355–360.

Schwartz, G. E., Fair, P. L., Salt, P., Mandel, M. R., & Klerman, G. L.   Facial expression and imagery in depression: An electromyographic study. *Psychosomatic Medicine*, 1976, *38*, 337–347. (a)

Schwartz, G. E., Fair, P. L., Salt, P., Mandel, M. R., & Klerman, G. L.   Facial muscle patterning to affective imagery in depressed and nondepressed subjects. *Science*, 1976, *192*, 489–491. (b)

Schwartz, G. E., & Weinberger, D. A.   Patterns of emotional responses to affective situations: Relations among happiness, sadness, anger, fear, depression, and anxiety. *Motivation and Emotion*, 1980, *4*, 175–191.

Sirota, A. D., & Schwartz, G. E.   Facial muscle patterning and lateralization during elation and depression imagery. *Journal of Abnormal Psychology*, 1982, *91*, 25–34.

Skinner, B. F.   *Science and human behavior*. New York: Macmillan, 1953.

Starr, A., McKeon, B., Skuse, N., & Burke, D.   Cerebral potentials evoked by muscle stretch in man. *Brain*, 1981, *104*, 149–166.

Strong, P.   *Biophysical measurements*. Beaverton, Ore.: Tektronix, Inc., 1970.

Sumitsuji, N., Matsumoto, K., & Kaneko, Z.   A new method to study facial expression using electromyography. *Electromyography*, 1965, *5*, 269–272.

Sumitsuji, N., Matsumoto, K., Tanaka, M., Kashiwagi, T., & Kaneko, Z.   Electromyographic investigation of the facial muscles. *Electromyography*, 1967, *7*, 77–96.

Sumitsuji, N., Matsumoto, K., Tanaka, M., Kashiwagi, T., & Kaneko, Z.   An attempt to systematize human emotion from EMG study of the facial expression. *Proceedings of the 4th Congress of the International College of Psychosomatic Medicine*, Kyoto, Japan, 1977.

Sunderland, J. W.   *A general systems philosophy for the social and behavioral sciences*. New York: Braziller, 1973.

Tarpy, R. M.   The nervous system and emotion. In D. K. Candland, J. P. Fell, E. Keen, A. I. Leshner, R. M. Tarpy, & R. Plutchik, *Emotion*. Monterey, Calif.: Brooks/Cole, 1977.

Tatsuoka, M. M.   *Multivariate analysis: Techniques for educational and psychological research*. New York: Wiley, 1971.

Teasdale, J. D., & Bancroft, J.   Manipulation of thought content as a determinant of mood and corrugator activity in depressed patients. *Journal of Abnormal Psychology*, 1977, *86*, 235–241.

Teasdale, J. D., & Rezin, V.   Effect of thought-stopping on thoughts, mood and corrugator EMG in depressed patients. *Behaviour Research and Therapy*, 1978, *16*, 97–102.

Tomkins, S. S.   *Affect, imagery, consciousness* (Vol. 1). *The positive affects*. New York: Springer, 1962.

Tomkins, S. S.   *Affect, imagery, consciousness* (Vol. 2). *The negative affects*. New York: Springer, 1963.

Tomkins, S. S.   The role of facial response in the experience of emotion: A reply to Tourangeau and Ellsworth. *Journal of Personality and Social Psychology*, 1981, *40*, 355–357.

Tourangeau, R., & Ellsworth, P. C.   The role of facial response in the experience of emotion. *Journal of Personality and Social Psychology*, 1979, *37*, 1519–1531.

Vaughan, K. B., & Lanzetta, J. T.   Vicarious instigation and conditioning of facial expressive and autonomic responses to a model's expressive display of pain. *Journal of Personality and Social Psychology*, 1980, *38*, 909–923.

Vaughan, K. B., & Lanzetta, J. T.   The effect of modulation of expressive displays on vicarious emotional arousal. *Journal of Experimental Social Psychology*, 1981, *17*, 16–30.

Velten, E.   A laboratory task for induction of mood states. *Behaviour Research and Therapy*, 1968, *6*, 473–482.

Vitti, M., & Basmajian, J. V.   Electromyographic investigation of procerus and frontalis muscles. *Electromyography and Clinical Neurophysiology*, 1976, *16*, 227–236.

Whatmore, G. B., & Ellis, R. M.   Some neurophysiologic aspects of depressed states. *Archives of General Psychiatry*, 1959, *1*, 70–80.

Whatmore, G. B., & Ellis, R. M.   Further neurophysiologic aspects of depressed states. *Archives of General Psychiatry*, 1962, *6*, 243–253.

Wilder, J.   The law of initial values in neurology and psychiatry: Facts and problems. *Journal of Nervous and Mental Disease*, 1957, *125*, 73–86.

Wolpe, J.   *Psychotherapy by reciprocal inhibition.* Stanford, Calif.: Stanford University Press, 1958.

CHAPTER 10

The Inner and Outer Meanings of Facial Expressions

Joseph C. Hager
University of California–San Francisco
Paul Ekman
University of California–San Francisco

INTRODUCTION

Investigators from a number of fields of psychology have been interested in facial expressions of emotion. Social psychologists studying person perception have often focused on the face. Recent research is examining the relative weight given to the face as compared to other sources of information, the relationship between encoding and decoding, and individual differences. Developmental psychologists are examining the age at which infants first show what can be considered an emotion, whether this age precedes or follows an infant's ability to recognize emotions, and the sequencing of expressions between caregiver and infant. Physiological psychologists have been concerned with the role of the right hemisphere in the recognition and, more recently, in the production of facial expression, and in the relationship between facial and autonomic measures of arousal. Many different investigators are studying the face in order to help answer the question of how we know how we feel.

These are but a few examples of the many divergent questions that involve consideration of facial expression. Most of these questions are not new. They were subject to considerable research a few decades ago, although sometimes the questions were phrased differently. Unfortunately, little progress was made. The most basic questions were not answered, and methods for measuring facial expression were not well developed. In the last decade, progress has been made both on methods and on a set of fundamental questions.

This chapter begins by reviewing the answers that have emerged to three basic questions about the face and emotion: Is there any relationship at all? Are facial expressions culturally bound or universal? And, are any universals in expression biologically based? Then we describe a new tool for measuring facial movement which has allowed more precise study of the face. We will report new findings that begin to clarify the nature of facial signals, and the degree to which they relate to different types of feelings.

Darwin (1872) argued that certain emotional expressions are innate and the same for all people. His evidence and arguments were largely ignored by scientists in the subsequent century. Instead, the view that facial expressions are not valid indicators of emotion was widely accepted even though the evidence was contradictory (Bruner & Tagiuri, 1954). Ekman, Friesen, and Ellsworth (1972, 1982) resolved this issue definitively by pointing out methodological problems that had confused other researchers. They showed that observers could agree on how to label both posed and spontaneous facial expressions in terms of either emotional categories or emotional dimensions. Much evidence, including reanalysis of negative studies, indicated that facial expressions can provide accurate information about emotion. The labels judges assigned to posed expressions tended to agree with the poser's intended message. For spontaneous expressions, judges selected labels consistent with emotions appropriate in the situations that elicited the expressions. These studies of spontaneous expression indicated that observers could distinguish pleasant from unpleasant emotions, but evidence was weak that observers could make finer distinctions about more specific categories of emotion, such as fear from anger. Also, there was no evidence about whether the face provided graded information about the intensity of any specific emotion (e.g., annoyance, anger, fury).

Unlike Darwin, anthropologists who endorsed cultural relativity argued that the meanings of expressions were arbitrary and specific to each culture, like symbols in a language (e.g., Birdwhistell, 1970; LaBarre, 1947). Recent evidence (e.g., Ekman, Sorenson, & Friesen, 1969; Izard, 1971) has indisputably shown that there are constants across cultures in the emotional meanings of certain facial expressions (for a detailed review of all the evidence, including studies of infants, the blind, and other primates, see Ekman, 1973). Ekman (1972) used a "neurocultural" theory to explain how cultural as well as biological influences could contribute to the meaning and use of facial expressions. A central concept in this theory is "display rules," which are an informal, nonverbal etiquette about socially acceptable ways to use and control expressions. Previous researchers had probably confused these culture specific modifications of emotional behaviors with the universals of expression. For example, Samurai women were reported to smile rather than to cry when hearing that their loved ones had died in battle (LaBarre, 1947). Although such observations were taken as evidence of cultural variability in the meaning of smiles, these smiles may not have been signs of grief, but rather could have been culturally required masks implementing the display rule to show joy and hide distress in this public situation (Ekman, 1973).

Evidence of universals in facial expression does not prove that they are innate, as Darwin believed. Universal connections between expressions and emotions could arise from learning which has a high probability of occurring in all cultures (Allport, 1924) or from a functional role of the movements in the emotional situation (Ekman, 1979). However, other evidence also supports the hypothesis that innate, biological factors mold some facial expressions. Oster (1978; Oster & Ekman, 1978) examined the expressions of neonates and found that certain spontaneous facial actions were not random, but rather were organized and temporally patterned. Since there was no opportunity to learn these patterns, some hardwired instructions underlie this organization. The relation of infant expressions to emotional behaviors has yet to be established, although some expressions, such as disgust, distress, and enjoyment, correspond to situations that can elicit these emotions in adults. Anencephalic neonates also have patterned facial responses to certain stimuli, such as disgust expressions to bitter-tasting substances and smiles to sweet tastes (Steiner, 1973). Studies of blind infants and children generally support the position that many facial expressions result from innate factors rather than depending on visual learning (Charlesworth & Kreutzer, 1973).

The evidence shows that facial expressions are related to emotion both biologically and culturally, but many other important questions remain. Until recently, all the evidence was based on observers' judgments of the face, which presumably reflect the expressions and messages the face provides. Few studies have tried to measure how the face conveys this information or precisely what the cues are for each emotion. Even fewer researchers have tried to measure every possible facial expression. Is it possible to describe and quantify every action the face can perform? If so, facial measurement can tell us about the universe of facial signals, and answer such questions as: How many different expressions are possible? Which of these expressions have emotional meanings and which have some other meanings? What muscles are involved in each emotion? Are there different muscles for each emotion, or do the same muscles play a role in more than one emotion? Can an emotion be shown by one muscle action, or does the expression of emotion require the combination of actions which are not meaningful singly?

THE FACIAL ACTION CODING SYSTEM

Ekman and Friesen's Facial Action Coding System (FACS) (1976, 1978) measures all visible facial movements. Ideally, FACS would differentiate every change in muscular action, but it is limited to what a user can reliably discriminate when movements are inspected repeatedly, in stopped and slowed motion. It does not measure invisible changes (e.g., certain changes in muscle tonus) or vascular and glandular changes produced by the autonomic nervous system. Limiting FACS measurement to visible movements was consistent with an interest in those behaviors which may be social signals, usually detected during social interactions. FACS can be applied to any reasonably detailed visual record of facial behavior. If the technique were to measure invisible or autonomic nervous system (ANS) activity, it would be limited to situations were sensors were attached (e.g., EMG electrodes) or special sensing and recording methods were used (e.g., thermography).

The primary goal in developing FACS was comprehensiveness, a technique that could measure all possible, visible discriminable facial actions. Comprehensiveness was important because many of the fundamental questions about the universe and nature of facial expressions cannot be answered if just a subset of behaviors is measurable. FACS was derived from an analysis of the anatomical basis for facial movement. A comprehensive system was obtained by discovering how each muscle of the face acts to change visible appearances. With this knowledge it is possible to analyze any facial movement into anatomically based, minimal action units.

Another consideration that guided the development of FACS was the need to separate description from inferences about the meanings of behaviors. Scoring is less likely to be biased if the observer does not have to evaluate or attach meanings to behaviors. Almost all the previous descriptive systems have included some inferential scores, such as "aggressive frown" (Grant, 1969), "lower lip pout" (Blurton Jones, 1971), and "smile tight—loose o" (Birdwhistell, 1970). Each of these actions could be described in noninferential terms.

By emphasizing measurement of the face in terms of muscle actions, inferences about meanings are minimized. The user of FACS learns the mechanics or muscular biasis of facial movement, not simply the consequences of actions or a description of static landmarks. FACS emphasizes patterns of movement: the movements of the skin, the temporary changes in size and location of the features, and the gathering, pouching, buldging, and wrinkling of the skin. As time passes, FACS users increasingly focus on behavioral description and are rarely aware of "meanings."

FACS's emphasis on movement and muscular action also helps overcome problems due to physiognomic differences between people. Individuals differ in the size, shape, and location of their features and in permanent wrinkles, bulges, or pouches. The particular shape of a landmark may vary from one person to another; for example, when the lip corner goes up, all people may not have the same angle, shape, or wrinkle pattern. If only the end result of movement is described, scoring may be confused by physiognomic variation. Knowledge of the muscular basis for actions helps deal with these differences.

FACS measures facial behaviors with "action units" (AUs), which indicate what muscles have contracted to produce the expression. Figure 10-1 illustrates the three AUs in the brow area and their combinations. Ekman and Friesen learned to contract each muscle separately and determined each AU based on the discriminability of their actions. In a few cases, more than one muscle was combined into one AU or more than one AU was derived from what most anatomists have described as one muscle.

After determining the single AUs, between 4000 and 5000 AU combinations were performed and examined. This total includes all the possible combinations of AUs in the upper regions of the face, all two-AU and three-AU combinations in the lower face, plus some of the four-, five-, six-, seven-, and eight-AU combinations in the lower face. Study of these combinations showed that most of the appearance changes were additive (i.e., each AU was clearly recognizable and virtually unchanged). There were a few AU combinations which were not additive, but instead showed new appearances. All of these distinctive combinations are described in FACS in the same detail as the single AUs.

FACS is a very elaborate system, much more comprehensive than any previous technique. There is no facial action described by other systems

FIGURE 10-1. The three FACS action units in the brow area and their combinations are illustrated. AU 1 (action of inner frontalis) raises the inner corners of the eyebrows, forming wrinkles in the medial part of the brow. AU 2 (action of the outer frontalis) raises the outer portion of the eyebrows, forming wrinkles in the lateral part of the brow. AU 4 (action of procerus, corrugators, and depressor supercilii) pulls the eyebrows down and together, forming vertical wrinkles between them and horizontal wrinkles near the nasion. The combinations of AUs show how these AUs can act together to form composites of the appearances each produces separately.

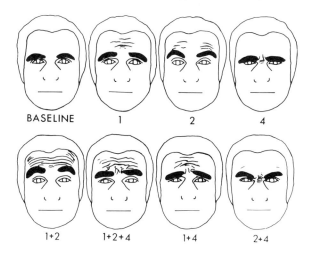

BASELINE　　1　　2　　4

1+2　　1+2+4　　1+4　　2+4

which cannot be described by FACS, and there are many behaviors described by FACS not previously distinguished. FACS allows for scoring asymmetries, either in terms of different AUs or different intensities. A means for measuring the intensity and the timing of actions is also detailed.

Reliability was a major concern in the development of FACS. Ekman and Friesen (1978) assessed several aspects of reliability, including describing the behavior verses locating it in time. Their studies have repeatedly shown good reliability even when the learner uses only the self-instructional FACS manual without direct guidance from FACS's authors. The evidence shows that FACS can successfully measure the visibly distinctive facial actions as its authors intended.

Besides being reliable, FACS has revealed the answer to many basic questions about expressions. From the single AUs and their combinations, Ekman and Friesen have estimated that there are several hundred thousand possible visibly distinguishable facial expressions, most of which are never seen on people's faces in everyday life. FACS has been used to score pictures of faces which observers have judged to express emotion and to score faces of people in emotionally arousing situations. Based on evidence from such scoring, the expressions produced by different combinations of AUs which convey emotional meanings appear to number in the hundreds, if not thousands. If the strength of muscular contraction and the timing or sequence of muscular recruitment were included, this number would be substantially increased. Of course, people do not have a different emotion name for each of these expressions. Instead, many emotional expressions are synonyms or convey different connotations of particular emotions. Further research is needed to determine the extent to which synonymous expressions with different AUs, strengths of contraction, or timing can be distinguished by naive observers and whether such distinctions are accompanied by additional messages. For example, different expressions which are judged as one emotion may be perceived as genuine, as an attempt to deceive, as artificial, or as a word-like symbol for an emotion. Observers also perceive differences in the intensity of emotion expressions which may be based on strength of muscular contraction, number of muscles recruited, or area of the face in which contractions occur. The number of expressions conveying emotional meanings is much greater than researchers have typically acknowledged, but it is much smaller than the number of possible expressions.

Every facial muscle can be involved in one or more emotional expressions, so there is no distinction between emotional and nonemotional muscles. Some muscles always signal a particular emotion, such as zygomatic major which produces a smile and is characteristic of happiness. It is never involved in a negative emotional expression without blending its own message. Other muscles, such as the corrugator, are involved in expressions which convey many different emotional messages and nonemotional messages. Some emotions, such as happiness and disgust, can be signaled by the action of only one muscle, but other emotions, such as sadness, need the action of more than one muscle to be signaled unambiguously.

Findings like those above cannot be obtained without the comprehensiveness of FACS. Consider other measurement systems which are not comprehensive, such as the Facial Affect Scoring Technique (Ekman, Friesen, & Tomkins, 1971) and Affex (Izard, 1980). Such noncomprehensive techniques consist of a limited number of expressions which the authors thought on a priori grounds were relevant to emotion. The problem with these techniques is that only the expressions included in the system can be studied; other possible expressions are ignored if they cannot be coded. These techniques can say little about the universe of expressions. Conclusions based on them are limited to only the expressions measured. Hypotheses about those expressions can be tested, but the possibility that other actions signal emotion cannot be discovered.

Researchers using electromyography (EMG) have measured facial activity without relying on an observer's ability to distinguish visible actions, but their efforts have not resulted in a comprehensive measurement system. It would be possible to construct a comprehensive measurement system by specifying the electrode placements which would measure all distinctive facial expressions. However, a surface electrode measures any muscular activity in its general area (see Basmajian, 1978, p. 26), eliminating distinctions that may be made visually. Thus, the researcher would have to use a pattern of surface electrode placements carefully configured to discriminate the activities of nearby muscles. An alternative solution might be to use a needle electrode which measures only the activity of the muscle in which it is inserted. If measuring all muscular activity in the face were the goal, either of these procedures might involve an impractical number of electrodes since each muscle or portions of muscles on both sides of the face would have to be monitored.

EMG has both advantages and disadvantages in respect to visible measurement of facial behavior. EMG units for measuring the activity of muscles are smaller and enable more precise measurement of the degree of activity than units of intensity based on visible distinctions. The often used procedure of averaging EMG over seconds loses information about the visually distinguishable timing of contractions. Also, the relation between EMG measurements and visible movement is ambiguous because EMG may measure inhibition of movement as well as actual movement. A distinct advantage of EMG is that it can measure invisible activity, but a distinct disadvantage is that the electrodes alert subjects to the observation of their faces, which may alter normal behavior (see the section on asymmetry of expressions). Although attaching electrodes to other parts of the body may or may not confuse the subject about the investigator's interest in the face, there is no doubt that EMG electrodes are intrusive and make it impossible to hide the very fact of observation and recording. (See Ekman, 1981, for a more detailed comparison and results on the relationship between EMG and the coding of visible facial movement.)

THE RELATION BETWEEN FACIAL EXPRESSIONS AND THE FEELINGS OF EMOTION

Facial measurement has answered questions about the universe of facial expression. It has also helped to discern the functions of facial expressions. Social psychologists have usually been interested in expressions as social signals, although they rarely measured the signal itself. Another function of facial expression may be as a signal to the self about one's own emotional state. The next several paragraphs discuss how some important theories of emotion view the relation between facial expressions and the feelings of emotion. This relation is only one of many which comprise the construct of emotion, but discussing these other relationships is beyond the scope of this chapter. Later, however, a brief look at the evidence for these theories emphasizes the mistake of assuming that these different relationships, such as those between facial expression and feelings versus those between physiological arousal and feelings, are interchangeable rather than possibly quite different and even apparently contradictory.

William James (1884) promoted the idea that the feelings of emotions arise from the perception of characteristic bodily changes. In an elaborate theory of emotion, Tomkins (1962, 1982) postulated that there are nine fundamental affects and affect auxiliaries, each having a characteristic and innate facial, vocal, and physiological expression. These expressions provide feedback which when consciously perceived gives rise to the feelings of affect. Each innate expression has inherently different feedback which underlies each emotional feeling. In recent statements, Tomkins (1982) regarded the feedback from the skin of the face, altered by blood flow and muscle movements, as most important for the feelings of affect. Although the number of affects is limited, the variety of feelings experienced is great because affects can blend and because other inputs to consciousness influence emotional experience. According to Tomkins, emotional feelings can also arise in the absence of facial expressions if there are memories that can substitute for them.

In contrast to the theories that emphasize peripheral changes in the body are theories that specify cognitive or inferential decisions as the source of emotional feelings. Schachter and Singer (1962) promulgated one of the first cognitive social theories of emotion in a widely cited experiment. In their theory, the important determinants of the quality of emotional feelings are cognitions about physiological arousal. Arousal that has no apparent explanation creates a need to label the feeling it produces in emotional terms. Situational and social cues provide a basis for inferring an appropriate category of emotion, and this decision underlies the qualitative differences in emotional feelings. Arousal itself is probably undifferentiated (i.e., the same across all emotions), but if different patterns exist, they are unimportant factors. This theory was intensely criticized, in part, because it did not explain how arousal itself was elicited, the results of the experiment were not as predicted and were rationalized with post hoc explanations, and the experiment has not replicated (e.g., Izard, 1971; Leventhal, 1974; Marshall & Zimbardo, 1979; Maslach, 1979). Nevertheless, this theory became the dominant model of emotion for social psychologists, in part because of its emphasis on cognition.

Mandler (1975) also emphasized autonomic arousal and cognitive interpretation as the important factors in determining the feelings of emotion. Arousal is probably undifferentiated and determines only the visceral character and intensity of emotion. Interpretation determines the quality and category of the experience. Mandler discussed the role of facial expression in this kind of model. Facial expressions may be biologically tied to certain events or situations which, in turn, have a high probability of eliciting particular cognitions about emotion. Also, expressions may generate automatic cognitions which contribute to the interpretative process. Rather than an inherent, direct link to feelings, these automatic cognitions depend on cognitive interpretation to influence emotional feelings. The role of cognition in emotion is so important that Mandler considers the belief in fundamental emotions "a human vanity."

Bem's (1972) self-perception theory also links emotional feelings to inferences based on behavioral cues. People may observe their own facial behaviors and use them as cues about emotion (Laird, 1974). The ability to use such cues depends on learning from the verbal community to make the discriminations. Unlike Mandler, Bem's theory does not explain why the same connections between particular facial expressions and emotions are found universally across widely differing cultures.

The dispute over the source of emotional feelings is difficult to resolve empirically, in part because conceptions like Mandler's "automatic cognitions" and Tomkins's "consciousness of facial feedback" generate many similar predictions. One approach is to examine how closely distinct facial expressions are associated with different emotional feelings. If the differences are merely between positive and negative emotions, they cannot be the substrates for emotional feelings as hypothesized by facial feedback models. Conversely, subtle, intimate relations between expressions and feelings would challenge the cognitive theories, especially if these relations are too subtle for an ordinary observer to detect or to teach to expressors.

None of the past studies which have shown that the face can provide accurate information about emotion measured felt experience. Some did provide indirect evidence of a relation between expressions and feelings. For example, in many studies of posed expressions, subjects were asked to make their face look like they felt an emotion, and these expressions were distinctive enough for judges to identify the intended emotion. Only recently have studies directly assessed the relation between feelings and expression.

In his review of this issue, Buck (1980) distinguished two versions of the hypothesis that feedback from facial expression underlies the feelings of emotion. The "between-subjects version" specifies individual differences in emotion (e.g., less expressive people have less intense emotions), and the "within-subjects version" specifies that for any given person, the degree of expressiveness is positively related to intensity of emotion. Looking at the evidence for each version separately, Buck rejected the between-subjects version based on evidence showing an inverse, rather than a positive relation between facial expression and physiological arousal (e.g., Buck, Miller, & Caul, 1974; Notarius & Levenson, 1979). However, a recent study by Levenson and Mades (1980) suggested that this inverse relationship may arise only between "true-low-anxious" versus "repressor" subjects. None of these studies directly addressed the central issues of the facial feedback model proposed by Tomkins (1962) and reiterated by Izard (1971). They did not examine the evidence crucial to this model—the relation between facial expression and the subjective experience of emotion. Instead, they examined the relation between expression and autonomic activity. There is no reason to presuppose that ANS activity and facial expression are related the same way as subjective experience and facial expression. Still another problem with these studies is that they lumped together quite diverse expressions, failed to measure expressions directly, and only counted activities, not the type of activity (e.g., whether the expressions were emotional or not).

Two substantive issues concern a relation between facial expression and emotional feelings: (1) distinctive expressions correspond to different feelings, and (2) intensities of expressions and feelings correlate. Two methodological approaches are possible. One is to manipulate facial expression experimentally and 'measure feelings to show that changes in expression alter feelings. This approach can provide a direct test of the facial-feedback models of emotional feelings, but it is difficult to design such a study without introducing artifacts.

Several studies have manipulated the degree of spontaneous smiling to films and measured the effect on evaluation of the films (e.g., Fuller & Sheehy-Skeffington, 1974; Leventhal & Mace, 1970). Generally, conditions that produced greater smiling also produced evaluations that the content of the films was more humorous, although this relation may not hold for men (Leventhal, 1974). Regrettably, these studies did not assess whether there was a greater experience of humor. The implications of such findings for the facial-feedback models is unclear because the relationship between evaluations of films and felt emotion is not straightforward (Leventhal, 1974). Evaluating the humor in a film may depend, for example, not only on evaluating the emotional feelings one has in response to it, but also on evaluating how funny it was in respect to other films, how easily one responds to humor in respect to other people, how tasteful the humorous devices in the film were, and so on. In other words, evaluating films is more cognitively complex than evaluating how one feels. Lanzetta, Cartwright-Smith, and Kleck (1976) manipulated the intensity of pain expressions and assessed the effect on self-reports of pain in response to electric shock. Conditions that affected intensity of pain expressions altered self-reports of shock painfulness. Although this finding fits with the facial-feedback hypothesis, most of its proponents (e.g., Izard, 1971; Tomkins, 1962) do not think that pain is an emotion.

Several studies have tried to show that manipulating the face into simulacrums of emotion expressions produces emotion. Laird (1974) had subjects frown or smile and concluded that these movements altered self-reports of aggression and elation. He theorized that expressions influence feelings by a process of tacit inference, but he did not explain why subjects inferred that the expressions were relevant to emotion if they were clearly prescribed by the experimenter. Rhodewalt and Comer (1979; Comer & Rhodewalt, 1979) and McArthur, Solomon, and Jaffe (1980) used a procedure similar to Laird's and obtained similar results concerning the relations between manipulated frowns or smiles and self-reports of feelings. Their results indicated that individual differences (e.g., weight and field dependence) influence this relation. A problem for interpreting these studies is that in the McArthur *et al.* study, only the frown appeared to alter reports of feelings. The other two studies did not permit assessing which expression was effective.

Tourangeau and Ellsworth (1979) conducted a similar but more elaborate study than those described above. Like the others, they claimed to have manipulated facial expressions without alerting subjects to their emotional meanings. Subjects ma.le either fear or sad expressions, or a grimace unrelated to emotion. They watched either a fear, sad, or neutral film and reported their emotional feelings. The experiment revealed no effect of facial expression on self-report, either for producing a corresponding feeling or for inhibiting other feelings aroused by the film. Nor did the investigators find a correlation between observers' ratings of the intensity of expression and self-reports of feelings.

Three articles criticized the Tourangeau and Ellsworth experiment, but many of the criticisms also apply to other studies which have experimentally manipulated facial expressions whether their results confirmed or disconfirmed a relation between expressions and feelings. Hager and Ekman (1981) argued that the experiment was an inadequate test of the hypothesis, partly because of inadequate facial measurement. Tomkins (1981) explained that the experiment had nothing to do with his theory of emotion because artificial expressions are not related to emotional feelings, as are spontaneous expressions. In his comments on methodological and conceptual problems, Izard (1981) referred to his own studies of this issue (Kotsch, Izard, & Walker, 1979). They gave little evidence that such artificial expressions can produce emotional feelings. Izard argued that making extreme voluntary facial movements can increase self-reports of anger, a view that suggests a reinterpretation of the studies using Laird's procedure. In general, the studies of manipulated expressions have not provided much evidence for an association between facial expression and emotion.

The other approach to demonstrating a relation between expressions and feelings is to create conditions which elicit different emotions, measure the feelings and expressions, and determine the relations between them. This approach also has problems. For example, retrospective reports may be distorted by memory. The alternative procedure of interrupting the emotional experience to obtain self-reports may create artifacts, especially if done repeatedly.

Several recent studies have examined how facial expressions are related to the experience of emotion, but for the most part, they have only replicated established findings. Schwartz, Fair, Salt, Mandel, and Klerman (1976), for example, found that EMG activity was different when subjects imagined different emotions. The contribution of this study was using EMG to measure low or invisible levels of facial activity. It is not clear, however, just what processes are involved in imagining emotion. They may be little different than posing, and many studies from 1930 to 1960 (reviewed by Ekman et al., 1972) have shown that facial expressions differ when people pose different emotions. The question remains whether expressions differ among more spontaneous emotions. Buck and his colleagues (e.g., Buck et al., 1974) showed observers videotapes of subjects who viewed pleasant or unpleasant slides. They found that observers' ratings of subjects' pleasant–unpleasant feelings were correlated with the subjects' own ratings. Again, many studies decades ago showed that facial expressions differed for this simple pleasant–unpleasant distinction. What is needed is to go beyond this distinction and determine whether spontaneous facial expressions vary with more specific aspects of emotional experience.

Ekman, Friesen, and Ancoli (1980) conducted such a study. The faces of 35 women were videotaped without their knowledge. The women viewed a positive film with three segments, of which two had elicited mostly happiness and one, mostly relaxation in previous studies. They also viewed a negative film which showed two industrial accidents. Subjects reported their emotional reactions on a questionnaire which had separate unipolar scales for interest, anger, disgust, fear, happy, pain, sadness, surprise, and arousal.

The experiment was conducted individually for each subject. After a baseline period in which subjects relaxed, they reported their feelings on the questionnaire. They then saw the positive and the negative films in a counterbalanced order. Between the two films was another baseline period and a questionnaire for it. After the positive film, subjects filled out the questionnaire once for each of the three segments. They also reported their emotions for each accident after the negative film.

FACS was used to measure the activity of the face during the films. The investigators looked for signs of positive affect in the two happy segments of the positive film. It may seem obvious that smiles are the signs of positive affect, but some observers (e.g., Birdwhistell, 1970) claimed that the smile can be a sign of negative affect. The term "smile" may be too imprecise to distinguish behaviors with different meanings. Other researchers (e.g., Brannigan & Humphries, 1972; Grant, 1969) distinguished more than one type of smile (e.g., upper smile, broad smile, tight smile), but they rarely specified the same number of smiles or which ones, if any, are signs of positive affect.

FACS distinguishes many more types of smiles than other measurement systems have. A smiling appearance in which the lip corners are pulled upward and laterally can be produced by the action of zygomatic major, zygomatic minor, buccinator, risorious, and caninus muscles. FACS can score each of these actions, their combinations, and their combinations with other facial actions. Ekman, Friesen, and Ancoli (1980) found, as they predicted, that the specific smiling action of zygomatic major was related to subjects' self-reports of happiness, but other smiling actions were not. Second, the relation between this one action and felt experience was so precise that its activity accurately reflected during which film segment each subject felt happier. Third, measures of the extent of this muscular activity were related to the intensity of felt happiness. The authors also reported that other facial actions correlated as predicted with the intensity of felt negative emotions. Finally, actions predicted to be signs of disgust (levator labii superioris) correlated with reports of disgust feelings but not with the reports of other negative emotions.

ASYMMETRY OF FACIAL ACTIONS

Facial actions are not limited to spontaneous emotional expressions. In addition to posed expressions, there are false expressions which are put on to convince others that an emotion not actually felt is being experienced. There are also many facial actions which bear little relationship to any type of emotion: facial gestures such as the wink, and facial emphasis and question marks (see Ekman, 1978, 1979, for a description of various facial signals). Our analyses of recent studies of facial asymmetry, and a new study we then conducted, suggest that symmetry of facial action may be informative about whether a facial action is an expression of a felt emotion or is not felt but purposefully made.

Most researchers have used observers' judgments to assess facial asymmetry. Thus, evidence that observers rate one side of the face as happier, angrier, and so on, has been interpreted to show that this side expresses the emotion more intensely. This logic assumes that judgments are based on facial cues that express emotion, but they may not be. The face provides many cues which are irrelevant to the expression of emotion, but which observers sometimes confuse with emotional cues. For example, people who have thick eyebrows set low in relation to their eyes may appear to be frowning perpetually and give the impression of anger to observers, regardless of the true emotional state. Such physiognomic features and other features which change slowly over time (e.g., wrinkles) are known to be asymmetrical (e.g., Gorney & Harries, 1974), and these asymmetries may be lateralized. For example, Burke (1971) found that in a group of children, the maxillary skin surface area tended to be greater on the left side. Artificially created cues may also be asymmetrical, as in hair combing and applying some cosmetics (e.g., to emphasize moles or hide blemishes).

Using observers' judgments to index asymmetry in the intensity of emotional expression creates a significant problem for interpretation. The influence on judgments of the muscle movement cues which signal emotion cannot be separated from physiognomic or artificial cues which are irrelevant to emotion. If intensity judgments of the sides of the face differ due to asymmetries in cues irrelevant to emotion, it would be a mistake to conclude that emotions are expressed more intensely on one side. Only if judgments are based on cues relevant to emotion expression would such a conclusion be warranted. The problem is increased when still photographs are used as stimuli because there are fewer cues for judges to distinguish static features from muscle actions.

An example of this problem is a study by Sackeim, Gur, and Saucy (1978). To obtain stimulus faces, they printed one photograph normally and one mirror-reversed photograph by turning the negative over. They cut these photographs down the midline and rearranged the halves to produce faces in which each side was an image of the other (i.e., either a right or a left composite). Observers judged on rating scales how intensely the composite faces expressed emotion. The left composite pictures were judged as more intense than the right composites in five of the six emotion categories. The authors stated that "emotions are expressed more intensely on the left side of the face."

Nelson and Horowitz (1980) showed that there were asymmetries in the sizes of the faces used by Sackeim *et al.* and argued that this variable might have influenced their findings. Spinrad (1980) noted that artificial cues produced by different lighting on the two sides might have been responsible. Such alternative explanations can be eliminated by measuring the facial movement cues of emotion directly.

Whether observers' judgments or direct measurement are used to assess asymmetry, the researcher must determine whether the expressions are emotional or not, or more generally, the type of facial movement must be distinguished. Ekman (1980) criticized the Sackeim *et al.* study because they did not distinguish carefully enough the type of facial movements they studied. He explained that they failed to recognize that they had studied at least two types of facial movements and that there was a difference in judged asymmetry between these two types. Ekman noted that the expressions which were judged as more intense on the left were not genuine emotional expressions, but rather were deliberately produced movements, carefully directed by the photographer, who gave instructions to move particular muscles, such as "raise your upper lip." Sackeim *et al.* did not find left composites more intense for the one expression (happy) which spontaneously occurred during the photographic session.

Other studies of asymmetry have studied ambiguous types of facial movements. Some have recorded conversations (e.g., Moscovitch & Olds, 1979), but the types of movements during conversation are especially varied. For example, although some expressions are spontaneous in the sense that they have not been requested, the speaker can initiate deliberate movements. Movements that signal emotion may be spontaneous emotional expressions or emblems that refer to emotion but do not involve emotional experience (Ekman, 1978).

Some studies have examined the movements of subjects who posed emotion (e.g., Borod & Caron, 1980), but subjects can adopt a variety of performance strategies to produce different types of movements. Ekman, Roper, and Hager (1980) noted that when people are asked to pose an emotion or to imitate an expression, they could use at least two methods to solve the problem. Subjects could self-induce the emotion and allow the expression to emerge, as in method acting. Alternatively, subjects could deliberately produce movements without emotion. Situations like conversation and posing an emotion are not conducive for observing one specific type of movement.

Another circumstance that creates ambiguity about the type of movement produced is when subjects know or suspect that their face is being scrutinized. Once aware of observation, subjects may become self-conscious and alter their facial behaviors (Ekman, 1972; Kleck, Vaughan, Cartwright-Smith, Vaughan, Colby, & Lanzetta, 1976). In studies of natural, spontaneous movements, self-consciousness can be minimized by recording behaviors in a manner that does not draw attention to the observation.

Ekman, Hager, and Friesen (1981) showed that, indeed, the pattern of asymmetry depends on the type of movement examined. They reduced ambiguity about the type of movement by carefully choosing circumstances that would elicit particular types. The two sets of records chosen for asymmetry scoring were collected in other studies and had been scored by FACS previously. To score asymmetry, each action was again viewed repeatedly in slowed and real time. At the apex of each action, the movements were scored as symmetrical or asymmetrical, with greater intensity on the left or the right side.

One set of records was from a study of the development of the ability to imitate facial movements (Ekman, Roper, & Hager, 1980). Boys and girls ($n = 36$) imitated a series of facial actions shown to them one at a time on a television monitor. Their performances of six actions were selected for symmetry scoring. In addition, spontaneous movements of zygomatic major were located and scored on most children's faces. These smiles occurred in response to the experimenter's jokes and praise.

A contrast between the deliberate and spontaneous emotional use of zygomatic major showed different patterns of asymmetry. Asymmetrical movements were significantly more frequent in deliberate imitations than in spontaneous smiles. Deliberate asymmetrical movements were more frequently greater on the left than the right side of the face. This laterality of movement was not apparent for spontaneous smiles. The deliberate imitations of the five other muscles scored were as frequently asymmetrical as deliberate smiles, and these asymmetrical movements were more often greater on the left than the right.

The other set of records (from Ekman, Friesen, & Ancoli, 1980) showed women spontaneously expressing both positive and negative emotions. Like children's spontaneous smiles, the smiles of women during a humorous film were rarely asymmetrical and did not manifest laterality. Asymmetries of negative emotional movements during a stress film also were not lateralized, but they were often asymmetrical. The small number of these negative movements made these findings tentative.

Taken together, these results indicate that asymmetry of facial actions is a function of the type of movement. Spontaneous movements that occurred in an emotional context were rarely asymmetrical and were not stronger on one side more frequently than on the other. Lynn and Lynn (1943) reported results for spontaneous happy expressions entirely consistent with this finding. Deliberate imitative actions were more often asymmetrical and these asymmetries were lateralized, with the left side stronger. Campbell (1978) and Chaurasia and Goswami (1975) reported similar results for the deliberate movements they studied.

The evidence that symmetry differs between spontaneous, emotional movements and deliberate nonemotional movements suggests that the symmetry of facial movements may be related to the felt experience of emotion. Since the nonemotional movements in the studies discussed above were more frequently asymmetrical than the emotional movements, one prediction is that the more symmetrical the expression, the more likely it is that the person actually experiences the emotion. Our attempts to verify such hypotheses with post hoc analyses have been inconsistent. Contrary to the prediction, women with greater asymmetry of zygomatic major reported more happiness during the second humorous film segment, although there was an insignificant trend in the predicted direction during the first segment. Consistent with the prediction, zygomatic major smiles that occurred during pleasant films were more symmetrical than such smiles which occurred during unpleasant films, but additional aspects of the smiles differed between film conditions, such as the actions that co-occurred with the zygomatic action. Our preliminary observations of conversational facial movements which do not involve emotion indicate that they are often asymmetrical.

DISCUSSION AND SUMMARY

The evidence on the universe of facial expression indicates that it is a large and complex set. The relation of spontaneous expressions to emotion is precise and refined with different expressions corresponding to distinct emotions. Even subtle differences in one expression (i.e., intensity, duration, frequency) correspond to differences in the feelings of the corresponding emotion. The symmetry of expression may reveal whether it is spontaneous and emotional or more deliberate and cortically mediated. What are the implications of these findings for the face as a signal system and for theories of emotion?

Whether the information revealed by careful facial measurement can be detected by untrained observers has yet to be determined. It is likely that the characteristic spontaneous expressions of different emotions can be seen and understood by the naive observer, as indicated by studies using posed expressions. More research on spontaneous expression is needed to verify this point. On the other hand, some aspects of expression, such as differences in intensity and asymmetry, typically appear too subtle for untrained observers to detect or too insignificant for attaching meaning.

Our findings do not allow us to pick the one correct theory of emotion, but they are more consistent with some theories than others. First, the evidence of a close association of several aspects of facial expression to the experience of emotions creates difficulties for theories, like Schachter and Singer's, which view the bodily changes during emotions as undifferentiated. Also, the subtlety of some of these relations argues against theories, such as Bem's, which state that culture teaches the distinctions among emotions, because it is unlikely that people learn or teach such relations. It is also unlikely that people are aware of such subtle qualities in their own expressions, so that if the inferential processes proposed by cognitive theories are based on such cues, they must be made outside of awareness. Of course, there are obvious differences among emotions in facial expressions which people could be aware of and use to make conscious inferences about their own feelings. On the other hand, there mày be even more subtle differences in facial activity among emotions that cannot be scored with visible measurement. Simple associations cannot prove that facial expressions provide a basis for emotional feelings, but the close association between feelings and subtle, varied aspects of expression as well as gross differences in expression among emotions show that such a relation is possible. Whether this relation is mediated by inferences such as Mandler's automatic cognitions or more directly as proposed by Tomkins is an issue as yet unresolved.

R E F E R E N C E S

Allport, F. H. *Social psychology.* Boston: Houghton Mifflin, 1924.

Basmajian, J. V. *Muscles alive: Their functions as revealed by electromyography* (4th ed.). Baltimore: Williams & Wilkins, 1978.

Bem, D. J. Self-perception theory. In L. Berkowitz (Ed.), *Advances in experimental social psychology* (Vol. 6). New York: Academic, 1972.

Birdwhistell, R. L. *Kinesics and context.* Philadelphia: University of Pennsylvania Press, 1970.

Blurton Jones, N. G. Criteria for use in describing facial expressions of children. *Human Biology,* 1971, *41,* 365–413.

Borod, J. C., & Caron, H. S. Facedness and emotion related to lateral dominance, sex, and expression type. *Neuropsychologia,* 1980, *18,* 237–241.

Brannigan, C. R., & Humphries, D. A. Human non-verbal behavior, a means of communication. In N. Blurton Jones (Ed.), *Ethological studies of child behavior.* Cambridge: Cambridge University Press, 1972.

Bruner, J. S., & Tagiuri, R. The perception of people. In G. Lindzey (Ed.), *Handbook of social psychology.* Reading, Mass.: Addison-Wesley, 1954.

Buck, R. Nonverbal behavior and the theory of emotion: The facial feedback hypothesis. *Journal of Personality and Social Psychology,* 1980, *38,* 811–824.

Buck, R., Miller, R. E., & Caul, W. F. Sex, personality, and physiological variables in the communication of affect via facial expression. *Journal of Personality and Social Psychology,* 1974, *30,* 587–596.

Burke, P. H. Stereophotogrammetric measurement of normal facial asymmetry in children. *Human Biology,* 1971, *43,* 536–548.

Campbell, R. Asymmetries in interpreting and expressing a posed facial expression. *Cortex,* 1978, *14,* 327–342.

Charlesworth, W. R., & Kreutzer, M. A. Facial expression of infants and children. In P. Ekman (Ed.), *Darwin and facial expression: A century of research in review.* New York: Academic, 1973.

Chaurasia, B. D., & Goswami, H. K.   Functional asymmetry in the face. *Acta Anatomica*, 1975, *91*, 154–160.

Comer, R., & Rhodewalt, F.   Cue utilization in the self-attribution of emotions and attitudes. *Personality and Social Psychology Bulletin*, 1979, *5*, 320–324.

Darwin, C.   *The expression of the emotions in man and animals*. London: Murray, 1872.

Ekman, P.   Universals and cultural differences in facial expressions of emotion. In J. Cole (Ed.), *Nebraska Symposium on Motivation, 1971*. Lincoln: University of Nebraska Press, 1972.

Ekman, P.   Cross-cultural studies of facial expression. In P. Ekman (Ed.), *Darwin and facial expression: A century of research in review*. New York: Academic, 1973.

Ekman, P.   Facial signs: Facts, fantasies, and possibilities. In T. A. Sebeok (Ed.), *Sight, sound and sense*. Bloomington: Indiana University Press, 1978.

Ekman, P.   About brows: Emotional and conversational signals. In M. von Cranach, K. Foppa, W. Lepenies, & D. Ploog (Eds.), *Human ethology*. Cambridge: Cambridge University Press, 1979.

Ekman, P.   Asymmetry in facial expression. *Science*, 1980, *209*, 833–834.

Ekman, P.   Methods for measuring facial action. In K. Scherer & P. Ekman (Eds.), *Handbook of methods in nonverbal behavior research*. New York: Cambridge University Press, 1981.

Ekman, P., & Friesen, W. V.   Measuring facial movement. *Environmental Psychology and Nonverbal Behavior*, 1976, *1*, 56–75.

Ekman, P., & Friesen, W. V.   *The facial action coding system*. Palo Alto, Calif.: Consulting Psychologists Press, 1978.

Ekman, P., Friesen, W. V., & Ancoli, S.   Facial signs of emotional experience. *Journal of Personality and Social Psychology*, 1980, *39*, 1125–1134.

Ekman, P., Friesen, W. V., & Ellsworth, P.   *Emotion in the human face*. Elmsford, N.Y.: Pergamon, 1972.

Ekman, P., Friesen, W. V., & Ellsworth, P.   Research foundations. In P. Ekman (Ed.), *Emotion in the human face* (2nd ed.). Cambridge: Cambridge University Press, 1982.

Ekman, P., Friesen, W. V., & Tomkins, S. S.   Facial Affect Scoring Technique: A first validity study. *Semiotica*, 1971, *3*,(1), 37–58.

Ekman, P., Hager, J. C., & Friesen, W. V.   The symmetry of emotional and deliberate facial actions. *Psychophysiology*, 1981, *18*, 101–106.

Ekman, P., Roper, G., & Hager, J. C.   Deliberate facial movement. *Child Development*, 1980, *51*, 886–891.

Ekman, P., Sorenson, E. R., & Friesen, W. V.   Pan-cultural elements in facial displays of emotion. *Science*, 1969, *164*, 86–88.

Fuller, R. G. C, & Sheehy-Skeffington, A.   Effects of group laughter on responses to humorous material, a replication and extension. *Psychological Reports*, 1974, *35*, 531–534.

Gorney, M., & Harries, T.   The preoperative and postoperative consideration of natural facial asymmetry. *Plastic and Reconstructive Surgery*, 1974, *54*, 187–191.

Grant, E. C.   Human facial expression. *Man*, 1969, *4*, 525–536.

Hager, J. C., & Ekman, P.   A methodological criticism of Tourangeau and Ellsworth's study of facial expression and emotion. *Journal of Personality and Social Psychology*, 1981, *40*, 358–362.

Izard, C. E.   *The face of emotion*. New York: Appleton-Century-Crofts, 1971.

Izard, C. E.   Differential emotions theory and the facial feedback hypothesis of emotion activation: Comments on Tourangeau and Ellsworth's "The role of facial response in the experience of emotion." *Journal of Personality and Social Psychology*, 1981, *40*, 350–354.

Izard, C. E., & Dougherty, L. M.   *A system for identifying affect expressions by holistic judgments (Affex)*. Newark: University of Delaware, Instructional Resources Center, 1980.

James, W.   What is emotion? *Mind*, 1884, *9*, 188–204.

Kleck, R. E., Vaughan, R. C., Cartwright-Smith, J., Vaughan, K. B., Colby, C. Z., & Lanzetta, J. T.   Effects of being observed on expressive, subjective, and physiological responses to painful stimuli. *Journal of Personality and Social Psychology*, 1976, *34*, 1211–1218.

Kotsch, W. E., Izard, C. E., & Walker, S. *Experimenter manipulated facial patterns and emotion experience.* Unpublished manuscript, 1979.

LaBarre, W. The cultural basis of emotions and gestures. *Journal of Personality*, 1947, *16*, 49–68.

Laird, J. D. Self-attribution of emotion: The effects of expressive behavior on the quality of emotional experience. *Journal of Personality and Social Psychology*, 1974, *29*, 475–486.

Lanzetta, J. T., Cartwright-Smith, J., & Kleck, R. E. Effects of nonverbal dissimulation on emotional experience and autonomic arousal. *Journal of Personality and Social Psychology*, 1976, *33*, 354–370.

Levenson, R. W., & Mades, L. L. *Physiological response, facial expression, and trait anxiety: Two methods for improving consistency.* Paper presented at the Society for Psychophysical Research, Vancouver, British Columbia, 1980.

Leventhal, H. Emotions: A basic problem for social psychology. In C. Nemeth (Ed.), *Social psychology: Classic and contemporary integrations.* Chicago: Rand McNally, 1974.

Leventhal, H., & Mace, W. The effect of laughter on evaluation of a slapstick movie. *Journal of Personality*, 1970, *38*, 16–30.

Lynn, J. G., & Lynn, D. R. Smile and hand dominance in relation to basic modes of adaptation. *Journal of Abnormal and Social Psychology*, 1943, *38*, 250–276.

Mandler, G. *Mind and emotion.* New York: Wiley, 1975.

Marshall, G. D., & Zimbardo, P. G. Affective consequences of inadequately explained arousal. *Journal of Personality and Social Psychology*, 1979, *37*, 970–988.

Maslach, C. Negative and emotional biasing of unexplained arousal. *Journal of Personality and Social Psychology*, 1979, *37*, 953–969.

McArthur, L. Z., Solomon, M. R., & Jaffe, R. H. Weight differences in emotional responsiveness to proprioceptive and pictorial stimuli. *Journal of Personality and Social Psychology*, 1980, *39*, 308–319.

Moscovitch, M., & Olds, J. *Asymmetries in spontaneous facial expressions and their possible relation to hemispheric specialization.* Paper presented at the International Neuropsychology Society, The Netherlands, June 1979.

Nelson, C. A. & Horowitz, F. D. Asymmetry in facial expression. *Science*, 1980, *209*, 834.

Notarius, C. I., & Levenson, R. W. Expressive tendencies and physiological response to stress. *Journal of Personality and Social Psychology*, 1979, *37*, 1204–1210.

Oster, H. Facial expression and affect development. In M. Lewis & L. Rosenblum (Eds.), *The development of affect.* New York: Plenum, 1978.

Oster, H., & Ekman, P. Facial behavior in child development. *Minnesota Symposiam on Child Psychology*, 1978, *11*, 231–276.

Rhodewalt, F., & Comer, R. Induced-compliance attitude change: Once more with feeling. *Journal of Experimental Social Psychology*, 1979, *15*, 35–47.

Sackeim, H. A., Gur, R. C., & Saucy, M. C. Emotions are expressed more intensely on the left side of the face. *Science*, 1978, *202*, 434–436.

Schachter, S., & Singer, J. Cognitive, social and physiological determinants of emotional state. *Psychological Review*, 1962, *69*, 379–399.

Schwartz, G. E., Fair, P. L., Salt, P., Mandel, M. R., & Klerman, G. L. Facial muscle patterning to affective imagery in depressed and non-depressed subjects. *Science*, 1976, *192*, 489–491.

Spinrad, S. I. Asymmetry in facial expression. *Science*, 1980, *209*, 834.

Steiner, J. E. The gustofacial response: Observation on normal and anencephalic newborn infants. In J. F. Bosma (Ed.), *Fourth symposium on oral sensation and perception.* Bethesda, Md.: U.S. Department of Health, Education and Welfare, 1973.

Tomkins, S. S. *Affect, imagery, consciousness* (Vol. 1). *The positive affects.* New York: Springer, 1962.

Tomkins, S. S. The role of facial response in the experience of emotion. *Journal of Personality and Social Psychology*, 1981, *40*, 355–357.

Tomkins, S. S. Affect theory. In P. Ekman (Ed.), *Emotion in the human face* (2nd ed.). Cambridge: Cambridge University Press, 1982.

Tourangeau, R., & Ellsworth, P. C. The role of facial response in the experience of emotion. *Journal of Personality and Social Psychology*, 1979, *37*, 1519–1531.

CHAPTER 11

Facial Asymmetry and the Communication of Emotion

Harold A. Sackeim
New York University and
New York State Psychiatric Institute

Ruben C. Gur
University of Pennsylvania

The sides of the human face differ in their display of emotional expression (e.g., Sackeim, Gur, & Saucy, 1978; Wolff, 1943). People are also characterized by lateral biases in their processing of human faces. For most people, one side of the human face is more salient than the other side (e.g., Gilbert & Bakan, 1973; Sackeim & Gur, 1978; Wolff, 1943). These phenomena have been investigated principally within the context of neuropsychology and are thought to be outcomes of functional brain asymmetry (e.g., Gilbert & Bakan, 1973; Sackeim & Gur, 1978). In this chapter we concentrate on the findings concerning asymmetry in the production of facial emotional expression. In the first section we raise a variety of conceptual and methodological issues in the study of facial asymmetry. In the second section we examine differences between the sides of the human face in voluntary, spontaneous, and "resting" emotional expressions. We note that different patterns of asymmetry may characterize these types of emotional expression, reflecting, we suggest, differences in their neural regulation. In the third section we integrate the findings in these areas and indicate how current theories of lateralization in the regulation of emotion may account for them. We raise here some of the implications of facial asymmetry and perceiver biases in regard to the interpersonal communication of emotion.

FACIAL ASYMMETRY: CONCEPTUAL AND METHODOLOGICAL ISSUES

The recent discovery that the sides of the human face differ in emotional expression has received considerable scientific and popular attention. That this is so may not be surprising. Patterns of facial expressive asymmetry may provide inroads for investigation of neural control of emotion. Such patterning may be helpful in uncovering the psychological and physiological processes that underlie emotional expression. Further, such patterning is likely to be of particular consequence for the study of how emotion is communicated. At the least, the discovery of consistent facial expressive asymmetry reveals a ubiquitous, but intimate, characteristic about ourselves that, for the most part, had gone unnoticed.

The rapid increase in studies of facial asymmetry has occurred with relatively little discussion of the particular conceptual and methodological problems that pertain to this field of research. Owing to space limitations, we can only summarize some of these issues here.

Spontaneous and Voluntary Expression

There is separate neural control of voluntary and spontaneous facial movements (e.g., Crosby & DeJonge, 1963). Loss of voluntary facial movement, one form of facial paralysis, is not uncommon in cases of supranuclear (above the level of the facial nerve nucleus) corticobulbar lesions (damage along a pathway that originates in motor cortex and terminates at the motor nucleus in the pons). Spontaneous emotional expression may remain unaltered and, in cases of pseudobulbar palsy (weakness or paralysis of muscles innervated by cranial nerves due to supranuclear corticobulbar lesion) may in fact be exaggerated (e.g., Kuypers, 1958). Conversely, weakness or paralysis of spontaneous emotional expression (mimic or mimetic paralysis) is seen at times without loss of voluntary movement. Therefore, brain-damaged patients may lose the ability to simulate deliberately emotional expression or to express emotion spontaneously, or both.

This double dissociation between mimic paralysis and paralysis of voluntary facial movement and the fact that mimic palsy is not obtained with corticobulbar lesions indicate that the neural control of spontaneous emotional expression in the face involves a different supranuclear pathway than the corticobulbar tract (Monrad-Krohn, 1924; Peele, 1961). Given this, it is necessary to evaluate findings concerning facial asymmetry in regard to whether they pertain to voluntary or spontaneous affective displays.

Orthogonal to the distinction between spontaneous and voluntary emotional expression is the distinction between tonic facial expression (the "resting" face) and phasic facial displays of emotion. Similar to phasic displays, the expressive features of the resting face may contain spontaneous and/or voluntary components. Discrete spontaneous phasic expressive displays may be released (disinhibited) naturally by destructive lesions (e.g., Davison & Kelman, 1939; Sackeim, Greenberg, Weiman, Gur,

Hungerbuhler, & Geschwind, 1982) or irritative lesions (e.g., Daly & Mulder, 1957; Sackeim *et al.*, 1982); and experimentally by electrical (e.g., Delgado, 1970) or chemical (e.g., Grossman, 1970) stimulation. As with normal motor reflexes, the tonic absence of spontaneous expressive displays must involve a balance between excitatory and inhibitory processes. The inhibition of displays may be naturally occurring, that is, spontaneous, and/or it may be voluntarily produced. For instance, Campbell (1978, 1979a, 1979b), in a set of studies on asymmetry in the resting or "neutral" face, asked subjects to display a relaxed expression. Such instructions presumably encouraged voluntary control of facial expression, and the results obtained with such instructions might differ considerably from those obtained in studies where the resting face is covertly photographed, with no instructions concerning facial expression.

Facial Asymmetry: Neural Control

For the study of facial asymmetry to be a feasible paradigm by which to investigate functional differences between the sides of the brain in the regulation of emotion, there must be lateralization in the neural control of facial movement. Both neuroanatomic and clinical data indicate that such lateralization exists in the case of voluntary facial movement.

Various parts of the face are represented in the cortical motor strip in the precentral gyrus of each hemisphere. A corticobulbar tract that subserves voluntary facial movement extends without synapse from the motor cortex of each hemisphere to the nuclei of the facial or VIIth nerve in the pons. The ventral (anterior) portion of each nucleus receives bilateral (from each side of the brain) projections from the motor cortex, whereas the dorsal (posterior) portion of each nucleus receives only contralateral (from the opposite side) projections (e.g., Crosby & DeJonge, 1963; Diamond & Frew, 1979). The ventral portions innervate muscles in the upper part of the face (e.g., frontalis and periorbital). The dorsal subnuclei innervate muscles in the lower two-thirds of the face. Therefore, each hemisphere has predominant control over voluntary movement in the contralateral lower two-thirds of the face. Clinical findings concerning patterns of facial paralysis support this view. Unilateral supranuclear lesions result in inability to perform voluntary facial movement in the contralateral lower two-thirds of the face (e.g., Dyken & Miller, 1980).

Neural control of spontaneous emotional expression is more complex and less clearly understood. A number of cortical and subcortical areas have been implicated in the regulation of spontaneous facial expression (e.g., Crosby & DeJonge, 1963). Stimulation studies, principally with monkeys, have produced facial movements with placements in frontal, parietal, and temporal cortex, the island of Reil, the cingulate area, the hippocampus, and the amygdala (e.g., Baldwin, Frost, & Wood, 1956;

DeJonge & Crosby, 1960; Foerster, 1931; Frontera, 1956; Penfield & Rasmussen, 1950; Showers, 1959). Paralysis of spontaneous facial movement in humans is commonly associated with lesions in frontal cortex and in thalamic areas. Lesions, widely differing in location, may produce uncontrollable, spontaneous outbursts of laughing and/or crying (Sackeim et al., 1982). In contrast to voluntary expression, where the corticobulbar pathways extend without synapse from motor cortex to the pons, it is generally accepted that pathways involved in spontaneous expression are multisynaptic and have several courses. Some have referred to the distinction in neural control of voluntary and spontaneous expression as involving, respectively, pyramidal (corticospinal and corticobulbar tracts that project to motor neurons without synapse) and extrapyramidal (other motor tracts outside the pyramidal network) systems (e.g., Ekman, 1980). However, as Diamond and Frew (1979) pointed out, the distinction between pyramidal and extrapyramidal systems is becoming less clear and these terms are being abandoned. It is probably also mistaken to distinguish voluntary and spontaneous neural regulation of emotional expression by associating exclusively cortical control with the former and limbic or subcortical control with the latter (e.g., Ekman, Hager, & Friesen, 1981). We noted that stimulation and ablation in cortical areas can profoundly alter spontaneous emotional expression.

Clinical data suggest that there is some degree of lateralization in neural pathways regulating spontaneous facial movement. Brain-damaged patients may present paralysis of spontaneous facial movement on only one side of the face. Indeed, there are case reports (e.g., Davison & Kelman, 1939) of patients who display paralysis for voluntary and spontaneous movement on opposite sides of the face. The fact that unilateral mimic paralysis may occur in the absence of paralysis of voluntary movement on the same side indicates that damage in such cases is above the level of the motor nuclei of the facial nerve. Otherwise, unilateral paralysis for both types of movement would be expected, as in cases of Bell's palsy. Clinical data alone are not informative, however, of direction and degree of consistency in lateralization in the neural control of spontaneous facial movement.

Only one study to date has attempted to address these issues. Remillard, Andermann, Rhi-Sausi, and Robbins (1977) collected a sample of 50 temporal lobe epilepsy patients. Patients and neurologically intact controls were photographed at rest, during the voluntary performance of a facial movement, and while laughing in response to jokes. Degree of asymmetry in expression was assessed for each condition. Of the patients with unilateral foci, contralateral lower facial weakness was observed in one or more of the conditions in 73%, 13% had ipsilateral weakness, and only 13% were judged symmetric. This pattern was consistent for all three types of facial expression. However, contralateral facial weakness appeared to be most frequent and most severe during the emotional expression of laughing. The control group evidenced a significantly lower rate of asymmetric expressions in all conditions. Remillard *et al.* concluded that contralateral facial weakness was a common occurrence in temporal lobe epilepsy and was particularly apparent during emotional expression.

Although the Remillard *et al.* data support the view that there is predominant contralateral cortical control over spontaneous emotional expression, this evidence is only suggestive. Remillard *et al.* did not spell out their criteria for assessing facial asymmetry, nor did they report the reliability of these judgments. It is not known whether lack of facial movement was required for weakness to be ascribed to a side of the face or whether only a difference in intensity of expression was sufficient. This issue is of consequence because epileptogenic lesions could conceivably produce greater intensity of expression on the ipsilateral facial side, rather than diminishing expression on the contralateral side. Furthermore, since subjects were aware of being photographed, the expressions obtained of laughing in response to jokes are likely to have contained a voluntary element. Although there is suggestive data of greater contralateral neural control of spontaneous facial expression, further investigation is required. In particular, studies of the effects of lateralized stimulation (e.g., visual half-field presentation) in eliciting asymmetric spontaneous emotional expressions would be helpful.

Even if it were established that spontaneous emotional expression, like voluntary movement, is under predominantly contralateral control, it could not be claimed with assurance that control of muscle tonus in the resting face is also predominantly contralateral. Expression in the resting face is an outcome of both excitation and inhibition of facial movement, as we described above. Studies relevant to the issue of lateralization in the neural control of spontaneous emotional expression are for the most part concerned with identifying regions involved in the excitation or disinhibition of facial movement. This is clearly the case in research using electrical or chemical stimulation to elicit facial expression (e.g., Delgado, 1970; Grossman, 1970). On the other hand, different neural centers, possibly with distinct patterns of lateralization, may control the inhibition of spontaneous facial movements, and a different set of neurological disorders may reflect excessive inhibition of facial movement. For example, the fixed facies or facial rigidity observed in Parkinsonism gives the face a mask-like appearance. Some have thought that the fixed facies derive from irritation of inhibitory pathways regulating spontaneous facial movement (e.g., Hausman, 1958). Stimulation of some cortical areas is known to result in facial rigidity (e.g., Crosby & DeJonge, 1963). Until the nature of lateralization is understood both in terms of excitatory and inhibitory pathways, the nature of asymmetry in the neural control of the resting face will be at issue.

This summary of the evidence concerning lateralization in the neural control of facial expression suggests that probably the most fruitful area to begin investigation of facial asymmetry in emotional expression is with expressions that are voluntarily produced. This is not to say, however, that significant asymmetry does not exist in regard to spontaneous emotional expression and in the emotional expression of the "spontaneous" resting face. Indeed, in these two cases were such asymmetry to be demonstrated and found to be independent of peripheral factors, such as facial size disparity, there would be grounds for claiming that there is lateralization in the neural control of these types of expression, whatever its direction.

The Problem of Midline

Studies of facial asymmetry, whether concerned with emotional expression, size or area, or motility of facial movement must all confront the fact that the face does not contain a clearly demarcated midline. In studies using the technique of comparing photographic composites made up of the left and right sides of the face (e.g., Gilbert & Bakan, 1973; Rubin & Rubin, 1980; Sackeim & Gur, 1978), this problem is explicit in that criteria must be established to cut original and reversed photographs of the full face at some midline to construct the composites. In studies in which judgments are obtained of asymmetry when raters view full faces (e.g., Borod & Caron, 1980; Ekman et al., 1981), raters must adopt their own implicit criteria of what constitutes a midline. Variability in such decisions, coupled with perceiver biases in weighting information from one side (e.g., displacing midlines more to one side), presumably add considerable noise to data when ratings are obtained from the full face in original orientation.

It is noteworthy that most investigators who have used the split-face composite technique have not reported their criteria for determining facial midline (Campbell, 1978, 1979a, 1979b; Gilbert & Bakan, 1973; Rubin & Rubin, 1980; Sackeim et al., 1978). The issue of criteria choice is of consequence because some landmarks may deviate systematically to the left or right, possibly producing artifactually asymmetry in the size of composites that, in turn, may influence other dimensions of asymmetry.

Sutton (1963, 1968) reported an association between direction and degree of deviation of the tip of the nose and direction and strength of handedness. Owing to methodological problems, this finding must be viewed with caution.[1] Nonetheless, Sutton's data highlight the fact that systematic deviation of landmarks is possible.

1. We examined lateral deviation of the tip of the nose in a sample of 53 right-handed male undergraduates, with faces at rest. Deviation was measured relative to midline, independently for original- and reverse-orientation photographs. No consistent direction of asymmetry was observed. Data from this sample on asymmetry in size and area of facial regions and on asymmetry in resting face emotional expression are presented below. Midline criteria are described in footnote 2.

Various criteria have been used in establishing facial midline in radiological studies of asymmetry of hard tissue and in anthropometric studies of asymmetry on the facial surface. Sutton (1968) suggested, for instance, the line bisecting the line connecting the two most lateral points in the frontal plane of the face, at the level of the zygions (cheekbone). In contrast, in our work, a set of landmarks are used more central in the frontal plane.[2] If there is consistent asymmetry in facial width, the use of extreme lateral landmarks will displace the midline toward the wider part of the face. The use of more central landmarks, for which there is no evidence of consistent lateral deviation, minimizes the influence of asymmetry in width of midline determination.[3]

2. In our laboratory at New York University we use four points on the face to define midline: the intersection of two arcs drawn upward (above the head) 30° with the internal canthi as origins, the intersection of two arcs drawn downward (toward the mouth) 30° with the internal canthi as origins, the midpoint of the nasal base at the level of the nasofrontal suture corresponding to nasion, and the vertex of the indentation on the upper lip corresponding to philtrum and approximating the intermaxillary suture. A best-fitting line is determined for these points. When composites are constructed, midline determination is independently made for original- and reverse-orientation photographs.

3. Another methodological problem in studies of facial asymmetry concerns head position when faces are photographed or observed. Frequently, investigators have not reported methods for ensuring that photographs were strictly frontal plane and/or they permitted head movement. Composites constructed off frontal view, like laterally displaced midlines, will artifactually distort asymmetry in facial size and possibly influence judgments of asymmetry in other dimensions. Control of head position is particularly important given the evidence of consistent lateral deviation of the head and/or eyes as a function of cognitive task (e.g., Kinsbourne, 1972), affective state (e.g., Ahern & Schwartz, 1979; Tucker, Roth, Arneson, & Buckingham, 1977), and individual differences in personality (e.g., R. E. Gur & Gur, 1977). There is no method available that can guarantee absolute frontal-plane head position across individuals. A technique that has been commonly used in radiography is to insert rods an equal distance into the external acoustic meati, that is, into the ear holes (e.g., Broadbent, 1931). Problems with this technique are that displacement may be produced around the vertical axis of the head when the meati differ in anterior–posterior position and displacement may be produced horizontally when meati differ upward–downward or when the angles of penetration are not equal (e.g., Cheney, 1952). Since this technique fixes head position with extreme lateral points in the frontal plane, distortion of asymmetry will be magnified most for central facial landmarks. Instead, we have developed a method for fixing head position that incorporates both distal and medial facial landmarks, as well as the contour of the posterior basal portion of the skull. The back of the head is rested against a firm "midline" support, with padded rods, extending equal lengths, supporting the head at the level of the temples. The center of the upper base of the nose, approximately corresponding to nasion, is then adjusted to fall at the center of the crosshairs of a camera lens. We use this technique in photographing and videotaping faces at rest and during voluntary emotional displays. We adapt the technique using only back and side head restraint for spontaneous emotional expression studies. For the latter, a cover story is used as to why head position must remain fixed and subjects are photographed or taped covertly.

Asymmetry in Facial Regional Size, Shape, and Area

Given the suggestion of lateral deviation in a central facial landmark (Sutton, 1963) and the fact that asymmetry in sheer size of the face may influence judgments of composites, it may be questioned whether differences in expressiveness on the sides of the face are simply a consequence of asymmetry in total size or of asymmetries in the size and/or shape of particular physiognomic features. For instance, one side of an individual's face may appear as more frightened, passive, or sad because it is smaller, thinner, or more angular. Therefore, the question has been raised (e.g., Ekman, 1980; C. A. Nelson & Horowitz, 1980) whether asymmetry in emotional expression is an outcome of consistent asymmetry in facial morphology.

The issue of asymmetry in size or area of facial hard tissue has been studied extensively in anthropometric investigations across various cultural groups by taking measurements from human skulls (e.g., Harrower, 1928a, 1928b; Pearson & Woo, 1935; Woo, 1931, 1937) and in dental and orthodontic radiographic studies of normal and abnormal craniofacial structure and growth (e.g., Harvold, 1951, 1954; Letzer & Kronman, 1967; Posen, 1958; Shah & Joshi, 1978; Vig & Hewitt, 1974). There has been considerably less investigation devoted exclusively to asymmetry in the soft facial tissue, skin, fatty deposits, and muscles (e.g., Sutton, 1969). However, there has been some study of asymmetry in size of facial regions using photographic techniques or measurement on live faces that necessarily combine size differences attributable to hard and soft tissue asymmetry (e.g., Burke, 1971; Figalova, 1969; Haga, Ukiya, Koshihara, & Ota, 1964; Sackeim & Gur, 1980).

The results of these investigations on hard tissue, soft tissue, and surface feature asymmetry indicated that there is little, if any, consistent lateral asymmetry in facial regional size, area, or volume. Across studies, mean asymmetries were typically less than 1% of the size of the regions under consideration. The absence of consistent asymmetry was supported by the fact that those investigators who examined facial size disparities developmentally observed no increase with age in the mean asymmetries of facial regions, despite marked facial growth during childhood (e.g., Burke, 1971; Harvold, 1954; Mulick, 1965). Further, those investigators who examined hard-tissue asymmetry in the face and other parts of the skull noted marked and systematic asymmetries in cranial bones, but not in the face (Pearson & Woo, 1935; Woo, 1931; cf. LeMay, 1977). Degree of size homology between regions on the left and right sides of the face was noted to be consistently high and greater than that found for cranial regions. Some have commented that the face appears structurally to be of unusual symmetry and perhaps the most symmetric part of the body (e.g., Harvold, 1951; Pearson & Woo, 1935).

A drawback of this research was that most investigators took relatively few measurements in isolated facial regions. None of the studies was concerned with total area or volume asymmetry. Further, the material used to study hard- and soft-tissue asymmetry (skulls, computerized-axial-tomography scans, X rays, live faces, and contour maps of faces), was never the same material as that used to study expressive asymmetry (photographs and videotapes). At issue is whether there are consistent asymmetries in size of facial surface regions or in facial surface area in the type of material used to examine expressive asymmetry and whether size and/or area asymmetries are associated with expressive asymmetry. Two studies (Sackeim & Gur, 1980; Sackeim & Weiman, in preparation) have addressed these issues.

Sackeim et al. (1978) constructed left-side and right-side composites from the set of emotional expressions supplied by Ekman and Friesen (1976). With the exception of some instances of happiness (Ekman, 1980), the expressions were voluntarily produced. Sackeim et al. found that intensity of expression was greater in left-side than in right-side composites. Sackeim and Gur (1980) reported data on asymmetry for two measures of facial width taken in these same stimuli. There were no relations between asymmetry in width and asymmetry in emotional intensity, as the correlations were essentially zero.

Sackeim and Weiman (in preparation) photographed the resting face of 53 right-handed males. In addition to examining asymmetry in emotional expression, 11 linear measurements were taken of size of various facial regions. The measures taken are displayed in Figure 11-1. Four of the measures (2, 4, 6, 7) were completely independent of midline. Sensitivity of measurement was to the .01 mm. Each measurement was taken independently four times, once for each side of the face in original and mirror-image orientation. Area of the facial sides was also measured. A line was drawn perpendicular to midline through the external canthus. This line determined the upper limit of the area, the midline a lateral boundary, and the contour of the face in the frontal place completed the form. Area was measured independently four times with a compensating planimeter to the .01 cm^2.

The measurements of regional size and facial area were extremely reliable. For each of the 11 linear measures, a repeated measures analysis of variance (Familial History of Left-Handedness $\times$ Sighting Dominance $\times$ Side of the Face) was conducted on mean regional size for each of the two sides of the face. No main effect of side of the face was obtained in any analysis. The largest mean asymmetry in the total sample, $[(R - L)/(R + L/2)]$, was only 1.24% of the mean size of the region assessed (for the 11 measures, range = .00068 − .0124; median = .00399). Of the 33 possible interactions in the analyses of variance, one was significant. Right-eyed subjects tended to have a larger distance on the right side from external

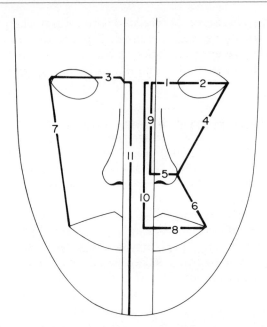

FIGURE 11-1. Eleven linear measurements taken independently from photographic composites of each side of the face. The regions are: 1, internal canthus to midline (perpendicular); 2, internal to external canthus; 3, external canthus to midline (perpendicular); 4, external canthus to lateral-most point of nostril; 5, lateral-most point of nostril to midline (perpendicular); 6, lateral-most point of nostril to corner of mouth; 7, external canthus to corner of mouth; 8, corner of mouth to midline (perpendicular); 9, length of midline at level of internal canthus to level of lateral-most point in nose; 10, length of midline at level of internal canthus to level of corner of mouth; 11, length of midline at level of internal canthus to level of lowest point of the chin.

canthus to the corner of the mouth (measure 7) than did left-eyed subjects ($p < .1$), while the two groups did not differ on the left side.

Mean asymmetry in facial area was .2% the mean area of a side of the face. A repeated-measures analysis of variance was conducted on the measures of area for each side of the face, with familial history of sinistrality and sighting dominance as between-subjects factors. For the total sample, the sides of the face did not differ in area. An interaction between family history and facial side emerged ($p < .05$). Subjects with positive and negative family histories did not differ in left-side area and those with positive history tended to have more area on the right side of the face ($p < .1$).

In contrast to the absence of notable differences between the sides of the face in regional size or in area, there was pronounced homology in these indices. The median correlation between homologous regional size measures was .85. The correlation between area on the left and right sides of the face was .90.

As described below, asymmetry in emotional expression was determined for this same set of resting faces. The various indices of asymmetry in regional size and area were correlated with emotional asymmetry scores. No significant relations were obtained. It would appear, therefore, that static structural size characteristics of the face are not the basis of, nor contribute to, the consistent asymmetries observed in emotional expression.

Facial Asymmetry in Motility of Movement

Another factor that may complicate interpretation of expressive asymmetries is the possibility of asymmetries in movement motility. Individuals differ in the degree to which they can carry out requested facial movements (Kwint, 1934), whether the movements are emotion related (e.g., raise up the corners of the mouth) or otherwise (e.g., wiggle the ears). Often the requested movements can be performed to a greater extent on one side of the face, and there may be consistent lateral differences in movement motility (Chaurasia & Goswami, 1975).

Chaurasia and Goswami (1975) in India conducted the only study to date to examine systematically asymmetries in movement motility. Their sample was composed of 300 right-handed adults (250 male, 50 female) and 30 left-handed adults (26 male, 4 female). Motility of movement was tested for lateral deviations of the angles of the mouth, winking, platysma (muscle extending from neck to mouth) contraction, raising and everting the upper lip with dilation of nostril, and vertical wrinkling of the forehead. The experimenter first noted the dominant side of spontaneous smiles during conversations and then asked subjects to perform each of the five types of unilateral movement in rapid succession. Movements were first demonstrated by the experimenter and then subjects performed each type 10 times on each facial side. Determination of asymmetry in performance was made purely by observation. Furthermore, judgments of asymmetry were based on "the fine performance, convenience and uniform rapidity of movements" (p. 55), as opposed to extent of movements, per se.

The vast majority of subjects demonstrated asymmetry, as few movements were performed equally well on both sides of the face. Right-handers tended to show greater motility on the left side, whereas left-handers had a reversed pattern. The association of side of asymmetry and handedness was significant for four of the five types of movement. Consistency in asymmetry was more marked among the left-handers than the right-handers. Across the five exercises, 59% of right-handers showed more motility on the left side of the face and 39% had greater motility on the right. For left-handers, 23% had greater left motility and 73% had greater right motility. In both groups, males and females did not differ in distribution.

Chaurasia and Goswami (1975) provided preliminary data suggesting lateral asymmetry in muscle motility for voluntary movement in the face. (They did not report data separately for lateral deviation of the angles of the mouth for voluntary movements and spontaneous smiles.) The fact that movements were first demonstrated by the experimenter and then assessed by the same individual was a serious methodological problem with the study. However, Moscovitch and Olds (1979), in line with our informal observations, reported that when right-handers can wink with only one eye, typically they wink with the left eye.

Depending on the processes that determine facial motility asymmetry, this dimension of facial behavior may be related to asymmetry of voluntary and/or spontaneous emotional expression. The fact that there is a developmental progression with age of increasing motility of movement across the face (Kwint, 1934), as perhaps with other motor skills, might suggest that a central brain process is involved and related primarily to the dimension of voluntary emotional expression. In right-handers, displaying a requested movement on the face, emotional or otherwise, may require greater involvement of right-hemisphere than left-hemisphere processes, just as in right-handers the right hemisphere is typically superior in recognition of unfamiliar faces (see Benton, 1980, for a review) and of emotional expressions (e.g., King & Kimura, 1972; Ley & Bryden, 1979; Suberi & McKeever, 1977). Motility asymmetry and asymmetry in voluntary emotional expression may both reflect lateralization in the cognitive processes necessary to translate requested or demonstrated facial actions into motor codes.

On the other hand, motility asymmetry might also contribute to spontaneous expressive asymmetries. Motility asymmetry may be a peripheral result of asymmetric use of facial muscles during emotional or other behaviors (e.g., chewing). Such asymmetry of use may itself be an outcome of functional brain asymmetry, producing peripherally greater exercise of muscles on one side and greater muscle contraction on that side upon any requested or spontaneous movement. Consistent facial asymmetry could then be expected during spontaneous sneezing, as well as during voluntary expression of sadness or during spontaneous crying. This last scenario highlights the "chicken and egg" problem in disentangling motility from emotional expressive asymmetry. Conceivably, either may be an outcome of the other.

No investigation has yet examined motility asymmetry in the same individuals in whom asymmetries in voluntary and spontaneous emotional expressions are known.[4] Without such investigations there is no direct evidence of the degree to which motility asymmetry is related to the effects obtained in various types of emotional expression. Indirect evidence

---

4. We are presently analyzing data on asymmetry in the spontaneous emotional expressions of newborns (in collaboration with Sara Weber) and adults (in collaboration with Laura Monserat). In the study on adults, data are also available on voluntary emotional displays and on facial motility. Relations among these three dimensions will be determined from data on the same indivduals.

is available to the extent that Chaurasia and Goswami's (1975) claims are valid—that is, that right-handers and left-handers show greater motility on opposite sides of the face and that the effect is more consistent among left-handers. Findings regarding emotional asymmetry that fit this pattern may reflect motility asymmetry; findings of emotional asymmetry that depart from this pattern are less likely to be an outcome of the same processes that determine motility of facial movement.

Perceiver Biases in the Processing of Facial Information

When viewing an unfamiliar face, most perceivers' impressions are determined more by the side of the poser's face to their left (typically the right side of the poser) than by the side to their right. Originally, Wolff (1943) and then McCurdy (1949) and Lindzey, Prince, and Wright (1952) presented subjects with full faces in original orientation (R/L), as well as the right- and left-side composites of those faces. Subjects were required to determine which composite looked more like the original orientation, full face. In all studies, right composites were chosen significantly more frequently.

These investigators questioned whether the predominance of the poser's right facial side in similarity judgments was related to attributes of the face or to aspects of the perceiver. The early studies lacked a critical methodological control to decide this issue. When full faces are presented only in original orientation, the right side of the poser's face is always to the perceiver's left. The phenomenon may be due either to a bias to select the right side or to a bias to select the side to the perceiver's left.

Gilbert and Bakan (1973) conducted a series of studies that partially resolved these issues. They presented raters with full faces either in original (R/L) or reversed, mirror-image (L/R) orientation. As before, right composites were chosen significantly more frequently for faces presented in original orientation. However, for reverse-orientation faces, left composites were chosen more frequently. The phenomenon appeared to be due to a lateral bias of the perceiver to find more salient the side of the full face to the left.

Since the face is asymmetric in emotional display, perceiver biases to weight information from one side of the face may strongly influence the communication of emotion. As we outline below, there were a number of methodological problems in previous research on perceiver biases. Before we could examine the role of such biases in influencing the communication of emotion, we thought it important to more rigorously establish the classic phenomenon of perceiver bias in the judgment of facial similarity.[5]

5. The data presented here on perceiver biases are part of a larger series of studies conducted at the NYU Neuropsychology Laboratory, in collaboration with Dennis Grega, Sigmound Hough, and Evelyn Sanchez.

We constructed a 16-mm movie that contains 30 test trials, half of male and half of female faces. Each trial was composed so that there is one frame containing a fixation point followed by six frames of a full face (in original or reversed orientation). After the full face, five frames of a computer-generated line pattern are presented, followed by a one frame fixation dot and then by 12 frames containing left and right composites of the face. The composites are aligned horizontally, with position to the left or right side random. In any given orientation of the movie, half the full faces are in original and half in reverse orientation. In the work discussed here, the movie was presented at a rate of one frame per second (fps), using a variable-speed control projector.

The movie provides a more rigorous test of the perceiver bias than in previous research. First, the full faces were originally photographed with shower caps to mask hairlines and gowns to cover clothing asymmetry. In previous studies (e.g., Gilbert & Bakan, 1973) hairlines were exposed, and since this feature is usually asymmetrically distributed, composites often appear bizarre. Further, the faces were photographed under the same conditions as in the research reported below on the resting face, with expressions "neutral." Therefore, the only asymmetric information subjects could use to manifest perceiver biases were characteristics of the resting face. Second, by imposing a delay and visual mask between full-face and composite presentations manifestation of the perceiver bias was dependent on memory. Third, and most important, the movie contains half original- and half reversed-orientation full faces, with order random. When the movie is shown left/right reversed (orientation B), each original face becomes a reversal or mirror image, and vice versa. This control is critical since it is only certain that Gilbert and Bakan (1973) included a reverse-orientation face condition. In fact, in three of their four studies original-versus reverse-orientation condition was a between-subjects factor. Since hairlines and extrafacial asymmetries were not masked, it was possible that subjects in the reverse-orientation condition realized they were presented with mirror-image faces. In their fourth study all subjects were presented with a set of original-orientation trials and then a set of reverse-orientation trials, also a questionable procedure. The randomization of original- and reverse-orientation full faces and the mirror imaging of these same faces by left/right reversal of the movie itself provides a powerful test of perceiver biases.

In an early study, we presented the movie to 212 subjects (106 male, 106 female); 108 subjects were presented with orientation A and 104 were presented with orientation B, the mirror image. Subjects were asked on each trial to judge which composite, the one to their left or right looked more like the previously presented full face. We computed for each subject the number of right composites chosen on each of the 15 trials when a full face was presented in original and in reverse orientation. In manifesting the standard perceiver bias, weighting the side of the face more to their left, subjects should choose right composites more during original-orientation than reverse-orientation trials. As is seen in Figure 11-2, this effect ($p < .001$) was obtained to an equal degree in both movie orientations. The equivalence of movie orientations is particularly significant since original-orientation trials in orientation A were reversals in orientation B, and vice versa. We have collected similar data with several hundred additional subjects and have obtained this effect consistently. The perceiver bias appears to be a highly reliable phenomenon.

In other work we have shown that perceiver biases influence not only judgments of similarity but also of emotionality. The first indication of an influence on perception of emotion was in our original study on facial asymmetry in voluntary emotional expression (Sackeim & Gur, 1978). In addition to rating the intensity of emotional expressions in slides of left composites, right composites, and full faces in original orientation, subjects were asked to report the emotion most expressed in each slide. Overall, raters were quite accurate in identifying emotions, and rates of correct identification did not differ among the three types of slides.

To examine whether perceiver bias influenced rates of identification, absolute differences were computed in the percentages of raters correctly identifying right composites and left composites relative to original-orientation full faces. The discrepancy between left composites and original faces was consistently greater than the discrepancy between right com-

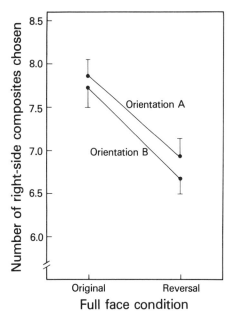

FIGURE 11-2. Mean number of right composites chosen as more similar to full faces when full faces were presented in original (R/L) or reversed (L/R) orientation. Lateral orientation of stimuli in film orientation A was the mirror image of that in film orientation B.

posites and original faces. Thus, the degree to which a given emotion was identified in an original-orientation face corresponded more with its rate of identification in right than left composites. We wished to examine these data further to determine whether the effect differed for positive and negative expressions. We could not perform this analysis since a ceiling effect was obtained for ratings of happy expressions across the three types of stimuli.

The findings of this first study suggested that when judging the emotion conveyed in a full face in original orientation, most individuals' impressions are influenced more by the expressive features on the right than on the left side of the face. In recent work we have attempted to determine whether the bias also influences judgments of emotional intensity and whether individuals who differ in direction of perceiver bias, as assessed by judgments of facial similarity, also differ in their judgments of emotional intensity.

In this research we have presented people with full-face slides (original and reversed orientation) in which one side of the face is known to be more intense in emotional expression. We have found that people who differ in direction of perceiver bias (as determined by facial similarity judgments) also differ in the side of the face they weight in assessing emotional intensity. This effect has been strongest for negative emotional expressions and we have tentative findings that the side of the face that is typically more salient reverses within the same individuals as a function of whether emotional expressions are negative or positive.[6]

It would seem, therefore, that perceiver biases are robust and influence the perception of facial similarity and emotionality. There are data sug-

6. In the study on perceiver bias effects on judgments of emotional intensity, subjects were classified as manifesting the standard perceiver bias (weighting the side of the face to their left, $n = 60$) or as showing an inverse bias (weighting the side to their right, $n = 30$) on the basis of judgments of facial similarity, using 16-mm film. They were then presented slides of full faces, in original and reversed orientation, displaying negative and positive emotional expressions and asked to rate emotional intensity. Asymmetry in intensity of expression previously had been determined for these slides (Sackeim & Gur, 1978). Subjects with the standard bias rated negative expressions as more intense when the more intense side of the face was to their left and rated positive expressions as more intense when the more intense facial side was to their right. An opposite pattern was obtained in the inverse perceiver bias group. We interpreted these effects as reflecting hemispheric asymmetry in the processing of positive and negative emotional information. As discussed below, there is evidence that most individuals display relatively greater right- than left-hemisphere activation when processing negative emotional information, whereas the reverse obtains when processing positive emotional information (e.g., Tucker, Stenslie, Roth, & Shearer, 1981; see Sackeim, Greenberg, Weiman, Gur, Hungerbuhler, & Geschwind, 1982, for a review). Asymmetric activation patterns may lead to a greater salience of the side of space opposite to the more active hemisphere. Further, to account for these initial findings, it should be the case that individual differences in direction of perceiver bias in judgments of facial similarity predict individual differences in direction of affective lateralization.

gesting that perceiver biases play an important role in aesthetic judgment and in the processing of visual stimuli other than faces (e.g., Levy, 1976; T. Nelson & MacDonald, 1971).

Perceiver biases are a major methodological issue in studies of facial expression where asymmetry ratings are obtained only from original orientation faces (e.g., Borod & Caron, 1980; Ekman et al., 1981). Observers weight information more from the side of the face, and the direction of this effect may vary as a function of emotional expression. The extent to which this confounds ratings of asymmetry may depend on complex interactions among the type of bias in raters, the emotion being rated, and the extent of asymmetry. It would seem a necessary precaution that, whenever full faces are rated to obtain judgments of asymmetry, ratings be made in both original and reverse orientations.[7] Similarly, in the social psychology literature, hundreds of studies have been reported in which judgments of facial expression have been obtained (e.g., Ekman & Oster, 1979; Izard, 1977). Lack of control over perceiver bias probably adds even more noise to such data since raters are rarely informed to examine deliberately both sides of the face when making judgments. This previously may not have seemed like much of a problem since we rarely are aware of noticeable asymmetry in the faces we encounter. However, perceiver biases to weight information from one side may account for this lack of awareness. Patterns of perceiver bias coupled with patterns of facial asymmetry may influence the communication of emotion. Before we discuss this issue, we review findings on facial asymmetry in the expression of emotion.

FACIAL ASYMMETRY IN EMOTIONAL EXPRESSION

Voluntary Emotional Expression

Consistent differences between the sides of the face in the voluntary expression of emotion have been demonstrated. The first study to examine this issue (Sackeim & Gur, 1978; Sackeim et al., 1978) compared intensity of six types of emotional expression in 14 posers (12 right-handers and two with unknown handedness). Left-side and right-side composites of the expressions (see Figure 11-3) were rated for emotional intensity. Across emotions there was a main effect of composite type. The left side of the face was judged to be more intense in its emotional expression.

This effect—greater left-side intensity in right-handers—has been obtained in every published study to date of facial asymmetry in voluntary emotional expression. Campbell (1978) photographed right-handers while they were requested to smile and found that the left facial side was rated

7. This can be done both for photographic and videotape stimuli. In our laboratory video monitors are equipped to reverse electronically left–right orientation of images.

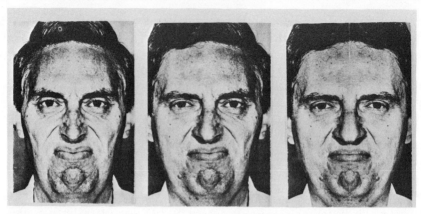

FIGURE 11-3. Example of a left-side composite (extreme left), original orientation (middle), and right-side composite of the same face expressing disgust. The photograph of the original face was obtained courtesy of P. Ekman. The set of three photographs appeared in "Emotions are expressed more intensely on the left side of the face" by H. A. Sackeim, R. C. Gur, & M. C. Saucy, *Science*, 1978, **202**, 434–436. Copyright 1978 by the American Association for the Advancement of Science. Reprinted by permission.

as happier. The same result was recently reported by Heller and Levy (1981). Borod and Caron (1979, 1980) had samples of right-handers and left-handers engaged in nine distinct emotional expressions. Across expression type, right-handers were rated as more expressive on the left side of the face. Rubin and Rubin (1980) asked 10 right-handed and 10 left-handed 8- to 10-year-old children to pose happy, neutral, sad, and angry expressions. Greater left-side intensity was found among the right-handers. For posing of smiles, Moscovitch, Strauss, and Olds (1980) found greater left-side intensity in right-handed graduate students but no asymmetry in right-handed children 2 to 5 years old. In children aged 5, 9, and 13, Ekman *et al.* (1981) found that asymmetric deliberate imitations of smiles and of negative facial expressions were frequently more pronounced on the left side than on the right side.

Two issues are of particular consequence in interpreting these findings: Is the effect of greater left-side intensity uniform across emotions? Is this effect produced by asymmetry in motility of facial movement?

The emotional expressions that appear to show the greater left-side intensity effect most consistently are of negative affects. Whether positive emotional expressions demonstrate this effect appears related to the contexts in which the expressions are elicited. In our original study (Sackeim *et al.*, 1978) significantly greater left-side intensity was obtained for disgust and anger. No effect was obtained for expressions of happiness. With the exception of some expressions of happiness, all other expressions were produced under conditions in which posers were shown examples of the facial actions to perform, knew the emotion they were to convey, and were coached so as to achieve the correct expression (Ekman & Friesen, 1975). We later learned that some of the expressions of happiness were produced while posers were actually amused (Ekman, 1980). Therefore, the difference we observed in patterns of asymmetry for positive and negative expressions might be attributed to the difference in spontaneous as opposed to voluntary production.

Under conditions where right-handed subjects are asked to smile deliberately or to imitate deliberately an expression of a smile, greater left-side intensity has been found consistently (e.g., Campbell, 1978; Ekman et al., 1981; Heller & Levy, 1981; Moscovitch et al., 1980). Borod and Caron (1979, 1980) had subjects, who were aware of being videotaped, imagine themselves in different emotional situations. Greater left-side intensity was found among right-handers across nine expressions. This effect was significant for four of six negative expressions (disappointment, disgust, grief, tough guy) and for none of the three positive expressions (clowning, flirting, greeting). It appears that regardless of whether a voluntary display of negative emotion is accompanied or not by expression-appropriate mood or imagery, in right-handers the left side of the face is more intense in expression. It may be that as voluntary expression includes more spontaneous components, positive emotions in right-handers manifest less asymmetry or, as we propose in the next section, reverse toward greater right-side intensity.

Given that there is evidence of consistent asymmetry of facial motility of movement, the degree to which asymmetry in voluntary emotional expression is related to this dimension should be ascertained. Chaurasia and Goswami (1975) found that right-handers displayed greater motility on the left side and left-handers displayed greater motility on the right side. In the absence of data directly comparing facial asymmetries in motility and in voluntary emotional expression in the same individuals, we can at least determine whether the effects of handedness appear similar for the two dimensions.

Four studies of asymmetry in voluntary facial expression have included left-handers. Campbell (1979b) instructed 24 left-handers "to smile for the camera" and obtained ratings of their left-side and right-side composites. Left-handers were judged to smile more with the left than right side of the face. In a small sample of left-handers ($n = 4$), Heller and Levy (1981) also obtained a left-side predominance for smiles. Rubin and Rubin (1980) found that left-handed and right-handed children differed significantly in intensity asymmetry. Seven of ten right-handers displayed marked left-side predominance. Among the left-handers, one was left-sided, five were indeterminant, and four were right-sided. Borod, Caron, and Koff (1981) conducted an extensive analysis of previous data (Borod & Caron, 1980) on facial asymmetry as a function of handedness, footedness, and eyedness. Across the nine expressions, left-handers displayed a nonsignificant degree of asymmetry, with the trend toward greater left-side expressiveness. They did not, however, differ significantly from right-handers. Borod *et al.* conducted a principal-component factor analysis on the facial asymmetry scores and found that eight of the nine expressions loaded highly on the first factor and the remaining expression, "tough guy," loaded highly on a second factor. Of note, the "tough guy" expression was the only display that required a unilateral movement, snarling on one side of the mouth. Right-handers and left-handers did not differ on the "emotion" factor (the eight expressions), but they did differ on the toughness expression, with right-handers displaying greater expressivity on the left side of the face. This last finding is of note, since Chaurasia and Goswami (1975) compared the performance of unilateral facial movements separately on each side of the face. Chaurasia and Goswami's effect may be particular to situations where unilateral movements are requested, and may not pertain to bilateral facial expressions.

In none of the four studies that examined asymmetry of voluntary emotional expression in left-handers did effects emerge for consistently greater expression on the right side of the face. Since Chaurasia and Goswami not only found greater right-side motility of movement in left-handers, but also greater consistency in this effect than in the greater left-side motility among right-handers, it would seem that different neuropsychological processes subserve facial asymmetry in these two dimensions. This conclusion should be regarded as tentative until the degree of association, or lack thereof, between the two dimensions is evaluated in the same group of individuals.

In light of our greater knowledge about lateralization in neural control of voluntary facial movement than about other types of emotional expression, it is not surprising that much of the research to date has concentrated on voluntary displays of emotion. This work has been of mixed quality in controlling for a number of the methodological issues we raised earlier. At times, head position has not been controlled, midline criteria not reported, videotapes have been rated by very small samples of judges only in original orientation, and so on. Nonetheless, the findings have been rather uniform. Across variable conditions, right-handers above the age of 5 years have been found to display voluntary negative emotional expressions more intensely on the left side. When smiles are obtained in the most deliberate circumstances, greater left-side intensity is also obtained.

Spontaneous Emotional Expression

Studies of neurologic, psychiatric, and normal populations have shown that there is substantial functional brain asymmetry in the regulation of positive and negative emotion. The findings suggest that in most individuals the left side of the brain subserves positive emotional states to a greater extent than the right side, whereas the reverse holds for negative emotional states (see Sackeim *et al.*, 1982, for a review; cf. Tucker, 1981). This pattern of lateralization appears consistent across both the experience of emotion (mood) and spontaneous emotional expression. For instance, the likelihood of manifestation of either of two contrasting mood changes, a euphoric-indifference reaction or a dysphoric-depressive reaction, following unilateral brain damage is in large part a function of side of lesion (e.g., Gainotti, 1972). Similarly, Sackeim *et al.* (1982) found that whether patients manifested uncontrollable, spontaneous outbursts of laughing or crying as a consequence of destructive or epileptogenic (giving rise to epileptic attacks) lesions was strongly related to predominant side of damage.

It is in the area of spontaneous emotional expression that one would expect this dimension of lateralization to be most manifest in studies on normal populations. In regard to facial asymmetry, we noted earlier that the available evidence suggests that there is at least a degree of lateralization in neural control of spontaneous facial movement, with greater contralateral than ipsilateral neural regulation (e.g., Remillard *et al.*, 1977). Therefore, our working hypothesis is that in most individuals there is greater intensity of spontaneous negative emotional expression on the left side of the face, as in voluntary expression, but greater right-side spontaneous positive emotional expression. As we shall see, at this time this view remains at the level of hypothesis. There has been no methodologically sound investigation of facial asymmetry in spontaneous emotional expression.

Wolff (1933, 1943) was the first investigator to compare emotional expression on the left and right sides of the face. He collected judgments for photographic composites of the lateral sides of the faces of children, normal adults, psychiatric groups, and cadavers. It appears from his reports that he examined asymmetry in spontaneous expressions and in the resting face. Unfortunately, Wolff did not provide details about his procedures or results. He did claim that there were consistent asymmetries in facial expression.

> The right-hand view [right side of the face] produces an effect of liveliness and individuality while the left-hand view produces one of remoteness from life. The right-hand view is described as full of vitality, sensual, smiling, frank, active, brutal, social, or full of emotion, while the left-hand face is described as being in a state of rigor, dead, concentrated, reticent, passive, ethereal, demoniac, solitary, and mask-like. (Wolff, 1933, p. 175)

Lynn and Lynn (1938, 1943) conducted two studies on "spontaneous" smiles. The first involved testing of 398 subjects varying in age from 4 to 80 years (60% of the sample were summer campers between the ages of 6 and 15). Smiles were observed by three raters during the course of conversation with the subjects and during the assessment of handedness and sighting dominance (eyedness). Asymmetry judgments were based on the relative lengths of lateral eye–mouth lines during smiles and there was only moderate interobserver agreement. (In 57.5% of cases, the three raters agreed in assessments as more dominant on the left, right, or symmetrical.) Lynn and Lynn's (1938) results pertained primarily to 105 subjects who the raters agreed had asymmetric smiles. In particular, they reported strong associations between personality factors and whether smiles were more pronounced on the side of the face ipsilateral or contralateral to the preferred hand. For instance, right-handers with asymmetric right-sided smiles were independently evaluated as manifesting greater initiative, self-confidence, aggressiveness, and so on, than those with left-sided smiles. Overall, the distributions of left- and right-side smiling in the 105 asymmetric subjects did not differ from chance. Lynn and Lynn claimed that direction of smile asymmetry was not related to handedness or eye dominance. However, they did not present data concerning these factors, and it cannot be determined whether they concurrently examined the role of handedness, eye dominance, and/or sex as possible moderating variables associated with direction of smile asymmetry (cf. R. E. Gur & Gur, 1977). The findings of their second investigation (Lynn & Lynn, 1943) suggested that their claim of independence may not have been valid.

In the second study, Lynn and Lynn related individual differences in smile asymmetry of 104 psychiatric patients to personality variables. They more objectively assessed smile asymmetry by unobtrusively filming 3 minutes of facial behavior as subjects reacted to a Walt Disney cartoon. They had noted that the absolute difference between the distances traveled by the right and left corners of the mouth during the upward motion of the smile was quite variable and influenced by factors such as breadth of smile and size of face. Instead, they developed a measure of asymmetry based on the initial phase of smiling. They found that in over 90% of smiles, one corner traveled farther and faster than the other corner during the initial upward motion. Following this observation, they used a smile asymmetry quotient of the absolute differences in the initial distance traveled by the two corners divided by total distance: $(R - L)/(R + L)$. Reliability of quotient scores for multiple smiles during the same sessions and over a 3-week period was moderate.

As in the first study, Lynn and Lynn (1943) reported significant associations between side of greater smile and personality characteristics. Patients who smiled more on the right side were rated by nurses on a set of 15 trait descriptions as more self-confident, dominant, aggressive, and so on, than left-side smilers. Right-side smilers were also rated as more "emotionally responsive" and, interestingly, they displayed seemingly more intense smiles. The total amount of upward motion of both corners of the mouth was greater in right-handed, right-side smilers than in right-handed left-side smilers. Overall, the distributions of subjects with left- and right-smile dominance did not differ from chance. There were few left-handers in the sample. Right-eyedness was associated with greater right-sided smiles. (Borod *et al.*, 1981, observed a similar effect on asymmetry scores for the eight voluntary expressions among right-handers.)

There are a number of problems in evaluating Lynn and Lynn's findings. Foremost among these is the issue of whether the smiles they obtained in the two studies were truly spontaneous and homogeneous expressions of positive mood states of happiness or amusement. It has often been pointed out that in the presence of others emotional expressions are subject to strong social display rules (e.g., Ekman & Oster, 1979). It should be seriously questioned whether smiles observed, for instance, in children and adolescents necessarily are spontaneous when they are elicited during conversation with and testing by three adults. Further, the nature of the smiles may be at issue. People smile when they are happy, embarrassed, or shy. Smiles accompany reports of negative affect. It is noteworthy that Lynn and Lynn's (1938, 1943) robust finding in normal children and in psychiatric patients was that those subjects rated as more shy, socially retiring, and timid showed left-sided smiles, whereas the more assertive, self-confident subjects smiled more on the right side. One might wonder whether the smiles manifested by both sets of subjects were, indeed, outward expressions of different moods.

The possibility that the smiles conveyed by the two asymmetry groups were distinct is supported by two observations. First, Lynn and Lynn (1943) themselves speculated that right-handers with left-sided smiles "develop a maximum of cortical inhibition of emotional drives" (p. 275), whereas the subjects with greater right-side smiles express emotional drives more directly. Second, and perhaps more critically, there was objective evidence that in the study with psychiatric patients the smiles of the two groups differed. In stating their rationale for the asymmetry quotient, Lynn and Lynn (1943) noted that not only did the smiles of patients involve greater movement when they were predominantly right-sided, but also that the absolute difference between the sides $(R - L)$ was greater in right-sided than in left-sided smiles. "The average of these initial measurements $[R - L]$ on subjects with a definite right initial millimeter lead was found to be one and one-half times greater than the average of the same measurements $[L - R]$ on left-faced subjects. Moreover, this quantitative difference in the two extreme smiledness groups extended also (and to a like degree) to the sum of the initial distances traveled by the right and left sides" (p. 259). It would therefore appear that by using the ratio score to control for intensity, Lynn and Lynn (1943) failed to highlight possibly strong findings that across subjects there was greater initial movement on the right than on the left side of the mouth during smiles and that right-sided smiles were also more intense.

One final methodological problem was evident in the Lynn and Lynn research. Their measure of smile asymmetry in the second study was based on the *initial* upward motion of the corners of the mouth. They noted that 91.5% of all the smiles they assessed were asymmetric. They also noted that after the first upward movement, "the initially slower mouth corner usually catches up with and often passes the mouth corner with led at first" (p. 259). Unlike deliberate or voluntary emotional expressions in which subjects fix a pose, spontaneous emotional expressions are more likely to be dynamic, with more changing patterns of involvement on the two sides of the face. This would suggest that when facial asymmetry for spontaneous expressions is studied such asymmetry be sampled over the course of expressions[8] and not statically only at the initiation or peak.

One recent investigation (Ekman *et al.*, 1981) examined facial asymmetry for spontaneous emotional expression. In the same study as on children's deliberate limitations of facial movement, Ekman *et al.* collected samples of spontaneous facial movement. Children were presented on a monitor with 15 facial movements they were to imitate. Their facial behavior was videotaped. Movements of the zygomatic major muscle occurring within 1 second of a joke or encouragement and not including movement of triangularis, mentalis, or orbicularis oris were considered instances of spontaneous happy expressions or smiles. Analyses of asymmetry were based on the ratings of one judge who scored the apex or peak of each movement from the videorecord viewed only in original orientation. In the first analyses of 78 "spontaneous smiles," only 5 (6%) were rated as asymmetric. Ekman *et al.* pointed out that with the selection procedure used, the possibility that nonspontaneous, social smiles were included could not be ruled out.

A second study was conducted on the facial behavior of female adults, the videotapes of whom had also been obtained for other purposes (Ekman, Friesen, & Ancoli, 1980). The subjects were videotaped surreptitiously as they watched brief pleasant and unpleasant films. The method of analyzing asymmetry was the same as that used in the study on children. A total of 110 muscle movements thought to be indicative of positive affect were obtained and only 4 (4%) were judged asymmetric. Only 24 movements believed to be indicative of negative emotion were observed, and 6 (25%) were rated as asymmetric. By these analyses it appeared that there was simply not much asymmetry to spontaneous emotional expression. The direction of asymmetry could not be examined.

---

8. In an ongoing study of spontaneous adult expressions, we have timed the duration of expressions and are obtaining asymmetry ratings for video frames at three fixed points in time (e.g., 1/4, 1/2, and 3/4 points in the duration of the expressions).

No facial expression, spontaneous or otherwise, is symmetric in an absolute sense. Perhaps recognizing that sensitivity of measurement was at issue, Ekman *et al.* had the facial movements of children and adults rated for what they termed "trace" asymmetry, more subtle differences between the sides of the face in emotional expression. Rates of asymmetry were enhanced for both the positive and negative deliberate expressions of children (48%, 46%), the "spontaneous" positive expressions of children (29%), and the adult positive and negative spontaneous expressions (24%, 46%). Ekman *et al.* contended that greater left-side intensity was maintained in the children for voluntary productions, while in the children and adults no consistent direction of asymmetry was observed in the spontaneous conditions. Ekman *et al.* concluded that, unlike deliberate expression, spontaneous displays are characterized by little asymmetry, irrespective of direction.

The number of asymmetric expressions observed in any of the spontanous conditions, whether the original or "trace" analyses were used, was low. Subjects did not contribute equal numbers of asymmetric expressions. For example, in the largest group of asymmetric spontaneous expressions (trace asymmetry for adult positive expressions) there were only 26 instances contributed by an unknown number of subjects. No information was collected on subjects' handedness. In this circumstance one cannot draw any conclusions about the direction of asymmetries.

At issue, then, is only the claim that spontaneous asymmetric expressions are relatively rare, particularly in relation to deliberate facial movements. Ekman *et al.* (1981) stated that "Lynn and Lynn (1938, 1943) forty years ago reported results for spontaneous happy expressions entirely consistent with ours" (p. 105). However, we noted that in both studies Lynn and Lynn reported high rates of asymmetric expressions when ratings were either based on observer's global judgments or on measurement of facial movement. Indeed, they claimed (1943) that by the latter method over 90% of spontaneous smiles were asymmetric. Why the discrepancy?

The methodological problems that characterized the Ekman *et al.* study may account for their observing little asymmetry. First, they examined asymmetry at the apex of expressions. It is likely that expressions will appear most intense when both sides contribute than at the outset when one side may predominate. Their sampling method, therefore, may have been biased toward judgments of symmetry. Second, there is little doubt that deliberate imitations of movements are likely to be more intense than the spontaneous expressions one usually obtains in a laboratory when subjects watch films or are given encouragement. No analyses were reported as to whether, for instance, the deliberate and spontaneous zygomatic major movements of children were of equal intensity. If rates of asymmetry in these movements were to be compared, the dimension of intensity should have been controlled. Third, analyses were based on the ratings of a single judge who viewed full faces only in original orientation. We have observed repeatedly that marked asymmetry in emotional expression, easily seen when contrasting left-side and right-side composites, is not easily discernible when viewing the full face. This may be evident by examining Figure 11-3. Part of the reason for this appears to be that individuals weight information more from one side of the face than the other. As indicated earlier, we have obtained data that suggest that the side of the face that has greater impact on impressions is determined in part by whether the emotional expression is positive or negative. Ratings of asymmetry obtained under the conditions used by Ekman *et al.* (1981) are likely to be strongly influenced by perceiver biases. Weighting of information from the less intense side of the face will result in overestimation of symmetry. Finally, it appears that in neither of the studies was an attempt made to control for head movement. When heads are off center, one side of the face will be more prominent. Ahern and Schwartz (1979) reported that right-handers tend to move their eye to the left following negative emotional questions and to the right following positive emotional questions (cf. Ehrlichman & Weinberger, 1978, for a discussion of problems in eye movement studies). We (unpublished data) have obtained the same effect for head movement following presentation of unpleasant and pleasant emotional slides.[9] If the less intense side of the face is more prominent, expressions may appear symmetric.

Findings in two related areas of research should be mentioned briefly. Schwartz, Fair, Salt, Mandel, and Klerman (1976) demonstrated differences in patterning of facial electromyographic (EMG) activity as a function of type of affective state (cf. Oliveau & Willmuth, 1979). EMG activity was assessed on only one side of the face. Recently, Schwartz, Ahern, and Brown (1979) measured EMG bilaterally from zygomatic and corrugator regions while subjects responded to questions that varied in emotional content. From the zygomatic region, they obtained a significant interaction between emotion type (positive or negative) and side of the face. Greater relative activity on the right side of the face was found following positive emotional questions and greater relative activity was obtained on the left side following negative emotional questions. The magnitude of the effects appeared larger in the negative emotion condition. Subjects were also asked to display deliberately expressions of happiness, excitement, sadness, and fear. Across emotion expression type, greater relative left-side EMG

---

9. Twelve right-handed males were presented with slides of positive, neutral, and negative emotional content and videotaped surreptitiously while viewing. There was significantly more head movement to the left following presentation of negative slides compared to both neutral and positive slide conditions. There were significantly fewer left head turns in the positive than in the neutral condition.

activity was obtained during the voluntary expressions. Schwartz *et al.* interpreted their findings as suggesting greater activation in left-side muscles during deliberate emotional expression and during spontaneous experiences of negative affect. They suggested that spontaneous positive affect was associated with greater right-side muscle activity.

This pattern of findings fits neatly with our view that in right-handers deliberate expressions are more intense on the left side of the face, while side of greater intensity is likely to reverse during spontaneous positive expressions. However, the Schwartz *et al.* findings should be regarded as tentative. Most at issue was whether the facial behavior following emotional questioning was a consequence of spontaneous changes in affective state or was more cognitively based (e.g., Ekman *et al.*, 1981). Patterns of asymmetry in bilateral EMG need to be examined as a function of standard mood manipulations. It is of note that, using EEG measures, both Davidson, Schwartz, Saron, Bennett, and Goleman (1979) and Tucker, Stenslie, Roth, and Shearer (1981) found that positive and negative affective states, induced by having subjects reflect on relevant personal experiences, were associated with heightened activation in left and right frontal lobes, respectively. Linking asymmetries in hemispheric activation during mood states using electrocortical or regional cerebral blood flow measures (e.g., R. C. Gur & Reivich, 1980) to patterns of facial asymmetry in EMG and emotional expression would provide potent tests of the role of functional brain asymmetry in subserving these asymmetries.

Moscovitch and colleagues (Moscovitch & Olds, 1979; Moscovitch *et al.*, 1980) investigated asymmetry in spontaneous facial gestures that accompany speech. In a series of studies, unilateral facial movements were assessed in children and adults as they related sad, funny, or frightening experiences. Since subjects directly faced a videocamera and were engaging in conversation with an experimenter, the degree to which facial movements were truly spontaneous is uncertain. Further, unilateral facial gestures (e.g., raised eyebrow) as well as emotional expressions were not distinguished. Across studies, right-handed subjects above the age of 5 years exhibited more left-sided than right-sided movements. Left-handers did not display consistent asymmetry. Moscovitch replicated Kimura's (1973) finding that during speech right-handers gesture more with the right hand. However, this effect held only when hand gestures were not accompanied by a facial gesture or expression.

There has been no extensive or methodologically adequate investigation of facial asymmetry in spontaneous emotional expression. That such asymmetry exists was established in the work of Lynn and Lynn (1938, 1943) on smiles. Similarly, we are in the process of analyzing data on spontaneous positive and negative facial expressions of newborns and adults. Marked asymmetry in expression is a frequent observation. This in itself suggests that there is some degree of lateralization in the neural control of spontaneous expression, a necessary condition for the study of spontaneous facial asymmetry to reveal more about brain lateralization in the regulation of emotion. It would appear that the fundamental issues will be whether there is consistency in direction of such asymmetry and whether the direction is a function of the emotion expressed. Based on research on brain lateralization in the regulation of emotion, we suggested that it is likely that in most individuals the right side of the face is more expressive of positive affect and the left of negative affect. Wolff's (1933, 1943) characterization that the right side is alive and vital, while the left is moribund, Lynn and Lynn's (1943) finding that initial asymmetry was more marked for right-side smiles and that right-side smiles were more intense, and the tentative EMG data relating greater activation on the right and left sides with positive and negative affective states, respectively —all provide hints that the hypothesis may have merit.

Facial Asymmetry of the Resting Face

Largely because of the issue of facial asymmetry in motility of movement, the determination of whether there are consistent asymmetries in the emotional expression of the face at rest is of particular interest. Since by definition muscle movement is minimized in the resting face, asymmetry in motility is less likely to contribute to expressive asymmetry. But unlike voluntary and spontaneous emotional expression, where expressive asymmetries are likely to be an outcome of inequalities in extent of muscle contraction, one wonders what the determinants might be of expressive asymmetries in the resting face.

The first possibility that comes to mind concerns asymmetry in static facial structure. If one side of the face were consistently thinner or more angular, this might produce asymmetry in emotional expression. However, as we indicated above, over 50 years of research on size, shape, and area asymmetry has failed to yield consistent patterns of asymmetry in these dimensions. Further, when we (Sackeim & Weiman, in preparation) took measurements of 11 facial regions and of facial area, none of the asymmetries in these measures or in statistically derived principal components were associated with expressive asymmetries in the same set of male resting faces.

We offer two theoretical possibilities as to factors that contribute most to resting-face expressive asymmetry. First, asymmetries in relative hemispheric activation may influence patterns of muscle tonus in the face. Birdwhistell (1970) proposed that there are reliable individual differences in patterns of muscle tonus in the resting face. Systematic investigation of this notion using EMG measurement rarely has been conducted (e.g., Shipman, Heath, & Oken, 1970; Smith, 1973). The hypothesis seems reasonable given that resting faces appear to differ considerably in the types of affect they convey. Presuming lateralization in neural control of resting facial muscle tonus, consistent lateral differences in both tonus and expression would also seem reasonable. Following this, it would be likely that variation in experimental conditions that influence patterns of relative hemispheric activation that obtain when resting faces are examined could lead to variation in direction and type of asymmetries.

Second, emotional expression in the resting face may be determined in part by the sequelae of facial movement, emotional or otherwise. Facial features show marked, relatively enduring changes with age, as exemplified by wrinkling. These rather static properties may contribute significantly to patterns of facial asymmetry. For instance, lateral disparities in extent of "laugh lines" or "crow's-feet" are commonly observed. Characteristic asymmetry in phasic emotional movement may alter patterns of facial contours, resulting in consistent asymmetry in the emotional expression of the resting face.

A number of investigators examined lateral differences in resting-face emotional expression. Lindzey *et al.* (1952) had observers rate left- and right-side composites of 16 male undergraduates on seven bipolar adjective scales. Handedness of posers was unknown. Subjects with marked facial asymmetry had been dropped and during the development of photographs "any striking marks on either side of the face were eliminated" (p. 71). Nonetheless, right-side composites were rated as more vital (passive–vital) than left-side composites. There was also a trend for the right side to be evaluated as more intelligent.

Seinen and van der Werff (1969) had subjects evaluate their own sides of the face on 17 adjective scales. One side of full-face photographs was covered up during the ratings. They claimed that the right side of the face was evaluated more favorably than the left side, but quantitative analyses were not reported. In a control study, subjects were presented with mirror-image photographs and again one side was covered up. Seinen and van der Werff observed the same direction of effects (i.e., more favorable evaluation of the right side), but the differences appeared unreliable. Further, in a study where observer ratings were obtained, they did not find consistent differences.

Karch and Grant (1978) constructed composites of the resting faces of 11 right-handed male naval cadets. These faces were chosen from a pool of 37 photographs on the basis of being "most symmetrical in construction" (p. 729). Observer ratings on nine bipolar adjective scales were collected. In addition to an overall difference between the sides of the face across the scales (MANOVA), left composites were judged significantly more healthy, strong, masculine, hard, active, excitable, and bad.

Campbell (1978), as well as examining asymmetry in posed smiles, collected photographs of right-handed male and female subjects when requested to relax. Left-side composites of smiling faces were found to be rated as happier than right-side composites. Left-side composites of relaxed expressions were rated as more miserable than right-side composites. In further work with right-handers, Campbell (1979a) found that the effect of greater unhappiness associated with the left side of the face held only for females. Campbell (1979b) conducted a similar study in a group of 24 left-handers. Like right-handers, the posed smile was more intense on the left side. On the other hand, in the "relax" condition the right facial side of the left-handers was consistently judged as being more unhappy.

Rappoport and Friendly (1978) constructed composites of the resting faces of 76 right-handers and 16 left-handers. Each composite was rated on the dimension of pleasant–unpleasant by a large group (231) of raters. Seventy-nine percent of faces were found to be significantly asymmetric in expression. Contrary to Campbell (1978, 1979a, 1979b), in both right- and left-handers the left-side composite was rated as more pleasant. The handedness groups differed significantly in the consistency of this effect. Of the 16 left-handers, in none was the right side judged as significantly more pleasant, while right-handers were more variable.

We recently completed a study on the emotional expression in the resting faces of 53 right-handed male undergraduates (Sackeim & Weiman, in preparation). Subjects were photographed with head position fixed and with instructions to look directly at the camera. Composites were constructed using the midline criteria described earlier. In addition to assessments of handedness, familial history of sinistrality (left-handedness), and sighting dominance, predominant direction of conjugate lateral eye movements was determined. The latter is believed to be an index of asymmetry in resting level of preferred hemispheric activation (e.g., R. E. Gur & Gur, 1977) and has been found to predict resting-level asymmetry in hemispheric blood flow on the basis of radioisotopic clearance rates (R. C. Gur & Reivich, 1980).

Each composite was rated by groups of 20 right-handers on 20 7-point bipolar scales (see Table 11-1). Acceptable split-half reliabilities were demonstrated for the scale ratings of both left and right composites. Mean scale scores were subject to a principal-components factor analysis, separately for ratings of left and right composites. Both factor analyses yielded four principal-component factors that accounted for 82% (left composite) and 80% (right composite) of the variance. The loadings of the scales on the first two factors in each analysis are presented in Table 11-1. The scale loadings were highly congruent. Scores on scales that loaded .70 or above on the same factor in each analysis were summed to yield two principal-component factor scores for each composite. The first factor was labeled as pleasant–unpleasant and the second as strong–weak.

Three main findings emerged in this portion of the study. First, subjects with characteristic left conjugate lateral eye movement, who are thought to evidence greater relative right-hemispheric activation, were rated as displaying more unpleasant resting faces than right-movers. Scores of left-movers on the unpleasantness factor were higher on both sides of

TABLE 11-1. Emotion Scale Loadings on First Two Principal Components in Factor Analyses of Ratings of Left-Side and Right-Side Composites of 53 Male Resting Faces

BIPOLAR SCALE	FIRST FACTOR—UNPLEASANTNESS		SECOND FACTOR—WEAKNESS	
	LEFT COMPOSITE	RIGHT COMPOSITE	LEFT COMPOSITE	RIGHT COMPOSITE
1. Friendly-angry*	.91	.87	-.22	-.29
2. Calm-nervous	.50	.59	.56	.42
3. Honest-dishonest*	.79	.82	-.41	-.41
4. Sensitive-insensitive	.06	.64	-.35	-.27
5. Happy-sad*	.83	.82	.14	.10
6. Strong-weak†	.17	-.07	.88	.90
7. Logical-intuitive	.52	.44	.12	.46
8. Sane-crazy*	.76	.80	.05	.13
9. Extraverted-introverted	.69	.58	.40	.38
10. Masculine-feminine†	.01	-.05	.84	.80
11. Intelligent-unintelligent*	.74	.72	.08	.30
12. Pleasant-unpleasant*	.96	.96	-.12	-.12
13. Kind-cruel*	.88	.85	-.39	-.44
14. Mature-immature	.64	.52	.24	.62
15. Verbal-nonverbal*	.79	.73	-.11	.10
16. Not disgusted-disgusted	.71	.47	-.28	-.39
17. Likable-unlikable*	.93	.94	-.18	-.12
18. Active-passive	.28	.14	.60	.70
19. Unafraid-afraid†	.31	.43	.84	.74
20. Emotional-unemotional	-.29	-.41	.39	.54

*Bipolar scale loads above .70 on the first factor for analyses of both left- and right-composite ratings.
†Bipolar scale loads above .70 on the second factor for analyses of both left- and right-composite ratings.

338 BASIC SOCIAL PSYCHOPHYSIOLOGICAL RESEARCH

the face. This effect was confirmed by having another group of judges rate unpleasantness for full faces in original and reserved (mirror) orientations. This finding supports the hypothesis that the right side of the brain subserves negative affect to a greater extent than the left side (e.g., Sackeim *et al.*, 1982; Sackeim & Weber, 1982). It is of interest that no effect of side of the face emerged in this analysis.

The second finding concerned the absence of consistent facial asymmetry in the total sample of right-handed males. Scores did not differ significantly on either of the two emotion factors as a function of facial side. No significant effects were apparent on any of the 20 scales taken individually. In contrast to prior studies, therefore, we did not observe consistent facial asymmetry in the resting face of right-handers when they were examined as a group.

The third finding was that consistent asymmetry emerged for the pleasant–unpleasant dimension when family history of sinistrality and sighting dominance were taken into account. As is seen in Figure 11-4, the interaction between these variables was significant. It is of interest that sighting dominance or eyedness contributed to the effect. The individual difference factor has rarely been examined in studies of cognitive lateralization (e.g., Bryden, 1973; Gottlieb & Wilson, 1965). Yet Lynn and Lynn (1943) and Borod *et al.* (1981) found respectively that eyedness was related to facial asymmetry for spontaneous smiles and for voluntary emotional expressions.

The pattern of findings has certainly been inconsistent in studies of facial asymmetry in the emotional expression of the resting face. This inconsistency contrasts with the uniform set of results for voluntary emotional expression. Some methodological and theoretical considerations may account for this discrepancy.

Although it is the case that some individuals display noticeable disparities in emotional expression on the two sides of the resting face, our impressions are that for the most part in young adults asymmetry is far less marked for the resting face than for voluntary and spontaneous emotional expression. Given a phenomenon of smaller magnitude, extra care is needed to determine its consistency.

On a procedural level, any lateral bias in the photographing or construction of composites is likely to confound results. For instance, Campbell (1978, 1979a, 1979b) constructed composites of subjects while they wore hats, eyeglasses, makeup, and so on. Such extrafacial characteristics are hardly ever symmetrical and can produce distortions in ratings of emotional expression.[10] In a number of the studies it is unclear whether

10. This issue is of particular consequence in studies of the female resting face. Cosmetics undoubtedly influence resting-face emotional expression. Given perceiver bias and handedness factors, cosmetics may be applied to the face consistently asymmetrically. There already are indications of sex differences in asymmetry of resting-face expression (e.g., Campbell, 1979b). The possible confound of cosmetics has not been controlled in any work to date.

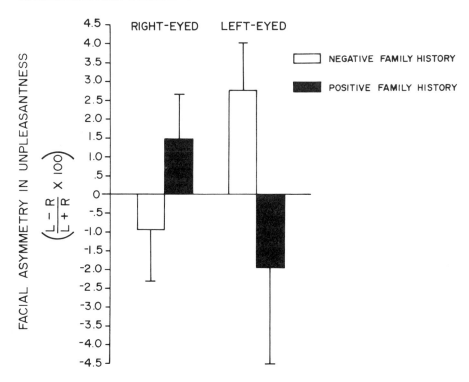

FIGURE 11-4. Mean facial asymmetry in unpleasantness as a function of family history of sinistrality and sighting dominance. Positive scores indicate greater unpleasantness associated with the left relative to the right side of the face.

lighting was homogeneous and it is likely that investigators differed considerably in their choice of midline criteria, possibly introducing artifactual size asymmetries in the construction of composites.

On a more theoretical note, the inconsistencies in results may also be due to variation in the conditions under which photographs of resting faces were obtained. We noted earlier that the expression of the resting face may reflect voluntary and/or spontaneous inhibition of facial movement. Patterns of asymmetry may differ when subjects are told to produce a relaxed expression (Campbell, 1978) or when they are not given instructions about facial display (Sackeim & Weiman, in preparation). Further, conditions that lead to variation in hemispheric activation may influence asymmetry in the resting face. For example, whether or not there are consistent asymmetries in the alpha band of the resting EEG has been a controversial issue with inconsistent patterns of findings (see Butler & Glass, 1976, for a review). Butler and Glass (1976) suggested that the presence or absence of consistent asymmetry varied as a function of whether subjects were tested in conditions where there was a possibility of hearing or partaking in conversation or in conditions where subjects were isolated in soundproof chambers. They suggested that the possibility of language processing was associated with greater left-side activation in right-handers. Similarly, patterns of asymmetry in the resting face may depend on various factors that constitute the "resting" state and which influence patterns of hemispheric activation.

We suggested that both asymmetries in hemispheric activation and in facial features such as wrinkles and laugh lines contribute to asymmetry in resting-face emotional expression. Systematic investigation is called for of both these possible determinants. The activation factor may be examined by manipulating conditions (e.g., mood states) under which resting faces are obtained and relating facial asymmetry in expression both to the manipulations and directly to measures of activation asymmetry [EEG or regional cerebral blood flow (rCBF)]. We are initiating a set of studies that concentrate on the second factor. It is noteworthy that all the reports to date on the resting face used principally young adult subjects. Facial features such as wrinkling increase with age and if there are systematic lateral effects one would expect that longitudinally facial asymmetry in emotional expression of the resting face becomes increasingly manifest. Therefore, the study of such asymmetry in geriatric samples seems particularly attractive. The second area we are concentrating on attempts to remove the influence of resting-level asymmetry in brain activation on resting-face emotional asymmetry. One way to do this is to study facial asymmetry in cadavers. Although this population introduces a special set of methodological challenges (e.g., rigor mortis), the absence of any brain activation in such samples can aid in identifying the relative contributions of the two sets of determinants to resting-face asymmetry in emotional expression.

We noted earlier in this chapter that asymmetry in the resting face was particularly problematic. The facts that tonic expression involves a balance of inhibitory and excitatory processes, that these processes may be under relative degrees of both spontaneous and voluntary control, and that the extent and direction of lateralization in neural control of some of these processes is unknown all complicate investigation of resting-face asymmetry. The findings in this area suggest that there are significant asymmetries in the emotional expression of the resting face. The fact that we have found such asymmetry to be independent of size and area disparities (Sackeim & Weiman, in preparation) suggests that other factors are determinative. Variation in resting-face emotional asymmetry has been found to be a function of handedness (Campbell, 1978, 1979b; Rappoport & Friendly, 1978), familial history of sinistrality, and sighting dominance (Sackeim & Weiman, in preparation). Such findings suggest that this dimension of facial asymmetry, like voluntary emotional expression, is related to functional brain asymmetry. It is also the case that the findings of expressive asymmetry in the resting face, while significant within studies, are contradictory across studies. We have suggested that this state of affairs has been brought about in part by lack of standardization of techniques and by methodological inadequacies. Perhaps more critically, the inconsistencies may only highlight the fact that the term "resting face" is a euphemism for facial displays of minimal muscular contraction or movement. Studies differed considerably in the conditions used to obtain stimuli of faces at rest, leading, we suggest, to variation in patterns of neural activity and in patterns of facial asymmetry.

FACIAL ASYMMETRY: INTEGRATION OF FINDINGS

We have seen that different patterns of findings emerged in regard to facial expressive asymmetry depending on whether voluntary emotional expression, spontaneous expression, or the expression of the resting face was examined. In our view this specificity most likely reflects differentiation in the neuropsychological processes subserving the expression of emotion. Indeed, the study of facial asymmetry provides an opportunity to obtain greater understanding of these processes.

Originally, we hypothesized that the greater intensity of voluntary emotional expression on the left facial side reflected greater relative involvement of the right side of the brain in voluntary emotional expression (Sackeim & Gur, 1978; Sackeim et al., 1978). We indicated that this pattern may or may not generalize to spontaneous expression, given the differences in neural control of the two types of facial behavior. Since then this hypothesis has received considerable support.

Asymmetries in size, shape, and area of facial regions (hard and/or soft tissue) are not at issue. If they exist at all, they are minor in extent and have been found to be unrelated to expressive asymmetries (Sackeim & Gur, 1980; Sackeim & Weiman, in preparation). Despite considerable variation in procedures for obtaining voluntary expression, all studies to date of right-handers older than 5 years obtained the greater left-side intensity effect, using composite-construction techniques (e.g., Campbell, 1978; Rubin & Rubin, 1980; Sackeim et al., 1978) or ratings of full faces (Borod & Caron, 1980; Ekman et al., 1981). Choice of midline criteria or other technical factors does not appear critical in establishing this effect, and the finding appears to be neither an outcome of peripheral facial size factors nor of a number of possible confounds related to stimulus construction. On the other hand, individual difference variables known to predict direction and/or extent of brain lateralization in the cognitive domain (e.g., handedness, eyedness) have been related to facial asymmetry in voluntary emotional expression (Borod et al., 1981; Rubin & Rubin, 1980).

In specifying the processes underlying this effect, the findings in the literature on hemispheric asymmetry in the comprehension of emotion may be useful. Heilman and colleagues (Dekosky, Heilman, Bowers, & Valenstein, 1980; Heilman, Scholes, & Watson, 1975; Tucker, Watson, & Heilman, 1977) have demonstrated that patients with unilateral right-side damage in temporoparietal areas and who present left unilateral neglect are deficient in recognizing or identifying emotions conveyed in human voices or faces. In the Heilman *et al.* (1975) study such patients performed at chance level in recognizing affects conveyed in voices and the deficit was termed "auditory affective agnosia." Tucker *et al.* (1977) demonstrated that when such patients were instructed to convey voluntarily affect in their own voices, judges were at chance level in recognizing the emotions that were to be conveyed. Two patients with right-side supra-Sylvian infarctions (tissue death due to inadequate blood flow in areas above the Sylvian fissure) were recently described (Ross & Mesulam, 1979) as having lost the ability to express affect both in speech and facially, despite intact experiences of mood. Studies of normal, neurologically intact subjects have also highlighted right-hemisphere superiority in the recognition of emotion. Left-sensory-field advantages in both dichotic tasks (e.g., Carmon & Nachson, 1973; Haggard & Parkinson, 1971; King & Kimura, 1972) and tachistoscopic-viewing tasks (e.g., Ley & Bryden, 1979; Suberi & McKeever, 1977) have been found consistently for the recognition of emotion.

We suggest that both the recognition and voluntary expression of affect are dependent on a lateralized template-matching procedure. To recognize or identify affect on the basis of paralinguistic cues, multimodal sensory inputs (e.g., auditory, visual) may be matched against internal representations or templates of particular emotions (e.g., happiness, fear). In the voluntary production of emotion, these templates must be matched with or translated into motor codes to convey particular facial or vocal affective expressions. The right side of the brain appears to be superior in the recognition and voluntary production of emotional expressions either because of lateralization in the loci of template storage, lateralization in characteristics of the templates, and/or because of lateralization in the cognitive processes necessary to carry out the matching procedures.

This dimension of lateralization may not only underlie facial asymmetry in the voluntary expression of emotion, but could also be related to facial asymmetry in motility of muscular (nonemotional) movement. We noted that Chaurasia and Goswami (1975) observed notably greater dexterity of facial movement on opposite sides of the face in left- and right-handers. This pattern has not been obtained in studies of asymmetry for voluntary emotional expression, where left-handers as a group have shown either no consistent asymmetry (Rubin & Rubin, 1980) or weaker consistent asymmetries in the same direction as right-handers (Borod & Caron, 1980; Borod *et al.*, 1981; Campbell, 1979b). In the area of cognitive lateralization, left-handers typically display either no consistent asymmetries or patterns similar to right-handers (e.g., Hécaen & Albert, 1978). Findings of consistent lateral behavior in left-handers that is opposite in direction to and more consistent than the right-handers' pattern is highly unusual. Although it would appear that the asymmetry in movement motility observed by Chaurasia and Goswami (1975) is at least partially independent of voluntary emotional expressive asymmetry, a proviso should be added. Aside from using a flawed method, Chaurasia and Goswami examined asymmetry for requested unilateral movements. Borod *et al.* (1981) found that asymmetry for their one requested unilateral emotional expression (i.e., a sneer) loaded on a distinct factor than that of asymmetry for eight bilateral emotional expressions. Voluntary unilateral expressions may require not only movement on one side of the face, but also voluntary inhibition of the contralateral side, involving a different set of neural processes. Asymmetry in motility for nonemotional bilateral facial movements (e.g., suck in the cheeks and pucker the lips) has not been examined. To the extent that the production of such bilateral nonemotional movements also requires the proposed template-matching procedure, we would expect these movements to manifest the same pattern of asymmetry as in voluntary emotional expression.

We hypothesized that patterns of facial asymmetry differ for some voluntary and spontaneous expressions of emotion. We proposed that to the extent that there is predominantly contralateral neural control of spontaneous emotional expression, in right-handers negative affect is more intensely expressed on the left side and positive affect on the right side. The qualification concerning lateralization in neural control is critical, since little is known about the neural mechanisms regulating spontaneous expression, and unless there is lateralization in pathways from higher centers to the nuclei of the facial nerve, consistent facial asymmetry would not be expected for spontaneous expression. It is curious that the one recent study (Ekman *et al.*, 1981) of spontaneous expressive asymmetry did not raise this issue.

The available evidence is suggestive that some degree of lateralization characterizes neural control of facial spontaneous expression (e.g., Remillard *et al.*, 1977) and that this control is primarily contralaterally mediated. Further, we indicated that there are hints in the literature supportive of our hypothesis that positive and negative emotions differ in the sides of the face on which they are most intensely expressed. Wolff's (1943) characterization of the affective characteristics of the sides of the face, Lynn and Lynn's (1943) findings that asymmetry in spontaneous right-sided smiles was of greater magnitude than in left-sided smiles and that the former group were also more extreme smiles, and the Schwartz *et al.* (1979) EMG data all point in this direction. Nonetheless, the data on spontaneous expression are far from complete and our hypothesis is offered as just that—a hypothesis.

The suggestion that different patterns of asymmetry obtain with voluntary and spontaneous expression reflects a belief that distinct neuropsychological processes subserve their production. A number of spontaneous emotional expressions are observed from birth or very early in development (e.g., Oster, 1978). Spontaneous and integrated emotional expressions such as laughing and crying may be released by irritative or destructive lesions (e.g., Sackeim et al., 1982). At least some expressions are observed in other primates (e.g., Darwin, 1872/1955; Redican, 1975), appear to be universal across human cultures (Ekman, 1972; Ekman & Friesen, 1971), and are manifested to some degree by the congenitally blind (e.g., Charlesworth & Kreutzer, 1973). These facts suggest that at least some spontaneous emotional expressions are hardwired, innate action patterns.

Recent work has shown that the manifestation of positive or negative spontaneous emotional expressions as a consequence of brain insult is determined by the predominant side of damage (see Sackeim & Weber, 1982, for a review). Uncontrollable outbursts of laughing (pathological laughing) are associated with predominantly right-side destructive (non-epileptogenic) lesions, whereas uncontrollable crying (pathological crying) is linked with predominantly left-side destructive lesions (Sackeim et al., 1982). Similar associations have been reported for the effects of unilateral electroconvulsive therapy (ECT) on emotional expression. In the phase immediately following unconsciousness, patients who receive unilateral ECT manifest greater relative ipsilateral suppression of brain activity, as indexed by slowing in the EEG and side-appropriate cognitive deficits (e.g., dysphasia with left ECT) (e.g., d'Elia, Lorentzson, Raotma, & Widepalm, 1976; d'Elia & Perris, 1970; Warrington & Pratt, 1973). Deglin (1973), using a within-patient design, reported a change toward facial expressions of happiness after right ECT and toward negative or depressed facial expression following left ECT.

These associations are also consistent with the mood changes associated with unilateral destructive lesions. Right-side damage is associated with a euphoric-indifference reaction, while a dysphoric reaction is more common after left-side insult (e.g., Gainotti, 1972; Hommes, 1965). Sackeim et al. (1982) suggested that manifestation of these expressive and mood changes associated with unilateral destructive insult was most often a consequence of disinhibition of affective centers on the contralateral side of the brain. This view was supported by findings concerning side of epileptic foci in patients presenting outbursts of uncontrollable laughing during seizures (ictal outbursts of laughing or gelastic epilepsy). Ictal manifestations have consistently been related to hyperexcitability in regions comprising epileptogenic neuronal aggregates. Foci in cases of gelastic epilepsy were more than twice as likely to be left-sided as right-sided. This pattern of findings would suggest that excitation or release in the left side of the brain results in certain spontaneous positive emotional displays, whereas excitation or release in the right side is associated with certain spontaneous negative displays.

Given these findings, lateralization of brain function would seem to play a different role in spontaneous and voluntary expression. In the case of spontaneous expression, patterns of facial asymmetry should be determined by the type of affect expressed, with the asymmetry reflecting the functional differences between the sides of the brain in subserving particular hardwired action patterns and mood states. In contrast, we suggested that facial asymmetry for voluntary emotional expression is independent of the affect conveyed and probably reflects functional asymmetry in template matching. The latter asymmetry may be cognitively based, itself a product of right-hemispheric superiority in nonsequential, synthetic, and/or multimodal processing.

Earlier we suggested that asymmetry in hemispheric activation and in relatively static facial contours such as laugh lines and other wrinkles are likely to be critical in determining asymmetry of the resting face. Admittedly, suggesting simply that a dimension of hemispheric activation is of importance leaves much unanswered. The expressive features of the face at rest (i.e., when there is minimal muscular movement) may reflect an admixture of voluntary and spontaneous control of movement, which in turn is produced by balance between inhibitory and excitatory neural processes. Less is known about the tonic inhibition of facial expression than about phasic release. In suggesting that predominantly unilateral destructive lesions disinhibit expressive displays and mood states primarily subserved by the contralateral side of the brain, Sackeim *et al.* (1982) argued that in normal individuals there are inhibitory relations between each side of the brain and the contralateral affective centers. The absence of a spontaneous smiling expression may be due, therefore, to relative inactivation in regions whose excitation is associated with smiling and/or to relative overactivation of presumably contralateral centers that normally inhibit this expression. Further, it is not known whether the pathways projecting from spontaneous inhibitory networks to the nuclei of the facial nerve are crossed, ipsilateral, or are not lateralized. The particular brain regions subserving the release or inhibition of expressive displays are also unknown, for the most part. It would seem then that while findings of asymmetry in the emotional expression of the resting face may implicate lateralized neural processes, the nature of these processes is likely to be at issue for some time to come.

CONCLUDING REMARKS

The investigation of facial asymmetry in the expression of emotion is of consequence not only because it provides inroads to examine neural regulation of affect. The face is a prime source in the nonverbal communication of emotion. We have seen that signals presented in the face may display complex lateralized disparities. It is also the case that perceivers are biased in weighting information more from one side of the face than the other. The demonstration of both consistent facial asymmetry in emotional expression and perceiver biases in processing human faces raises a special set of issues. The very fact that naive observers can consistently weight information from one side of the face, when all extrafacial asymmetries have been removed and facial expression is neutral, indicates that even in such circumstances there is considerable asymmetry in facial features.

At present it is not known whether and to what extent familiarity with faces influences perceiver biases. Neuropsychological data indicate that deficits in memory for familiar faces (prosopagnosia) and in memory for unfamiliar faces are dissociable disorders, probably reflecting disruption of different neuropsychological processes (e.g., Benton, 1980). It has been shown, however, that people familiar with an individual prefer original-orientation photographs of the person, whereas people prefer reverse-orientation photographs of themselves (Mita, Dermer, & Knight, 1977). This effect was attributed to preference for the orientation to which individuals are most accustomed. We have asked subjects to choose whether original- or reverse-orientation full faces and whether left and right composites look more like themselves. Mirror-orientation full faces and left composites were both chosen significantly more frequently. Importantly, there was a significant association between choice of composite and choice of full orientation. Subjects who chose reverse-orientation full faces were also likely to select left composites. This would suggest that perceiver biases influence visual impressions of ourselves. We mostly see ourselves mirror-reverse. The standard perceiver bias to view the side to the perceiver's left as more like the full face appears to result in greater salience of the left facial side in self-impressions. Interestingly, acquaintances and possibly friends should be more likely to have their impressions of us weighted by the opposite side of the face.

We have seen that in voluntary displays of emotion the left side of the face is most often more intense. We hypothesized that this effect is maintained for spontaneous negative displays and may reverse for spontaneous positive displays. Patterns of perceiver bias, coupled with these patterns of facial asymmetry, may lead to characteristic distortions in the communication of emotion. The faces that we perceive, other than our own, are almost always in original orientation. Our data suggest that at least for negative affects most individuals weight the right side of the unfamiliar face they are viewing when identifying type of emotion and assessing emotional intensity. This is the side of the face that for negative affect, we believe, is less intense in expression. Our initial data also indicate that most individuals weight the left side of the face when assessing intensity of happy expressions. For spontaneous displays, this is also the side we hypothesize to be less intense. Individuals with reverse direction of perceiver bias for judgments of facial similarity also appear to show reverse patterns in judgments of emotionality. This would suggest that individuals with standard perceiver bias may observe consistently less intensity in the emotional displays of others compared to people with reverse biases. One wonders whether this difference has an impact on individual differences in personality and, in particular, on sensitivity to nonverbal cues and beliefs about the emotionality of others.

Finally, we may speculate about the relations between individual patterns of facial asymmetry and of perceiver bias. Consider the situation of the therapist and patient, or husband and wife, face to face, where one may typically express emotion most on the side of the face that is less salient according to the bias of the other. We could expect that nonverbal communication of affect would be subject to more missed cues and misinterpretation than in contexts where expressive asymmetry and direction of bias are harmonious.

ACKNOWLEDGMENTS

The research reported here was supported in part by NIMH Grants MH 34494 and MH 35636, by a grant from the Spencer Foundation, and by a grant from the Research Challenge Fund of New York University. We thank our collaborators, Dennis Grega, Sigmund Hough, Evelyn Sanchez, and Andrew Weiman, for contributing some of the findings reported here. We also thank Betty Brewer, Shirley Chalke, Maureen Kanzler, and Sara Weber for comments and editorial assistance.

REFERENCES

Ahern, G. L., & Schwartz, G. E.   Differential lateralization for positive versus negative emotion. *Neuropsychologia*, 1979, *17*, 693–698.

Baldwin, M., Frost, L. L., Wood, C. D.   Investigation of the primate amygdala: Movements of the face and jaws. 2. Effect of selective cortical ablation. *Neurology*, 1956, *6*, 288–293.

Benton, A. L.   The neuropsychology of facial recognition. *American Psychologist*, 1980, *35*, 176–186.

Birdwhistell, R. L.   *Kinesics and context.* Philadelphia: University of Pennsylvania Press, 1970.

Borod, J. C., & Caron, H. S.   *Facial asymmetry during emotional experience.* Paper presented at the meeting of the International Neuropsychology Society, New York, 1979.

Borod, J., & Caron, H.   Facedness and emotion related to lateral dominance, sex, and expression type. *Neuropsychologia*, 1980, *18*, 237–242.

Borod, J., Caron, H., & Koff, E.   Asymmetry of facial expression related to handedness, footedness, and eyedness: A quantitative study. *Cortex*, 1981, *17*, 381–390.

Broadbent, B. H.   A new x-ray technique and its application to orthodontia. *Angle Orthodontist*, 1931, *1*, 45–66.

Bryden, M. P.   Perceptual asymmetry in vision: Relation to handedness, eyedness and speech lateralization. *Cortex*, 1973, *9*, 419–435.

Burke, P. H.   Stereophotogrammetric measurement of normal facial asymmetry in children. *Human Biology,* 1971, *43,* 536–548.

Butler, S. R., & Glass, A.   EEG correlates of cerebral dominance. In A. H. Rissen & R. F. Thompson (Eds.), *Advances in psychobiology* (Vol. 3). New York: Wiley, 1976.

Campbell, R.   Asymmetries in interpreting and expressing a posed facial expression. *Cortex,* 1978, *14,* 327–342.

Campbell, R.   *Cerebral asymmetries in looking at faces and in facial movements.* Unpublished doctoral dissertation, University of London, 1979.(a)

Campbell, R.   Left-handers' smiles: Asymmetries in the projection of a posed expression. *Cortex,* 1979, *15,* 571–579. (b)

Carmon, A., & Nachson, I.   Ear asymmetry in perception of emotional nonverbal stimuli. *Acta Psychologica,* 1973, *37,* 351–357.

Charlesworth, W. R., & Kreutzer, M. A.   Facial expression of infants and children. In P. Ekman (Ed.), *Darwin and facial expression.* New York: Academic, 1973.

Chaurasia, B. D., & Goswami, H. K.   Functional asymmetry in the face. *Acta Anatomica,* 1975, *91,* 154–160.

Cheney, E. A.   The influence of dentofacial asymmetries upon treatment procedures. *American Journal of Orthodontics,* 1952, *38,* 934–945.

Crosby, E. C., & DeJonge, B. R.   Experimental and clinical studies of the central connections and central relations of the facial nerve. *Annals of Otology, Rhinology, & Laryngology,* 1963, *72,* 735–755.

Daly, D. D., & Mulder, D. W.   Gelastic epilepsy. *Neurology,* 1957, *7,* 189–192.

Darwin, C.   *The expression of emotion in man and animals.* New York: Philosophical Library, 1955. (Originally published, 1872.)

Davidson, R. J., Schwartz, G. E., Saron, C., Bennett, J., & Goleman, D.   Frontal versus parietal EEG asymmetry during positive and negative affect. *Psychophysiology,* 1979, *16,* 202–203.

Davison, C., & Kelman, H.   Pathological laughing and crying. *Archives of Neurology and Psychiatry,* 1939, *42,* 595–643.

Deglin, V. L.   A clinical study of unilateral electroconvulsive seizures. *Zhurnal Nevropatologii i Psikhiatrii,* 1973, *73,* 1609–1621. (Russian)

DeJonge, B. R., & Crosby, E. C.   The supplementary motor function of the temporal lobe. *Transactions of the American Neurological Association,* 1960, 171–176.

Dekosky, S. T., Heilman, K. M., Bowers, D., & Valenstein, E.   Recognition and discrimination of emotional faces and pictures. *Brain and Language,* 1980, *9,* 206–214.

Delgado, J. M. R.   Modulation of Emotions by Cerebral Radio Stimulation. In P. Black (Ed.), *Physiological correlates of emotions.* New York: Academic, 1970.

d'Elia, G., Lorentzson, S., Raotma, H., & Widepalm, K.   Comparison of unilateral dominant and non-dominant ECT on verbal and non-verbal memory. *Acta Psychiatrica Scandinavica,* 1976, *53,* 85–94.

d'Elia, G., & Perris, C.   Comparison of electroconvulsive therapy with unilateral and bilateral stimulation: I. Seizure and past-seizure electroencephalographic pattern. *Acta Psychiatrica Scandinavica,* 1970, *Suppl. 215,* 9–29.

Diamond, C., & Frew, I.   *The facial nerve.* New York: Oxford University Press, 1979.

Dyken, P., & Miller, M. D.   *Facial features of neurologic syndromes.* St. Louis: Mosby, 1980.

Ehrlichman, H., & Weinberger, A.   Lateral eye movements and hemispheric asymmetry: A critical review. *Psychological Bulletin,* 1978, *85,* 1080–1101.

Ekman, P.   Universals and cultural differences in facial expressions of emotion. In J. Cole (Ed.), *Nebraska Symposium on Motivation, 1971.* Lincoln: University of Nebraska Press, 1972.

Ekman, P.   Asymmetry in facial expression. *Science,* 1980, *209,* 833–834.

Ekman, P., & Friesen, W. V.   Constants across cultures in the face and emotion. *Journal of Personality and Social Psychology,* 1971, *17,* 124–129.

Ekman, P., & Friesen, W. V.   Unmasking the face. Englewood Cliffs, N.J.: Prentice-Hall, 1975.

Ekman, P., & Friesen, W. V. *Pictures of facial affect.* Palo Alto, Calif.: Consulting Psychologists Press, 1976.

Ekman, P., Friesen, W. V., & Ancoli, S. Facial signs of emotional experience. *Journal of Personality and Social Psychology*, 1980, *39*, 1125–1134.

Ekman, P., Hager, C. J., & Friesen, W. V. The symmetry of emotional and deliberate facial actions. *Psychophysiology*, 1981, *18*, 101–106.

Ekman, P., & Oster, H. Facial expressions of emotion. *Annual Review of Psychology*, 1979, *30*, 527–554.

Figalova, P. Asymmetry of the face. *Anthropologie (Paris)*, 1969, *7*, 31–34.

Foerster, O. The cerebral cortex in man. *Lancet*, 1931, *2*, 309–312.

Frontera, J. G. Preliminary report on the results of electrical stimulation of the cortex of the Island of Reil in the brain of the monkey (*Macaca mulatta*). *Journal of Comparative Neurology*, 1956, *105*, 365–394.

Gainotti, G. Emotional behavior and hemisphere side of the lesion. *Cortex*, 1972, *8*, 41–55.

Gilbert, C., & Bakan, P. Visual asymmetry in perception of faces. *Neuropsychologia*, 1973, *11*, 355–362.

Gottlieb, G., & Wilson, I. Cerebral dominance: Temporary disruption of verbal memory by unilateral electroconvulsive shock therapy. *Journal of Comparative and Physiological Psychology*, 1965, *60*, 368–372.

Grossman, S. P. Modification of emotional behavior by intracranial administration of chemicals. In P. Black (Ed.), *Physiological correlates of emotions.* New York: Academic, 1970.

Gur, R. C., & Reivich, M. Cognitive tasks effects on hemispheric blood flow in humans: Evidence for individual differences in hemispheric activation. *Brain and Language*, 1980, *9*, 78–92.

Gur, R. E., & Gur, R. C. Correlates of conjugate lateral eye movements in man. In S. Harnad, R. W. Doty, L. Goldstein, J. Jaynes, & G. Krauthamer (Eds.), *Lateralization in the nervous system.* New York: Academic, 1977.

Haga, M., Ukiya, M., Koshihara, Y., & Ota, Y. Stereophotogrammetric study of the face. *Bulletin of the Tokyo Dental College*, 1964, *5*, 10–24.

Haggard, M. P., & Parkinson, A. M. Stimulus and task factors as determinants of ear advantages. *Quarterly Journal of Experimental Psychology*, 1971, *23*, 166–177.

Harrower, G. A biometric study of one hundred and ten Asiatic mandibles. *Biometrika*, 1928, *20*, 279–293. (a)

Harrower, G. A study of the crania of the Hylam Chinese. *Biometrika*, 1928, *20*, 245–278. (b)

Harvold, E. The asymmetries of the upper facial skeleton and their morphological significance. *Transactions of the European Orthodontics Society*, 1951, 63–39.

Harvold, E. Cleft lip and palate: Morphologic studies of the facial skeleton. *American Journal of Orthodontics*, 1954, *40*, 493–506.

Hausman, L. *Clinical neuroanatomy, neurophysiology and neurology.* Springfield, Ill.: Charles C Thomas, 1958.

Hécaen, H., & Albert, M. L. *Human neuropsychology.* New York: Wiley, 1978.

Heilman, K. M., Scholes, R., & Watson, R. T. Auditory affective agnosia. *Journal of Neurology, Neurosurgery, and Psychiatry*, 1975, *38*, 69–72.

Heller, W., & Levy, J. Perception and expression of emotion in right-handers and left-handers. *Neuropsychologia*, 1981, *19*, 263–272.

Hommes, O. R. Stemminsanomalien als neurologisch symptoom. *Nederlands Tijdschrift voor Geneeskunde*, 1965, *109*, 588–589. (Dutch)

Izard, C. E. *Patterns of emotion.* New York: Academic, 1977.

Karch, G. R., & Grant, C. W. Asymmetry in perception of the sides of the human face. *Perceptual and Motor Skills*, 1978, *47*, 727–734.

Kimura, D. Manual activity in right-handers associated with speaking. *Neuropsychologia*, 1973, *11*, 45–56.

King, F. L., & Kimura, D.   Left-ear superiority in dichotic perception of vocal sounds. *Canadian Journal of Psychology*, 1972, *26*, 111–116.

Kinsbourne, M.   Eye and head turning indicates cerebral lateralization. *Science*, 1972, *176*, 539–545.

Kuypers, H. G. J. M.   Corticobulbar connexions to the pons and lower brain-stem in man. *Brain*, 1958, *81*, 364–388.

Kwint, L.   Ontogeny of motility of the face. *Child Development*, 1934, *5*, 1–12.

LeMay, M.   Asymmetries of the skull and handedness. *Journal of the Neurological Sciences*, 1977, *32*, 243–253.

Letzer, G. M., & Kronman, J. H.   A posteroanterior cephalometric evaluation of craniofacial asymmetry. *Angle Orthodontist*, 1967, *37*, 205–211.

Levy, J.   Lateral dominance and aesthetic preference. *Neuropsychologia*, 1976, *14*, 431–445.

Ley, R. G., & Bryden, M. P.   Hemispheric differences in processing emotions and faces. *Brain and Language*, 1979, *7*, 127–139.

Lindzey, G., Prince, B., & Wright, H. K. A.   A study of facial asymmetry. *Journal of Personality*, 1952, *21*, 68–84.

Lynn, J. G., & Lynn, D. R.   Face-hand laterality in relation to personality. *Journal of Abnormal and Social Psychology*, 1938, *33*, 291–322.

Lynn, J. G., & Lynn, D. R.   Smile and hand dominance in relation to basic modes of adaptation. *Journal of Abnormal and Social Psychology*, 1943, *38*, 250–276.

McCurdy, H. G.   Experimental notes on the asymmetry of the human face. *Journal of Abnormal and Social Psychology*, 1949, *44*, 553–555.

Mita, T. H., Dermer, M., & Knight, J.   Reversed facial images and the mere-exposure hypothesis. *Journal of Personality and Social Psychology*, 1977, *35*, 397–601.

Monrad-Krohn, G. H.   On the dissociation of voluntary and emotional innervations in facial paresis of central origin. *Brain*, 1924, *47*, 22–45.

Moscovitch, M., & Olds, J.   *Asymmetries in spontaneous facial expressions and their possible relation to hemispheric specialization.* Paper presented to the International Neuropsychological Society, Amsterdam, 1979.

Moscovitch, M., Strauss, E., & Olds, J.   *Children's production of facial expressions.* Paper presented at the annual meeting of the American Psychological Association, Montreal, 1980.

Mulick, J. F.   An investigation of craniofacial asymmetry using the serial twin-study method. *American Journal of Orthodontics*, 1965, *51*, 112–129.

Nelson, C. A., & Horowitz, F. D.   Asymmetry in facial expression. *Science*, 1980, *209*, 834.

Nelson, T., & MacDonald, G.   Lateral organization, perceived depth and title preference in pictures. *Perceptual and Motor Skills*, 1971, *33*, 983–986.

Oliveau, D., & Willmuth, R.   Facial muscle electromyography in depressed and nondepressed hospitalized subjects: A partial replication. *American Journal of Psychiatry*, 1979, *136*, 548–550.

Oster, H.   Facial expression and affect development. In M. Lewis & L. A. Rosenblum (Eds.), *The development of affect*. New York: Plenum, 1978.

Pearson, K., & Woo, T. L.   Further investigation of the morphometric characters of the human skull. *Biometrika*, 1935, *27*, 424–465.

Peele, T. L.   *The neuroanatomic basis for clinical neurology*. New York: McGraw-Hill, 1961.

Penfield, W., & Rasmussen, T.   *The cerebral cortex of man: A clinical study of localization of function.* New York: Macmillan, 1950.

Posen, A. L.   Vertical height of the body of the mandible and the occlusal level of the teeth in individuals with cleft and non-cleft palates. *Journal of the Canadian Dental Association*, 1958, *24*, 211–217.

Rappoport, M., & Friendly, M.   *Facial asymmetry in emotion: Observer and stimulus differences.* Paper presented at the annual meeting of the Canadian Psychological Association, Ottawa, 1978.

Redican, W. K.   Facial expressions in nonhuman primates. In L. A. Rosenblum (Ed.), *Primate behavior* (Vol. 4). New York: Academic, 1975.

Remillard, G. M., Andermann, F., Rhi-Sausi, A., & Robbins, N. M.   Facial asymmetry in patients with temporal lobe epilepsy. *Neurology*, 1977, 27, 109–114.

Ross, E. D., & Mesulam, M.-M.   Dominant language functions of the right hemisphere? Prosody and emotional gesturing. *Archives of Neurology*, 1979, 36, 144–148.

Rubin, D. A., & Rubin, R. T.   Differences in asymmetry of facial expression between left- and right-handed children. *Neuropsychologia*, 1980, 18, 373–377.

Sackeim, H. A., Greenberg, M. C., Weiman, A. L., Gur, R. C., Hungerbuhler, J. P., & Geschwind, N.   Hemispheric asymmetry in the expression of positive and negative emotions: Neurologic evidence. *Archives of Neurology*, 1982, 39, 210–218.

Sackeim, H. A., & Gur, R. C.   Lateral asymmetry in intensity of emotional expression. *Neuropsychologia*, 1978, 16, 473–481.

Sackeim, H. A., & Gur, R. C.   Asymmetry in facial expression. *Science*, 1980, 209, 834–836.

Sackeim, H. A., Gur, R. C., & Saucy, M. C.   Emotions are expressed more intensely on the left side of the face. *Science*, 1978, 202, 434–436.

Sackeim, H. A., & Weber, S.   Functional brain asymmetry in the regulation of emotion: Implications for bodily manifestations of stress. In L. Goldberger (Ed.), *Handbook of stress*. New York: Macmillan, 1982.

Sackeim, H. A., & Weiman, A. L.   *Asymmetry of the resting face: Size, expression, and psychopathology.* Manuscript in preparation.

Schwartz, G. E., Ahern, G. L., & Brown, S.   Lateralized facial muscle response to positive and negative emotional stimuli. *Psychophysiology*, 1979, 16, 561–571.

Schwartz, G. E., Fair, P. L., Salt, P., Mandel, M. R., & Klerman, G. L.   Facial muscle patterning to affective imagery in depressed and nondepressed subjects. *Science*, 1976, 192, 489–491.

Seinen, M., & van der Werff, J. J.   The perception of asymmetry in the face. *Netherlands Journal of Psychology*, 1969, 24, 551–558.

Shah, S. M., & Joshi, M. R.   An assessment of asymmetry in the normal craniofacial complex. *Angle Orthodontist*, 1978, 48, 141–148.

Shipman, W. G., Heath, H. A., & Oken, D.   Response specificity among muscular and autonomic variables. *Archives of General Psychiatry*, 1970, 23, 369–374.

Showers, M. H. C.   The cingulate gyrus: Additional motor area and cortical autonomic regulator. *Journal of Comparative Neurology*, 1959, 112, 231–301.

Smith, R. P.   Frontalis muscle tension and personality. *Psychophysiology*, 1973, 10, 311–312.

Suberi, M., & McKeever, W. F.   Differential right hemispheric memory storage of emotional and non-emotional faces. *Neuropsychologia*, 1977, 15, 757–768.

Sutton, P. R. N.   Handedness and facial asymmetry: Lateral position of the nose in two racial groups. *Nature*, 1963, 198, 909.

Sutton, P. R. N.   Lateral facial asymmetry: Methods of assessment. *Angle Orthodontist*, 1968, 38, 82–92.

Sutton, P. R. N.   Bizygomatic diameter: The thickness of the soft tissues over the zygions. *American Journal of Physical Anthropology*, 1969, 30, 303–310.

Tucker, D. M.   Lateral brain function, emotion, and conceptualization. *Psychological Bulletin*, 1981, 89, 19–46.

Tucker, D. M., Roth, R. S., Arneson, B. A., & Buckingham, V.   Right hemisphere activation during stress. *Neuropsychologia*, 1977, 15, 697–700.

Tucker, D. M., Stenslie, C. E., Roth, R. S., & Shearer, S. L.   Right frontal lobe activation and right hemisphere performance. *Archives of General Psychiatry*, 1981, 38, 169–174.

Tucker, D. M., Watson, R. T., & Heilman, K. M.   Discrimination and evocation of affectively intoned speech in patients with right parietal disease. *Neurology*, 1977, 27, 947–950.

Vig, P. S., & Hewitt, A. B.   Asymmetry of the human facial skeleton. *Angle Orthodontist*, 1974, 45, 125–129.

Warrington, E. K., & Pratt, R. T. C.   Language laterality in left-handers assessed by unilateral E.C.T. *Neuropsychologia*, 1973, *11*, 423–428.
Wolff, W.   The experimental study of forms of expression. *Character and Personality*, 1933, *2*, 168–176.
Wolff, W.   *The expression of personality.* New York: Harper & Row, 1943.
Woo, T. L.   On the asymmetry of the human skull. *Biometrika*, 1931, *22*, 324–352.
Woo, T. L.   A biometric study of the human malar bone. *Biometrika*, 1937, *29*, 113–123.

CHAPTER 12

The Perceptual–Motor
Theory of Emotion

Howard Leventhal
University of Wisconsin–Madison
Peter A. Mosbach
University of Wisconsin–Madison

INTRODUCTION

In his classic work, *Social Psychology*, William McDougall states that motives and emotions are "the mental forces, the sources of energy, which set the ends and sustain the course of all human activity—of which forces the intellectual processes are but the servants, instruments, or means—that must be clearly defined, and whose history in the race and in the individual must be made clear before the social sciences can build upon a firm psychological foundation" (see McDougall, 1928, p. 3). McDougall was convinced that psychology was the basic science among the social sciences and that emotion and motivation were the basic explanatory concepts of psychology. In McDougall's eyes, emotion and motivation were the central topics for psychological inquiry. Emotion was the motor and the director that pushed a passive sensory–motor apparatus toward specific behavioral ends.

Although McDougall was convinced of the importance of emotion, its study has clearly been of secondary importance in psychology. There are signs that this is changing. For example, the recent Carnegie-Mellon Symposium on Cognition and Emotion (Clark & Fiske, 1982) and this volume bring together research papers on emotion by investigators from virtually every area of contemporary psychology. In keeping with this new focus, the goal of this chapter is to present an update of our formulation of a comprehensive theory of emotional processes (Leventhal, 1980). This is no simple task. The word "emotion" refers to a wide variety of behaviors, subjective, expressive (facial, postural) and autonomic, and any theory that tries to account for these behaviors will necessarily be complex. We believe that such a theory must conceptualize emotion as the product of a multi-component, hierarchical set of mediating mechanisms that function as a unified system. To understand the mechanisms and their components, it will be necessary to understand their interaction in the creation of emotional behaviors. Emotion cannot be understood by theories that propose a single hypothesis or a single mechanism.

To achieve our objectives, we have divided our chapter into three main sections. The first section summarizes two major barriers to the study of emotion. These are (1) the nature of emotional phenomena, and (2) the tendency to explain emotional phenomena with nonemotional, rationalist concepts. The second section presents an overview of our perceptual–motor theory of emotion. In this model, emotions are constructed by a hierarchical processing system which is parallel to and partially independent of nonemotional (perceptual and cognitive) processes. In the third section we examine how the simultaneous activity and interactions between levels in the hierarchy generate a number of relevant outcomes that have been documented by a variety of investigators.

BARRIERS TO THE STUDY OF EMOTION

There appear to be two types of barriers to the study of emotion: (1) the nature of emotional phenomena, and (2) competition from nonemotional (cognitive) concepts. With respect to the nature of the phenomenon, three factors stand out. First, emotional experience is private, and like all private experience, is difficult to study. Second, emotion refers to operations at the neurophysiological, behavioral, and subjective levels (Izard, 1971; Lang, 1977; Tomkins, 1962). This adds a significant degree of complexity as three types of descriptive language and theory are involved in their study. Finally, emotions are unstable states of the organism, adding further to the difficulty of their study.

We do not believe that the three factors cited above are sufficient to account for the absence of more intensive study of emotion. Perceptions are like emotions in all these respects: they are private, involve multiple levels of function, and fluctuate rapidly with stimulus change. Konorski (1967) has also recognized this similarity. Emotions differ from perceptions with respect to their ties to stimuli. The stimuli that give rise to the perception of objects such as chairs, elephants, tables, horses, and cars are likely to do so for all perceivers. The same stimuli that give rise to emotions such as fear, joy, anger, and sadness are likely to differ across individuals and to differ for the same individuals at different times. There is more "noise" in the processing of emotional events. "Noise," however, can be dealt with by statistical measures such as increases in sample size. Once this is done, there is no reason why the study of emotion should not proceed as has the study of perception.

The emotion literature suggests that to a great degree this has happened. For example, studies show a substantial degree of consistency across cultures in the judgment of emotion from facial expressions (Ekman,

Friesen, & Ellsworth, 1972; Izard, 1971, 1977; Osgood, 1966; Woodworth & Schlosberg, 1954) and tones of voice (Davitz, 1970). There is also consistency in people's judgments of what emotion is likely to appear in simple social situations when the judges have information about the causes, consequences, and controllability of actions in these situations (Weiner, 1981). Combinations of expressive and social cues (Frijda, 1969) also lead to consistent judgments. These findings are matched by data showing a high degree of consistency in the way people encode or express emotion (Ekman *et al.*, 1972; Izard, 1971, 1977; Leventhal & Sharpe, 1965; Tomkins, 1962). Thus, although the study of emotion has not been on center stage, there is a growing data base from which to begin constructing a theory of emotional processing.

The second type of barrier is the use of nonemotional, rationalistic or cognitive concepts to account for emotional phenomena (Cofer, 1972). This is less easily dealt with. There is a strong and unfortunate tendency to use terms such as "evaluation," "preference," and "attitude," all of which imply stable appraisals of objects, as synonyms for emotion (see Clark & Fiske, 1982). Simon (1982) has suggested that many of the properties of emotion, such as the intensity of feeling, the variability, and the expressive component, are absent from these evaluative, rationalistic concepts. We agree. These terms refer to relatively stable memories of appraisals of objects which serve as anchors or stabilizers of a person's emotional reactions (Leventhal, 1980). Emotions, by contrast, are in constant flux and need not be consistent with evaluations. A father may be angry with his daughter one moment and joyful about her accomplishments the next, without any substantial change in his attitude toward her. He knows he loves her and knows she is a central figure in his life. If she were less important, we would expect less varied and less intense reactions to her behaviors. Therefore, the greater stability of preferences or attitudes is one important attribute differentiating them from emotions. The daughter, her behavior, and her reactions to her father are complex and multifaceted. They represent a domain of "objects" in contrast to being a "single" attitude object (Fishbein & Ajzen, 1974).

The separation of emotion and attitude raises the important question of when and how emotional experiences change evaluations or attitudes. Emotional reactions to an object may vary widely. It is unreasonable to assume that the parent in our example would evaluate his daughter by simply averaging these emotional responses. The child and his or her relationship to the parent forms a domain of meaning, or a set of differentiated contents and reactions which can arouse quite different (and intense) emotional reactions at different times. A wide range of questions respecting attribution, weighting, and so on, need to be addressed in order to understand how attitudes toward a complex object, such as a child, are altered when emotion is experienced in relation to this knowledge domain.

Differences in rate of change are only one of the factors that separate attitudes and preferences from emotions. A more significant difference is that attitudes and preferences are appraisals of objects and events, while emotions are ongoing appraisals of the state of the organism. Emotions reflect or meter the moment-by-moment states of the organism. When I tell you I am tired, I am reporting to you about my state of energy (that my body machinery has limited energy for work). If I tell you that I am distressed and feeling strained, I am telling you that my body machinery is working at its limit and that I am experiencing excessive pressure to perform. States such as pain–distress, fatigue–tiredness, anger–irritability, and nausea–disgust (Nowlis, 1965) are examples of this internal, "metering" function of emotion. The individual's emotional state also varies with moment-to-moment changes in the environment. Emotions tell us whether situations are making threatening, fatiguing, or joy-inducing demands on our system. Labels such as fear, sexual arousal, humor, interest, and depression can refer to emotions where the body state is closely linked to external realities (Janis & Leventhal, 1965). Therefore, the emotional state is a meter that can be accessed by both internal and external cues.

The perceptive reader may ask: "How do emotions compare with drives such as hunger and thirst, or with internal states such as fatigue and illness?" The answer is that they all share a "metering" function. Illness, for example, is a readout of one's body state, and is often confused with and combined with emotional experience (Leventhal, 1982; Mechanic & Volkart, 1961; Zola, 1973). Drives share this readout function with emotions. Tomkins (1962) argues that internal needs such as hunger, thirst, and sexual desires are experienced as drives because the need signal they communicate is coupled with an emotional response. Drives may be integrations of information signals such as gut activity or dryness of the mouth with emotion.

Emotions differ from rationalistic concepts such as goals, preferences, and attitudes in yet another way. They are fluid and may enter the stream of behavior or consciousness at almost any point in time. This can take place during gaps or breaks in a task, during the task itself, or at the end of a task. Freud (1930/1962) commented on this varied and fluid relationship of emotion to other behaviors. He stated that emotions, in contrast to other psychological structures, could travel freely between the id, ego, and superego. Emotional reactions are constructed by a multilevel hierarchical system. Emotion can be generated by activity at any one (or more) of the levels of the system while other levels are involved with nonemotional processes such as perception, problem solving, and action. Therefore, it makes sense that emotion is experienced during gaps in performance. If the emotion appeared during a task, it might disrupt performance by redirecting attention or by interfering with motor output. This is especially likely to happen when a task is not overlearned. Experiencing emotion during a pause in task performance may also provide an opportunity for appraising the worth of the task and its cost or benefit to oneself. Such opportunities may facilitate the formation of bonds between affect and task cognitions. This leads to the formation of attitudes and results in stable affective–cognitive bonds. In this context emotion can be seen as a stimulus to the reformulation of attitudes and preferences rather than just a stimulus for immediate, impulsive action (see Eysenck, 1967; Tomkins, 1962; and Tomkins & McCarter, 1964; for similar elaborations).

The suggestion that emotions are often most noticeable during gaps in task performance should not lead us to conclude that emotion is antagonistic to problem solving, and that emotion always has a disorganizing effect on structured, goal-oriented behavior (Leeper, 1948). Emotion can be integrated with organized behavior and become an integral part of action. Musical performance provides an excellent example of the congruence of emotion and task performance (Clynes, 1972). Musicians who play with technical virtuosity but omit feeling from their performance are often described as technicians. Skilled musicians incorporate emotional behaviors, both subjective and motor, into their performance. The integration of feeling and task performance in consciousness and in the face and fingers puts emotion into the sound and structure of the playing and influences the pulse and the tone of the music.

Summary

We have reviewed two sets of barriers presumed to interfere with the study of emotion. These are (1) the nature of emotional phenomena, and (2) the use of alternative, nonemotional concepts to account for these phenomena. We suggested that the difficulties in the study of emotion are similar to those found in the study of perception. Therefore, these problems can be overcome and cannot justify any further inattention to research on emotion. We then compared emotion to alternative concepts such as evaluation, preference, and attitude in order to identify properties of emotional behavior that cannot be readily understood by use of these rationalistic concepts. These phenomena include the rapid fluctuation of emotion, its sensitivity to variations in the organism's state during person–situation interactions, and its appearance during gaps in task performance, integrated with task performance, and after the completion of a task. The next section outlines a hierarchically structured theory of emotional processing which we believe can account for and predict most if not all of these aspects of emotional behavior. It presents basic assumptions about the operation of the emotional system and its relationship to cognition at different levels of emotional processing. The section begins with a brief description of past theories of emotion, most of which attempt to account for emotional behavior using a single hypothesis. This historical review is included to demonstrate the consequences of postulating a primary mechanism for a theory of emotion.

PERCEPTUAL-MOTOR THEORY OF EMOTION

Antecedents

Theories of emotion can be divided into four broad classes. In the first group, the experience of a specific emotion (i.e., whether one *feels* anger, fear, joy, or some other affect) is a product of the pattern of autonomic activity (Ax, 1953; Davis, 1957; Funkenstein, King, & Drolette, 1957; James, 1890/1950; J. Schachter, 1957; Sternbach, 1966). In the second group, the experience of emotion is the product of the combination of undifferentiated autonomic feedback with a cognition (a perception or an idea). This is the cognition–arousal position (Russell, 1927; S. Schachter, 1964; S. Schachter & Singer, 1962; Sully, 1902). In the third group of theories, emotion is constructed from the interaction of specific "emotion" sites in the central nervous system. Cannon (1929) identified the thalamus and cortex as two such sites, while MacLean (1958) postulated an interaction between limbic structures such as the amygdaloid and septal bodies and the cortex as being the source of emotion.

The fourth group of emotion theories derives from Darwin's theory of emotion (Darwin, 1872/1904). Theorists such as Izard (1971, 1977; see also Fridlund & Izard, Chapter 9, this volume), Tomkins (1962, 1980), and Plutchik (1980) share with the central neural theorists the belief that emotion depends on activity in specific "emotion centers" of the central nervous system. These theorists have also assigned an important role to feedback from the face for creating specific, emotional experiences such as fear, anger, joy, and disgust. While there is reason to believe that feedback, either from the facial muscles or the skin, plays an important role in sustaining emotion (Tomkins, 1980), it is not clear that facial feedback is *necessary* for the experience of subjective emotional qualities. We believe that Tomkins is correct in hypothesizing that facial activity can both initiate and maintain emotional reactions. We also believe that facial motor activity is most often a consequence of the activation of central emotional processes and their accompanying emotional experiences. The latter processes, which include the experience of emotion, can take place with little or no facial participation. In our model, central motor activity rather than peripheral feedback is seen as the necessary element for arousing emotional experience (Leventhal, 1979, 1980).

The present hierarchical theory clearly aligns itself with the third group, since it assumes that the central nervous system has "noncognitive" centers that can generate emotional experience with or without the participation of autonomic nervous system activity. It also aligns itself with the fourth set of theorists because it sees nearly all emotional behavior as integrations of expressive–motor, cognitive, and central processes. Having adopted the position that emotions are differentiated behavioral and experiential events, and not merely a synthesis of autonomic and cognitive processes, we can proceed to examine our assumptions as to how the emotion system operates. When we have completed that task, we will define the mechanisms that we believe operate at different levels of the emotion-processing system.

Fundamental Assumptions about the Nature of the System

Hierarchical Processing

The concept of hierarchical processing is the fundamental notion under-lying our model. Since this processing system is hierarchical, every emotion must be composed of multiple components. The components must vary from emotion to emotion, and may also vary from moment to moment for the same emotion. The hierarchical nature of the system also accounts for the fact that emotion may appear to be independent of cognition or reason, and that emotion accompanies many types of cognition, including sensa-tions, perceptions, images, and ideas.

There are two hierarchies involved in emotional processing. First, the central nervous system forms a hierarchy with the peripheral machinery of the body. The central nervous system uses information from the body and the body's motor mechanisms for constructing emotional reactions. We agree with Neisser (1967) and Mandler (1975) that perception and emotion are the experiential products of complex, constructive activity. Second, within the central nervous system we postulate a hierarchical processing system consisting of at least three levels (Figure 12-1).

Expressive–Motor Level. The expressive–motor mechanism is the basic processor of emotional behavior and experience. It includes an innate set of central, neuromotor programs for generating a distinctive set of expres-sive reactions and feelings in response to specific releasing stimuli in the newborn and the developing child (Izard, 1971).

Schematic Level. The schematic mechanism is an automatic processing system which involves the coding of emotional experience in memory. It is not a memory about emotional reactions, it is the record of the reactions. The schematic system combines the subjective feelings and expressive motor reactions with stimulus inputs and other motor reactions, particu-

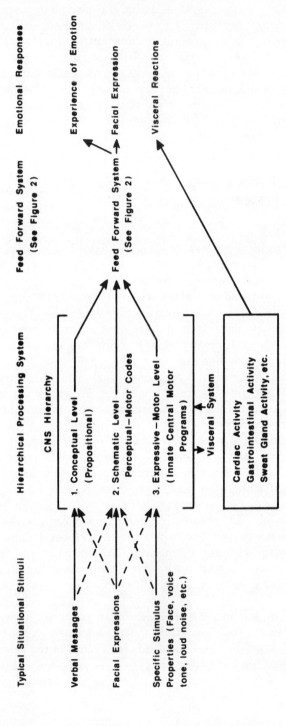

FIGURE 12-1. Model of the hierarchical processing system for the construction of emotional reactions: (1) the three levels of central neural processing (CNS) and (2) the relation of CNS to the visceral system.

larly autonomic responses. Instrumental reactions are less tightly linked to schemata than are autonomic or expressive motor responses. This system can be conceptualized as a record of conditioned emotional reactions.

Conceptual Level. The conceptual system includes a set of abstract propositions or rules about emotional episodes and a set of rules for voluntary responding to emotion-provoking situations and to emotions themselves. The rules or propositions that make up this system emerge from self-observation and variations in voluntary efforts to control subjective feelings. Rules or propositions for creating emotion are easy to verbalize. For example, we can observe and comment on our emotional reactions by making statements such as "The near miss with that car really upset me," or "I seem to feel butterflies in my stomach and shaky all over whenever I have a close call with danger."

The voluntary motor component of the conceptual system is separate from the motor system that is linked to automatic or schematic processing (Geschwind, 1975). It provides the individual with the capacity to perform voluntarily specific expressive and instrumental "feeling" responses. This system is crucial for developing voluntary control over emotional experience and behavior. The comparison between voluntary (intended) and automatic (unintended) expressive motor impulses is the key to feeling.

We have differentiated two hierarchical systems, one relating the central nervous system to the body machinery and the other within the central nervous system. In this model, emotional experience does not require feedback from peripheral or motor (autonomic or facial-motor) activity. This is true of the emotional experiences of both neonates and adults. Even though we claim that peripheral motor activity is not necessary for emotional experience and behavior, we are not suggesting that it is irrelevant to them. Peripheral motor activity typically feeds back into and is integrated with central emotional processing. These "subtleties" may seem academic, but they are critical in differentiating the perceptual–motor model from the cognition–arousal models proposed by S. Schachter and Singer (1962) and others. The cognition–arousal models argue that autonomic activity is necessary for emotion and that cognition without autonomic activity is cold or emotion-like but nonemotional. Our perceptual–motor position argues that genuine emotion can be experienced solely on the basis of central motor activity (although this may be an unusual case) and that autonomic activity is not necessary for emotion. It also argues that emotion can be independent of what we commonly call cognition or reason (if only expressive–motor activity is present) and that emotion can be associated with several types of cognition (perceptual, schematic, and conceptual). The perceptual–motor model also suggests that autonomic and other types of motor activity can arouse emotion when they have been associated with central neural emotional processes (Izard, 1971; Leventhal, 1974, 1979, 1980; Tomkins, 1962).

Simultaneous Action

All three processing mechanisms in the central neural hierarchy and the accompanying body machinery are active in emotion-provoking situations. Thus, one cannot separately observe conceptual, schematic, or expressive motor action. It is only possible to observe the product of their interaction. To study the contribution of a particular component to the total system, one has two choices: (1) to vary a factor that has its primary impact on the activity in one of the three levels, or (2) to develop an analytic model that links specific independent variables to responses (verbal expression, facial activity, etc.) presumed to reflect activity in a particular mechanism.

Although each of the levels is involved in every emotional response, the degree and the nature of their involvement may vary from occasion to occasion. They will also vary at different times in the life cycle, since the degree and type of conceptual involvement changes with development (Piaget, 1968). On the other hand, we hypothesize that the expressive-motor system changes very little over time.

Processing of Emotions in Meaning Domains

With experience, an individual develops an increasingly rich and differentiated store of knowledge which is linked to a wide variety of emotional memories and emotional experiences (Bower & Cohen, 1982; Mandler, 1962). The phrase "meaning domain" refers to specific content areas which include the self-system and its subareas (e.g., the self as child, student, father, etc.) as well as content areas such as illness, work, and sports. Each domain contains a history of emotional experience such as joy, interest, pain, and anxiety. The activation of a meaning domain or its components will activate the emotion integrated with it. For example, we can expect different emotional reactions from a woman hospitalized with uterine cancer and a woman in childbirth, even though each may experience the same sensations during a medical examination. The cancer patient may perceive the pain as confirming her terminal illness and may become severely frightened and anxious. The pregnant woman, in contrast, may feel happy and exhilarated as the same sensations remind her of the ensuing birth. It is for this reason that preparatory information about sensations that take place during an examination can be so important in reducing fear and distress (Janis, 1974; Johnson, 1975; Johnson & Leventhal, 1974).

Emotional reactions also define boundaries and can link into meaning domains various cognitive contents that would not otherwise be associated with one another. We believe that emotions do this by linking concrete perceptual memories to one another and then tying these memories to conceptual interpretations. For example, there are emotional meaning systems for depression (Beck, Rush, Shaw, & Emery, 1979), euphoria (Clark & Isen, 1982), and anger (Berkowitz, 1974, 1982). The activation of a specific emotion enhances the availability of content linked to that subjective feeling. Depressive feelings, for example, evoke a complex set of cognitive materials which have been characterized as a negative cognitive triad or a negative view of the self, world, and future (Beck *et al.*, 1979). Affect also generates biases in thought and selectivity in recall. Bower (1981) has suggested that the phenomenon of state-dependent memory (e.g., learning under the influence of drugs that can only be recalled during the drug-induced state) may be due to the presence of a state-specific emotion which activates a specific sector or domain within the mnemonic system.

Each meaning system or domain changes in structure or cognitive organization with development of the individual and with increased experience in specific content areas. The construction of emotion by expressive–motor processing is analogous to the child's sensory–motor assimilation of external reality. In the young child, undifferentiated wholes (the human face) or specific components (high-pitched tones of voice) may evoke prepared expressive reactions and subjective feelings. These expressive and subjective reactions may be conditioned to perceptual memories. The entire complex of perceptual memories, expressive reactions, and subjective feelings can then be tightly linked with autonomic reactions. Long exposures to such combinations, either over repeated occasions or from a single, long-lasting occasion, can lead to well-structured schematic memories which become a perceptual memory system for mediating emotional behavior. Well-structured systems of this type join feelings, expressions, and autonomic responses to perceptual memories, and form what Piaget termed a "concrete operational system" (Piaget, 1971). As an affective system grows to include conceptual and volitional rules or properties, it takes on the characteristics of a formal operational system. Since meaning domains are organized by specific contents or by specific emotions, they tend to be segregated. For example, an individual may be differentially mature in some domains but not in others, and be able to exert volitional control over anger and fear but not over joy and love.

Multiple Routes of Activation

The entire emotional system, including overt emotional reactions and subjective feelings, can be stimulated to activity by processing at any level of the system. The speed and clarity with which emotion will be experienced and the cognitive content that will accompany emotional arousal will vary according to which and how many levels of the system are active. For example, if an emotional sequence is initiated by activity at the visceral or autonomic level (from the bottom up in Figure 12-1), emotional behavior and experience may be relatively ambiguous as autonomic activity accompanies all types of vigorous or intense activity. The feeling state would become more distinct and be experienced as fear, anger, or joy, etc., when a central expressive motor program is activated by either external stimulation [e.g., seeing (S. Schachter & Singer, 1962), or imitating the behavior of a stooge (Walters & Parke, 1964)], or through cognitive activity that stimulates central expressive–motor activity. At some point, all levels of processing will be active, and expressive–motor processing will always play a central role in the active generation of feelings.

The possibility of a separate or independent activity at each of the processing levels suggests that emotion and cognition are independent. For example, we may smile and have a positive feeling in response to the smile of a person we do not like. Our emotion would be independent of our attitudes. This phenomenon was repeatedly illustrated in our early research on fear communications. Pictures of the end results of tetanus, long-term cigarette smoking, or poor dental hygiene would evoke powerful, negative emotions (through schematic processing) that had relatively little bearing on long-term conceptualizations of risk or on risk-reducing behaviors (Leventhal, 1970; Leventhal, Singer, & Jones, 1965). Rogers (Chapter 6, this volume) has convincingly demonstrated the validity of this conclusion through his careful research using verbal report and psychophysiological recording. Zajonc (1980) is a recent convert to the independence position in his suggestion that "preferences need no inferences," but has ignored both prior statements of the position and the research which generated and followed its initial presentation. As a consequence, he argues for a degree of independence of emotion and cognition which can only be defended if cognition is identified with only one type of cognitive activity —conscious, volitionally controlled thought. As Lazarus (1966, 1980) and one of us (Leventhal, 1974, 1979, 1980) have suggested, this position is unwarranted and requires too restrictive a definition of cognition. This issue is discussed in more detail in later sections of this chapter.

Evidence for the Processing Mechanisms

We have provided an overview of our assumptions regarding the fundamental structure and function of the emotion-processing system. The definition of terms and description of the processes were presented in abstract terms. The goal of the present section is to concretize these abstractions by tying them to observations. In this section we focus on data relevant to the expressive–motor, schematic, and conceptual levels of neural processing.

Expressive-Motor Processing

We have suggested that a central emotional–motor program generates both expressive action and feeling, and that this system is operative at birth. Although we have no way of testing this hypothesis in the newborn, we believe it plausible since so many central states, such as imagery, dreams, and thought during anticipation of exposure to counterattitudinal arguments, are accompanied by motor responses in adults (Cacioppo & Petty, 1981). Since there is continuity of emotional behavior from childhood to adulthood, it seems reasonable to believe that the same relationship of motor activity to subjective events would appear in infancy. This hypothesis seems highly plausible given the greater congruence between motor activity and experience in childhood. The presumed link between the feeling and motor response is the reason for labeling the system an expressive–motor system.

There is a wide range of data to support a hypothesis for a central motor mechanism that generates both innate expressive–motor reactions and subjective emotional experiences. First, there are data describing the structure and function of the facial musculature. This musculature is highly differentiated (Ekman *et al.*, 1972; Izard, 1971, 1977; Tomkins, 1962) and therefore able to express a full range of differentiated feelings (Leventhal, 1979, 1980). The face also has extensive connections to central neural areas implicated in emotional responding (Gellhorn, 1964). Second, there is considerable evidence showing that facial expressions of emotion are recognized with high accuracy both within and across cultures (Ekman & Friesen, 1971; see also Hager and Ekman, Chapter 10, this volume; Izard, 1971; Tomkins & McCarter, 1964). Third, there are data showing that expressive behavior develops in the blind as well as the normally sighted child (Eibl-Eibesfeldt, 1980). This demonstrates that expressive-motor behaviors are not learned. Fourth, emotional states seem to be sufficiently tied to expressive behavior to allow for predictions of subjective feelings from electromyograph recordings of facial muscle activity that is invisible to an unaided observer (Schwartz, Fair, Mandel, Salt, & Klerman, 1976). Facial muscle activity can also predict an observer's judgment of emotion (Ekman & Friesen, 1975) and, in some circumstances, the emotional experience of the person observed (Leventhal & Sharpe, 1965). Finally, there is abundant evidence to support the hypothesis that specific emotional states are keyed to particular eliciting cues. For example, nausea-disgust is related to upset of the gastrointestinal tract and taste (Garcia, 1981); pain–distress is related to noxious stimulation rather than threat; and fear is stimulated by specific visual and auditory cues such as a rapidly approaching shadow or an abrupt, loud sound.

This varied list of findings provides evidence for the existence of an innate expressive–motor system. More important, they point to a variety of functions and hypotheses respecting the operation of this system. For example, it is clear that infants' expressive–motor reactions serve important adaptive functions, such as reducing the possibility of harm by signaling the presence of danger. Thus an infant will produce cries of distress and vigorous face, head, and arm movements in response to the placement of a cloth over the face. Expressive responses also signal an infant's internal state, which allows the caregiver to remove threats and satisfy needs that an infant is unable to satisfy on his or her own. A third important function of expressive responses is to establish attachment of the infant to the caregiver and the caregiver to the infant. The infant's alerting and attention to high-pitched voices, and the mutual provocation of expressive responses and feelings during social contact from the adult, are ways of ensuring continued interaction and of developing schematic structures (perceptual memories joined to affect) in both parties. The sensitivity of the expressive–motor emotional mechanism to the expressive (visual and vocal) cues of others is a central factor in the development of mutual affective stimulation that serves as the base for more complex forms of imitative and modeling behaviors (Brazelton, Koslowski, & Main, 1974).

The stimulus specificity of different affective states is an extremely important aspect of emotional communication. It is evident that determining the relevance of cues to affect will be largely an empirical issue. It also seems that we can anticipate many of these stimulus–response specificities. Garcia (1981) indicates that there is nothing mysterious about the favored relationship of taste as a cue to the conditioning of nausea-disgust. The sensory organ involved—the mouth and tongue—is part of the biological system that forms the body component of that emotion complex. Pain–distress provides another obvious example in that distress is largely a response to injury or other noxious stimuli (Mandler & Kessen, 1959). Distress serves to inhibit responding to prevent further damage to injured body parts. It appears more difficult to detect the stimuli that are specific to emotions that are responsive to specific external events, but there has been some progress in this area and more will follow (see the review in Leventhal, 1980).

Most theorists who recognize the importance of facial expressions have hypothesized that sensory feedback from the facial muscles creates subjective feelings (Izard, 1971; Tomkins, 1962). We do not. We have theorized that a motor mechanism located in the central nervous system can create feelings in the absence of peripheral feedback (Leventhal, 1980). We discuss this mechanism in the section detailing the interactions between systems.

Schematic Processing

The schematic processing system begins as a record or memory of prior expressive–motor activity. Once the record is formed, schematic processes can be activated automatically. There is no need for deliberate, conscious processing of information in order to activate schematic activity. The entire schematic complex, including stimulus representation, motor reactions (expressive, autonomic, and postural), and subjective feelings can be activated by any stimulus element corresponding to its components. Schemata therefore consist of conditioned reactions. A package or set of responses is integrated by this conditioning. These packages have specific shapes or patterns, as they are built on a set of available expressive–motor templates with the stimulus preferences built into these templates.

As we have already suggested in our discussion of meaning domains, schematic structures change with development (Piaget, 1971). The cognitive component of emotional schemata in neonates is likely to include little more than sensory features (e.g., tastes for nausea–disgust, shadows, or approaching images for fear). The infant's attention to the stimuli eliciting his or her expressive–motor reactions may be close and prolonged. But once he or she codes the key image features and joins them with feeling and motor components, processing becomes rapid and automatic, with little or no need for the eliciting events to enter focal awareness. At later points in time, attention is required only to bring the stimulus into the receptor field in order to activate the schematic unit, which includes the motor components and subjective feelings. With time, the cognitive component becomes more complex, more of a structured perception, and eventually, more of a cognitive unit or concrete category. We believe that these concrete categories are closely tied to perception (Broadbent, 1977), and can structure perception under conditions of impoverished stimulation (Allport & Pettigrew, 1957).

Although we do not have a precise notion of the nature of the earliest schematic structures, it is useful to think of them as associative units whose components fall in a common cortical field or column. A column is a vertical section through the layers of the cortex that allows for a combination of sensory and motor events to be represented in their respective layers. We conceive of these cortical memory units as automatic activators of the expressive–motor and autonomic machinery. They are the discrete memory units that activate and arouse analog mechanisms in the nervous system and body. In short, the schematic unit is the high-speed detector and integrator of the growing affective perceptual–motor processing system.

There are several types of evidence which support the concept of schematic coding and processing of emotional information. Best known are the studies which show that imagery stimulates autonomic arousal, whereas verbalizations generally do not (Grossberg & Wilson, 1968; Lang, 1979). When words provoke emotional reactions, such as aggressive behavior, they do so more readily when they are concrete and high in perceptual value. Words equivalent in meaning but low in perceptual value fail to do so (Turner & Layton, 1976). Second, images of recent, vivid, disturbing experiences intrude on subsequent mental activity even if the individual tries to keep them out of mind (Horowitz, 1970). These images can be induced by exposure to threatening films and they will even intrude into the dream imagery of paradoxical sleep (Witkin & Lewis, 1967). It has also been observed that threats in later life can reactivate images of frightening situations from childhood, a phenomenon that has been labeled "unrepression" (Janis, 1974). This phenomenon seems to fit better the notion of state-dependent memory discussed previously. These observations reinforce the hypothesis of a symmetrical relationship between emotional reactions and imagery. Findings that show autonomic motor system arousal can provoke negative feeling states (Marshall & Zimbardo, 1979; Maslach, 1979) or add to existent emotional reactions (Zillmann, 1979; see also Chapter 8, this volume) also suggest that schemata are well-integrated image–motor units. These associative processes seem to occur automatically, which one would expect in schematic processing.

Data on dreaming provide another set of observations linking imagery to emotion. The vivid images occurring during paradoxical sleep are accompanied by eye movements, heightened cortical arousal, a variety of muscular changes, and appropriate emotional experience (Dement, 1972). Vivid sexual dreams have even been reported by paraplegics who no longer experience sexual arousal when awake (Money, 1960). Schematic processes appear to be sufficient to provoke sexual arousal during sleep. In contrast, during awake periods when the organism functions as an integrated whole, the individual is aware of the absence of peripheral autonomic feedback and this deprives him or her of a complete sexual experience. Dreams during nonparadoxical or slow-wave sleep are rich in body sensations and often accompanied by powerful emotions such as terror (Broughton, 1968).

Finally, there is a growing body of neuropsychological evidence on cerebral lateralization which provides support for a schematic processing system. These data support the hypothesis that right-hemisphere functions allow for the integration of holistic perceptual memories with motor (autonomic and expressive) functions. The right hemisphere is sensitive to emotional cues since it is able to detect facial expressions of emotion and expressive sounds (Carmon & Nachson, 1973; Haggard & Parkinson, 1971; Jaynes, 1976; King & Kimura, 1972; Ley & Bryden, 1979; Moscovitch, Scullion, & Christie, 1976; Safer, 1981; Safer & Leventhal, 1977; Suberi & McKeever, 1977), and is active during the expression of emotion (Sackeim & Gur, 1978). It is also very sensitive to motor information from the body (Davidson, Horowitz, Schwartz, & Goodman, 1981; Hécaen, 1969; Luria, 1973; Semmes, 1968). Data relevant to laterality and emotion have been reviewed by Davidson (1980), Galin (1974), Safer (1981), and Tucker (1981).

These five classes of evidence begin to converge on the conclusion that the emotional processing system makes use of a perceptual or image-like memory system that records events and attaches these perceptual patterns to visceral feedback, and to programs that evoke expressive-motor behavior. The schematic system is designed for conditioning, or formation of tight associative bonds between perceptual events (first simple features and then more complex patterns) and unconditioned, or primary, sensory–motor-generated emotional responses (e.g., disgust in response to aversive taste). This is an extremely important point which is developed at length in the final section, which focuses on interactions between the processing systems.

Finally, the phenomenon of phantom pain has played a crucial role in developing our concept of schematic processing (see discussions in Leventhal, 1980; Leventhal & Everhart, 1979; Melzack, 1973; Simmel, 1962). Phantom body parts are often experienced after amputation, and are frequently extremely painful. It is the occurrence of pain in the phantom which strongly suggests that emotions can be stored in perceptual (schematic) memory. The pain stored in a phantom is often closely related to a prior emotionally distressing experience. For example, a pain from an ankle sprain will appear in the phantom if the individual regards the sprain as responsible for the amputation. Emotional upset created by major, distressing life events may also reactivate a phantom that has been dormant for years (McKechnie, 1975). Studies by Bower and his collaborators (Bower, 1981; Bower & Cohen, 1981) and Clark and Isen (1982) provide further examples of the way emotion activates and organizes memory.

In addition to providing us with yet another source of data to support the notion of schematic processing, research on the neurophysiology of the pain system has greatly reinforced our belief in the plausibility of the perceptual–motor model. These studies show that the pain system is complex. It contains parallel branches for processing specific information about the features of the pain stimulus on the one hand, and for activating cortical functions and stimulating emotional reactions on the other (Casey, 1973). This organization into separate but parallel informational and activating systems suggests that perceptual information can be integrated in complex ways with cerebral activation and autonomic arousal for the formation of pain schemata. It also suggests that much of the affective organization is preattentive and occurs independent of conscious attention and decisional processes, although it may be affected by them. We will return to this in the final section.

Conceptual Processing

We have defined two components of conceptual processing: (1) one that stores information about past emotional episodes which can be accessed to talk about emotional experiences, and (2) one used for the voluntary performance of emotional acts. Both components make use of a propositional information network in which specific elements (e.g., snake, fear, me) are logically related. Propositions are comprised of discrete meaning elements which are logically organized (e.g., I am fearful of snakes). Propositional storage is more abstract than schematic storage and protects the representation from excessive change after exposure to a new experience. Propositional storage also permits more flexible (thoughtful) response to emotional situations. Thus, conceptual storage aids in the short- and long-term control of emotional experience. Conceptual processing is also effortful and makes demands on conscious attentional capacity (Carver & Scheier, 1981; Clark & Isen, 1982; Posner & Snyder, 1975). Conceptual processing can affect the total emotional processing system because of its role in the interpretation of instructions, the direction of attention, and the initiation of behavior. For example, by orienting attention toward or away from particular parts of a stimulus field, one can intensify or minimize encounters with emotion-provoking events. Many attentional tactics are generalized as abstract commonsense rules for the control of emotional reactions. When these rule-bound actions become habitual they can be identified as cognitive styles or ego defenses. Unlike ego defenses, they seem to be accessible to consciousness. People are often aware that they are using them and will defend doing so when criticized. For example, distraction or avoidance is seen by many people as the most effective tactic for coping with stressful life events, while paying attention to a stressful event is seen as producing greater pain and distress, despite evidence to the contrary (Leventhal & Everhart, 1979).

Conceptual structures for emotional processing develop from repeated practice in coping with (expressing and controlling) emotional states, and from observational learning and practice in social communication. Studies of sex differences in emotional response provide one source of evidence for the development of conceptual emotional processing. Compared to males, females are more likely to display and talk about emotional experience, to have expressive models, and to express rather than surpress feelings. This difference in socialization is expected to generate structures that make women more skilled in the voluntary encoding (expressing) and decoding (detecting) of emotional responses. Two different sets of data, one on fear, the other on humor, show that women exhibit greater consistency than men among the verbal, expressive, and autonomic components of emotion. This difference may reflect greater practice in females. For example, Lang and his associates (Lang, 1979; Lang, Kozak, Miller, Levin, & McLean, 1980) found that judgments of fear and autonomic responses were more consistent for female subjects than for male subjects. They also reported that males became consistent after rehearsing concrete images of themselves as emotionally (i.e., autonomically) active. In a second example, data from our laboratory showed that judgments of funniness and facial expressions of mirth were more consistent for female than for male subjects (Cupchik & Leventhal, 1974; Leventhal & Cupchik, 1976; Leventhal & Mace, 1970). These findings have been replicated by others (Svebak, 1975). Sex differences also appear in studies on lateralization of emotional processing. The evidence suggests that they may be due to differences in prior practice or rehearsal of emotional behavior. The relationship of practice to hemispheric involvement has also been shown for musical performance. Skilled musicians show equal left- and right-hemisphere activity during musical performances, whereas novice performers show stronger right-hemisphere involvement (Bever & Chiarello, 1974). Thus, practice appears to enhance left-hemisphere (volitional or conceptual) processing. Safer (1981) found that females were equally accurate in identifying facial expressions of emotion in the left and right visual fields (right and left hemispheres). Males could match females in accuracy only in the left visual field (right hemisphere). Therefore, females can as readily decode briefly exposed expressions of emotion with either schematic (right-hemisphere) or volitional (left-hemisphere) codes. This skill was specific to emotional decoding, as both sexes were better at identifying faces (a pattern perception task) in the left visual field. Taken as a whole, the sex-difference data suggest that it is reasonable to distinguish perceptual or schematic codes on the one hand, and conceptual or volitional codes on the other. The data suggest that practice is critical in the development of skilled volitional emotional performances.

Simultaneous Action of the Levels in the System Framework

Our basic theme is that emotional behavior is the product of a complex, multilevel processing system. The system operates at the visceral, expressive–motor, schematic, and conceptual levels. Each level may contribute more or less to an emotional reaction at specific points in time. We can learn more about the operation of each level by relating its activity to each of the others, but we can learn the most by examining occasions where the individual levels generate discrepant emotional reactions.

Discrepancies are most likely to be observed between the volitional, conceptual processes on the one hand, and the automatic, expressive–motor, and schematic on the other. The discrepancies arise because each level is organized and operates differently from each other level. Thus, the individual levels use different types of information for emotional processing. For example, we have suggested that conceptual processing is propositionally organized and its informational nodes are retrieved in logical sequences. Autonomic and expressive–motor activity, by contrast, is stimulated by expressive and contextual cues, and is spatially organized. In addition, it is graded in intensity and best described in analog terms as being continuously variable in strength.

These differences between the levels of the system are responsible for the frequency with which people experience emotions as being beyond voluntary control. They cannot activate or inhibit emotional reactions as easily as they can activate or inhibit instrumental, task-oriented movements by means of propositionally organized self-statements and voluntary acts. Hence, efforts to control emotions are often indirect rather than direct. For example, if I want to reduce my anxiety and lower my heart rate while giving a talk, I can go to the lectern, take a deep breath to slow my heart rate (a voluntary response that acts as an unconditioned stimulus to the unconditioned response of lowered heart rate), and look at the faces and seats in the room as I do so. By repeating this strategy, I can condition slowing of my heart rate to cues in the lecture hall. Furedy and Riley (Furedy & Riley, 1982; Riley & Furedy, in press) argue that teaching self-control with biofeedback involves the very type of control described above. Information is used to control instrumental or operant behaviors (a propositional system), which then influence unconditioned (expressive–motor) and conditioned (schematic) responses that are part of an automatic motor skill system. This represents but one type of control of automatic processes by conceptual processes. There are also a variety of other ways in which expressive–motor and schematic processes can influence or control the conceptual level of processing. These will be discussed next.

CONCEPTUAL CONTROL OF EXPRESSIVE–MOTOR AND SCHEMATIC PROCESSING

It is likely that the majority of our emotional reactions are initiated by external stimulation that activates schematic processing or provokes unconditioned expressive–motor reactions. These reactions are provoked whether or not we expect or "want" to feel the specific emotions. This is the source of most of the inconsistency that we experience between how we feel and how we want to feel! Think how easy it would be to diet if we felt hunger at the sight of carrots, salads, and celery, and disgust at the sight of ice cream, caramels, and cream puffs, or how little divorce there would be if we were always more strongly attracted to our spouses rather than anyone else! Since these automatic processes evoke feelings that are often discrepant with the demands of conceptual knowledge and our social roles, our worlds are filled with warnings and advice on how to diet, how to love, and how to express and control our fear and anger.

Conceptually directed processing uses two major sets of tactics to regulate and control the expressive–motor, schematic, and autonomic levels of functioning. These are (1) regulating stimulation, and (2) regulating motor responses. We will briefly discuss strategies in each of these areas.

Regulating Stimulation

Stimulation can be regulated by simple tactics such as approaching or avoiding situations that provoke automatic emotional responding. A neonate will strike out to remove an offending object, avert his or her gaze, push away distasteful food, and so on. These are avoidance tactics. Attending, pulling something toward oneself, and stuffing things in the mouth are assimilative or approach strategies. Both approach and avoidance behaviors regulate contact with stimuli that are primary elicitors of emotion. These tactics are transferred to mental representations as soon as they are performed and become stable response styles. Our model suggests these styles will be emotion specific, and that strategies of this sort may generalize across situations to different degrees in different emotions as a function of the way the individual voluntarily deploys his or her attention. For example, Clark and Isen (1982) suggest that people follow different rules in deploying attention during positive and negative feeling states. The rule for positive states is to think and act so as to enhance or maintain the state, while the rule for negative states is to avoid thinking about negative material so as to change the state. Cognitions that have accompanied positive moods during one's life history will thus become associated with one another regardless of their logical relatedness. Therefore, the arousal of positive moods will lead to the recall of a wide variety of positive past experiences. In contrast, the withdrawal of attention from environmental cues during negative emotions should facilitate the association of specific situational perceptions and memories with internal, autonomic reactions. Hence, autonomic arousal on subsequent occasions should lead to recall of a more limited range of specific negative experiences. This appears to correspond to the type of recall observed in phobics and hypochondriacs. The hypothesized difference in the relationship between positive and negative emotions with external events and internal, autonomic responses is consistent with the findings obtained by Maslach (1979) and Marshall and Zimbardo (1979) showing that autonomic activation was clearly biased toward recall of negative events.

The foregoing examples focus on the way in which attentional strategies affect the organization of the underlying automatic processing system. Attention influences the conditioning of the schematic structures by bringing a vast array of images and ideas into awareness during positive states, and by focusing cognition and images of threats during negative states. We have observed a number of these effects in our studies of pain. In our typical study, the subject is exposed to a noxious stimulus which produces ischemic pain. This is done by cutting off circulation in the arm with a blood pressure cuff or by immersing the hand in cold (2 or 7°C) water for a period of 6 to 7 minutes. The subject rates the amount of distress he or she is experiencing at 30-second intervals for the first 2 minutes, and at 1-minute intervals thereafter. Subjects are given different sets of instructions prior to the noxious exposure. Our studies have compared instructions that focus attention on the features of the stimulus (e.g., information about the component sensations of the stimulus and instructions to attend to them), with instructions to pay attention to slides, to think positive thoughts, or to instructions which inform the subject about the procedures to which they will be exposed (see Johnson, 1973; Leventhal, Brown, Shacham, & Engquist, 1979; Reinhardt, 1979; Shacham, 1979). The findings are quite consistent: Subjects who pay attention to and analyze the component features of the stimulus report substantial reductions in distress compared to control subjects. It is unlikely that this difference is due to response sets, as the subjects attending to specific sensations report equally high levels of distress during the first 1 to 2 minutes of exposure. The differences occur in the last half of the exposure period (the final 3 to 4 minutes). The sensation-monitoring procedure also carries over from the first to the second trial. Subjects who monitored during the first trial report very low levels of pain and distress on the second trial even when they are instructed not to monitor on that trial (Ahles, Blanchard, & Leventhal, in press; Shacham, 1979). In contrast, blocking or ignoring the noxious event produces a reduction in pain experience only during the time the subject actively tries to distract himself or herself. It does not carry over to later trials.

It is important to note that the effects of sensation monitoring are counterintuitive. Ahles et al. (in press) found that subjects regarded monitoring as a very poor way to adapt to a stressful event, and Reinhardt (1979) found that very few people spontaneously monitor sensations. Even after subjects have experienced the benefits of monitoring, they rate monitoring as an ineffective strategy (Reinhardt, 1979). These studies demonstrate that an attentional strategy can profoundly influence adaptation to a noxious experience without subjects accurately conceptualizing its effects. The changes appear to take place in the automatic, schematic processing of emotional distress. The consequences (reduced distress) of this are available to consciousness. The subjects report reductions in distress, but they do not accurately conceptualize the change because they have inadequate information. Since they have not been exposed to the noxious stimulus under both attentional sets, they are not able to abstract the correct rule respecting the relative effectiveness of attention and distraction. A number of rules respecting the conceptualization of pain experiences have been discussed elsewhere (Leventhal, 1982; Leventhal & Everhart, 1979).

Interpretive strategies form a second type of stimulus control. If a stimulus is given a benign rather than a threat interpretation, it will be less likely to provoke strong emotions. Interpretive defenses such as denial and intellectualization have been shown to reduce the intensity of verbal and psychophysiological indicators of fear in response to watching a stress-producing movie. This was demonstrated in several early experiments by Lazarus and his associates (Lazarus, 1966; Lazarus & Alfert, 1964) and in a replication by Holmes and Houston (1974). Barber and Hahn (1962) reported similar effects for cold-pressor stimulation. Subjects instructed to interpret the noxious experience as pleasant and cooling sensations on a very hot day were less distressed than subjects not using reinterpretations of this sort. Shacham's (1979) study points out a major limitation of reinterpretations of this sort; they are effective only when actively used. The reinterpretive strategy appears to stimulate a competing positive affect by provoking schematic processes contrary to those provoked by the noxious event. The subject must make continuing volitional efforts (e.g., self-talk) to sustain these competing reactions.

Regulating Motor Responses

Volitional, conceptual processes can be used to control automatic sensory-motor and schematic processing by regulating the motor component of the emotional system. The relationship between the volitional and the automatic motor systems, however, is extremely complex. At a simple level one can proceed to classify motor or performance strategies as blocking or assimilative. One can "wipe the smile" from one's own face, or tense up muscles to suppress feelings or pain–distress, or hum a happy tune to counter feelings of depression or fear. The major difficulty with suppressive strategies is they often increase the intensity of subjective feeling. For example, suppressing a smile elicited by the unexpected comment of a child on a solemn occasion may increase one's feeling of mirth and humor. This feature of expressive behavior is inconsistent with the hypothesis that facial-motor feedback is the primary cause of feelings.

Assimilative performance strategies also differ from assimilative stimulus-control strategies. These performance strategies involve more than a passive taking in of information. They involve practice and rehearsal of the motor movements of the emotional reaction. One can rehearse smiles, frowns, and head turning, and learn to perform and to anticipate one's own emotional expressions. The ability to perform expressive actions volitionally can cancel the emotional impact of the activation of the central neural expressive–motor programs (Leventhal, 1979, 1980). Our feed-forward model of central motor programs for emotional expression predicts both intensification of emotional experience when a volitional action suppresses an emotional response, and the diminution of an emotional experience when a volitional expression anticipates a spontaneous emotional expression (see Figure 12-2). The model suggests that automatically elicited motor programs generate the signals for emotional experience and emotional expression. These signals are assumed to feed forward both toward the facial motor apparatus and to the voluntary motor control system. Subjective feelings arise when the impulse feeds into the voluntary motor control system. The automatic motor impulse is felt as an emotion rather than as a movement when it is not anticipated or intended. This occurs

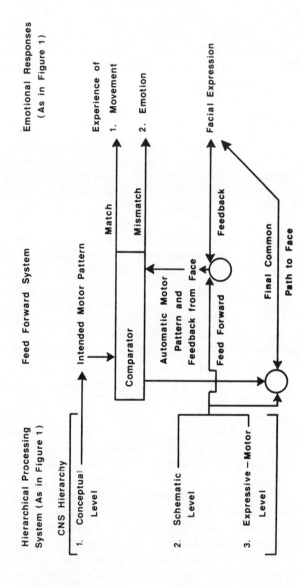

FIGURE 12-2. Feedforward system. Each of the three levels of the hierarchical processing system (see Figure 12-1) generates a motor pattern: the conceptual, an intentional motor pattern; the schematic and expressive-motor, an automatic motor pattern. The two types of patterns enter a comparator. If they match, the experience is of an intended movement. If they mismatch, the experience is of a spontaneous emotion. (The type of emotion depends on the motor pattern.) The intended and automatic patterns compete for control of overt expression via the final common path to the face. Facial feedback enters the feedforward loop, where it can initiate as well as intensify (its usual effect) emotional experience.

when no voluntary motor set or intention is present prior to the arrival of the automatic motor signal in the voluntary system: for example, if the impulse to laugh is provoked by a slapstick movie scene before I anticipate it, or before I am consciously ready to laugh. When a motor impulse is compared to an existing intention, it is felt as a planned movement, not as an emotion. When the intention is to suppress feeling, the automatic emotional impulse is compared to a nonemotional set, and can be felt more strongly. Whether one feels the emotion from the expressive–motor impulse or from the effort and strain of suppressing the impulse depends on their relative strength. An extremely intense effort at suppression could mask awareness of the feedforward signal from the expressive–motor system.

In summary, not all expressive activity is associated with subjective feeling. Voluntary movements, such as efforts to smile or to frown, do not need a subjective component. Efforts to smile when one is being stimulated by humorous material, or efforts to frown in anger when one is being provoked, may actually diminish the intensity of affect by canceling out the feeling induced by the spontaneous motor discharge. The hostess may smile to an exaggerated degree at her detested visitor, both to hide her animosity and to satisfy social graces, without feeling a positive affect that could accompany a spontaneous smile. It is clear that we have barely begun to explore the complexities of the interactions between expression of emotion and subjective feelings.

Influence of Automatic Processing on Volitional Systems

Any emotion system functions as a two-way, indeed a multiway street (Carver, 1979; Carver & Scheier, 1981). Influences occur from the upper to the lower levels of the system (conceptual to schematic and expressive motor), from the lower to the upper (autonomic and expressive motor to schematic and conceptual), and from the middle level both upward and downward.

One important "bottom-up" effect that we have previously mentioned is the tendency for autonomic activity to stimulate expressive–motor activity that provokes anxiety and fear (Marshall & Zimbardo, 1979; Maslach, 1979). Another is Zillmann's (1979) demonstrations of the generalization of arousal. High levels of arousal generated through exercise can enhance subsequent expressions of anger, overt expressions of joy (laughter), and sexual arousal (Zillmann, 1978, 1979; Zillmann, Katcher, & Milavsky, 1972). Mueller and Donnerstein (1981) have also demonstrated that exposure to emotionally arousing films can increase prosocial behavior. Generalization effects do not occur, however, if the subject is aware of the arousal and perceives its link to the prior exercise activity.

The findings noted above illustrate several important points about bottom-up effects. First, it is clear that activity at the visceral level can both stimulate and add to ongoing emotional processing at both the schematic and expressive–motor levels, and can do so for a variety of emotions. This is partly consistent with S. Schachter's (1964) hypothesis that autonomic activity may contribute to several emotional behaviors, but not completely consistent with it, as autonomic activity seems to contribute more easily to some emotional states than to others. For example, Erdmann and Janke (1978) found that autonomic arousal caused by injection of ephedrine added to situationally induced anger and happiness, but reduced situationally induced anxiety. There are a number of ways of dealing with these findings. First, it is fair to say that the experimental techniques used to activate the autonomic system are far too gross to detect links between specific autonomic patterns and particular emotions. Walters and Parke (1964), have argued that stimulants act to intensify motor activity and strengthen those emotions that involve either substantial levels of overt action, or actions that are compatible with situational constraints. This hypothesis is compatible with Cannon's view that autonomic activity was an essential component of action, not emotion.

An alternative hypothesis is that autonomic activity activates emotions by provoking those schematic memories to which it has been previously conditioned. If intense autonomic arousal has been linked to anger or to sexual behavior, activation of any critical component of autonomic activity could automatically trigger the schematic complex of which it is a part. A third alternative is that different autonomic patterns are associated with different emotions. This hypothesis has been suggested by investigators such as J. Schachter (1957), Ax (1953), Graham (1972), and others. It seems likely that different emotions may link to somewhat different patterns of visceral activity, as emotions may differ in the particular neurohumoral system they bring into play. For example, gastrointestinal activity may come into action with nausea–disgust and involve neurochemical systems somewhat different from those called into play by fear or anxiety (see McGeer & McGeer, 1980). Thus, the activation of the particular visceral system may bias expressive–motor and schematic memory so as to increase the likelihood of activation of specific emotions.

Finally, it is clear that activation of expressive–motor behavior can stimulate a wide range of schematic and conceptual processing. Audience laughter, for example, typically enhances the expressive activity and perceived humorousness of visual stimuli (Cupchik & Leventhal, 1974; Leventhal & Cupchik, 1976). Instructions have been used to promote emotional expression by encouraging subjects to laugh (Leventhal & Mace, 1970), or by instructing subjects to make it easier for others to judge their emotions (Zuckerman, Klorman, Larrance, & Spiegel, 1981). These strategies appear to add to the impact of humorous or noxious events. The degree to which an overt expressive reaction will generate or add to an existing emotional state is limited by the degree to which the expressive movements are automatic and unanticipated, or controlled and anticipated by the volitional motor system. According to our feedforward hypothesis, anticipating expressive movement (Cupchik & Leventhal, 1974), anticipating tickling (Weiskrantz, Elliott, & Darlington, 1971), or engaging in motor acts in a deliberate, voluntary manner (Tourangeau & Ellsworth, 1979) should limit their power to produce emotional experience. Anticipated, voluntary reactions are felt as movements, not as emotions.

Interpretations of Automatic, Emotional Reactions

There are two types of bottom-up effects which deserve separate discussion because of their extreme importance. The first involves the difficulty people have in distinguishing between visceral upset of an emotional nature and visceral upset due to illness. If visceral activity promotes expressive–motor reactions or evokes schematic structures for a specific emotion, the individual will experience an affective state or mood change. Alternatively, if the activity evokes a schema for illness (i.e., a structure that combines symptoms, emotional reactions, and perceptual memories and images of illness), the consequence is likely to be a decision to self-medicate or to seek medical care. For example, if visceral activity includes gastrointestinal distress together with cardiac activity, the individual may conclude that he or she is emotionally upset when actually suffering a heart attack. Deciding that the state is emotional could lead to actions to regulate emotion, such as taking a mild tranquilizer or an antacid, instead of attending to the medical emergency. If the same visceral activity is actually provoked by an external environmental event, interpreting it as illness can lead to the equally inappropriate decision to seek medical care when it is not needed. People presenting at primary-care settings often wonder whether they are ill or "just upset" (Robinson, 1971; Zola, 1973). There is abundant evidence that life stresses stimulate illness behavior in addition to provoking emotional distress (Mechanic, 1974; Mechanic & Volkart, 1961). The increase in the utilization of health services during times of emotional distress may lead to discoveries of a variety of chronic conditions which are not yet symptomatic. One possible conclusion that could be drawn from this contingency is that emotional stress leads to illness. The correct conceptualization would be that stress is influencing illness behavior.

The problem of differentiating illness from emotion illustrates how lower-level processes influence successively higher levels of the system, including the decision to seek medical care. Similar effects have been observed in our studies of the development of conditioned or anticipatory nausea in cancer patients receiving chemotherapy treatment. Nerenz,

Leventhal, and Love (1982) have found that patients who report tastes from their chemotherapy agents are more likely to develop conditioned nausea than are patients not noticing taste during the injections. The taste cue quickly links to nausea. The anticipatory nausea spreads to other cues, such as the sight of the nurse, the sight of the hospital, or the preparations to leave for the hospital. Each of these cues can evoke the taste response in certain patients. In a preliminary analysis of a sample of 125 patients, Nerenz and Leventhal found that the spread of taste to environmental cues occurred primarily in patients who also experienced anxiety at the time of the injection. While the visceral feeling of nausea readily attached to taste, as Garcia (1981) has found, the linkage of anxiety to the situation appeared to facilitate the spread of both taste and nausea to other perceptual cues and even to conceptual cues, including thinking about the treatment. The expressive–motor and schematic structure formed by the anxiety or fear at the time of injection served as a catalyst connecting the taste–nausea pair to perceptions and then to ideas.

The second important aspect of bottom-up effects concerns the degree to which subjective emotional states are used to draw conclusions about the self-system. Visceral activity, illness-induced fatigue and depression, and schematically provoked states of fear, anger, joy, and nausea are seen as signs that we are ineffective in problem solving and unable to alter our fates. This was dramatically illustrated by many patients showing conditioned or anticipatory nausea. They interpreted their symptoms as a sign that they were losing control of themselves and were experiencing a "nervous breakdown." They could not accept it simply as a "learned" phenomenon. Emotions, moods, and generalized mood changes induced by illness have powerful effects on self-appraisals of effectance (Bandura, 1977; Rosen, Terry, & Leventhal, 1982) and our appraisals of the quality of our lives. We believe that emotions contribute more to these judgments than do the experiences we accumulate in our attempts to influence or control outer reality.

CONCLUSION: EMOTIONS AS READOUTS
OF MEANING DOMAINS

We began our chapter by addressing Simon's (1982) question concerning the difference between emotions and goals and preferences. We have suggested two ways of distinguishing between these two sets of concepts: (1) Emotions are more volatile and changeable, and (2) emotions provide an ongoing readout of the moment-by-moment state of the organism as it is engaged in problem solving. Emotions are like pressure gauges, tachometers, and fuel gauges. They tell us of pressures within regions of the body system, of rates of activity in areas of the system, and of rates of energy utilization within the system. This definition allows us to include within the concept of emotion a broad range of states, including the typical primary emotions (fear, anger, disgust, joy, depression, etc.) as well as states such as fatigue–tiredness and pain–distress. All the labels tell us about the organism's state at a particular moment—a moment when it may be struggling with a specific, environmental problem.

We have described our multilevel processing model and discussed some of the ways in which processes at the conceptual level may be discrepant from those at the expressive–motor and schematic levels, and how visceral activity can affect all three central neural levels of processing. At this point the reader may well ask: "How can emotions provide a readout of organismic state with so much complex machinery in the emotion system?" How can emotions provide a readout of the organism's present state if they are brought into play by conditioned schematic responding and can be minimized or canceled by anticipating their expressive–motor displays? For example, an individual may suppress his or her fatigue or depression by blocking awareness of it by anticipating its expressive components. This can also be achieved by altering attention and continuing with the task at hand. This is the situation of the coronary-prone or Type A individual, who blocks emotional responding and problem solving at the expense of his cardiovascular system (Carver, Coleman, & Glass, 1976; Glass, 1977; Matthews, 1982; see also Scheier, Carver, & Matthews, Chapter 18, this volume).

Raising this question can help deepen our understanding of the emotional processing system. Underlying the question is the assumption that fatigue, pain–distress, fear, nausea–disgust, and so on, are valid representations of our biological states. This assumption is both true and false. It is false if the biological state is taken to mean the state of our system as measured by physical instruments. It is true if the biological state includes our memory systems. For example, pain in a phantom limb does not provide information about a current body injury. There is no limb; the pain is only a memory. Conditioned nausea in cancer chemotherapy patients does not indicate that contact with their nurse is distressing to their gastrointestinal systems. It is an associative memory of past internal upsets. Hence, emotions provide more than just a readout of the current state of the machine, but also of future states, based on schematically stored experience. Emotions do not just tell us how much nausea and disgust our body may be experiencing due to contact with nausea-producing substances, but can also anticipate future nausea based on past experiences. Emotion is *invalid* as a readout of some type of "absolute" biophysical criteria of our body states, but is *not invalid* as a readout of our organismic state when state is defined as *"the state of our psychological processing system."* The conceptual and schematic histories are as important a part of the processing system as the innate, expressive–motor, and visceral levels.

If emotions serve as ongoing signals regarding the status of our inner processing machinery, it is clear that they reflect meaning (Pribram, 1970). The emotions we experience when writing a manuscript from moment to moment and from day to day reflect the status of this meaning domain. This includes a variety of professional self-referents, interpersonal experiences, and the specific substantive contents of the sections, paragraphs, sentences, and words that make up the manuscript. The emotions of a parent in response to the problems of his or her child reflect the meaning of parenthood, childhood, and the past history of the relationship between the two. We agree with Mandler (1975, 1980) and Schwanenberg (1981) that emotions are experienced in relation to meaning domains or systems. We believe that emotional systems form meaning domains. Feelings are of the present, but they reflect the past and anticipate the future. In this sense feelings often become a separate set of goals or objectives for coping. We act to minimize, maintain, and otherwise alter feeling states in ways that are more often suited to maintaining internal self-regulation than meeting the "objective" demands of external reality. In this way emotions add a dimension of mystery and a predictable irrationality to our behavior.

ACKNOWLEDGMENT

The authors wish to thank Robert Hirschman for comments on the previous draft of this chapter.

REFERENCES

Ahles, T., Blanchard, E., & Leventhal, H. Cognitive control of pain: Attention to the sensory aspects of the cold pressor stimulus. *Cognitive Behavior Therapy*, in press.

Allport, G., & Pettigrew, T. F. Cultural influence on the perception of movement: The trapezoidal illusion among Zulus. *Journal of Abnormal and Social Psychology*, 1957, 55, 104–113.

Ax, A. The physiological differentiation between fear and anger in humans. *Psychosomatic Medicine*, 1953, 15, 433–442.

Bandura, A. Self efficacy: Toward a unified theory of behavioral change. *Psychological Review*, 1977, 84, 191–215.

Barber, T. X., & Hahn, K. W., Jr. Physiological and subjective responses to pain producing stimulation under hypnotically-suggested and waking-imagined "analgesia." *Journal of Abnormal and Social Psychology*, 1962, 65, 411–418.

Beck, A. T., Rush, A. J., Shaw, B. F., & Emery, G. *Cognitive therapy of depression*. New York: Guilford, 1979.

Berkowtiz, L. Some determinants of impulsive aggression: Role of mediated associations with reinforcement for aggression. *Psychological Review*, 1974, 81, 165–176.

Berkowtiz, L. The experience of anger as a parallel process in the display of impulsive "angry" aggression. In R. G. Geen & Edward Donnerstein (Eds.), *Aggression: Theoretical and empirical issues*. New York: Academic, 1982.

Bever, T. G., & Chiarello, R. J.   Cerebral dominance in musicians and nonmusicians. *Science,* 1974, *185,* 537–539.

Bower, G. H.   Mood and memory. *American Psychologist,* 1981, *36,* 129–148.

Bower, G. H., & Cohen, P. R.   *Emotional influences in memory and thinking: Data and theory.* Unpublished manuscript, Stanford University, 1981.

Bower, G. H., & Cohen, P. R.   Emotional influences on learning and cognition. In M. S. Clark & S. T. Fiske (Eds.), *Affect and cognition: The 17th Annual Carnegie Symposium on Cognition.* Hillsdale, N.J.: Erlbaum, 1982.

Brazelton, T. B., Koslowski, B., & Main, M.   The origins of reciprocity: The early mother–infant interaction. In M. Lewis & L. A. Rosenblum (Eds.), *The effect of the infant on its caretaker.* New York: Wiley, 1974.

Broadbent, D. E.   The hidden preattentive process. *American Psychologist,* 1977, *32,* 109–118.

Broughton, R.   Sleep disorders: Disorders of arousal. *Science,* 1968, *158,* 1070–1078.

Cacioppo, J., & Petty, R.   Electromyograms as measures of extent of affectivity of information processing. *American Psychologist,* 1981, *36,* 441–456.

Cannon, W. B.   *Bodily changes in pain, hunger, fear and rage.* New York: Appleton-Century, 1929.

Carmon, A. & Nachson, I.   Ear symmetry in perception of emotional nonverbal stimuli. *Acta Psychologica,* 1973, *37,* 351–357.

Carver, C. S.   A cybernetic model of self-attention processes. *Journal of Personality and Social Psychology,* 1979, *37,* 1251–1281.

Carver, C. S., Coleman, A. E., & Glass, D. C.   The coronary-prone behavior pattern and the suppression of fatigue in a treadmill test. *Journal of Personality and Social Psychology,* 1976, *33,* 460–466.

Carver, C. S., & Scheier, M. F.   *Attention and self-regulation: A control-theory approach to human behavior.* New York: Springer-Verlag, 1981.

Casey, K. L.   Pain: A current view of neural mechanisms. *American Scientist,* 1973, *61,* 194–200.

Clark, M. S., & Fiske, S. T. (Eds.).   *Affect and cognition: The 17th Annual Carnegie Symposium on Cognition.* Hillsdale, N.J.: Erlbaum, 1982.

Clark, M. S., & Isen, A. M.   Toward understanding the relationship between affect and behavior. In A. H. Hastorf & A. M. Isen (Eds.), *Cognitive social psychology.* New York: Elsevier/North-Holland, 1982.

Clynes, M.   The sentic cycles: Passion at your fingertips. *Psychology Today,* May 1972, pp. 59–60; 68; 70; 72.

Cofer, C.   *Motivation and emotion.* Glenview, Ill.: Scott, Foresman, 1972.

Cupchik, G., & Leventhal, H.   Consistency between expressive behavior and the evaluation of humorous stimuli: The role of sex and self-observation. *Journal of Personality and Social Psychology,* 1974, *30,* 429–442.

Darwin, C.   *The expression of emotions in man and animals.* London: Murray, 1904. (Originally published, 1872).

Davidson, R. J.   Consciousness and information processing: A biocognitive perspective. In J. M. Davidson & R. J. Davidson (Eds.), *The psychobiology of consciousness.* New York: Plenum, 1980.

Davidson, R. J., Horowitz, M. E., Schwartz, G. E., & Goodman, D. M.   Lateral differences in the latency between finger tapping and heart beat. *Psychophysiology,* 1981, *18,* 36–40.

Davis, R. C.   Response patterns. *Transactions of the New York Academy of Sciences,* 1957, *19,* 731–739.

Davitz, J. R.   A dictionary and grammar of emotion. In M. B. Arnold (Ed.), *Feelings and emotions: The Loyola Symposium.* New York: Academic, 1970.

Dement, W. C.   *Some must watch while some must sleep.* Stanford, Calif.: Stanford Alumni Association, 1972.

Eibl-Eibesfeldt, I.   Strategies of social interaction. In R. Plutchik & H. Kellerman (Eds.), *Emotion: Theory, research, and experience.* New York: Academic, 1980.

Ekman, P., & Friesen, W. V.   Constants across culture in the face and emotion. *Journal of Personality and Social Psychology,* 1971, *17,* 124–129.

Ekman, P., & Friesen, W. V.   *Unmasking the face: A guide to recognizing the emotions from facial clues.* Englewood Cliffs, N.J.: Prentice-Hall, 1975.

Ekman, P., Friesen, W. V., & Ellsworth, P.   *Emotion in the human face: Guidelines for research and an integration of the findings.* Elmsford, N.Y.: Pergamon, 1972.

Erdmann, G., & Janke, W.   Interactions between physiological and cognitive determinants of emotion: Experimental studies on Schachter's theory of emotions. *Biological Psychology,* 1978, *6,* 61–74.

Eysenck, H. J.   *Biological basis of personality.* Springfield, Ill.: Charles C Thomas, 1967.

Fishbein, M. & Ajzen, I.   Attitudes toward objects as predictors of single and multiple behavioral criteria. *Psychological Review,* 1974, *81,* 59–74.

Freud, S.   *The ego and the id.* London: Hogarth Press, 1962. (Originally published, 1930.)

Frijda, N. H.   Recognition of emotion. In L. Berkowitz (Ed.), *Advances in experimental social psychology* (Vol. 4). New York: Academic, 1969.

Funkenstein, D. H., King, S. H., & Drolette, M. E.   *Mastery of stress.* Cambridge, Mass.: Harvard University Press, 1957.

Furedy, J. J., & Riley, D. M.   Classical and operant conditioning in the enhancement of biofeedback: Specifics and speculations. In L. White & B. Tursky (Eds.), *Clinical biofeedback: Efficacy and mechanisms.* New York: Guilford, 1982.

Galin, D.   Implications for psychiatry of left and right cerebral specialization. *Archives of General Psychiatry,* 1974, *31,* 572–583.

Garcia, J.   Tilting at the paper mills of academe. *American Psychologist,* 1981, *36,* 149–158.

Gellhorn, E.   Motion and emotion: The role of proprioception in the physiology and pathology of the emotions. *Psychological Review,* 1964, *71,* 457–472.

Geschwind, N.   The apraxias: Neural mechanisms of disorders of learned movement. *American Scientist,* 1975, *63,* 188–195.

Glass, D. C.   *Behavior patterns, stress, and coronary disease.* Hillsdale, N.J.: Erlbaum, 1977.

Graham, D.   Psychosomatic medicine. In N. S. Greenfield & R. A. Sternbach (Eds.), *Handbook of psychophysiology.* New York: Holt, Rinehart & Winston, 1972.

Grossberg, J. M., & Wilson, H. K.   Physiological changes accompanying the visualization of fearful and neutral situations. *Journal of Personality and Social Psychology,* 1968, *10,* 124–133.

Haggard, M. P., & Parkinson, A. M.   Stimulus and task factors as determinants of ear advantages. *Quarterly Journal of Experimental Psychology,* 1971, *23,* 168–177.

Hécaen, H.   Aphasic, apraxic and agnostic syndromes in right and left hemisphere lesions. In P. J. Vinken & G. W. Bruyn (Eds.), *Handbook of clinical neurology* (Vol. 4). Amsterdam: North-Holland, 1969.

Holmes, D., & Houston, B. K.   Effectiveness of situation redefinition and affective isolation in coping with stress. *Journal of Personality and Social Psychology,* 1974, *29,* 212–218.

Horowitz, M. J.   *Image formation and cognition.* New York: Appleton-Century-Crofts, 1970.

Izard, C. E.   *The face of emotion.* New York: Appleton-Century-Crofts, 1971.

Izard, C. E.   *Human emotions.* New York: Plenum, 1977.

James, W.   *The principles of psychology* (Vol. 2). New York: Dover, 1950. (Originally published, 1890.)

Janis, I. L.   *Psychological stress.* New York: Academic, 1974.

Janis, I. L., & Leventhal, H.   Psychological aspects of physical illness and hospital care. In B. Wollman (Ed.), *Handbook of clinical psychology.* New York: McGraw-Hill, 1965.

Jaynes, J.   *The origins of consciousness in the breakdown of the bicameral mind.* Boston: Houghton Mifflin, 1976.

Johnson, J.   Effects of accurate expectations about sensations on sensory and distress components of pain. *Journal of Personality and Social Psychology,* 1973, *27,* 261–275.

Johnson, J. E.   Stress reduction through sensation information. In I. C. Sarason & C. D. Spielberger (Eds.), *Stress and anxiety* (Vol. 2). Washington, D.C.: Hemisphere, 1975.

Johnson, J. E., & Leventhal, H.   Effects of accurate expectations and behavioral instructions on reactions during a noxious medical examination. *Journal of Personality and Social Psychology,* 1974, *29,* 710–718.

King, F. L., & Kimura, D. Left-ear superiority in dichotic perception of nonverbal sounds. *Canadian Journal of Psychology*, 1972, *26*, 111–116.

Konorski, J. *Integrative activity of the brain: An interdisciplinary approach.* Chicago: University of Chicago Press, 1967.

Lang, P. Imagery in therapy: An information processing analysis of fear. *Behavior Therapy*, 1977, *8*, 862–886.

Lang, P. J. A bio-informational theory of emotional imagery. *Psychophysiology*, 1979, *16*, 495–512.

Lang, P. J., Kozak, M. J., Miller, G. A., Levin, D. N., & McLean, A. Emotional imagery: Conceptual structure and pattern of somato-visceral response. *Psychophysiology*, 1980, *17*, 179–192.

Lazarus, R. S. *Psychological stress and the coping process.* New York: McGraw-Hill, 1966.

Lazarus, R. S. *The stress and coping paradigm.* In C. Eisdorfer, D. Cohen, A. Klienman, & P. Maxim (Eds.), *Theoretical bases for psychopathology.* New York: Spectrum, 1980.

Lazarus, R. E., & Alfert, E. The short circuiting of threat by experimentally altering cognitive appraisal. *Journal of Abnormal and Social Psychology*, 1964, *69*, 195–205.

Leeper, R. W. A motivational theory of emotion to replace "Emotion as a disorganized response." *Psychological Review*, 1948, *55*, 5–21.

Leventhal, H. Findings and theory in the study of fear communications. In L. Berkowitz (Ed.), *Advances in experimental social psychology* (Vol. 5). New York: Academic, 1970.

Leventhal H. Emotions: A basic problem for social psychology. In C. Nemeth (Ed.), *Social psychology: Classic and contemporary integrations.* Chicago: Rand McNally, 1974.

Leventhal, H. A perceptual–motor processing model of emotion. In P. Pliner, K. Blankenstein, & I. M. Spigel (Eds.), *Perception of emotion in self and others* (Vol. 5). New York: Plenum, 1979.

Leventhal, H. Toward a comprehensive theory of emotion. In L. Berkowitz (Ed.), *Advances in experimental social psychology* (Vol. 13). New York: Academic, 1980.

Leventhal, H. The integration of emotion and cognition: A view from the perceptual–motor theory of emotion. In M. S. Clark & S. T. Fiske (Eds.), *Affect and cognition: The 17th Annual Carnegie Symposium on Cognition.* Hillsdale: N.J.: Erlbaum, 1982.

Leventhal, H., Brown, D., Shacham, S., & Engquist, G. Effect of preparatory information about sensations, threat of pain and attention on cold pressor distress. *Journal of Personality and Social Psychology*, 1979, *37*, 688–714.

Leventhal, H., & Cupchik, G. A process model of humor judgment. *Journal of Communication*, 1976, *26*, 190–204.

Leventhal, H., & Everhart, D. Emotion, pain and physical illness. In C. E. Izard (Ed.), *Emotions and psychopathology.* New York: Plenum, 1979.

Leventhal, H., & Mace, W. The effect of laughter on evaluation of a slapstick movie. *Journal of Personality*, 1970, *38*, 16–30.

Leventhal, H., & Sharpe, E. Facial expressions as indicators of distress. In S. S. Tomkins & C. E. Izard (Eds.), *Affect, cognition and personality.* New York: Springer, 1965.

Leventhal, H., Singer, R., & Jones, S. Effects of fear and specificity of recommendations upon attitudes and behavior. *Journal of Personality and Social Psychology*, 1965, *2*, 1965.

Ley, R. G., & Bryden, M. P. Hemispheric differences in processing emotions and faces. *Brain and Language*, 1979, *7*, 127–138.

Luria, A. R. *The working brain.* New York: Basic Books, 1973.

MacLean, P. D. Contrasting functions of limbic and neocortical systems of the brain and their relevance to psychophysiological aspects of medicine. *American Journal of Medicine*, 1958, *25*, 611–626.

Mandler, G. Emotion. In R. Brown, E. Galanter, E. H. Hess, & G. Mandler (Eds.), *New directions in psychology* (Vol. 1). New York: Holt, Rinehart & Winston, 1962.

Mandler, G. *Mind and emotion.* New York: Wiley, 1975.

Mandler, G. The generation of emotion: A psychological theory. In R. Plutchik & H. Kellerman (Eds.), *Emotion: Theory, research, and experience.* New York: Academic, 1980.

Mandler, G., & Kessen, W.   *The language of psychology*. New York: Wiley, 1959.

Marshall, G. D., & Zimbardo, P. G.   Affective consequences of inadequately explained physiological arousal. *Journal of Personality and Social Psychology*, 1979, *37*, 970–985.

Maslach, C.   Negative emotional biasing of unexplained arousal. *Journal of Personality and Social Psychology*, 1979, *37*, 953–969.

Matthews, K. A.   Psychological perspectives on the Type A behavior pattern. *Psychological Bulletin*, 1982, *91*, 293–323.

McDougall, W.   Emotion and feelings distinguished. In M. L. Reymert (Ed.), *Feelings and emotion*. Worcester, Mass.: Clark University Press, 1928.

McGeer, P. L., & McGeer, E. G.   Chemistry of mood and emotion. *Annual Review of Psychology*, 1980, *31*, 273–307.

McKechnie, R. J.   Relief from phantom limb pain by relaxation exercises. *Journal of Behavior Therapy and Experimental Psychiatry*, 1975, *6*, 262–263.

Mechanic, D.   Discussion of research programs on relations between stressful life events and episodes of physical illness. In B. Dohrenwend & B. Dohrenwend (Eds.), *Stressful life events: Their nature and effects*. New York: Wiley, 1974.

Mechanic, D., & Volkart, E. H.   Stress, illness behavior, and the sick role. *American Sociological Review*, 1961, *26*, 51–58.

Melzack, R.   *The puzzle of pain: Revolution in theory and treatment*. New York: Basic Books, 1973.

Money, J.   Phantom orgasm in dreams of paraplegic men and women. *Archives of General Psychiatry*, 1960, *3*, 373–383.

Moscovitch, M., Scullion, D., & Christie, D.   Early versus late stages of processing and their relation to functional hemispheric asymmetries in face recognition. *Journal of Experimental Psychology: Human Perception and Performance*, 1976, *2*, 401–416.

Mueller, C. W., & Donnerstein, E.   Film-facilitated arousal and prosocial behavior. *Journal of Experimental Social Psychology*, 1981, *17*, 31–41.

Neisser, U.   *Cognitive psychology*. New York: Appleton-Century-Crofts, 1967.

Nerenz, D. R., Leventhal, H., & Love, R. R.   Factors contributing to emotional distress during cancer chemotherapy. *Cancer*, 1982, *50*, 1020–1027.

Nowlis, V. L.   Research with the mood adjective checklist. In S. S. Tomkins & C. E. Izard (Eds.), *Affect, cognition and personality*. New York: Springer, 1965.

Osgood, C. E.   Dimensionality of the semantic space for communication via facial expression. *Scandinavian Journal of Psychology*, 1966, *7*, 1–30.

Piaget, J.   *Six psychological studies*. New York: Randon House, 1968.

Piaget, J.   *Mental imagery in the child: A study of the development of imaginal representations*. New York: Basic Books, 1971.

Plutchik, R.   *Emotion: A psychoevolutionary synthesis*. New York: Harper & Row, 1980.

Posner, M. I., & Snyder, C. R.   Attention and cognitive control. In R. Solso (Ed.), *Information process and cognition: The Loyola Symposium*. Hillsdale, N.J.: Erlbaum, 1975.

Pribram, K. H.   Feelings as monitors. In M. B. Arnold (Ed.), *Feelings and emotions: The Loyola Symposium*. New York: Academic, 1970.

Reinhardt, L. C.   *Attention and interpretation in control of cold pressor pain distress*. Unpublished doctoral dissertation, University of Wisconsin, Madison, 1979.

Riley, D. M., & Furedy, J. J.   Psychological and physiological systems: Modes of operation and interaction. In S. R. Burchfield (Ed.), *Stress: Psychological and physiological interaction*. Washington, D.C.: Hemisphere, in press.

Robinson, D.   *The process of becoming ill*. Boston: Routledge & Kegan Paul, 1971.

Rosen, T. J., Terry, N. S., & Leventhal, H.   The role of esteem and coping in response to a threat communication. *Journal of Research in Personality*, 1982, *16*, 90–107.

Russell, B.   *An outline of philosophy*. New York: Meridian Books, 1960. (Originally published, 1927.)

Sackeim, H., & Gur, R. C.   Lateral asymmetry in intensity of emotional expression. *Neuropsychologia*, 1978, *16*, 473–481.

Safer, M. A.   Sex and hemisphere differences in access to codes for processing emotional expressions and faces. *Journal of Experimental Psychology: General*, 1981, *110*, 86–100.

Safer, M. A., & Leventhal, H.   Ear differences in evaluating emotional tones of voice and verbal content. *Journal of Experimental Psychology: Human Perception and Performance*, 1977, *3*, 75–82.

Schachter, J.   Pain, fear and anger in hypertensives and normotensives: A psychophysiological study. *Psychosomatic Medicine*, 1957, *19*, 17–19.

Schachter, S.   The interaction of cognitive and physiological determinants of emotional state. In L. Berkowitz (Ed.), *Advances in experimental social psychology* (Vol. 1). New York: Academic, 1964.

Schachter, S., & Singer, J. E.   Cognitive, social, and physiological determinants of emotional state. *Psychological Review*, 1962, *69*, 377–399.

Schwanenberg, E.   Sozilaler affect: Konstrucktüberprüfung des Schachter-paradigmas. In W. Michaelis (Ed.), *Bericht über den 32. Kongress der Deutschen Gesellschaft für Psychologie, Zürich 1980*. Göttingen: Hogrefe, 1981.

Schwartz, G. E., Fair, P. L., Mandel, M. R., Salt, P., & Klerman, G. L.   Facial electromyography in the assessment of improvement in depression. *Psychosomatic Medicine*, 1976, *38*, 337–347.

Semmes, J.   Hemisheric specialization: A possible clue to mechanism. *Neuropsychologia*, 1968, *6*, 11–27.

Shacham, S.   *The effects of imagery monitoring, sensation monitoring and positive suggestion on pain and distress*. Unpublished doctoral dissertation, University of Wisconsin, Madison, 1979.

Simmel, M. L.   The reality of phantom sensations. *Social Research*, 1962, *29*, 337–356.

Simon, H. A.   Comments on Bower and Cohen's presentation on emotional influences on learning and cognition. In M. S. Clark & S. T. Fiske (Eds.), *Affect and cognition: The 17th Annual Carnegie Symposium on Cognition*. Hillsdale, N.J.: Erlbaum, 1982.

Sternbach, R. A.   *Principles of psychophysiology*. New York: Academic, 1966.

Suberi, M., & McKeever, W. F.   Differential right hemispheric memory storage of emotional and non-emotional faces. *Neuropsychologia*, 1977, *15*, 757–768.

Sully, J.   *An essay on laughter*. London: Longmans, Green, 1902.

Svebak, S.   Styles in humor and social self-images. *Scandinavian Journal of Psychology*, 1975, *16*, 79–84.

Tomkins, S. S.   *Affect, imagery, consciousness* (Vol. 1), *The positive affects*. New York: Springer, 1962.

Tomkins, S. S.   Affect as amplification: Some modifications in theroy. In R. Plutchik & H. Kellerman (Eds.), *Emotion: Theory, research, and experience*. New York: Academic, 1980.

Tomkins, S. S., & McCarter, R.   What and where are the primary affects? Some evidence for a theory. *Perceptual and Motor Skills*, 1964, *18*, 119–158.

Tourangeau, R., & Ellsworth, P. C.   The role of facial response in the experience of emotion. *Journal of Personality and Social Psychology*, 1979, *37*, 1519–1531.

Tucker, D. M.   Lateral brain function, emotion and conceptualization. *Psychological Bulletin*, 1981, *89*, 19–46.

Turner, C. W., & Layton, J. F.   Verbal imagery and connotation as memory induced mediators of aggressive behavior. *Journal of Personality and Social Psychology*, 1976, *33*, 755–763.

Walters, R. H., & Parke, R. D.   Social motivation, dependency, and susceptibility to social influence. In L. Berkowitz (Ed.), *Advances in experimental social psychology* (Vol. 1). New York: Academic, 1964.

Weiner, B.   *The emotional consequences of causal ascriptions*. Unpublished manuscript, University of California, Los Angeles, 1981.

Weiskrantz, L., Elliott, J., & Darlington, C.   Preliminary observations on tickling oneself. *Nature (London)*, 1971, *230*, 598–599.

Witkin, H. A., & Lewis, H. B.   Pre-sleep experiences and dreams. In H. A. Witkin & H. B. Lewis (Eds.), *Experimental studies of dreaming*. New York: Random House, 1967.

Woodworth, R. S., & Schlosberg, H.   *Experimental psychology* (rev. ed.). New York: Holt, 1954.

Zajonc, R. B. Feeling and thinking: Preferences need no inferences. *American Psychologist*, 1980, *35*, 151–175.

Zillmann, D. Attribution and misattribution of excitatory reactions. In J. H. Harvey, W. Ickes, & R. F. Kidd (Eds.), *New directions in attribution research* (Vol. 2). Hillsdale, N.J.: Erlbaum, 1978.

Zillmann, D. *Hostility and aggression*. Hillsdale, N.J.: Erlbaum, 1979.

Zillmann, D., Katcher, A. H., & Milavsky, B. Excitation transfer from physical exercise to subsequent aggressive behavior. *Journal of Personality and Social Psychology*, 1972, *8*, 247–259.

Zola, I. K. Pathways to the doctor—from person to patient. *Social Science and Medicine*, 1973, *7*, 677–689.

Zuckerman, M., Klorman, R., Larrance, D. T., & Spiegel, N. H. Facial, autonomic, and subjective components of emotion: The facial feedback hypothesis versus the externalizer–internalizer distinction. *Journal of Personality and Social Psychology*, 1981, *41*, 929–944.

C · INTERPERSONAL PROCESSES

The Psychophysiology of Extraversion–Introversion

Russell G. Geen
University of Missouri–Columbia

INTRODUCTION

Extraversion-introversion (E-I), as discussed by H. J. Eysenck (1957, 1967), is one dimension of a two-dimensional theory of personality that is somewhat unique among personality theories in that it is based on assumptions of individual differences in neurophysiology. The differences that one ordinarily observes between introverts and extraverts, such as the greater sociability of the latter, are traced by Eysenck to the hypothesized physiological differences. As a general introduction to the theory, it can be stated that introverts are more "arousable" than extraverts. If we assume that overly high levels of arousal are aversive and to be avoided, it follows that the introvert should seek out situations that provide relatively little stimulation, whereas the extravert should show stronger signs of stimulus need. It is for this reason that introverts tend to be less sociable than extraverts, more likely to wear clothing that is conservative in cut and color, better able to detect stimuli of low intensity, and less able to tolerate stimuli of high intensity (see H. J. Eysenck, 1967, for a review of findings on these matters). The variable of extraversion–introversion has, in fact, been found to correlate with another dimension of personality directly relevant to stimulus seeking, as measured by Zuckerman's Sensation-Seeking Scale (S. Eysenck & Zuckerman, 1978).

As the chapters of this book indicate, research in several areas of social psychology is based to some degree on an assumption that arousal processes mediate social behaviors. An individual difference variable founded on the arousal construct may therefore have some value for such research. Consideration of individual difference variables as possible moderators of situational effects plays an important role in current "interactionist" views of personality (Endler & Magnusson, 1976). Furthermore, Eysenck's extraversion–introversion variable consists of two components, one related to sociability and the other to impulsiveness, suggesting links to such social psychological processes as interpersonal attraction and decision making. Finally, research on influences of extraversion–introversion on behaviors such as signal detection and tolerance for stimulation indicates that the variable may be useful in personnel selection, job assignment, and related applications. For example, the relatively great sensitivity of introverts to weak or infrequent signals indicates that such persons might be admirably suited to jobs involving radar detection.

The other dimension in Eysenck's theory of personality is neuroticism (N), a variable conceptually similar to anxiety. Both the E-I and N have usually been measured by means of a personality inventory originally introduced by H. J. Eysenck (1962) as the Maudsley Personality Inventory (MPI), a 48-item paper-and-pencil self-report form. The MPI was followed by the Eysenck Personality Inventory (EPI), a 57-item test that added to the E-I and N items a Lie subscale for detection of dissimulation (H. J. Eysenck & Eysenck, 1968b). Most of the studies reviewed in this chapter involved use of either the MPI or the EPI for assessment of E-I and N. A few did not, however, and they will be described in footnotes to Tables 13-1 and 13-2, which indicate the measure of E-I used in each study reviewed.

Extraversion–introversion and neuroticism were originally derived as higher-order traits from factor analysis of case histories, interview data, and scores on personality inventories (H. J. Eysenck, 1957). The first attempt to explain their bases in terms of underlying physiological processes was built on the Pavlovian concepts of excitation and inhibition. The extravert was defined as one in whom hypothetical excitatory potentials develop slowly, dissipate rapidly, and are relatively weak, whereas inhibitory potentials develop rapidly, dissipate slowly, and are relatively strong. The exact opposite in each case was said to characterize the introvert. In his later writing, H. J. Eysenck (1967) has related both E-I and N to specific structures in the nervous system. Extraverts are now described as showing relatively high thresholds for activity in the ascending reticular activating system (ARAS), and introverts as showing relatively low thresholds for activity in that structure. The neurological foundation of neuroticism is located in the limbic system, with persons high in N showing low thresholds for limbic arousal and persons low in N showing correspondingly high thresholds. The E-I and N variables are not independent of each other, because various ascending and descending pathways link the ARAS with the hypothalamus (see Figure 1-4). The ARAS thus connects with both the cerebral cortex and the limbic system. The latter point is important to note because it forms the basis for using measures of "emotional" arousal mediated by the autonomic nervous system as indicators of individual differences in E-I. A modification of Eysenck's model has been advocated by Gray (1972), who proposed that the neurological foundation of E-I includes not just the ARAS, but also the hippocampus, a limbic structure, and the orbital frontal cortex and medial septal area, both of which connect to the limbic system. Gray's model thus appears to have the advantage of providing for a more direct description of the reported autonomic differences between introverts and extraverts than does Eysenck's, although both give adequate accounts of the data. Both also support the generalization that introverts are more arousable than extraverts in terms of both cortical and autonomically mediated activity.

In the review to follow, the N variable will be mentioned only in connection with the few studies that have reported E-I effects to be moderated by neuroticism. Most experiments on E-I do not deal with N as a source of variance, but instead control for it in sampling subjects.

Considerable evidence pertaining to the hypothesis of greater arousability in introverts has come from psychophysiological studies. The purpose of the present chapter is to review this evidence, which has been organized along four topical lines. We review studies of (1) cortical arousal, (2) habituation of the orienting reflex (OR), (3) autonomic activation outside the context of OR habituation, and (4) reversal of the extravert-introvert difference at high levels of stimulation.

EXTRAVERSION–INTROVERSION AND CORTICAL AROUSAL

If extraversion–introversion is related to individual differences in activity within the reticular–hypothalamic system, we might expect that it would manifest itself in predictable differences in arousal in the cerebral cortex. Specifically, extraverts should show lower levels of cortical activity than introverts. The data do not permit such a simple conclusion, however. For one thing, as most of the studies cited will show, extravert–introvert differences in psychophysiological activity often depend on the precise experimental conditions imposed and tasks used. For another, "cortical arousal" may refer to any of several indicators of cortical activity, and studies sometimes find evidence of E-I differences for one measure but not others. In this section we review studies on three measures of cortical activity: the EEG, the evoked potential, and contingent negative variation.

EEG

The electroencephalogram (EEG) is a complex waveform consisting of several frequencies. Four bandwidths are usually studied: delta (1.5 to 4.5 Hz), theta (4.5 to 6.5 Hz), alpha (7.5 to 13.5 Hz), and beta (13.5 to 20.0 Hz). Most of the studies on E-I differences in the EEG reviewed here have involved measurement of alpha, and several different measures of alpha activity have been reported. Besides frequency, the most common descriptor has been amplitude, which describes the area under the tracing of the waveform. In general terms, large alpha amplitude and low frequency are associated with relatively low cortical arousal, whereas low amplitude and high frequency indicate high arousal. Displacement of the former by the latter is termed alpha blocking. In addition, two other measures are sometimes reported. One describes the area under the waveform curve associated with a particular frequency over a fixed period of time, and is designated as alpha abundance. The other refers to the proportion of time occupied by alpha activity within a given period, and is called the alpha index.

More data have been reported on E-I differences in the EEG than on any other measure of cortical activity. Most of this literature is summarized in an excellent review by Gale (1973), who discusses 13 studies reported between 1938 and 1972.[1] It would be redundant to re-review these studies. The reader is therefore advised to consult Gale's paper to learn not only the outcomes of the major studies but also the major flaws in the research reported to that time. Briefly stated, Gale found that the existing evidence allowed no firm conclusions regarding the role of E-I in EEG activity. Of the 13 studies, three indicated that extraverts were more aroused than introverts (Broadhurst & Glass, 1969; McAdam & Orme, 1954; Mundy-Castle, 1955), four showed extraverts as less aroused (Gale, Coles, & Blaydon, 1969; Gottlober, 1938; Marton & Urban, 1971; Savage, 1964), and six showed no evidence of extravert–introvert differences (Claridge & Herrington, 1963; Fenton & Scotton, 1967; Gale, Coles, Kline, & Penfold, 1971; Gale, Harpham, & Lucas, 1972; Henry & Knott, 1941; Winter, Broadhurst, & Glass, 1972). Nine of the 12 studies thus reported findings inconsistent with the simple prediction of greater cortical arousal in introverts.

All in all, the data reviewed by Gale offer little indication that E-I is related to EEG activity in the simple manner suggested in the beginning of this section. Much of the inconsistency in the findings may, of course, be due to variable procedures, the use of different EEG measures, selection of subjects, experimenter instructions, and many other variables. Table 13-1 gives a summary of the 13 studies reviewed by Gale and of two more recent experiments. Some of the difficulties involved in drawing general conclusions from a heterogeneous mix of studies are obvious from this summary.

Evoked Potentials

Presentation of a stimulus such as a tone or a light may elicit a low-voltage response that occurs against the background of higher-voltage EEG activity. These evoked potentials (EPs) are extracted from the EEG records by a technique of averaging across a large number of such responses. Several

---

1. A fourteenth study reviewed by Gale (Nebylitsyn, 1963) is of questionable relevance to E-I, as Gale has noted.

TABLE 13-1. Summary of EEG Studies

STUDY	MEASURE OF E-I	TASK OR CONDITION	MAIN MEASURE	OUTCOME
Gottlober (1938)	Nebraska Personality Inventory (NPI)*	Resting	Alpha index	E's less aroused than I's
Henry & Knott (1941)	NPI	Resting	Alpha index	No E-I difference
Mundy-Castle (1955)	Primary–secondary function†	Resting	Alpha frequency	E's more aroused than I's
McAdam & Orme (1954)	Structured interview	Resting	Alpha index	E's more aroused than I's
Savage (1964)	Maudsley Personality Inventory (MPI)	Resting	Alpha abundance	E's less aroused than I's
Claridge & Herrington (1963)	MPI	Observation of Archimedes spiral	Alpha abundance	No E-I difference
Fenton & Scotton (1967)	MPI	Resting	Alpha index	No E-I difference
Broadhurst & Glass (1969)	MPI	Performance of mental arithmetic	Alpha index and amplitude	E's more aroused than I's
Gale, Coles, & Blaydon (1969)	Eysenck personality Inventory (EPI)	Eyes open and closed on command	Alpha abundance	E's less aroused than I's
Gale, Coles, Kline, & Penfold (1971)	EPI	Resting	Alpha abundance	No E-I difference
Marton & Urban (1971)	Not specified	Weak auditory stimulation	Alpha frequency and index	E's less aroused than I's
Gale, Harpham, & Lucas (1972)	EPI	Resting	Alpha abundance	No E-I difference
Winter, Broadhurst, & Glass (1972)	EPI	Eyes open and closed, mental arithmetic	Alpha amplitude	No E-I difference
Deakin & Exley (1979)	EPI	Resting	Alpha amplitude	E's less aroused than I's
Gilliland, Andress, & Bracy (1981)	EPI	Resting	Alpha index	E's less aroused than I's

*Guilford & Guilford (1936)

†P-S function (Biesheuvel, 1949) is considered to be practically synonymous with E-I by H. J. Eysenck (1953).

variables influence evoked potentials, including stimulus intensity, the sense modality stimulated, rate and regularity of stimulus presentation, age, sex, overall arousal levels, and attention (Tecce, 1972). Extraversion–introversion may also moderate the amplitude of the evoked potential, although few data relevant to the relationship can be marshaled and the findings are not entirely consistent with each other. Rust (1975) found no E-I differences in auditory potentials elicited by a tone. Two other studies have reported E-I differences in amplitude of the auditory evoked response, but for different components of the reaction.

Friedman and Meares (1979) found that extraverts showed greater amplitude of the late (P_2N_2) component of the evoked auditory potential[2] than did introverts when a tone of 1000 Hz was presented at an intensity of 55 dB. They also found a slight tendency toward a larger amplitude of the earlier N_1P_2 component in introverts than in extraverts. The visual evoked responses of extraverts and introverts revealed a similar effect for the late component: larger amplitude in extraverts than introverts. Extraverts and introverts did not differ in amplitude of the N_1P_2 component of the evoked visual response, however.

The findings of Friedman and Meares (1979) are generally consistent with those of Stelmack, Achorn, and Michaud (1977), who studied amplitude of the earlier N_1P_2 component of the auditory evoked potential. These investigators found greater amplitude in introverts than in extraverts in response to a relatively low-frequency (500 Hz) tone presented at either 55- or 80-dB intensity, but no E-I differences at either intensity to a tone of 8000-Hz frequency. Tones presented at an intensity of 40 dB at either high or low frequency did not elicit reliable E-I differences. Thus, in terms of the component of the EP analyzed in both studies (N_1P_2), introverts were found to be more cortically aroused than extraverts by both Friedman and Meares (1979) and Stelmack et al. (1977). Extraverts may be more aroused in terms of the later component of the EP, however. It is difficult to compare the two studies with any greater precision, however, because they differ in more than one way. Not only did Stelmack et al. (1977) use tones of a wider range of intensities and quantify the AEP over a narrower period of time than Friedman and Meares (1979), but they also used tones of different frequencies. Much of the confusion could be cleared up by a single study in which tones of variable frequency are used and EP is quantified across the entire period of the response. A more recent study by Andress and Church (1981) suggests that stimulus intensity may also be a variable moderating extravert–introvert differences in the auditory evoked potential. Measuring evoked potentials at the level of the brainstem, these investigators found evidence of greater inhibition in extraverts than introverts when clicks at 80-dB intensity were used, but no E-I differences in response to clicks at three lower levels of intensity. However, Campbell, Baribeau-Braun, and Braun (1981) also recorded auditory EP in response to auditory clicks of varying intensity at the level of the brainstem and found no E-I differences. It is difficult to generalize across such contradictory data. We must conclude that the findings on evoked potentials support Eysenck's hypothesis that introverts are more arousable than

2. The evoked auditory potential is described by a complex waveform composed of an early positive peak (about 50 to 100 msec after the stimulus), an early negative peak (100 to 150 msec), a late positive peak (150 to 200 msec), and a late negative peak (250 to 300 msec). These four peaks are referred to, respectively, as P_1, N_1, P_2, and N_2.

extraverts only when an early component of the potential is analyzed. The relationship may not hold, or even be reversed, when a late component is studied. Nothing in Eysenck's theory predicts or accounts for such possible fine-grained differences between introverts and extraverts. Of course, we must be extremely cautious in drawing conclusions on the basis of such a mere handful of studies. Nevertheless, future attempts to link E-I differences to evoked potentials will have to take into account exactly where in the brain such differences become manifest, as Campbell *et al.* (1981) have suggested.

Contingent Negative Variation

In addition to the brief positive and negative components of the evoked potential, another, slower potential has been observed in studies involving the association of two successive stimuli. This has been called contingent negative variation (CNV), and it is generally found in connection with an experimental paradigm in which the subject receives a warning stimulus followed within a short time by a signal requiring a motor response. The CNV has been discussed in terms of a number of variables (Tecce, 1972), and has recently been studied as a concomitant of extravert–introvert differences. Two experiments have tested differences between extraverts and introverts in CNV amplitude under conditions of either high stimulation (white noise) or low stimulation (no noise). In both studies (Janssen, Mattie, Plooij-Van Gorsel, & Werre, 1978; Plooij-Van Gorsel & Janssen, 1980) it was shown that extraverts showed greater CNV amplitude than introverts under conditions of noise, but essentially no difference under normal stimulation.

It has been suggested by some investigators (e.g., Knott & Irwin, 1973) that the resting dc level of the brain becomes more negative under stressful or arousing conditions. It has also been shown that the baseline or resting brain dc level is negatively related to CNV amplitude (Low, 1969). A person who is highly aroused in general would therefore be expected to show a CNV of smaller amplitude than one who is generally less aroused. The relatively small CNV shown by stimulated introverts may therefore be due to their higher overall level of arousal. Such reasoning is consistent with Eysenck's point of view.

EXTRAVERSION–INTROVERSION AND HABITUATION OF THE ORIENTING RESPONSE

If introverts are generally more arousable than extraverts, we would expect them to generate less inhibition during repeated presentations of a stimulus and hence to habituate more slowly. With few exceptions, studies

TABLE 13-2. Summary of Psychophysiology Studies

STUDY	E-I MEASURE	TREATMENT	MEASURE	OUTCOME*
Rust (1975)	PEN†	1000-Hz, 55/75/95-dB tones	Auditory EP	No support
Friedman & Meares (1979)	EPI	1000-Hz, 55-dB tone	Auditory and visual EP	Partial support
Stelmack, Bourgeois, Chien, & Pickard (1979)	EPI	1000- or 8000-Hz tone at 40, 55, or 80 dB	Auditory EP	Partial support
Andress & Church (1981)	EPI	80-dB auditory clicks	Auditory EP	Support
Campbell, Baribeau-Braun, & Braun (1981)	EPI	20-, 30-, 50-, 70-dB clicks	Auditory EP	No support
Janssen, Mattie, Plooij-Van Gorsel, & Werre (1978)	MPI‡	400-Hz, 64-dB tone; 12-lux light; background noise 58 dB or no noise	CNV	Support
Plooij-Van Gorsel & Janssen (1980)	MPI	750-Hz, 60-dB tone; 12-lux light; background noise 60 dB or no noise	CNV	Support
Crider & Lunn (1971)	MMPI§	1000-Hz, 90-dB tone	GSR habituation	Support
Coles, Gale, & Kline (1971)	MPI	1000-Hz, 65-dB tone	GSR habituation	No support
Koriat, Averill, & Malmstrom (1973)	EPI	1000-Hz, 75-dB tone	Spontaneous GSR and HR habituation	Partial support
Stelmack, Bourgeois, Chien, & Pickard (1979)	EPI	Colors and verbal stimuli	GSR and HR habituation	Support
Mangan & O'Gorman (1969)	EPI	1000-Hz, 60-dB tone	GSR habituation	Support
Sadler, Mefford, & Houck (1971)	EPI	Verbal stimuli	GSR habituation	Support
Wigglesworth & Smith (1976)	EPI	1000-Hz, 80/100-dB tone	GSR habituation	Partial support
Smith & Wigglesworth (1978)	EPI	1000-Hz, 60/80/100-dB tone	GSR habituation	Partial support
Smith, Wilson, & Rypma (1981)	EPI	1000-Hz, 90-dB tone; over-habituation trials at 60/100/140 dB	GSR habituation	Partial support
Purohit (1966)	MPI	500-Hz, 120-dB tone	GSR and HR conditioning	No support
Hastrup (1979)	EPI	1000-Hz, 65-dB tone	SC fluctuation	No support
Feij & Orlebeke (1974)	MPI	Spiral aftereffect	SC	No support
Gange, Geen, & Harkins (1979)	EPI	Signal detection	SC and HR	Support
Thackray, Jones, & Touchstone (1974)	EPI	Serial reaction time	HR variability	Partial support
Hinton & Craske (1977)	EPI	Stressful examination	HR	Support
Holmes (1967)	MPI	Light from 100-W bulb	Pupillary response	Support

TABLE 13-2. (*Continued*)

STUDY	E-I MEASURE	TREATMENT	MEASURE	OUTCOME*
Stelmack & Mandelzys (1975)	EPI	Neutral and taboo words	Pupillary response	Support
Hinton & Craske (1976)	PEN	Tones varying from 40 to 14,000 Hz and light flashes (no intensity given)	MAP	Support
Fine & Sweeney (1968)	MPI	Cold stress	Secretion of catecholamines	No support
Seagraves (1970)	MPI and PEN	Normal daily routine	Secretion of adrenal cortico-steroids	No support
Keister & McLaughlin (1972)	EPI	Signal detection	Percent correct	Support
Geen (1981)	EPI	Verbal learning	GSR and HR	Support
Revelle, Amaral, & Turriff (1976)	EPI	Verbal task and caffeine	Verbal perform-ance	Partial support
Gilliland (1980)	EPI	Verbal task and caffeine	Verbal perform-ance	Partial support
Smith, Rypma, & Wilson (1981)	EPI	1000-Hz, 100-dB tone and caffeine	GSR habituation	Support
Fowles, Roberts, & Nagel (1977)	Ego control and resiliency scales‖	Noise and task; 1000-Hz, 83/103-dB tone	GSR	Support

*Support/no support for hypothesis of greater arousability in introverts.

†Psychoticism–extraversion–neuroticism scale (H. J. Eysenck & Eysenck, 1968a).

‡Dutch equivalent.

§(-R) scale from Minnesota Multiphasic Personality Inventory.

‖Block (1965).

of E-I and habituation have involved measures of skin conductance within a single experimental session.[3] The evidence from these studies has been inconclusive. Crider and Lunn (1971) found that extraverts habituated more readily to a 90-dB, 1300-Hz tone than did introverts. However, Coles, Gale, and Kline (1971) found no evidence of extravert–introvert differences in habituation of the electrodermal orienting response (OR) to

3. The typical paradigm for studying the electrodermal OR consists of (1) a baseline measure; followed by (2) measurement of the response to the initial presentation of a standard stimulus; (3) repeated presentation of the standard stimulus until some criterion for habituation has been reached; (4) measurement of the response to a test stimulus of the same intensity as the standard, but of a different frequency; and (5) measurement of the response to the standard

a 65-dB, 1000-Hz tone. They did find, however, that introverts emitted more spontaneous skin conductance responses during the habituation series than did extraverts. Another failure to show E-I effects on habituation was reported by Koriat, Averill, and Malmstrom (1973) in a study that included measures of both skin conductance and heart rate.

By contrast, Stelmack, Bourgeois, Chien, and Pickard (1979) reported convincing evidence of extravert–introvert differences in an experiment that involved both multiple physiological measures and two different habituation stimuli presented in two sessions. Introverts were found to habituate more slowly to both chromatic and verbal stimuli, with both GSR and vasomotor activity used as measures. Neither type of stimulus revealed a personality difference for heart rate. In a follow-up experiment Stelmack and his colleagues also found that introverts responded with greater skin conductance amplitude to the initial presentation of the habituation stimulus than did extraverts.

It is obvious from the studies cited here that making comparisons across experiments is hampered by lack of uniformity in the choices of stimuli used for habituation. Further difficulties arise from different ways in which the variable of neuroticism (N) is treated. Theoretically, neuroticism should be associated with individual differences in activation only under conditions of emotional excitement and thus should not have any effect on habituation in studies using simple stimuli of moderate intensity. Nevertheless, habituation of the OR has been shown to be related to neuroticism by Coles et al. (1971), whereas, as already noted, it was not related to E-I. Other investigators have suggested that N interacts with E-I to influence habituation of the OR, but the precise nature of the interaction is unclear. Mangan and O'Gorman (1969) found that introverts who were also low in N habituated more slowly to a tone than both high-N introverts and low-N extraverts. No data on high-N extraverts were reported. Thus, the only comparison possible between E's and I's with N controlled revealed the expected slower habituation for Is under conditions of low N. Consistent with this finding, Sadler, Mefferd, and Houck (1971) reported slower habituation in introverts than in extraverts when both were low in N. However, Sadler et al. found that E-I and N interacted, so that under conditions of high N, extraverts showed slower habituation than introverts. It should also be noted that Stelmack et al. (1979) used only subjects who had N scores comparable to the high N's in the studies by Mangan and O'Gorman (1969) and Sadler et al. (1971), yet they found predictable E-I

---

stimulus, reintroduced one time. The latter measure allows an inference of the degree to which the novel test stimulus has produced dishabituation to the standard. Dishabituation may be defined in operational terms as the reoccurrence of a previously habituated response following the interposition of a novel stimulus.

differences. Finally, Smith and Wigglesworth (1978; Wigglesworth & Smith, 1976) made neuroticism a variable in two studies and found that it did not interact with E-I on any dependent variables. It would appear, therefore, that neuroticism may be involved in habituation of the electrodermal OR to simple stimuli, but the exact nature of that involvement is yet to be stipulated.

Considerable variability in results characterizes other studies that generally support the hypothesis of E-I differences in habituation. The findings of these studies may be summarized in terms of three dependent variables: amplitude of response to the initial presentation of the stimulus, the rate of habituation, and reactivity following the habituation series (see footnote 3).

Initial Response

Extraverts and introverts have been shown not to differ in response to the first stimulus presentation when the stimulus is a 1000-Hz tone of 60-dB intensity (Mangan & O'Gorman, 1969; Smith & Wigglesworth, 1978). When the 1000-Hz tone is of 80-dB intensity, introverts sometimes respond with higher conductance levels than extraverts, indicating greater arousability (Wigglesworth & Smith, 1976), but sometimes are equal to extraverts in response (Smith & Wigglesworth, 1978). The fact that such contradictory evidence was reported from the same laboratory, in two studies that were presumably run under comparable conditions, must make us wonder about the reliability of the finding. Furthermore, when the habituation stimulus is presented at an intensity level of 90 dB, again no differences are found between introverts and extraverts in response to the first presentation (Smith, Wilson, & Rypma, 1981). Finally, when the stimulus is presented at an intensity of 100 dB, extraverts show greater electrodermal reactivity than do introverts (Wigglesworth & Smith, 1976). This finding may indicate that the greater arousability of introverts may hold only at low to moderate levels of stimulation, and that at higher levels introverts begin to show a decline in reactivity while extraverts are still generating excitation. This matter is discussed at greater length in the final section of the chapter. We should note, however, that in a study subsequent to the one cited here (Smith & Wigglesworth, 1978) a 100-dB tone did not elicit different responses in introverts and extraverts.

Habituation Rate

Stimulus intensity levels may also play a part in the habituation rates of extraverts and introverts. Wigglesworth and Smith (1976) found no E-I differences with tones of either 80- or 100-dB intensity, whereas Smith

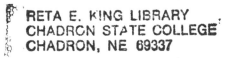

and Wigglesworth (1978) found that introverts habituated more slowly than extraverts to a 100-dB tone but not to a tone of either 60 or 80 dB. Matters are further complicated by the finding of Smith, Wilson, and Rypma (1981) of no E-I differences in habituation where the tone was presented at an intensity level of 90 dB.

Posthabituation Arousal

The most consistent findings relating E-I to physiological change in the habituation experiment pertain to events that follow the habituation series. Dishabituation is one such effect, as shown in studies by Wigglesworth and Smith (1976) and Smith and Wigglesworth (1978). The procedure followed in both studies consisted of repeated presentation of a 1000-Hz tone at a specified intensity either for a fixed number of times or until some stated criterion for GSR habituation was attained. This was followed by a single presentation of a test stimulus of a different frequency from that of the standard stimulus. Finally, the standard stimulus was presented again to test for effects of dishabituation produced by the interposition of the test stimulus. In both experiments Smith and Wigglesworth found that introverts dishabituated more than extraverts. If we assume that speed of dishabituation is a function of arousability, this finding supports Eysenck's viewpoint.

Extraversion–introversion has also been shown to be related to over-habituation. Sokolov (1963) has noted that repeated presentation of the stimulus past the point at which the subject becomes habituated to it may produce a paradoxical return of sensitivity. The reason for this, Sokolov argues, is that overhabituation (i.e., repetitious presentation of the stand-ard stimulus after habituation has occurred) induces cortical inhibition, which in turn leads to a release of lower centers from cortical control. In addition, Sokolov has proposed that overhabituation training, and the inhibition that builds up as a result, should enhance the novelty of a test stimulus that follows the series, so that the longer the overhabituation series, the greater the magnitude of the response to the test stimulus.

In a study designed to test these hypotheses, and to extend them to individual differences in E-I, Smith, Wilson, and Rypma (1981) first habituated subjects to a 90-dB, 1000-Hz tone, then continued presenting this tone for either 60, 100, or 140 additional trials. A test stimulus (90 dB, 7000 Hz) was then given. The paradoxical Sokolov effect was found: Both extraverts and introverts showed increased frequency of skin conductance responses during overhabituation as a function of the number of trials involved (Figure 13-1). Extraverts were somewhat more aroused after 60 trials than introverts, but introverts were the more aroused after both 100 and 140 trials, so that overall slope of the function relating GSR frequency to number of overhabituation trials was steeper for introverts

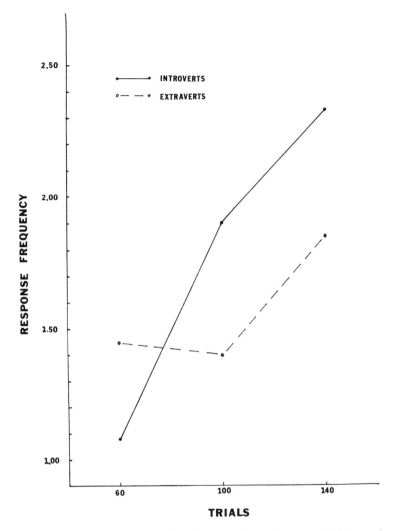

FIGURE 13-1. Changes in frequency of specific conductance responses with increasing over-habituation training. Data from Smith, Wilson, and Rypma, (1981).

than for extraverts. Extraverts showed a weaker conductance response than introverts to the test stimulus when the latter came after 60 trials, but were equal to the introverts in response strength following 100 or 140 trials (Figure 13-2). This finding can be attributed to generation of stronger cortical inhibition in extraverts over a prolonged series of overhabituation trials than over a shorter series, and a consequently greater sensitivity to stimulus change. This finding raises problems of interpretation for the E-I

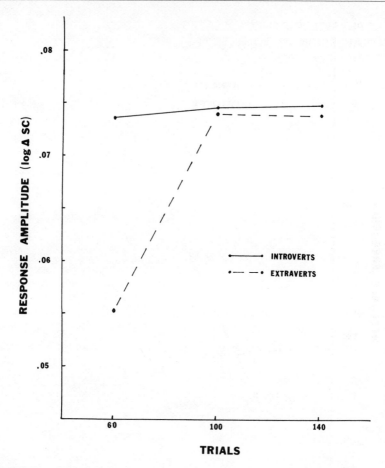

FIGURE 13-2. Changes in amplitude of the conductance response to test stimulus with increasing overhabituation training. Data from Smith, Wilson, and Rypma (1981).

difference during overhabituation, however. If extraverts equal introverts in responsivity to the test stimulus after 100 or 140 trials, why are they less reactive in specific response frequencies over those ranges of dishabituation trials? Furthermore, if H. J. Eysenck (1967) is correct, and extraverts generate inhibition more rapidly than introverts, we would expect extraverts to show greater autonomic arousal during overhabituation than introverts, which was not the case.

In summarizing the data on E-I differences in habituation of the OR, we would have to conclude that such differences are strongly suggested but as yet not firmly established. The work of Smith and his colleagues represents the best attempt at a systematic approach to the issue but replicability of findings has not been the rule even within this carefully controlled program.

PSYCHOPHYSIOLOGICAL CORRELATES OF EXTRAVERSION–INTROVERSION: ADDITIONAL FINDINGS

Skin Conductance

Despite the prominence given to autonomic processes in Eysenck's theory of E-I, the number of experiments designed to investigate such processes is surprisingly small. Most of the work that has been done has been concerned with the electrodermal OR, and this research was reviewed in the preceding section. A small handful of studies has been designed to investigate conductance differences in other settings, but the results of these studies are not conclusive. Purohit (1966) tested for differences between extraverts and introverts in GSR activity during classical autonomic conditioning, but found none. Other investigators have reported a similar failure to find E-I differences in conductance across a range of experimental conditions (Feij & Orlebeke, 1974; Hastrup, 1979). Overall, opinions regarding the validity of a relationship between E-I and electrodermal activity range from negative (Stern & Janes, 1973) to moderately positive (O'Gorman, 1977).

Two experiments have reported extravert–introvert differences in electrodermal conductance consistent with those predicted from Eysenck's theory. Gange, Geen, and Harkins (1979) tested male subjects in either a visual vigilance task or one of two control conditions. The vigilance task required that the subject report the occurrence of occasional signals (blips on a cathode-ray oscilloscope) over a period of 42 minutes. In one of the control conditions, subjects received the same visual display used in the vigilance task but were not required to respond to signals. In the other control condition, subjects received no visual presentation but merely waited for an equal amount of time. Introverts emitted a greater number of skin conductance responses than did extraverts to both signals and the trial markers that set off the periods in which signals occurred. In addition, introverts had a higher rate of spontaneous conductance responses than did extraverts. The finding that E-I did not interact with the treatment variable indicates that introverts were more aroused than extraverts across three conditions that differed in arousal potential. Nielsen and Petersen (1976) also found negative correlations between extraversion and the number of conductance responses elicited by a series of tones, the amplitude of the responses, and the rate of recovery to baseline levels.

Heart Rate

Few studies have been designed to measure the relationship of E-I to heart rate. Not surprisingly, given the paucity of data, results are not conclusive. In their study of OR habituation in which E-I differences were found in conductance and vasomotor variables, Stelmack et al. (1979) found no comparable difference in heart rate. Thackray, Jones, and Touchstone (1974) found that extraversion was correlated with variability in both performance and heart rate during a monotonous serial reaction time task. Heart rate variability was also correlated with the sociability subscale of the EPI, but not with the impulsivity subscale. The authors offered no explanation for this finding, but one seems plausible. Extraverts may have become prone to spells of inattention on the isolated and boring task because of their sociability. If there is a causal connection between attention and heart rate as some have supposed (e.g., Lacey & Lacey, 1974), variation in attention to the task would probably be accompanied by fluctuation in heart rate.

Three studies have reported differential heart rates in extraverts and introverts consistent with Eysenck's theory. Hinton and Craske (1977) observed larger increases in heart rate under stress among introverts than among extraverts. A similar difference has been reported by Orlebeke (1973), who suggested that the higher heart rate in introverts may be part of a defensive reaction against stimulation. This explanation would be consistent with the viewpoint that heart rate and attention processes (such as "taking in" or "shutting out" stimulation) are related, as noted above. Gange et al. (1979), in an experiment already described, found that introverts had higher heart rates than extraverts in all three treatment conditions, even the one involving no stimulation. However, these investigators found no E-I differences in baseline heart rate. It is therefore possible that their "no stimulation" condition may have been somewhat aversive to subjects and that the higher heart rate of introverts in that condition was related to a defensive response. It hardly seems necessary to note that considerably more data are required before any conclusions can be drawn regarding the relationship of E-I to heart rate and the possible significance of such a relationship for attentional processes.

Other Measures

Pupillary construction–dilation has been the subject of two studies on E-I differences. Holmes (1967) found that persons showing relatively slow pupil constriction were more extraverted than were rapid constrictors. Stelmack and Mandelzys (1975) measured pupil size in response to auditory presentation of words that were either neutral in nature, affectively toned, or taboo (sexual or scatological). Introverts were found to show greater pupillary dilation than extraverts during all phases of the experiment and also to dilate more in response to taboo words. "It is significant," the authors note, "that changes in pupil size to sensory or emotional stimuli are understood in terms of changes in thalamo-hypothalamo-cortical activity (Lowenstein & Loewenfeld, 1969), since Eysenck (1967) and Gray (1970) propose that individual differences in this system constitute the biological basis for individual differences in degree of extraversion" (Stelmack & Mandelzys, 1975, p. 539). This conclusion may be somewhat misleading. In both Eysenck's model and Gray's, the thalamus and hypothalamus are not *directly* related to the E-I variable. Presumably, however, they do articulate with structures described by Eysenck and Gray as part of the neural substrate of E-I.

The results of three other isolated studies yield no support for an assumption of physiological differences between extraverts and introverts. Hinton and Craske (1976) measured muscle action potential (MAP) from the right-side neck trapezius muscle of subjects who were engaged in tasks of locating sounds and judging brightness of lights. They found that although psychoticism as measured by the Eysenck Personality Questionnaire was correlated with MAP, E-I and neuroticism were not. Two studies investigated possible E-I correlation with psychoendocrine activity. Fine and Sweeney (1968) reported no correlation between extraversion and catecholamine output during stressful exposure to cold, while Seagraves (1970) discovered no relationship between extraversion and level of secretion of adrenal corticosteroids. The latter was detected from samples of urine collected during the course of normal activity.

Before drawing conclusions about E-I and arousal, however, we must consider a point of methodology. In almost all of the research reported to date a paradigm is used whereby introverts and extraverts are stimulated at some level or levels chosen by the experimenter. In addition, ambient stimulation is constant for the two personality groups. It is possible, therefore, that the customary E-I differences reported in the literature are due to general understimulation in the extraverts. If this is the case, it should be possible to manipulate stimulation in the laboratory to create levels at which the E-I differences disappear.

Keister and McLaughlin (1972) showed that the relationship of E-I to arousal-relevant performance is moderated by the level of stimulation. These investigators measured auditory vigilance in subjects who had first ingested either a capsule of caffeine, a placebo, or no drug. Under the placebo and no-drug conditions, the percent of signals detected by introverts remained relatively constant over the 48 minutes of the task, whereas among extraverts the percent of signals detected diminished sharply over the final 16 minutes, leading to a superiority in performance among introverts for that period. When the task followed administration of caffeine, however, the performance of neither extraverts nor introverts varied over the 48 minutes, nor did the two groups significantly differ in performance. The administration of caffeine therefore had little impact on introverts but greatly improved the performance of the normally underaroused extraverts.

Another way in which we might attenuate E-I differences in arousal would be to let subjects select their own levels of stimulation. We know that extraverts prefer higher levels of stimulation than do introverts (e.g., Brebner & Cooper, 1978; Philipp & Wilde, 1971). This finding suggests that extraverts and introverts may both seek some preferred level of arousal and that extraverts attain such a state under stronger stimulation than do introverts. It would follow from Eysenck's theory that given free choice of stimulus levels, extraverts and introverts should become more nearly equal in arousal than they are under conditions more or less forced by the experimenter. In a recent experiment, Geen (1981) tested this idea by allowing subjects in one condition to select the intensity of bursts of white noise they would receive just before and during part of a verbal task. As expected, extraverts selected noise of a higher mean intensity than did introverts. Measures of skin conductance and pulse rate were taken during a 2-minute pretask period and also during the first 2 minutes of a verbal task. Extraverts and introverts who heard noise of an intensity chosen by each group did not differ from each other in either pulse rate or in emission of specific skin conductance responses (see Tables 13-3 and 13-4).

The experiment included two additional conditions which controlled for possible effects of choice on arousal. In one, extraverts and introverts were yoked, respectively, to persons of the same personality type who had exercised choice, and were assigned noise at a level identical to that chosen by the yoked partners. In the other, extraverts and introverts were yoked to partners of opposite personality types from the choice condition. As Tables 13-3 and 13-4 show, the mere fact of choice had no effect on arousal, because persons assigned noise at a level chosen by those similar in personality did not differ from those who chose. Comparison between the two groups of subjects who were assigned noise equal to that chosen by their yoked partners of the opposite personality type reveals results more familiar to students of extraversion–introversion. At low levels of stimulation (those chosen by introverts), extraverts were significantly less aroused than introverts in terms of both conductance and pulse measures.

TABLE 13-3. Pulse Rate (Beats per Minute) of Extraverts and Introverts in Three Treatment Conditions

	PERSONALITY TYPE	
TREATMENT	EXTRAVERT	INTROVERT
Choice	74.7_{bc}	75.0_{bc}
Assigned—same type	73.1_{bc}	76.0_{b}
Assigned—other type	67.8_{c}	83.8_{a}

Note. Cells having common subscripts are not different from each other (.05 level) by a Duncan multiple-range test.

TABLE 13-4. Mean Number of Skin Resistance Responses Emitted by Extraverts and Introverts in Three Treatment Conditions

TREATMENT	PERSONALITY TYPE	
	EXTRAVERT	INTROVERT
Choice	13.3_{abc}	14.6_{ab}
Assigned—same type	12.1_{bc}	13.9_{ab}
Assigned—other type	7.9_c	18.1_a

Note. Cells having common subscripts are not different from each other (.05 level) by a Duncan multiple-range test.

At high levels (those chosen by extraverts), extraverts were again less aroused on both measures.

The time has come to summarize what we have reviewed so far, and to attempt an answer to the question of whether E-I differences are reflected in differences at the level of cortical and/or autonomic activation. The findings on EEG differences support the hypothesis to some extent, but the wide range of methods used in the studies makes generalization difficult, and the majority of studies reported so far fail to give support. The data from investigations on evoked potentials are mixed at best, and suggest the need for a more detailed theory that will specify what portion of the EP is related to E-I. The findings on contingent negative variation offer a promising start to supporting the Eysenck position, but the phenomenon has been related to E-I in only a few studies. Studies on E-I differences in habituation of the OR likewise present mixed and sometimes contradictory findings, even though some support for Eysenck's position can be found. A small collection of studies investigating such variables as heart rate, muscle action potential, and the pupillary response generally support the theory, but replications are badly needed.

EXTRAVERSION AND STRENGTH OF THE CENTRAL NERVOUS SYSTEM

A theory similar to Eysenck's in that it relates individual difference variables to arousability has been proposed by investigators in the USSR. According to this theory, as reviewed by Gray (1964), individuals are classified into a Pavlovian typology along various hypothetical dimensions of the nervous system, one such dimension being strength–weakness. Up to a point a "weak" nervous system reacts to stimulation with more excitation in general than a "strong one." At relatively low levels of stimulation the relation of stimulus to responsiveness is direct, but beyond a particular level of stimulation the relationship reverses, so that the weak nervous system becomes progressively less reactive as stimulation increases. The transition point (at which the relationship changes from positive to negative) is called the "threshold of transmarginal inhibition" (TTI). The TTI for strong nervous systems is at a still higher stimulus intensity (see Figure 13-3). A relationship of Pavlovian strength–weakness to extraversion–introversion has been suggested (Gray, 1967), introverts being equated with those individuals possessing weak nervous systems. As we have seen, there is evidence that introverts generate arousal more readily than do extraverts over the ranges of stimulation used in most of the studies reviewed. However, if introverts are in fact similar to "weaks," they should also decline in excitation at higher levels of stimulation. Such a finding has been shown in studies involving both behavioral and physiological measures.

Revelle, Amaral, and Turriff (1976) used a combination of caffeine and time constraints to place subjects under differing levels of stress while performing a complex test of verbal ability. Among introverts, subjects who were both timed for the task and given caffeine (and were presumably aroused by both treatments) performed more poorly than those who were merely timed. The latter, in turn, performed more poorly than introverts

FIGURE 13-3. Hypothesized relationship of reactivity to stimulus intensity for weak and strong nervous systems, showing thresholds of transmarginal inhibition for each type.

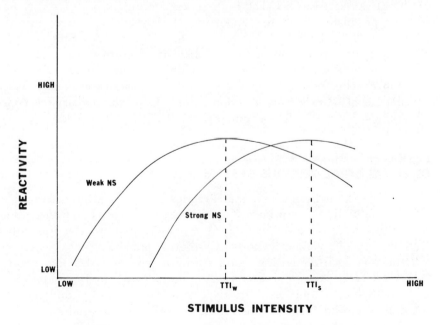

who worked under relaxed conditions. The performance of extraverts across the three conditions showed an opposite trend. Extraverts who were timed and also given caffeine performed better than those who worked under relaxed or timed-only conditions. The results can be interpreted as showing that introverts and extraverts were on opposite sides of their respective thresholds of transmarginal inhibition at the outset of the task and that whereas the increments in stimulation still continued to arouse the normally underaroused extraverts, they had the opposite effect on the overaroused introverts.

A subsequent experiment by Gilliland (1980) showed the effects of caffeine even more clearly. Using the same type of task as that used by Revelle *et al.* (1976), Gilliland first administered caffeine in two doses adjusted to the body weight of each subject, while giving no drug to subjects in a third condition. The results clearly indicated a curvilinear relationship between stimulation and performance in introverts. Compared to introverts who received no caffeine, those who received a small amount (2 mg/kg body weight) showed superior verbal performance. Introverts who received a larger amount of caffeine (4 mg/kg) performed no better than those given no stimulant at all. Extraverts, on the other hand, showed progressively better verbal performance as the amount of caffeine was increased.

That the normal arousal difference between introverts and extraverts may be reversed under conditions of high stimulation has been shown in two psychophysiological studies. Smith, Rypma, and Wilson (1981) observed the effects of caffeine on habituation of the electrodermal OR. The initial conductance amplitudes of introverts were greater than those of extraverts when a placebo was first given. Tonic conductance levels just prior to the test stimulus showed the same difference between extraverts and introverts. These findings support others cited in an earlier section on habituation of the OR. However, among subjects in the Smith, Rypma, and Wilson (1981) study who first received caffeine, the conductance levels of extraverts were higher than those of introverts both in response to the initial presentation of the standard stimulus and also just prior to the test stimulus. Caffeine increased conductance in extraverts but decreased it in introverts, a finding in accord with the hypothesis that introverts who receive caffeine will show decreased sensitivity to increasing stimulation. Their reactions are therefore similar to those shown by subjects with "weak" nervous systems in the Soviet research (Gray, 1964).

The results of a study by Fowles, Roberts, and Nagel (1977) add further support to the hypothesis that under high levels of stimulation introverts may show a decrease in arousal as stimulus intensity increases. Just prior to administering a series of tones, Fowles and his associates gave subjects a paired-associates learning task arranged to be either difficult or easy. It was assumed that working on a difficult task would arouse subjects more than working on a simple one. After a brief rest period, subjects were then stimulated with a series of tones at 1000-Hz intensity and either 83- or 103-dB intensity. Skin conductance levels during the presentation of the tones revealed a marginally significant interaction among E-I, difficulty of the PA task, and tone intensity. Figure 13-4 is redrawn from the data of Fowles *et al.* (1977). Treating difficulty of the PA task and intensity of the tones as additive sources of stimulation, we obtained the four data points on the *x* axis. The results clearly illustrate the curvilinear effect of stimulation levels upon conductance in introverts.

FIGURE 13-4. Skin conductance level as a function of overall stimulation in introverts and extraverts. **Note.** 83 and 103 refer to intensity of noise stimuli. S refers to "stimulation" (i.e., a difficult preliminary paired-associates task) and NS refers to "no stimulation" (i.e., an easy PA task). There is no theoretical reason for treating the S 83 condition as less stimulating than the NS 103. The order shown here was chosen only to facilitate exposition of the data. Data from Fowles, Roberts, and Nagel (1977).

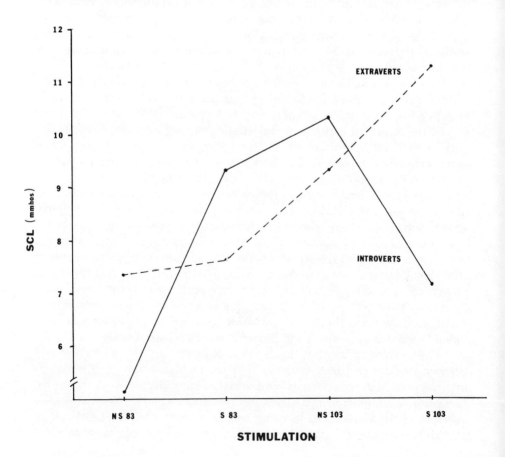

SUMMARY

Studies on the possible psychophysiological correlates of extraversion–introversion indicate that the hypothesis linking introversion to relatively higher arousability is generally true, but an oversimplification. Situational variables play an important moderating role in the relationship of E-I to arousal, and under certain conditions extraverts may be equal to, or even greater than, introverts in autonomic activity. Thus, the intensity of external stimulation must be considered. Unfortunately, replicability of findings across studies in which stimulus intensities have been varied is not encouraging. Furthermore, there is some question as to what E-I differences in arousal mean, and whether these differences have any functional significance. In only two of the several areas of research reviewed in this chapter do we have anything more than a handful of studies on which to base conclusions, and in both these areas (E-I differences in EEG activity and habituation of the electrodermal OR) there is still considerable uncertainty as to how extraverts and introverts differ. Probably the best conclusion to be drawn at present is that the hypothesis of greater arousability in introverts is tentatively supported, subject to considerable refinement in subsequent research.

R E F E R E N C E S

Andress, D. L., & Church, M. W. Differences in brainstem auditory evoked responses between introverts and extraverts as a function of stimulus intensity. *Psychophysiology*, 1981, *18*, 156–157.

Biesheuvel, S. An observational technique of temperament and personality assessment. *Bulletin of the National Institute of Personnel Research*, 1949, *1*, 9–27.

Block, J. *The challenge of response sets.* New York: Appleton-Century-Crofts, 1965.

Brebner, J., & Cooper, C. Stimulus- or response-induced excitation: A comparison of the behavior of introverts and extraverts. *Journal of Research in Personality*, 1978, *12*, 306–311.

Broadhurst, A., & Glass, A. Relationship of personality measures to the alpha rhythm of the electro-encephalogram. *British Journal of Psychiatry*, 1969, *115*, 199–204.

Campbell, K. B., Baribeau-Braun, J., & Braun, C. Neuroanatomical and physiological foundations of extraversion. *Psychophysiology*, 1981, *18*, 263–267.

Claridge, G. S., & Herrington, R. V. An EEG correlate of the Archimedes spiral aftereffect and its relationship with personality. *Behaviour Research and Therapy*, 1963, *1*, 217–229.

Coles, M. G. H., Gale, G., & Kline, P. Personality and habituation of the orienting reaction: Tonic and response measures of electrodermal activity. *Psychophysiology*, 1971, *8*, 54–63.

Crider, A., & Lunn, R. Electrodermal lability as a personality dimension. *Journal of Experimental Research in Personality*, 1971, *5*, 145–150.

Deakin, J. F., & Exley, K. A. Personality and male–female influences on the EEG alpha rhythm. *Biological Psychology*, 1979, *8*, 285–290.

Endler, N. S., & Magnusson, D. (Eds.). *Interactional psychology and personality.* Washington, D.C.: Hemisphere, 1976.

Eysenck, H. J. *The structure of human personality.* London: Methuen, 1953.

Eysenck, H. J. *The dynamics of anxiety and hysteria.* New York: Praeger, 1957.

Eysenck, H. J.   *The manual of the Maudsley Personality Inventory.* San Diego: EdITS/Educational and Industrial Testing Service, 1962.

Eysenck, H. J.   *The biological basis of personality.* Springfield, Ill.: Charles C Thomas, 1967.

Eysenck, H. J., & Eysenck, S. B. G.   A factorial study of psychoticism as a dimension of personality. *Multivariate Behavioral Research*, Special Issue, 1968, 15–31. (a)

Eysenck, H. J., & Eysenck, S. B. G.   *The manual of the Eysenck Personality Inventory.* San Diego: EdITS/Educational and Industrial Testing Service, 1968. (b)

Eysenck, S., & Zuckerman, M.   The relationship between sensation-seeking and Eysenck's dimensions of personality. *British Journal of Psychology*, 1978, *69*, 483–487.

Feij, J. A., & Orlebeke, J. F.   Spiral aftereffect duration as a correlate of impulsiveness. *Journal of Research in Personality*, 1974, *8*, 189–197.

Fenton, G. W., & Scotton, L.   Personality and the alpha rhythm. *British Journal of Psychiatry*, 1967, *113*, 1283–1289.

Fine, B. J., & Sweeney, D. R.   Personality traits, situational factors, and catecholamine excretion. *Journal of Experimental Research in Personality*, 1968, *3*, 15–27.

Fowles, D. C., Roberts, R., & Nagel, K.   The influence of introversion/extraversion on the skin conductance response to stress and stimulus intensity. *Journal of Research in Personality*, 1977, *11*, 129–146.

Friedman, J., & Meares, R.   Cortical evoked potentials and extraversion. *Psychosomatic Medicine*, 1979, *41*, 279–286.

Gale, A.   The psychophysiology of individual differences: Studies of extraversion and the EEG. In P. Kline (Ed.), *New approaches to psychological measurement.* London: Wiley, 1973.

Gale, A., Coles, M. G. H., & Blaydon, J.   Extraversion–introversion and the EEG. *British Journal of Psychology*, 1969, *60*, 209–223.

Gale, A., Coles, M., Kline, P., & Penfold, U.   Extraversion–introversion, neuroticism, and the EEG: Basal and response measures during habituation of the orienting response. *British Journal of Psychology*, 1971, *62*, 533–543.

Gale, A., Harpham, B., & Lucas, B.   Time of day and the EEG: Some negative results. *Psychonomic Science*, 1972, *28*, 269–271.

Gange, J. J., Geen, R. G., & Harkins, S. G.   Autonomic differences between extraverts and introverts during vigilance. *Psychophysiology*, 1979, *16*, 392–397.

Geen, R. G.   *Optimal stimulation levels and performance in introverts and extraverts.* Paper presented at the annual convention of the Midwestern Psychological Association, Detroit, April 1981.

Gilliland, K.   The interactive effect of introversion–extraversion with caffeine induced arousal on verbal performance. *Journal of Research in Personality*, 1980, *14*, 482–492.

Gilliland, K., Andress, D., & Bracy, S.   Differences in EEG alpha index between extraverts and introverts. *Psychophysiology*, 1981, *18*, 156.

Gottlober, A. B.   The relationship between brain potentials and personality. *Journal of Experimental Psychology*, 1938, *22*, 67–74.

Gray, J. A.   *Pavlov's typology.* Oxford: Pergamon, 1964.

Gray, J. A.   Strength of the nervous system, introversion–extraversion, conditionability and arousal. *Behaviour Research and Therapy*, 1967, *5*, 151–169.

Gray, J. A.   The psychophysiological basis of introversion–extraversion. *Behaviour Research and Therapy*, 1970, *8*, 249–266.

Gray, J. A.   The psychophysiological nature of introversion–extraversion: A modification of Eysenck's theory. In V. D. Nebylitsyn & J. A. Gray (Eds.), *Biological bases of individual behavior.* New York: Academic, 1972.

Guilford, J. P., & Guilford, R. B.   Personality factors S, E, and M, and their measurements. *Journal of Psychology*, 1936, *2*, 109–127.

Hastrup, J. L.   Effects of electrodermal lability and introversion on vigilance decrement. *Psychophysiology*, 1979, *16*, 302–310.

Henry, L. E., & Knott, J. R.   A note on the relationship between "personality" and the alpha rhythm of the electroencephalogram. *Journal of Experimental Psychology*, 1941, *28*, 362–366.

Hinton, J., & Craske, B. A relationship between Eysenck's P scale and change in muscle action potentials with attention to perceptual tasks. *British Journal of Psychology*, 1976, *67*, 461–466.

Hinton, J. W., & Craske, B. Differential effects of test stress on the heart rates of extraverts and introverts. *Biological Psychology*, 1977, *5*, 23–28.

Holmes, D. S. Pupillary response, conditioning, and personality. *Journal of Personality and Social Psychology*, 1967, *5*, 98–103.

Janssen, R. H. C., Mattie, H., Plooij-Van Gorsel, P. C., & Werre, P. F. The effects of a depressant and a stimulant drug on the contingent negative variation. *Biological Psychology*, 1978, *6*, 209–218.

Keister, M. E., & McLaughlin, R. J. Vigilance performance related to extraversion-introversion and caffeine. *Journal of Experimental Research in Personality*, 1972, *6*, 5–11.

Knott, J. R., & Irwin, D. A. Anxiety, stress, and the contingent negative variation. *Archives of General Psychiatry*, 1973, 29–39.

Koriat, A., Averill, J. R., & Malmstrom, E. J. Individual differences in habituation: Some methodological and conceptual issues. *Journal of Research in Personality*, 1973, *7*, 88–101.

Lacey, B. C., & Lacey, J. I. Studies of heart rate and other bodily processes in sensorimotor behavior. In P. A. Obrist, A. H. Black, J. Brener, & L. V. DiCara (Eds.), *Cardiovascular psychophysiology*. Chicago: Aldine, 1974.

Low, M. Discussion of "brain" potentials relating to expectancy: The CNV. In E. Donchin & D. B. Lindsley (Eds.), *Averaged evoked potentials: Methods, results, and evaluations*. Washington, D.C.: NASA, 1969.

Lowenstein, O., Loewenfeld, I. E. The pupil. In H. Davson (Ed.), *The eye* (2nd ed., Vol. 3). New York: Academic, 1969.

Mangan, G. L., & O'Gorman, J. Initial amplitude and rate of habituation of orienting reaction in relation to extraversion and neuroticism. *Journal of Experimental Research in Personality*, 1969, *3*, 275–282.

Marton, M., & Urban, Y. An electroencephalographic investigation of individual differences in the process of conditioning. In H. J. Eysenck (Ed.), *Readings in extraversion–introversion* (Vol. 3). New York: Wiley, 1971.

McAdam, W., & Orme, J. E. Personality traits and the electroencephalogram. *Journal of Mental Science*, 1954, *100*, 913–921.

Mundy-Castle, A. C. The relationship between primary–secondary function and the alpha rhythm of the electroencephalogram. *Journal of the National Institute of Personnel Research*, 1955, *6*, 95–102.

Nebylitsyn, U. D. An electroencephalographic investigation of the properties of strength of the nervous system and equilibrium of the nervous processes in man using factor analysis. In B. M. Teplov (Ed.), *Typological features of higher nervous activity in man* (Vol. 3). Moscow: Academy of Pedagogical Science, RSFSR, 1963.

Nielsen, T. C., & Petersen, K. E. Electrodermal correlates of extraversion, trait anxiety, and schizophrenia. *Scandinavian Journal of Psychology*, 1976, *17*, 73–80.

O'Gorman, J. Individual differences in habituation of human physiological responses: A review of theory, method, and findings in the study of personality correlates in nonclinical populations. *Biological Psychology*, 1977, *5*, 257–318.

Orlebeke, J. F. Electrodermal, vasomotor, and heart rate correlates of extraversion and neuroticism. *Psychophysiology*, 1973, *10*, 211. (Abstract)

Philipp, R. L., & Wilde, G. J. Stimulation seeking behavior and extraversion. *Acta Psychologica*, 1970, *32*, 269–280.

Plooij-Van Gorsel, P. C., & Janssen, R. H. C. Contingent negative variation (CNV) and extraversion in a psychiatric population. In C. Barber (Ed.), *Evoked potentials: Proceedings of an international evoked potentials symposium*. Lancaster, England: MTP Press, 1980.

Purohit, A. P. Personality variables, sex-differences, G.S.R. responsiveness, and G.S.R. conditioning. *Journal of Experimental Research in Personality*, 1966, *1*, 166–173.

Revelle, W., Amaral, P., & Turriff, S.   Introversion/extraversion, time stress, and caffeine: Effect on verbal performance. *Science*, 1976, *192*, 149–150.

Rust, J.   Cortical evoked potential, personality, and intelligence. *Journal of Comparative and Physiological Psychology*, 1975, *89*, 1220–1226.

Sadler, T. J., Mefferd, R. B., & Houck, R. L.   The interaction of extraversion and neuroticism in orienting response habituation. *Psychophysiology*, 1971, *8*, 312–318.

Savage, R. D.   Electro-cerebral activity, extraversion, and neuroticism. *British Journal of Psychiatry*, 1964, *110*, 98–100.

Seagraves, R. T.   Personality, body build, and adrenocortical activity. *British Journal of Psychiatry*, 1970, *117*, 405–411.

Smith, B. D., Rypma, C. B., & Wilson, R. J.   Dishabituation and spontaneous recovery of the electrodermal orienting response: Effects of extraversion, impulsivity, sociability, and caffeine. *Journal of Research in Personality*, 1981, *15*, 233–240.

Smith, B. D., & Wigglesworth, M. J.   Extraversion and neuroticism in orienting reflex dishabituation. *Journal of Research in Personality*, 1978, *12*, 284–296.

Smith, B. D., Wilson, R., & Rypma, C. B.   Overhabituation and dishabituation: Effects of extraversion and amount of training. *Journal of Research in Personality*, 1981, *15*, 475–487.

Sokolov, A. N.   *Perception and the conditioned reflex*. Oxford: Pergamon, 1963.

Stelmack, R. M., Achorn, E., & Michaud, A.   Extraversion and individual differences in auditory evoked response. *Psychophysiology*, 1977, *14*, 368–374.

Stelmack, R. M., Bourgeois, R., Chien, J. Y. C., & Pickard, C.   Extraversion and the OR habituation rate to visual stimuli. *Journal of Research in Personality*, 1979, *13*, 49–58.

Stelmack, R. M., & Mandelzys, N.   Extraversion and pupillary response to affective and taboo words. *Psychophysiology*, 1975, *12*, 536–540.

Stern, J. A., & Janes, C. L.   Personality and psychopathology. In W. F. Prokasy & D. C. Raskin (Eds.), *Electrodermal activity in psychological research*. New York: Academic, 1973.

Tecce, J. J.   Contingent negative variation and psychological processes in man. *Psychological Bulletin*, 1972, *77*, 73–108.

Thackray, R. I., Jones, K. N., & Touchstone, R. M.   Personality and physiological correlates of performance decrement on a monotonous task requiring sustained attention. *British Journal of Psychology*, 1974, *65*, 351–358.

Wigglesworth, M. J., & Smith, B. D.   Habituation and dishabituation of the electrodermal orienting reflex in relation to extraversion and neuroticism. *Journal of Research in Personality*, 1976, *10*, 437–445.

Winter, K., Broadhurst, A., & Glass, A.   Neuroticism, extraversion, and EEG amplitude. *Journal of Experimental Research in Personality*, 1972, *6*, 44–51.

CHAPTER 14

Empathic Motivation of Helping Behavior

C. Daniel Batson
University of Kansas

Jay S. Coke
U.S. Army Research Institute
Fort Sill, Oklahoma

INTRODUCTION

Around 1965 several tragic cases of failure to help caught the attention of social psychologists. In these cases, people watched but did nothing while another person suffered or even died. The question uppermost in the minds of the social psychologists trying to account for these tragedies was well expressed in the title of the classic little volume by Bibb Latané and John Darley, *The Unresponsive Bystander: Why Doesn't He Help?* (1970). Answers to this question posed by Latané and Darley and by other social psychologists focused on situational pressures that inhibit the bystander's impulse to help—diffusion of responsibility, cost of helping, ambiguity of need, and so on (see Rushton & Sorrentino, 1981, and Staub, 1978, for reviews). But as the list of inhibiting situational pressures grew longer and longer, another question came to the fore. This question was well expressed in the title of a widely circulated paper by Jane and Irving Piliavin, "The Good Samaritan: Why *Does* He Help?" (1973; see also Huston & Korte, 1976). This question raised an important issue not considered in the earlier research on situational inhibitors, the issue of motivation. The models developed to account for situational inhibition of helping (e.g., the well-known Latané and Darley decision tree) were cognitive; they were designed to answer the question of when a person would decide to help and, more important, not to help. They typically did not address the question of why the person should ever help at all.

The question of motivation for helping is of considerable importance on both a practical and a theoretical level. Practically, if we can understand what motivates people to help, we may be able to adjust our socialization practices to increase this motivation (see Aronfreed, 1970, and Hoffman, 1975, 1976, 1981a, for examples of such a strategy). Admittedly, attempting to change people's motivation is an ambitious undertaking, but if we desire a more caring, humane society, it may be worth trying. Indeed, it may be more practical than identifying situational inhibitors of helping. For as Latané and Nida (1981) have recently noted, even though social psychologists have been quite successful in demonstrating the power of situational inhibitors, this success has not produced any practical ideas for how to increase helping. Presumably, this is because one cannot easily control the relevant characteristics of need situations, such as the ambiguity of the need or the presence of other bystanders (although there is some evidence that simply knowing about situational inhibitors may diminish their effect —Beaman, Barnes, Klentz, & McQuirk, 1978). Attacking the problem of how to encourage helping at the level of motivation may yield more practical results.

Potentially, the theoretical implications of understanding the motivation for helping are immense, for it may even change our view of human nature. To ask why people help reintroduces a basic issue that was of central concern to nineteenth-century social philosophers and to early social psychologists interested in helping (e.g., McDougall, 1908; Mill, 1863), the issue of egoism versus altruism. This issue could be and was finessed by researchers looking for situational inhibitors (cf. Latané & Darley, 1970; Macaulay & Berkowitz, 1970). But it has become central once again for researchers considering why people help (cf. Batson, Darley, & Coke, 1978; Coke, Batson, & McDavis, 1978; Hoffman, 1981b; Krebs, 1975). Given the pervasiveness among psychologists of the assumption that all human behavior is motivated by self-interest, even to suggest that some helping might be truly altruistic (i.e., directed toward the end-state goal of increasing another's rather than one's own welfare) amounts to proposing a paradigm shift (Kuhn, 1962) in our understanding of human motivation.

Why, then, *do* people help? Obviously, there are many reasons. Although one might seek an answer by focusing on the relative rewards in helping situations (personal benefits minus costs) and the reinforcement history of the helper, the approach that has attracted the most interest among social psychologists is to focus on the helper's emotional response to witnessing the victim's distress. The Piliavins (1973) suggested that witnessing another person in distress produces emotional arousal in the potential helper, that this arousal is aversive, and that the potential helper acts to reduce it—either by helping and so removing the cause or by escaping from the situation and so diminishing contact with the cause. The Piliavins assumed that the various emotions experienced by the potential helper (shock, disgust, shame, fear, and empathy) summated to produce aversive arousal. But this assumption has been challenged. We and other researchers (Batson & Coke, 1981; Batson *et al.*, 1978; Coke *et al.*, 1978; Davis, 1981) have suggested that although many emotions resulting from witnessing another's distress may affect the motivation to help as the Piliavins suggest, empathy does not. We have suggested that instead of producing a state of aversive arousal which the potential helper is egoistically motivated to reduce, empathy produces motivation directed toward the end-state goal of reducing the victim's distress—that is, truly altruistic motivation (Batson & Coke, 1981; Batson *et al.*, 1978; Batson, Duncan, Ackerman, Buckley, & Birch, 1981).

Before we can even consider whether empathy is a source of altruistic motivation for helping, several more basic issues must be addressed. We must be clear what we mean by empathy; we must be sure that it exists, and we must be sure that it motivates helping. These are the issues that we address in this chapter.

THE PHENOMENON OF EMPATHIC EMOTION

For a relatively new term (apparently coined by Titchener in 1909 to translate the German *Einfühlung*), empathy has seen a wide range of definitions (cf. Wispé, 1968). Not only has its meaning varied, but its relation to associated concepts such as sympathy has also varied. Because empathy has been used by different people in contradictory ways, it would be impossible to propose a definition that would capture its essence. We can only try to make clear what we mean by the term.

Empathy as Congruent Emotion

Empathy, as we shall use the term, is *an emotional state elicited by and congruent with the perceived welfare of someone else*. This definition is built upon Heider's (1958, Chap. 11) discussion of reactions to the lot of another person. Empathy has often been defined as an emotional response to the emotion of another. We have chosen to focus instead on emotional response to the perceived welfare of another because, although the other's welfare is often reflected in his or her emotional state, it is not always (as, for example, when an accident victim is unconscious). We believe that to feel concern and compassion in response to the perceived distress of an unconscious victim, as presumably the Good Samaritan did, should be included in our definition of empathy.

We are employing Schachter's (1964) concept of emotion; to experience a given emotion an individual must perceive himself or herself to be physiologically aroused and must give this arousal an appropriate cognitive label. Thus, for empathic emotion to occur, observing another's condition must produce vicarious physiological arousal in the observer and this vicarious arousal must be cognitively labeled in a manner congruent with the perceived welfare of the other (Stotland, 1969).

When we say that empathic emotion is *congruent* with the perceived welfare of the other, we mean that empathy involves experiencing positive emotion when the other's lot is desirable and negative emotion when it is undesirable. A similar relationship exists for anticipated changes in the lot of the other. Empathic emotion should become more positive to changes that one perceives the other to desire and more negative to changes the other wants to avoid. In our view, empathy typically does not involve experiencing the same lot as the other, only a congruent reaction to that lot. Someone else's triumph is not likely to evoke a sense of triumph but a more subdued sense of happiness; another's suffering and distress is not likely to evoke the same sense of suffering or pain but feelings such as compassion or concern. As Solomon Asch put it: "It is because we become aware of the situation and experience of others that we can feel *with* them. The mere duplication of an observed reaction may in fact be a sign of an inadequate social relation. There are times when the sight of suffering merely reminds a person of his own suffering; when this is so, he has simply lost social contact" (1952, p. 172, italics in original).

Our conception of empathy does not always permit a clear distinction between empathy and sympathy. Empathy as we are defining it includes congruent reactions to another's pleasure as well as to another's pain. Sympathy is not usually applied to congruent emotional reactions to another's pleasure, but it is often applied to reactions to another's pain. So congruent emotion elicited by witnessing another in distress in a helping situation could appropriately be called sympathy instead of empathy, as for example Heider (1958) has done. Our reason for preferring the term "empathy" is that it has typically been the term used by social psychologists during the past decade.

We must also admit that our conception of empathy does not always permit a clear determination of whether an emotional reaction is empathic. In those cases in which the other's lot is clearly desirable and the emotional reaction is positive, or clearly undesirable and the emotional reaction is negative, we may say with confidence that the emotional reaction is congruent and therefore empathic. But as the lot of the other or the emotional response becomes more ambiguous, we enter a large gray area in which it is difficult to say whether or to what degree the reaction is empathic. On the other side of this gray area are reactions that clearly are not congruent and so not empathic, as for example when one feels negative emotion in reaction to another's triumph (jealousy or envy) or positive emotion in reaction to another's tragedy (malicious joy). Researchers studying empathy have sought to work with situations in which the lot of the other is clearly desirable or clearly undesirable, allowing them to infer with some confidence whether an emotional reaction to this lot is congruent and so empathic.

Evidence That Empathic Emotion Exists

Of course, to provide a definition carries no assurance that what is defined actually exists. Before we can say that empathy as we have defined it exists, we must be satisfied (1) that perceptions of the welfare of another person can trigger vicarious emotional responses, and (2) that these vicarious emotions are congruent with the presumed welfare of the other. To provide evidence for the first of these two criteria, it is necessary to show that witnessing a target person having a desirable or undesirable experience can cause an emotional reaction in an observer, even when it is clear that the stimuli causing the target's experience are not, and will not be, impinging on the observer.

To provide such evidence, Berger (1962) had people observe a target person performing a task and led them to believe that following the onset of a visual signal the target person either was receiving electric shock (electric shock condition) or was not receiving electric shock (no-shock condition). Further, the target person either jerked his or her arm following the visual signal (movement condition) or did not (no-movement condition). All research participants were told that they themselves would not be shocked during the study.

Berger reasoned, first, that both a painful stimulus in the environment (shock) and a distress response (movement) were necessary for an observer to infer that the target person was experiencing pain. He reasoned, second, that if participants in his experiment were responding vicariously, they should display a physiological reaction to watching the target person only when they inferred that he or she was experiencing pain. Therefore, Berger predicted that participants in the shock–movement condition would display the most physiological arousal, because only they would infer that the target person was experiencing pain and so only they would show a vicarious emotional response. For participants in each of the other three conditions, either the painful stimulus or the target's distress response was missing. Results followed the predicted pattern. Consistent with the assumption that people can experience vicarious emotion as a result of perceiving another in pain, participants in the shock–movement condition evidenced more skin resistance responses (SRRs) while observing the target person than participants in the other three conditions. Subsequent research (Bandura & Rosenthal, 1966; Craig & Lowrey, 1969; Craig & Wood, 1969; Lazarus, Opton, Nomikos, & Rankin, 1965) has provided additional evidence for this first criterion, including evidence that people can experience vicarious emotion (reflected in measures of electrodermal activity) as a result of perceiving another in a desirable as well as an undesirable state (Krebs, 1975; Stotland, 1969).

Subsequent research has also provided evidence (Bandura & Rosenthal, 1966; Hygge, 1976; Krebs, 1975; Milgram, 1963; Staub, 1978; Stotland, 1969) for the second criterion, that the vicarious emotions experienced are typically, although not always, congruent with the current and anticipated perceived welfare of the target person. Stotland and Sherman (reported in Stotland, 1969) found that people who responded with vicarious emotion to witnessing another undergoing what they perceived to be a painful experience reported their own emotional state to be one of increased tension and nervousness; they were also more likely than people in control conditions to report that they found participating in the study a relatively unpleasant experience. In contrast, people who responded vicariously to another undergoing what they perceived to be a pleasurable experience reported, relative to controls, that they found participating in the study to be a pleasant experience. Similarly, Krebs (1975) found that observers reported feeling relatively badly when watching someone whom they thought was about to receive an electric shock and relatively good when watching someone about to receive a reward.

Although self-reports of the sort used in these studies might easily result from a desire to *appear* empathic rather than from a true empathic response, it is important to note that in both the Stotland and Sherman and the Krebs studies these reports occurred in conjunction with evidence of increased vicarious emotion on physiological measures. In control conditions in which it would have been just as desirable to appear empathic, neither the physiological measures nor the self-reports provided evidence of an empathic response. This convergence of physiological and self-report data provides reasonably strong evidence that participants in these studies actually were experiencing emotions congruent with the perceived welfare of the other, and not simply saying that they were. Empathy as we have defined it apparently can exist.

An Alternative Conception of Empathy: Perspective Taking

Still, our conception of empathy as an emotional response is not the only possibility; there is an alternative view. The alternative is that empathy is a cognitive process (Borke, 1971; Regan & Totten, 1975; Shantz, 1975). According to this conception, empathy involves taking another person's perspective and seeing the world as he or she sees it. Like empathy defined as an emotion, empathy as perspective taking has been proposed as a possible instigator of helping (Rubin & Schneider, 1973; but see also Emler & Rushton, 1974; Krebs, 1981; Krebs & Stirrup, 1974; Rushton & Wiener, 1975; and Waxler, Yarrow, & Smith, 1977). Taking the perspective of a

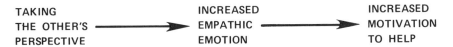

FIGURE 14-1. Two-stage model of the interaction of cognitive and emotional factors in empathic motivation for helping.

person in need, it is proposed, increases the likelihood of recognizing the need and acting to reduce it. Although advocates of the cognitive view recognize that taking another's perspective may sometimes lead to an emotional response (cf. Regan & Totten, 1975), they tend to consider the helper's emotional state to be unimportant for understanding the behavioral consequences of empathy. As long as one takes the perspective of the other, any emotions that may accompany this cognitive state are assumed to be epiphenomenal.

Feshbach (1975) has suggested that if we are to understand the behavioral consequences of empathy it may be a mistake to focus exclusively on either empathic emotion or cognitive perspective taking. In line with this suggestion, we would propose that the cognitive and emotional processes interact to produce empathic motivation for helping.

EMPATHIC MOTIVATION OF HELPING: A TWO-STAGE MODEL

Stotland (1969) and Krebs (1975) have suggested that taking another person's perspective should increase the intensity of empathic emotion in response to that person's distress. Building on their suggestion, we would like to propose a two-stage model of empathic mediation of helping. This model, presented in Figure 14-1, hypothesizes that (1) taking the perspective of a person in need tends to increase one's empathic emotional response, and (2) empathic emotion in turn increases motivation to see that person's need reduced.[1] Since helping is often the most effective way to see the other's need reduced, this motivation should increase the likelihood that one will help.

This model does not assume that taking the perspective of the other is the source of empathic emotion, only that perspective taking increases empathy. Moreover, it does not assume that cognitive perspective taking is the only factor that increases empathic emotion, only that it is one factor that does. In spite of these nonrestrictive assumptions, the model makes some explicit, restrictive predictions. For example, although the model postulates that perspective taking and empathic emotion both contribute

1. This two-stage model was introduced by Coke, Batson, and McDavis (1978); the present discussion is an expansion of that initial presentation. A similar model has recently been proposed by Weiner (1980).

to the motivation to help, it predicts that perspective taking affects helping only as a result of its effect on empathy. But is the model correct?

Evidence for Stage One: Perspective Taking Increases Empathic Emotional Response

The first stage of the two-stage model predicts that taking the perspective of a person in distress will increase one's empathic emotional response. To test this prediction Stotland (1969) and Krebs (1975) exposed people to target persons supposedly responding to painful, pleasurable, or neutral stimuli. In some studies Stotland manipulated perspective taking directly by instructing participants either to take the perspective or to observe the movements of a target person. In other studies he manipulated perspective taking indirectly by varying participants' perceived similarity to the target person, reasoning that among its other effects (e.g., increased liking) greater perceived similarity would lead to increased perspective taking. Krebs, in his study, also manipulated perspective taking indirectly by varying perceived similarity.

Both Stotland's (1969) and Krebs's (1975) results supported the hypothesis that taking another's perspective increases empathic response to that person's pleasure or pain. When observing a target presumed to be experiencing pain, persons instructed to take the target's perspective were more physiologically aroused than persons instructed to observe the target's movements, and those led to believe that they were similar to the target were more physiologically aroused than those led to believe that they were dissimilar. Further, self-reports by participants in both Stotland's and Krebs's research indicated that arousal experienced under these conditions tended to be labeled in a manner congruent with the perceived state of the other. If the other was perceived to be in pain, participants tended to describe their own emotional state as one of tension, nervousness, and unpleasantness; if the other was perceived to be having a pleasurable experience, participants were likely to describe themselves as experiencing a good, pleasant emotional state.

Perhaps, however, the increased arousal of participants in these studies was not due to an empathic response to the target's welfare but to the participants imagining how they would themselves react in the situation. If so, their increased arousal would not really be evidence of empathy. Steffan Hygge (1976) conducted an experiment to examine this possibility. He had people observe a female target person as she was exposed to auditory tones delivered through headphones. In a 2×2 factorial design participants were led to believe either that they themselves would experience pain if exposed to the tones or that they would not experience pain.

Further, participants were led to believe either that the target was experiencing pain when exposed to the tones or that she was not experiencing pain.

Consistent with the expectation that perspective taking increases empathic emotional response and not simply one's ability to imagine one's own response to the stimulus, vicarious arousal (reflected in frequency and magnitude measures of skin conductance responses but not in measures of skin conductance levels) was greater for those who thought that the tones were causing pain to the target. There was no effect on these measures for participants' belief that they themselves would or would not find the tones painful. Hygge's experiment, in combination with the research of Stotland and of Krebs, leads us to conclude that perspective taking does indeed increase empathic emotional response to the inferred emotional state of another person. Stage one of the two-stage model has received support.

Evidence for Stage Two: Empathic Emotion Increases Motivation to Help

The second stage predicts that empathic emotion increases motivation to see the other's need reduced, that is, that it increases motivation to help. As might be expected, testing this hypothesis has proven more difficult than testing the hypothesis that perspective taking increases empathy. To test the hypothesis that empathy leads to helping, one cannot simply manipulate the strength of the painful stimulus impinging on a target person or the strength of the target's apparent distress response. For although the research reported above suggests that such manipulations should affect the strength of a bystander's empathic response, they may also affect the bystander's perception of the magnitude of the target person's need. And perceived need might affect helping through mechanisms other than empathy (such as norms stipulating that you should help more when a person is in greater need—Berkowitz, 1972; Schwartz, 1977). Similarly, one cannot simply manipulate perspective taking and observe its effect on helping. For although the research reported above suggests that perspective taking affects the strength of the empathic response, perspective taking might also affect helping quite independently of its effect on empathic emotion. If so, any empathic emotion caused by perspective taking might not be the cause of increased helping following perspective taking (cf. Rubin & Schneider, 1973).

To test the effect of empathic emotion on helping, it is necessary somehow to vary the level of empathy while exposing all participants to the same need situation and controlling for their degree of perspective taking. In other words, it is necessary to vary the level of empathic emotion directly so that empathy is not confounded with other variables

426 BASIC SOCIAL PSYCHOPHYSIOLOGICAL RESEARCH

that might, by themselves, affect helping. With this criterion in mind, let us examine the research that has explored the empathy–helping relationship.

A number of studies (Aderman & Berkowitz, 1970; Aronfreed & Paskal, cited in Aronfreed, 1968; Krebs, 1975) have provided results consistent with the hypothesis that empathy leads to helping, but because they were not designed to test this specific hypothesis, they have not satisfied the criterion necessary to provide a direct test. Aderman and Berkowitz (1970) and Aronfreed and Paskal (cited in Aronfreed, 1968) manipulated variables that, in theory, should have affected the strength of individuals' empathic response to a person in need, and both pairs of researchers found that those people who theoretically should have responded more empathically were more helpful. In these studies, however, empathy was neither directly manipulated, as required by the criterion stated above, nor even measured. Thus, we cannot be sure that the manipulations actually increased empathy as we have defined it, or that even if they did, empathy was the variable that actually led to helping. An additional problem in interpreting Aderman and Berkowitz's study is that participants were not given an opportunity to help the person who evoked their empathic response, but someone else. A priori it is not clear that empathy for one person should generalize to a second, unrelated person.

By taking physiological and self-report measures of empathy, Krebs (1975) provided more convincing evidence that a relationship exists between empathic emotion and helping. All participants in his study observed a target person exhibit exactly the same sequence of behaviors. Some participants, though, were given information about the target's situation that led them to believe that his or her experience was sometimes positive and sometimes negative (high-affect condition); others were led to believe that his or her experience was affectively neutral (low-affect condition). Further, some participants were led to believe they were similar to the target person (similar condition); others were led to believe that they were dissimilar (dissimilar condition).

Krebs reasoned that only people in the high-affect conditions were exposed to a situation capable of eliciting empathy, for only they should have inferred that the target was experiencing pleasure or pain. Further, among people in the high-affect conditions, those in the similar condition should have been more likely to take the target's perspective. Thus, Krebs predicted that people in the high-affect–similar condition would experience more empathy and be more likely to help the target person than would people in the other three conditions.

Krebs's (1975) results tended to follow this predicted pattern. Relative to people in the other three conditions, those in the high-affect–similar condition tended to show more physiological arousal (as assessed using measures of SCL, vasoconstriction, and heart rate) while observing the target person, reported identifying with the target person to a greater extent, reported feeling worse while waiting for the target to experience pain, and gave more help to the target person.[2] Even Krebs's results, though, did not demonstrate a causal relation between empathic emotion and helping—only that the two were affected similarly by the same independent variables. Moreover, the manipulations used in this experiment to evoke empathy might also have increased perceived need and perspective taking, variables that might themselves increase helping.

A study by Harris and Huang (1973) provided more direct evidence that some form of emotion produces motivation to help, although it was not clear that the emotion was empathy. While participants were working on math problems, a confederate with a bandaged knee limped into the experimental room, tripped over a chair, and crying out in apparent pain, fell to the floor. Some participants were induced to misattribute arousal caused by this incident to an aversive noise; others were not. Harris and Huang based their prediction on Schachter's (1964) theory of emotions. If a bystander's emotinal response is important in motivating helping, and emotions consist of physiological arousal and cognitive labels, then leading people to attribute the arousal produced by witnessing the victim's distress to a stimulus other than the distress should reduce helping. Consistent with this prediction, participants induced to misattribute their arousal to the noise offered less help to the confederate than participants not so induced. Further, although it was not possible to measure perceived need in this study, there was no difference in reported emotional arousal between the two experimental conditions; there was only a difference in the degree to which the arousal was attributed to the noise. Harris and Huang interpreted their results as evidence that empathic emotion motivates helping.

Using misattribution to a placebo rather than to noise, Gaertner and Dovidio (1977, Experiment 2) provided a conceptual replication of Harris and Huang's study (including some interesting extensions not relevant to the present discussion). First, in Experiment 1, using a measure of heart rate, they confirmed that witnessing another person in distress produced increased cardiac activity. In Experiment 2, they found that people induced to misattribute any felt physiological arousal to a placebo were slower to help than those not so induced. Moreover, the Gaertner and Dovidio design permitted a measure of the perceived severity of the distressed person's need, and they reported no differences between the two placebo conditions on this measure.

The studies by Harris and Huang (1973) and Gaertner and Dovidio (1977) seem to meet the criterion for manipulating participants' self-

---

2. It should be noted that the data from the measures of heart rate and vasoconstriction were not in complete accord with the predicted arousal pattern.

perceived emotional state in a manner unconfounded with other variables that might affect helping, and their results indicate that emotional response to another's distress can lead to motivation to help. But it is not clear that the emotional response that led to helping in their studies was empathic. As Piliavin and Piliavin (1973) have observed, many emotions may be experienced when witnessing someone in distress: startle, shock, fear, disgust, and curiosity, as well as empathy. Neither Harris and Huang (1973) nor Gaertner and Dovidio (1977) clearly identified the emotions evoked in research participants when witnessing the target's distress. Participants in these experiments may have experienced one or more nonempathic emotions, and since these emotions would likely be aversive, participants may have been motivated to escape them. Given constraints in these experiments against escaping by leaving the need situation, the most effective means of escaping this aversive arousal may have been to help (cf. Piliavin & Piliavin, 1973).

Coke *et al.* (1978) reported two experiments in which they manipulated empathy in a more controlled manner. In both experiments participants learned of a victim's plight by listening to a taped radio broadcast. It was assumed that such a procedure would minimize startle, fear, and other nonempathic emotions that might be confounded with empathy in a face-to-face emergency. In addition, as they listened to the broadcast, participants were not aware that they would subsequently be given an opportunity to help.

In Experiment 1 reported by Coke *et al.* (1978), participants listened to a tape recording of a radio newscast designed to be emotionally arousing. The newscast presented the situation of a young college senior, Katie Banks, who had recently lost her parents in a tragic automobile wreck. Employing Stotland's (1969) technique for manipulating perspective taking, Coke *et al.* instructed participants either to imagine how Katie felt about her situation (imagine her condition) or to observe the broadcasting techniques used in the newscast (observe condition). Just before participants heard the newscast, they were given a capsule in the context of another experiment. Half of them were told that the capsule—actually a placebo—would relax them (relax condition); the others were told that it would arouse them (arouse condition). After hearing the newscast, all participants were unexpectedly given an opportunity to help Katie by offering to run errands, care for her brother and sister, and so on.

Coke *et al.* (1978) reasoned that since perspective taking increases empathic emotional response, people in the imagine conditions should have been more empathically aroused by the newscast than people in the observe conditions. People in the imagine–arouse condition, however, should have had a salient alternative explanation for this arousal; they had just taken a capsule that would arouse them. Only people in the imagine–relax condition were expected both to experience empathic arousal and cognitively to label that arousal as a response to Katie's plight; therefore, following Schachter (1964), only these participants were expected to experience empathic emotion. Results revealed that, as predicted, people in the imagine–relax condition offered significantly more help to Katie than did people in any of the other three conditions. Nor could this difference be accounted for by differences in perceived need; participants in the imagine–relax condition actually perceived Katie's need to be slightly less than did participants in the other three conditions. These findings were entirely consistent with the hypothesis that empathic emotion motivates helping.

In Experiment 2, Coke *et al.* (1978) used a different strategy for manipulating empathic emotion; they artificially increased perceived empathy through the use of a false feedback of arousal paradigm (Valins, 1966). Unlike Experiment 1, the need situation presented in the broadcast in Experiment 2 was designed to be intrinsically unarousing: A graduate student in education was seeking volunteers to paticipate in her master's thesis research. All participants were instructed to imagine, while listening to the broadcast, how the graduate student felt about her situation. While listening, some participants received false physiological feedback indicating that they were not aroused (low-arousal condition); others received false feedback indicating that they were highly aroused (high-arousal condition). Prior to unexpectedly being confronted with an opportunity to help the victim, all participants were asked to indicate the degree to which they had experienced a number of emotions while listening to the broadcast.

Coke *et al.* (1978) predicted that people in the high-arousal condition would perceive themselves to be experiencing more empathy than people in the low-arousal condition and that the greater empathy experienced by people in the high-arousal condition would lead to more helping. Results supported this prediction. Participants in the high-arousal condition indicated that they felt more empathic emotion while listening to the broadcast (more empathic, concerned, warm, softhearted, and compassionate) than participants in the low-arousal condition. Participants in the high-arousal condition also offered more help to the graduate student. Further, a path analysis suggested that the effect of the false-feedback manipulation on helping was mediated by self-perceived empathic emotion. Once again, there was no evidence that these effects were due to differences in perceived need.

The two experiments reported by Coke *et al.* (1978) appear to have met the criterion of directly manipulating empathic emotion in a manner unconfounded with other variables, such as perceived need and perspective taking, that might, by themselves, affect helping. Differences in perceived need could not account for the results of either experiment. Perspective taking was held constant in Experiment 2; in Experiment 1 it was manipulated but by itself did not increase helping; it did so only when participants attributed the arousal caused by perspective taking to the victim's plight.

When people misattributed the arousal to a placebo, perspective taking did not lead to helping. If the experiments reported by Coke *et al.* are considered together with the other studies that have provided results consistent with the hypothesis that empathy leads to helping, the support for this hypothesis now appears quite strong.

Evidence for the Causal Chain

Our two-stage model not only predicts that perspective taking increases empathic emotion and empathic emotion increases helping, it also makes a third prediction, that perspective taking affects helping as a result of its effect on empathic emotion. The only evidence directly relevant to this prediction comes from Experiment 1 reported by Coke *et al.* (1978), and that evidence supports the prediction. If perspective taking had a direct effect on helping, individuals in each of the imagine conditions should have offered more help than individuals in the observe conditions. This was not the case. By itself, imagining the victim's feelings was not sufficient to increase helping; people in the imagine–arouse condition offered no more help to the victim than did people in the observe–arouse condition. But if the observational set manipulation was not sufficient, by itself, to affect helping, neither was the attribution manipulation. People in the observe–relax condition did not offer more help than people in the observe–arouse condition. Apparently, without perspective taking there was no vicarious arousal to label. As predicted by the two-stage model, perspective taking did not affect helping directly; rather, it increased vicarious arousal, and when this arousal was labeled as empathic, it increased helping.

CONCLUSIONS

The basic issue addressed in this chapter is whether empathic emotion can motivate helping. We believe that the available empirical evidence suggests that it can. Consistent with the proposed two-stage model, there is evidence that perspective taking increases empathic emotion, that empathic emotion motivates helping, and that the effect of perspective taking on helping is mediated by empathic emotion. Still, the evidence is not always as extensive as one would like. This is especially true for the causal chain implied by the two-stage model; in only one experiment has this assumption been tested.

But one can always wish for more evidence, and on the strength and consistency of the evidence already assembled it seems reasonable to draw the tentative conclusion that empathic emotion can motivate helping. This conclusion does not, of course, mean that empathic emotion is the *only* motivator of helping or that empathic emotion motivates only *helping*. Other motivators of prosocial behavior may include anticipated rewards (including self-reward), norms, and internalized values. Empathy may also motivate other behaviors; for example, it seems possible that empathy could motivate escape from the need situation rather than helping if the costs involved in helping were extreme (cf. Piliavin & Piliavin, 1973).

Nor does the conclusion that empathy can motivate helping mean that all the important questions concerning the role of empathy as a motivator of helping have been answered. Quite the contrary, it invites a host of further questions. For example:

> 1. Where does the empathic response originate? To what degree, if at all, is it genetically built into our organismic structure; to what degree is it a product of socialization patterns that may vary from culture to culture? Hoffman (1981b) has provided some intriguing suggestions relevant to this question.
> 2. To whom do we respond empathically; to everyone, or only those with whom we have a particular relationship? If the latter (as seems likely), what is the nature of this relationship? It is based on kinship, on similarity, on prior interaction, on attachment, on dependency, on some combination of these, or on some unnamed factors? Said another way, is the appropriate analogy for a relationship in which empathic responding occurs one of brother and sisterhood, of reference-group membership, of acquaintance, of friendship, or of parenting? (See Hornstein, 1976.)
> 3. Do some of us respond empathically to the distress of a wider range of people than others? Presumably some do (cf. Davis, 1981; Mehrabian & Epstein, 1972; Stotland, Matthews, Sherman, Hansson, & Richardson, 1978), but there is much still to learn about what determines individual differences in the range of empathic responding.

These are only a sample of the fascinating questions still to be answered before we understand how and why empathy motivates helping. For now, we must be content to have at least one plausible answer to the question of why people help. At least at times it is because witnessing another's distress evokes a vicarious physiological response that is labeled as concern, and this congruent emotional response produces motivation to see that person's distress reduced. This answer does not allow us to answer the question of the nature of this motivation, whether it might be truly altruistic. But it does allow us to *ask* that question, as we have done elsewhere (see Batson & Coke, 1981; Batson *et al.*, 1981).

R E F E R E N C E S

Aderman, D., & Berkowitz, L.   Observational set, empathy, and helping. *Journal of Personality and Social Psychology*, 1970, *14*, 141–148.

Aronfreed, J. M.   *Conduct and conscience: The socialization of internalized control over behavior.* New York: Academic, 1968.

Aronfreed, J. M.   The socialization of altruistic and sympathetic behavior: Some theoretical and experimental analyses. In J. Macaulay & L. Berkowitz (Eds.), *Altruism and helping behavior.* New York: Academic, 1970.

Asch, S. E.   *Social psychology.* New York: Prentice-Hall, 1952.

Bandura, A., & Rosenthal, T. L.   Vicarious classical conditioning as a function of arousal level. *Journal of Personality and Social Psychology,* 1966, *3,* 54–62.

Batson, C. D., & Coke, J. S.   Empathy: A source of altruistic motivation for helping. In J. P. Rushton & R. M. Sorrentino (Eds.), *Altruism and helping behavior.* Hillsdale, N.J.: Erlbaum, 1981.

Batson, C. D., Darley, J. M., & Coke, J. S.   Altruism and human kindness: Internal and external determinants of helping behavior. In L. Pervin & M. Lewis (Eds.), *Perspectives in interactional psychology.* New York: Plenum, 1978.

Batson, C. D., Duncan, B. D., Ackerman, P., Buckley, T., & Birch, K.   Is empathic emotion a source of altruistic motivation? *Journal of Personality and Social Psychology,* 1981, *40,* 290–302.

Beaman, A. L., Barnes, P. J., Klentz, B., & McQuirk, B.   Increasing helping rates through information dissemination: Teaching pays. *Personality and Social Psychology Bulletin,* 1978, *4,* 406–411.

Berger, S. M.   Conditioning through vicarious instigation. *Psychological Review,* 1962, *69,* 450–466.

Berkowitz, L.   Social norms, feelings, and other factors affecting helping and altruism. In L. Berkowitz (Ed.), *Advances in experimental social psychology* (Vol. 6). New York: Academic, 1972.

Borke, H.   Interpersonal perception of young children: Egocentrism or empathy? *Developmental Psychology,* 1971, *5,* 263–269.

Coke, J. S., Batson, C. D., & McDavis, K.   Empathic mediation of helping: A two-stage model. *Journal of Personality and Social Psychology,* 1978, *36,* 752–766.

Craig, K. D., & Lowrey, J. H.   Heart rate components of conditioned vicarious autonomic responses. *Journal of Personality and Social Psychology,* 1969, *11,* 381–387.

Craig, K. D., & Wood, K.   Psychophysiological differentiation of direct vicarious affective arousal. *Canadian Journal of Behavioural Science,* 1969, *1,* 98–105.

Davis, M. H.   *Empathy, moods, and helping: The role of individual differences in cognitive and emotional factors.* Paper presented at the annual meeting of the Eastern Psychological Association, New York, April 1981.

Emler, N. P., & Rushton, J. P.   Cognitive-developmental factors in children's generosity. *British Journal of Social and Clinical Psychology,* 1974, *13,* 277–281.

Feshbach, N. D.   Empathy in children: Some theoretical and empirical considerations. *The Counseling Psychologist,* 1975, *5,* 25–30.

Gaertner, S. L., & Dovidio, J. F.   The subtlety of white racism, arousal, and helping behavior. *Journal of Personality and Social Psychology,* 1977, *35,* 691–707.

Harris, M. B., & Huang, L. C.   Helping and the attribution process. *Journal of Social Psychology,* 1973, *90,* 291–297.

Heider, F.   *The psychology of interpersonal relations.* New York: Wiley, 1958.

Hoffman, M. L.   Developmental synthesis of affect and cognition and its implications for altruistic motivation. *Developmental Psychology,* 1975, *11,* 607–622.

Hoffman, M. L.   Empathy, roletaking, guilt, and development of altruistic motives. In T. Lickona (Ed.), *Moral development and behavior.* New York: Holt, Rinehart & Winston, 1976.

Hoffman, M. L.   Development of the motive to help another. In J. P. Rushton, & R. M. Sorrentino (Eds.), *Altruism and helping behavior.* Hillsdale, N.J.: Erlbaum, 1981. (a)

Hoffman, M. L.   Is altruism part of human nature? *Journal of Personality and Social Psychology,* 1981, *40,* 121–137. (b)

Hornstein, H. A.   *Cruelty and kindness: A new look at aggression and altruism.* Englewood Cliffs, N.J.: Prentice-Hall, 1976.

Huston, T. L., & Korte, C.   The responsive bystander: Why he helps. In T. Lickona (Ed.), *Moral development and behavior: Theory, research, and social issues.* New York: Holt, Rinehart & Winston, 1976.

Hygge, S.   Information about the model's unconditioned stimulus and response in vicarious classical conditioning. *Journal of Personality and Social Psychology,* 1976, *33,* 764–771.

Krebs, D. L. Empathy and altruism. *Journal of Personality and Social Psychology*, 1975, *32*, 1134–1146.

Krebs, D. L. Role taking and moral judgment. In J. P. Rushton & R. M. Sorrentino (Eds.), *Altruism and helping behavior*. Hillsdale, N.J.: Erlbaum, 1981.

Krebs, D. L., & Stirrup, B. *Role-taking ability and altruistic behavior in elementary school children*. Paper presented at the annual meeting of the American Psychological Association, New Orleans, August 1974.

Kuhn, T. S. *The structure of scientific revolutions*. Chicago: University of Chicago Press, 1962.

Latané, B., & Darley, J. M. *The unresponsive bystander: Why doesn't he help?* New York: Appleton-Century-Crofts, 1970.

Latané, B., & Nida, S. Ten years of research on group size and helping. *Psychological Bulletin*, 1981, *89*, 308–324.

Lazarus, R., Opton, E. M., Nomikos, M. S., & Rankin, N. O. The principle of short-circuiting of threat: Further evidence. *Journal of Personality*, 1965, *33*, 622–635.

Macaulay, J., & Berkowitz, L. *Altruism and helping behavior: Social psychological studies of some antecedents and consequences*. New York: Academic, 1970.

McDougall, W. *Introduction to social psychology*. London: Methuen, 1908.

Mehrabian, A., & Epstein, N. A measure of emotional empathy. *Journal of Personality*, 1972, *40*, 525–543.

Milgram, S. Behavioral study of obedience. *Journal of Abnormal and Social Psychology*, 1963, *67*, 371–378.

Mill, J. S. *Utilitarianism*. London: Parker, Son, & Bourn, 1863.

Piliavin, J. A., & Piliavin, I. M. *The Good Samaritan: Why does he help?* Unpublished manuscript, University of Wisconsin, 1973.

Regan, D. T., & Totten, J. Empathy and attribution: Turning observers into actors. *Journal of Personality and Social Psychology*, 1975, *32*, 850–856.

Rubin, K. H., & Schneider, F. W. The relationship between moral judgment, egocentrism, and altruistic behavior. *Child Development*, 1973, *44*, 661–665.

Rushton, J. P., & Sorrentino, R. M. (Eds.). *Altruism and helping behavior*. Hillsdale, N.J.: Erlbaum, 1981.

Rushton, J. P., & Wiener, J. Altruism and cognitive development in children. *British Journal of Social and Clinical Psychology*, 1975, *14*, 341–349.

Schachter, S. The interaction of cognitive and physiological determinants of emotional state. In L. Berkowitz (Ed.), *Advances in experimental social psychology* (Vol. 1). New York: Academic, 1964.

Schwartz, S. H. Normative influences on altruism. In L. Berkowitz (Ed.), *Advances in experimental social psychology* (Vol. 10). New York: Academic, 1977.

Shantz, C. U. The development of social cognition. In E. M. Hetherington (Ed.), *Review of child development research* (Vol. 5). Chicago: University of Chicago Press, 1975.

Staub, E. *Positive social behavior and morality* (Vol. 1). New York: Academic, 1978.

Stotland, E. Exploratory investigations of empathy. In L. Berkowitz (Ed.), *Advances in experimental social psychology* (Vol. 3). New York: Academic, 1969.

Stotland, E., Matthews, K. E., Sherman, S. E., Hansson, R. O., & Richardson, B. Z. *Empathy, fantasy, and helping*. Beverly Hills, Calif.: Sage, 1978.

Valins, S. Cognitive effects of false heart-rate feedback. *Journal of Personality and Social Psychology*, 1966, *4*, 400–408.

Waxler, C. Z., Yarrow, M. R., & Smith, J. B. Perspective-taking and prosocial behavior. *Developmental Psychology*, 1977, *13*, 87–88.

Weiner, B. A cognitive (attribution)–emotion–action model of motivated behavior: An analysis of judgments of help giving. *Journal of Personality and Social Psychology*, 1980, *39*, 186–200.

Wispé, L. G. Sympathy and empathy. In D. L. Sills (Ed.), *International encyclopedia of the social sciences* (Vol. 15). New York: Free Press, 1968.

CHAPTER 15

Social Facilitation: A Psychophysiological Analysis

Danny L. Moore
University of Florida

Robert S. Baron
University of Iowa

HISTORY OF THE PROBLEM

Starting with Triplett's (1898) initial report that cyclists raced faster when paced by another rider, a good deal of early research indicated that the presence of a coworker or an audience facilitated performance on a wide variety of tasks (e.g., nest building, copying, vigilance, weight lifting, pursuit rotor). Moreover, these *social facilitation effects* were found over a wide variety of species. For example, ants work more rapidly building nests when a coworking ant is physically present (Chen, 1937), and even cockroaches run a simple maze faster when an audience of fellow cockroaches is present (Zajonc, Heingartner, & Herman, 1969). Despite these data, it became apparent by the 1930s that for certain tasks social conditions hampered performance. For example, Allee and Masure (1936) reported that parakeets and cockroaches solved some mazes more slowly in pairs than when working alone.

Zajonc (1965) offered a theoretical resolution of this apparent contradiction. Zajonc argued that the physical presence of species mates elevated an organism's drive or arousal level. He pointed out that according to Hull–Spence drive theory, high drive should facilitate simple, well-learned, and/or instinctual responses, and impair difficult, poorly learned, and counterinstinctual responses.[1] Zajonc therefore argued that prior studies re-

---

1. Stated differently, drive should facilitate that response which is dominant in the response hierarchy.

porting social facilitation probably employed tasks that required instinctual, simple, or well-learned responses, whereas studies finding social impairment probably focused on tasks requiring more difficult or poorly mastered responses.

Social facilitation research[2] in the last 15 years has provided further corroboration of Zajonc's speculation (see Geen & Gange, 1977, for a more extensive review). Specifically, the recent work on social facilitation indicates that the presence of species mates produces a variety of effects on task performance that are predicted by drive theory. These include indications that social conditions (1) facilitate performance on simple, well-learned tasks while impairing performance on complex tasks; (2) interfere with initial learning of difficult materials but facilitate performance after this same material is mastered; (3) impair short-term recall in paired-associate learning but facilitate long-term recall[3]; and (4) restrict the range of cues used in problem solving (see Geen & Gange, 1977). Finally, there is some physiological evidence that arousal is heightened under social conditions (e.g., Chapman, 1974; Geen, 1979; Martens, 1969a, 1969b). Unfortunately, these data are sparse and not completely consistent. As noted below (see Table 15-1), some eight studies find heightened physiological activation under social conditions, 13 find null effects, and one reports lower physiological activation under social conditions. The fact that only eight of 22 studies provide physiological support for the drive view is somewhat disconcerting given that drive/arousal has been a central mediating concept in this literature for at least 15 years.[4] Nevertheless, the confluence of *nonphysiological* evidence favoring a drive/arousal interpretation of social facilitation is impressive and was sufficient to lead Geen and Gange, in a recent review, to conclude that Zajonc's drive view "provides the most parsimonious explanations of the findings" (1977, p. 1283). Indeed, most theoretical points currently at issue concern *why* the presence of others elevates drive rather than whether it does so (e.g., Geen, 1981; Markus, 1981; Sanders, 1981). These theories and several nondrive explanations are described in the following section.

2. In this chapter references to social facilitation research and social facilitation phenomena are intended to include the impairment of poorly learned tasks under social conditions.

3. Audience presence in this research is manipulated during study trials only. On recall trials subjects are alone.

4. In this respect, research on social facilitation closely parallels the research attempting to distinguish dissonance theory from self-perception theory. Although a variety of ingenious techniques have been utilized to test the mediating role of arousal in dissonance-like phenomena, direct physiological evidence that dissonance heightens arousal is thin (Kiesler & Pallak, 1976; Zanna & Cooper, 1976).

CURRENT THEORETICAL ISSUES

The Mere Presence Hypothesis

One aspect of Zajonc's position that has become somewhat controversial is his contention that the *mere presence* of species mates is sufficient to trigger social facilitation effects. According to Zajonc (1980, pp. 42–43), audiences need not be highly evaluative and coactors need not be actively competing with the subject for their presence to heighten arousal. Competition and evaluation may produce even more arousal yet, but nonevaluative/non-competitive others, just by their presence, are thought to be enough to produce drive effects. Given the provocative nature of this hypothesis and the importance of psychophysiological measurement for its evaluation, our discussion of it will be fairly detailed.[5]

Zajonc's original statement of the mere presence hypothesis in 1965 suggested a number of interesting possibilities. Early evidence favoring the mere presence notion seemed to suggest that arousal could occur from such a seemingly benign condition as the mere presence of others. If this were true, long periods of exposure to crowded conditions could potentially result in long-term physiological changes. Indeed, Zajonc cited evidence that animals exposed to crowded conditions exhibit higher levels of adrenal activity (Morrison & Thatcher, 1969). Thus, at least one reason to be concerned with the mere presence hypothesis was its implications for the deleterious effects of crowding (Freedman, Klevansky, & Ehrlich, 1971). In addition, the mere presence hypothesis was a provocative notion in itself. Arguing that active competition or evaluation can elevate motivational states such as arousal, drive, anxiety, or fear is not very counterintuitive; however, to claim that the passive presence of species mates also produces

5. Zajonc's (1965) paper did not draw a distinction between drive and arousal. Whether such a distinction can be drawn has been a persistent source of controversy. Whereas some theorists treat drive as a hypothetical construct with no explicit physiological concomitants (e.g., Sanders, 1981; Spence, 1956), others treat drive as an intervening variable related to the activity of the central and autonomic nervous system (Duffy, 1962, 1972, Hebb, 1955; Malmo, 1959). Although a thorough discussion of this controversy is beyond the scope of this chapter, it seems clear that most social facilitation researchers tacitly assume a close link between drive and psychophysiological activity (e.g., Geen & Gange, 1977; Zajonc, 1965). Although we agree with the general notion that drive and physiological activity are closely related, we also realize that increased drive is unlikely to cause a simple, unidimensional increase in physiological activity (cf. Lacey, 1967, Chap. 1). However, we feel that increased drive will have *some* measurable physiological concomitants. If so, physiological measures would provide one method of avoiding a common problem in social facilitation research. Specifically, most researchers infer that drive mediates social facilitation phenomena because task performance is facilitated for simple tasks and impaired for complex tasks. That is, verifying that drive mediates social facilitation simply depends on demonstrating that social facilitation occurs. To avoid such tautological reasoning requires increased attention to measurement of mediating mechanisms. In this respect, psychophysiological measures may provide a method of exploring the processes mediating social facilitation effects.

such effects is a rather nonobvious prediction. Yet this seems to be Zajonc's position. In a recent paper (Zajonc, 1980), he reiterates the mere presence hypothesis and explains it further. According to Zajonc, species mates are such important and unpredictable stimuli that their presence triggers a variety of uncertainties. "Hence, in the presence of others, some degree of alertness or preparedness for the unexpected is generated—simply because one never knows, so to speak, what sort of responses—perhaps even novel or unique—might be required of the individual in the next few seconds" (Zajonc, 1980, p. 50). This alertness and preparation presumably elevates drive.

It is unfortunate for those of us who treasure the counterintuitive finding that the mere presence hypothesis has received at best only inconsistent support. Many studies that manipulate such factors as competitive set, availability or suitability of competitive cues, ability or interest of the audience to evaluate performance, find that the mere presence of others (in nonevaluative/noncompetitive settings) does not produce significant facilitation or impairment of task performance compared to alone control cells (Bray & Sugarman, 1980; Carment & Latchford, 1970; J. L. Cohen, 1980; Cottrell, Wack, Sekerak, & Rittle, 1968; Henchy & Glass, 1968; Innes, 1972; Innes & Young, 1975; Klinger, 1969; Martens & Landers, 1972; Paulus & Murdock, 1971; Sanders, Baron, & Moore, 1978; Sasfy & Okun, 1974; Seta, Paulus, & Schkade, 1976). For example, in a classic study, Cottrell *et al.* (1968) found that a blindfolded audience did not produce facilitation effects. Similarly, when Sanders *et al.* (1978) had subjects work on different tasks so that competitive cues and competitive motivation were irrelevant, no facilitation effects occurred; on the other hand, when subjects worked on the same task, facilitation effects were observed. In short, the mere presence of others has not reliably been found to be a sufficient condition for social facilitation effects.

In fairness, there are also many studies that lend some support to the mere presence hypothesis. In audience research, two replications of Cottrell's blindfold procedure find that the presence of blindfolded people does significantly facilitate task performance (Haas & Roberts, 1975—mirror tracing; Rajecki, Ickes, Corcoran, & Lenerz, 1977—hand maze). A related audience study by Markus (1979) finds that when people are struggling to change clothing, drive-like behavioral effects occur even when the audience is not associated with the study and has his or her back to the subjects (i.e., is nonevaluative). Rittle and Bernard (1977) also report that performance on a word construction task is facilitated when an experimenter sits with his or her back to the subject. In coaction research, a few studies find that the presence of *coactors* facilitates performance speed even when subjects are told that the setting is noncompetitive (Carment, 1970b; Dashiell, 1930). In an additional coaction study, Scott and McCray (1967) find that when dogs run for food and petting reward, they do not run faster if they are competing for the reinforcer than when both animals are reinforced. Finally, Zajonc, Wolosin, Wolosin, and Loh (1970) find that dominant tendencies in a light guessing task are enhanced by coactors although they are separated by cubicles (thereby minimizing competitive social comparison cues). One problem with all these studies as support for the mere presence view is that it is difficult to be sure when evaluative or competitive concerns are truly absent. Several researchers have argued that there may be a well-learned tendency to compete or worry about evaluation (when others are present in a task setting) that carries over into settings where competition and evaluation are deemphasized or not necessary. That is, the presence of others in a task setting may often be a discriminative stimulus for eliciting competitive behavior and concerns over evaluation, regardless of whether or not the experimenter constructs the setting to be evaluative or competitive[6] (cf. Crandall, 1974; Geen, 1980, p. 71; Rittle & Bernard, 1977). Certainly in three of the four coaction studies favoring mere presence described just above (Carment, 1970b; Dashiell, 1930; Scott & McCray, 1967),[7] it was easy enough for subjects in the "noncompetitive" cells to compete if they wished to, since the relative progress of their coactors was easily discernible, providing an accurate basis for social comparison.[8] Indeed, in other research, when social comparison cues are unavailable or inappropriate, coactors generally do not produce drive-like effects on performance (Carment, 1970a; Klinger, 1969; Sanders et al., 1978; cf. Geen & Gange, 1977, and Geen, 1980). This, of course, runs counter to the mere presence view.

This "conditioned evaluation" explanation seems particularly feasible since in almost every study in this area, subjects work on behavioral

6. It is possible, of course, that in some settings evaluative/competitive concerns may be truly minimal. Our point is only that it is hard to be sure when this is so because of the possibility of conditioned evaluation. If conditioned evaluation is, in fact, a problem in some settings and not others, this might explain the inconsistency between those studies that find social facilitation effects under manipulations purported to create low evaluation and those that find null effects under such conditions. The former studies would be those eliciting conditioned evaluation while the latter studies would be those minimizing such concerns. Such factors as the status of the audience, whether it is possible to compete (even if it is unnecessary), and the similarity to past evaluative settings might affect whether conditioned evaluation occurs.

7. Scott and McCray admit that the strain of dog used in their study "readily compete over" food. This suggests that even when competition was not required, these animals were reacting to the competitive cues of other animals because of innate tendencies to compete. This is not a mere presence effect. The latter would require that the passive presence of a noncompetitive animal also heightened response speed.

8. It is hard to determine whether subjects had competitive cues in the study by Zajonc et al. In that study subjects worked in cubicles and received chips for accurate light guessing. Although subjects could not *see* the earnings of their coactors, they may have used the auditory cues of chips being dropped in bowls as a basis for comparison and competition (Quarton, 1969).

tasks during the experimental session. This may heighten associations with past evaluative settings. One obvious means of circumventing this problem is to assess the impact of audiences and coactors without relying on behavioral–cognitive measures. This represents one use for which psychophysiological methodology seems well suited.

In one illustration of this approach, Chapman (1974) took electromyographic (EMG) readings of the frontalis muscle as subjects listened to a recorded story as they lay on their backs. EMG activity was elevated above alone control levels either when an experimenter was present reading a book or in a "concealed audience" cell where the experimenter glanced repeatedly at the one-way mirror in the subjects' room. These data are certainly consistent with Zajonc's views; however, there is a troublesome artifact. Although subjects may not have felt much evaluation apprehension regarding the listening task, they quite possibly were apprehensive about how they appeared lying fully prone with surface silver–silver chloride electrodes above their eyebrows and on their neck, particularly so in the concealed audience cell where the nature of the audience is unknown. Subjects could have been most concerned with embarrassment here, thinking that they must look particularly silly to strange people they have not met who may not even know about the purpose and importance of the research. Thus, the embarrassing nature of this form of physiological measurement detracts from this particular study as evidence favoring a mere presence view.[9] Admittedly, if one obtained a similar outcome with a relatively nonreactive, nonthreatening, or nonembarrassing measure, the data would represent good support for the mere presence view. Some of the measures of palmar sweat discussed below seem well suited for such a purpose. Note a very similar argument regarding embarrassment could be made about Markus's clothes changing study. That is the "mere presence" of an uninvolved, uninformed bystander may have heightened her subjects' concern over possible embarrassment while donning a second pair of socks, size 12 tennis shoes, and an oversized lab coat. As a result, we would argue that as of yet there is little compelling support for Zajonc's provocative notion that the mere presence of others heightens arousal. Our views, though, are by no means universal. A number of authors still subscribe to the mere presence notion, and there is no denying that there is some empirical support for this view. As the discussion above implies, psychophysiological measurements may be useful in clarifying these and related issues. The sections below amplify these possibilities.

9. These comments apply equally well to an earlier study by Chapman (1973) which assessed frontalis electromyograms as subjects lay on their backs, eyes open, listening to a humorous Shelley Berman tape. This study did not include an alone control group and therefore is not relevant to the mere presence controversy, but clearly a good deal of observed frontalis tension could have been atypically high because of embarrassment and uneasiness concerning appearance.

The Evaluation Apprehension Hypothesis

Cottrell (1968, 1972) offered one of the earliest alternatives to Zajonc's mere presence hypothesis. He argued that because social stimuli frequently have been paired with positive and negative events in an organism's learning history, they should become cues eliciting learned drive (e.g., incentive motivation—Spence, 1956). Cottrell argued that for humans, the association between social stimuli and positive or negative outcomes should be particularly strong in evaluative and competitive settings. As a result, he argued that evaluative/competitive cues comprised one class of stimuli that would heighten social facilitation effects. Consistent with this proposal, Cottrell *et al.* (1968) found that social facilitation occurred only when evaluative cues were present. As noted in the preceding section, there are at least 13 studies that replicate this basic finding and at least 8 that contradict it. Although there seems a good deal of controversy regarding whether competition/evaluation are necessary for social facilitation effects, there is little doubt that they enhance such effects (cf. Geen, 1980).

There are, however, some credible arguments suggesting that evaluation apprehension or competition cannot be the sole mediator of social facilitation phenomena. Zajonc (1980) points out that social facilitation occurs on tasks where there are no right or wrong answers (i.e., no evaluation possible), while several other studies have found that evaluative pressure per se is not always a sufficient condition to trigger social facilitation effects (e.g., Sanders *et al.*, 1978). Sanders *et al.* told subjects in alone cells that *they* were evaluating a practice task (low-evaluation cell). Subjects in coaction cells were told that they were being evaluated on the basis of task performance (high evaluation). These coaction subjects either worked on similar tasks or on noncomparable tasks. High evaluation did not produce social facilitation effects in the noncomparable cells. Social facilitation occurred only when subjects worked on similar tasks (where social comparison was possible). The fact that evaluative cues failed to produce social facilitation effects in certain coaction settings clearly runs counter to the notion that evaluation apprehension is necessary for social facilitation. In short, there are a number of theoretical and empirical loose ends characterizing the learned drive or evaluation apprehension hypothesis, and as such it is still the focus for a good deal of current research (e.g., Geen, 1979).

The Distraction/Conflict Hypothesis

Distraction/conflict theory offers a third account of why social conditions may heighten drive or arousal (e.g., Baron, Moore, & Sanders, 1978; Moore, 1977; Sanders *et al.*, 1978). This theory assumes that the presence of others distracts subjects from their task, placing subjects in attentional conflict. According to the distraction/conflict view, a major reason others are distracting is because by attending to competitors and audiences, subjects gain crucial social comparison information about the adequacy of their performance. Since subjects in social facilitation research are almost invariably under time pressure, attending to others directly conflicts with the attentional demands of the task. The resulting attentional conflict is closely akin to cognitive overload described by such writers as Milgram (1970), Kahneman (1973), and S. Cohen (1978). As such, it could enhance drive or arousal for several reasons. Kahneman argues that when people face overload, they attempt to compensate for the strain on capacity by increasing their expenditure of effort, this, in turn, elevating arousal. Similarly, a number of drive theorists argue that various forms of conflict heighten drive (Brown & Farber, 1951; Kimble, 1961).

Note that according to distraction/conflict theory, the mere presence of others will not invariably heighten drive as predicted by Zajonc (1980). If others do not provide useful information to subjects regarding the adequacy of their performance, they may be ignored, thereby minimizing the attentional conflict. Distraction/conflict theory predictions can also be distinguished from those of the learned drive or evaluation apprehension view. In particular, Cottrell's (1968) learned drive hypothesis predicts that some degree of evaluation apprehension is necessary for social facilitation phenomena. Distraction/conflict theory, on the other hand, suggests that social facilitation effects can appear even when evaluation apprehension is absent. If the subject desires or needs to perform a task and if cues from others compete for attention, then social facilitation effects should occur even when no evaluation apprehension is present. On the other hand, if task demands are minimal (such that the task can be easily ignored) or absent, the presence of others should not lead to conflict or overload and, consequently, should not heighten drive. Thus, according to distraction/ conflict theory, *the very behavioral measures commonly used to detect arousal or drive in social facilitation settings may be crucial elements creating the arousal they are supposed to measure!*[10] One method of addressing this issue is to examine psychophysiological indices when subjects are not required to work on a task in the presence of others provided, of course, that the physiological measure in question seems unlikely to affect subjects' physiological activity.[11]

10. This point is related to the fact that distraction/conflict theory does *not* simply say that if others are noticed they will cause arousal and that if they are not noticed they will not. Rather, arousal is thought to occur when attending to others conflicts with other attentional demands. Thus, there should be settings where others will be noticed and even attended to quite closely without causing elevations in physiological activity.

11. Of course, many physiological measurement procedures may alter the physiological activity they are designed to measure. This may be especially so when the procedures involve disfiguring electrode placement, intimidating equipment, mild pain, and/or unfamiliar procedures (cf. Christie & Todd, 1975; and McHugo & Lanzetta, Chapter 23, and Cacioppo,

Nondrive Interpretations of Social Facilitation/Impairment Effects

Self-Awareness Theory

Wicklund and Duval (1971), and more recently, Wicklund (1975), proposed that the presence of others affects task performance by increasing objective self-awareness. Social conditions are assumed to direct attention inward upon the self and thereby increase the individual's motivation to perform up to their ideals. Since it is likely that objectively self-aware persons will perceive a discrepancy between their actual performance and their ideal performance, they should try to reduce this discrepancy by improving performance. There are several problems with the self-awareness view. First, this explanation is hard-pressed to account in any straightforward way for impaired complex performance in social conditions. Second, this view is also unable to account for facilitation of dominant responses that are not more correct or socially appropriate than other responses (e.g., J. L. Cohen & Davis, 1973; Goldman, cited in Zajonc, 1980). Third, it is hard to apply self-awareness theory to nonhuman social facilitation data. Finally, a pivotal assumption of the self-awareness view is that both the presence of others and standard manipulations of self-awareness (e.g., a mirror) should produce similar effects. Available data indicate little support for this crucial assumption (Geen & Gange, 1977; Innes & Young, 1975; Paulus, Annis, & Risner, 1978; Rajecki et al., 1977).

Attentional Overload

S. Cohen (1978) has derived an explanation of attentional overload effects on task performance that represents a nondrive counterpart to the distraction/conflict formulation. Cohen relies heavily on the work of Kahneman (1973) and points out that there are data indicating that when individuals experience attentional overload, they restrict their attention to cues that are most relevant or central to task demands. Cohen argues that on many tasks, this restricted focus will facilitate performance. However, certain tasks require the processing of a wide range of cues. On these

---

Marshall-Goodell, & Gormezano, Chapter 24, this volume). Psychophysiological procedures may affect task performance in a social facilitation setting by either (1) distracting subjects from task performance or (2) embarrassing or frightening subjects. These reactive effects of psychophysiological measurement would create serious interpretive problems in social facilitation research only if they interacted with audience or coaction treatments. One could test for such interactive effects in the following design. Subjects would work on a drive-sensitive task either alone or in the presence of an audience or group of coactors. Half of the subjects in the alone and social presence conditions would receive physiological measures while the remaining half would not receive such measures. If physiological measures interact with social presence effects, task performance should vary as a function of both the presence or absence of others and the presence or absence of physiological procedures.

tasks, overload and restricted focus should impair performance. As a result, if social conditions do overload the organism as distraction/conflict theory suggests, then social facilitation effects could be due to perceptual changes (i.e., a reallocation of attention) rather than motivational changes.

Summary of Theoretical Issues

A variety of theoretical perspectives are currently available in the social facilitation literature. Although most of these involve drive as a central concept, at least two do not. Drive interpretations vary in terms of what conditions are thought to elicit arousal or drive. Clearly, one contribution psychophysiology can make in this literature is (1) to document whether and when social conditions have an arousal-like impact on various psychophysiological measures, and (2) to provide some way of elevating our sophistication regarding whether such psychophysiological effects can be confidently characterized as arousal. These issues are treated in the following sections.

APPLICATIONS OF PSYCHOPHYSIOLOGY TO SOCIAL FACILITATION/IMPAIRMENT RESEARCH
Some Conceptual Issues Concerning Arousal

An obvious issue concerning the application of psychophysiological techniques to social facilitation research involves testing Zajonc's (1965) assertion that the presence of others elevates an organism's arousal level. In his paper, Zajonc cited indirect evidence for the arousing properties of social presence stemming primarily from studies of crowding and active social interaction. However, social facilitation research since 1965 has not yielded very consistent results regarding the effects of audiences or coactors on physiological activity. In the present and following sections we attempt to review and reconcile these conflicting findings and suggest future directions for research.

Before discussing the physiological data related to social facilitation phenomena, it will be useful to first specify what the term "physiological arousal" usually implies in the social facilitation literature. The position taken in Zajonc's paper, and in subsequent social facilitation research, most closely resembles an activation theory approach such as Duffy's (1962, 1972) formulation, in which arousal represents the release of energy into various internal physiological systems through metabolic activity. According to this view, almost any physiological response can be considered an indicator of the degree of activation or arousal. Consequently, the concept of arousal has been linked to a variety of physiological changes such as increases in heart rate, blood pressure, muscle tension, sweating, body temperature, respiration, electroencephalograph readings, and adrenal activity (see Duffy, 1967, for a historical account of the activation concept). According to this view, if the presence of others increases arousal, one or more of the physiological changes listed above should be observed in comparisons of audience and coaction conditions with alone conditions. This simple view is represented in a good deal of social facilitation theory and research. However, as noted below (see also Cacioppo & Petty, Chapter 1, this volume), such a unidimensional view of arousal is problematic in several respects: Emerging evidence indicates that various "arousing" stimuli do not always produce similar patterns of physiological response; activity on one physiological measure is often poorly correlated with activity on others [indeed, negative correlations (i.e., directional fractionation) sometimes occurs] and task features often obscure or produce artifactual physiological changes (Fowles, 1980; Hassett, 1978; Lacey, 1967; Obrist, 1976; Shapiro & Crider, 1969). This discussion foreshadows our concern with developing methods of examining the arousing properties of social presence that are independent of task performance and stimuli-specific artifacts.

Psychophysiological Effects of Social Presence: A Review

The following review of psychophysiological research is organized around various physiological measures that have been used in social facilitation research. It will soon become apparent that the psychophysiological data are indeed complex and often conflicting. A summary of the relevant research is shown in Table 15-1. Studies concerning the influence of social conditions on a particular physiological variable are listed underneath the measure in Table 15-1. The reader will note that all studies listed in Table 15-1 involve audience manipulations. This is because at this writing there simply are no studies that report the effect of coaction on physiological activity. Social facilitation tasks are categorized as either motor or cognitive in this table. These categories were derived from a general concern with the potential influence of different types of activity on physiological responses. Although it seems clear that such physiological measures as cardiovascular activity will show increases as *motor activity* increases (Obrist, 1976), cognitive–perceptual tasks (i.e., tasks that do not require motor activity) may elicit *either increased or decreased* cardiovascular activity, depending on the amount and type of information processing activities induced by the task (Cacioppo & Petty, 1982). Therefore, we believe that in assessing the effects of social conditions on physiological activity, one must be cognizant of the particular motor and cognitive requirements of the task. From an activation theory standpoint, social conditions should elevate physiological activity relative to alone conditions for both motor and cognitive tasks. Finally, in the last column of Table 15-1, the physio-

TABLE 15-1. Summary of Psychophysiological Investigations of Social Facilitation

PHYSIOLOGICAL MEASURE	TYPE OF TASK*	EFFECT OF SOCIAL CONDITIONS ON PHYSIOLOGICAL ACTIVITY
Palmar sweating		
Martens (1969a)	M (coincident timing)	+
Martens (1969b)	M (coincident timing)	+
J. L. Cohen & Davis (1973)†	C (hidden word)	− peer, + expert
		0 evaluate, + observed
Geen (1976)	C (anagram task)	+ mere presence and + evaluation apprehension
Bargh & Cohen (1978)†	M and C	0
J. L. Cohen (1979)†	C (hidden word)	0
J. L. Cohen (1980)	C (hidden word)	0
Carver & Scheier (1981)	M (copy German task)	+ before task, 0 during task
Skin conductance levels		
Henchy & Glass (1968)	C (pseudorecognition)	0 nonexpert, 0 expert
Moore (1977)	M (reaction time)	0
Geen (1979)	C (paired-associates learning)	0
Borden, Hendrick, & Walker (1976)	C (listen to persuasive communication)	0
Skin resistance responses		
Geen (1979)	C (paired-associates learning)	+
Heart rate		
Henchy & Glass (1968)	C (pseudorecognition)	0
Borden, Hendrick, & Walker (1976)	C (listen to persuasive communication	0
Moore (1977)	M (reaction time)	0
Geen (1979)	C (paired-associates learning)	0
Musante & Anker (1972)	M (inhibit movement)	0
Muscular tension		
Chapman (1973)	C (listen to humorous story)	+ evaluative audience
Chapman (1974)	C (listen to dramatic story)	+
Musante & Anker (1972)	M (inhibit movement)	0 before task, − during task
Voice recordings		
Brenner (1974)	M and C (read poetry aloud)	+

*M, motor; C, cognitive.

†No audience was present in these studies. Subjects were instructed that they would be observed by an audience concealed by a one-way mirror or that videotapes of their performance would be examined at a future time.

logical activity in social conditions relative to alone conditions is compared for each study: A "+" signifies heightened activity in social conditions, a "0" indicates no difference between social and alone conditions, and a "−" denotes decreased activity in social conditions.

Palmar Sweating

Palmar sweating is by far the most popular physiological technique in social facilitation research. Two procedures for measuring palmar sweating have been developed. The first, referred to as the Palmar Sweat Index (PSI), provides a count of the number of active sweat glands at the measurement site (usually a fingertip)—see Dabbs, Johnson, and Leventhal (1968) and Johnson and Dabbs (1967) for a description of the PSI. A second, more recent method of measuring palmar sweating has been developed by Strahan, Todd, and Inglis (1974). Their technique involves measuring the conductivity of distilled water that has been placed in contact with the skin for a few seconds: The more sweat that collected in the sweat bottle, the greater the conductivity of the bottle's contents. Both the PSI and sweat bottle techniques provide relatively unobtrusive methods of assessing autonomic activity that are easy to administer and easy to score. However, it is important to note that the PSI and sweat bottle techniques do not correlate highly and may reflect different physiological components of palmar sweating (Strahan et al., 1974).

Social facilitation research utilizing palmar sweating measures has produced mixed results. Of eight relevant studies, only four have shown increased palmar sweating in social conditions. Table 15-1 also shows that motor tasks were used in three of the studies reporting increased palmar sweating in audience conditions. Martens (1969a, 1969b), for instance, gave subjects a coincident timing task which required them to move a cursor so that it hit a moving target. In both studies, Martens found that PSI was higher in audience than in alone conditions for PSI measures collected between trials of the task. Carver and Scheier (1981) also report increased PSI in audience conditions when subjects performed a motor task (i.e., copying German prose). However, they found that PSI was only greater in audience than in alone conditions before the task. During the copying task, Carver and Scheier found that there were no differences between the audience and alone conditions on the PSI measure. Moreover, palmar sweating actually decreased during the copying task. In the Carver and Scheier study, a mirror condition was included to test the self-awareness theory of social facilitation. Their results indicated that both the audience and mirror conditions produced facilitation of copying compared to an alone, control condition. This finding would seem to indicate that social facilitation effects might be mediated by increased objective self-awareness. However, Carver and Scheier also report that subjects in the mirror conditions, unlike those in the audience conditions, did not show significant elevations of PSI. Thus, audience and mirror conditions do not produce similar physiological effects (see also Paulus, Annis, & Risner, 1978). This, of course, suggests that social facilitation manipulations and objective self-awareness (OSA) manipulations are not producing parallel effects, as would be the case if increased self-awareness were mediating social facilitation phenomena.

The palmar sweating data for experiments utilizing cognitive tasks that do not require motor activity do not provide unequivocal support for the drive/arousal interpretation of social facilitation. J. L. Cohen and Davis (1973), for instance, found that an evaluative audience produced higher PSI than a nonevaluative audience under live conditions, but an opposite pattern occurred when the audience could only evaluate videotapes of subjects' performance. Geen and Gange (1977) suggested that the reason why Cohen and Davis did not find unequivocal support for the drive interpretation of social facilitation was because an audience was not physically present. However, a more recent study by J. L. Cohen (1980) in which an audience was physically present during task performance also indicates that neither merely present nor evaluative audiences increase palmer sweating as measured by the sweat bottle technique. Geen (1976), however, reports that subjects exhibit higher PSI in mere presence and evaluation apprehension conditions than in an alone condition when performing a complex anagram task. Clearly, the data on PSI are still inconsistent, but at this point it does not seem to be a simple function of whether the audience is visible or not. This seems particularly true when one considers that J. L. Cohen and Davis (1973), Bargh and Cohen (1978), and J. L. Cohen (1979) all show that hidden audiences affect *behavioral* measures while having no effect on PSI. If hidden audiences failed to heighten PSI because they simply were not salient, no behavioral effects should occur.

Electrodermal Activity

Two measures of the electrical activity of the skin have been used to assess physiological activity in social and nonsocial conditions. The first of these measures examines changes in the *level* of electrodermal activity over relatively long periods of time (tonic activity), while the second examines the frequency of short duration *responses* (phasic activity) (see Chapter 1 for more discussion).

Four studies have compared skin conductance levels in social and alone conditions. All these studies examine the influence of passive audiences and report no differences in tonic skin conductance levels between audience and alone conditions. Henchy and Glass (1968), for instance, found that neither expert nor nonexpert audiences elevated tonic skin conductance levels above an alone condition when subjects worked on a cognitive task (i.e., pseudorecognition). Moore (1977) utilized a motor task (i.e., reaction time) and also found that between-trial tonic skin conductance levels in audience and alone conditions did not differ. Similarly, Geen (1979) reported no difference in the tonic level of electrodermal activity when subjects performed a paired-associates learning task alone or in the presence of others. Finally, Borden, Hendrick, and Walker (1976) found that listening to a persuasive communication in the presence of an audience did not elevate tonic skin conductance levels above alone conditions. All these studies reported task performance differences between alone and audience conditions.

The results for tonic electrodermal activity (skin conductance levels) seem perplexing given the marginal support for the arousal view obtained with palmar sweating measures. That is, if both palmar sweat measures and skin conductance reflect sweating on the palms, why do they show different responses to social conditions? There are two potential answers to this question. First, palmar sweating measures and skin conductance tap different components, as well as similar components, of sweat gland responses (Edelberg, 1972).[12] While the PSI technique measures the number of active sweat glands, skin conductance also reflects the level of sweat within the gland duct. Thus, skin conductance may increase as sweat travels up the gland duct but is not secreted on the skin. Second, there seem to be peripheral physiological limitations on skin conductance which renders this measure less sensitive to conditions that elicit frequent responses. Specifically, repeated elicitation of responses by such stimuli as noise, shock, or task requirements causes skin conductance levels to rise to a maximum (Fowles, 1980; Fowles & Schneider, 1974, 1978; Schneider & Fowles, 1978). This suggests that skin conductance level will be less sensitive to the effects of social presence because it is subject to ceiling effects.

An alternative measure of electrodermal activity which does not seem to be subject to the physiological constraints of skin conductance level involves counting the number of spontaneous skin resistance responses (SSRRs) in a given time period. These phasic responses are termed spontaneous in that they cannot be associated with a particular stimulus. Geen (1979) found that just after performing a paired-associates task subjects had greater SSRRs in audience conditions than in alone conditions following failure feedback. Since drive effects carry over for up to 30

---

12. Several studies report high correlations between counts of the number of active sweat glands and skin conductance levels (Catania, Thompson, Michalewski, & Bowman, 1980; Juniper, Blanton, & Dykman, 1967; Thomas & Korr, 1957). Since the corneum is a low-conductance pathway to the epidermis, one would expect high correlations between sweat gland counts and skin-conductance-level measures (Edelberg, 1977). However, there are physiological reasons to expect lower correlations between level and count measures for older subjects and for subjects who do manual labor (see Catania et al., 1980). In addition, the high correlations between count and level measures in prior studies were observed for resting conditions. Hence, it is unclear whether or not such high correlations would be observed when subjects are actively engaged in task performance.

minutes following a drive induction, these data are consistent with Geen's argument that drive effects in social facilitation research involve some form of aversive motivation, such as embarrassment, guilt, or fear of failure (Weiss & Miller, 1971).

The use of SSRRs by Geen is interesting and adds a new measure to the list of psychophysiological measures used by social facilitation researchers. Such measures allow one to examine the effects of social conditions on phasic activity, as well as tonic activity. There is some evidence that tonic electrodermal levels and phasic electrodermal responses (SSRRs) are independent and reflect different dimensions. Kilpatrick (1972), for example, found that an IQ test elicited increases in skin conductance level without increases in spontaneous responses. When the IQ test was described as a measure of brain damage, both level and spontaneous responses increased. This suggests that SSRR reflects motivational processes such as threat, while skin conductance level reflects elevations in cognitive processing (see Hassett, 1978). This speculation may be useful to consider in future research (see Kilpatrick, 1972; Katkin, 1965, Fowles, 1980; and Bundy & Mangan, 1979, for discussions and some opposing points of view).

Heart Rate
The four studies examining the effects of social presence on skin conductance levels discussed above also reported heart rate data. As Table 15-1 shows, these studies failed to uncover differences in heart rate between alone and audience conditions. An experiment by Musante and Anker (1972) supplements these data and shows that the presence of an experimenter did not elevate heart rate above alone controls. In all cases, heart rate was measured during the task and should be classified as a tonic measure since in all cases heart rate was averaged across the task period.

Muscle Tension
Chapman (1974) has examined the influence of an audience on forehead (frontalis) muscle tension.[13] The results indicated that forehead muscle tension was highest in audience conditions followed by concealed audience and alone conditions, respectively. These results are often cited as good support for the notion that the mere presence of others is arousing (see Geen & Gange, 1977; Zajonc, 1980). There are, however, methodological problems in Chapman's study that necessitate a somewhat more cautious interpretation of his data. First, Chapman instructed his subjects to keep their eyes open while listening to the dramatic passage. However, he did

---

13. An earlier study (Chapman, 1973) examines some related issues, but since it did not include an alone control, it is not discussed. Many of our comments regarding Chapman (1974) also apply to Chapman (1973).

not monitor whether subjects actually obeyed his instructions in all conditions. Since the experimenter was present in the audience condition and absent in the concealed audience and alone conditions, it is possible that subjects in the alone and concealed audience conditions felt less compelled to follow Chapman's instructions. If this were so, one would expect forehead muscle tension to be higher in the audience condition simply because subjects in this condition kept their eyes open. Davis, Brickett, Stern, and Kimball (1978) demonstrate that recording procedures such as those used in Chapman's study are influenced by the tension in nearby ocular muscles. Future research could easily control for this alternative interpretation of Chapman's data by providing manipulation checks to determine whether subjects follow the task instructions. The second problem concerns potential embarrassment caused by having subjects wear facial electrodes while laying fully prone (see the discussion of the mere presence hypothesis in the second section of this chapter). This is a crucial problem with any study using such measures. The obtrusive and disfiguring nature of the measure makes it poorly suited to detecting audience effects. As with some of the behavioral measures we discussed, this particular measure could be *causing* the very effect it is only supposed to be detecting.

An interesting study by Musante and Anker (1972) also reports data concerning the influence of social conditions on forehead muscle tension. Rather than examining the heightening of motor activity in social conditions, Musante and Anker asked subjects to inhibit movement. Consider the following instructions given to subjects in the Musante and Anker study: "You will hear three sounds. Remain in the same position. Do not respond to the sounds. Concentrate on being deaf to the sounds; concentrate on disregarding the sounds. Be sure not to move any part of your body" (p. 903). Clearly, the task in this case is to inhibit movement following a tone. If audience conditions are arousing, one might expect that subjects in these conditions would have higher muscle tension even though they are attempting to inhibit movement. This, however, did not occur in Musante and Anker's study. Instead, subjects who performed before the experimenter (i.e., the audience condition) exhibited *lower* muscle tension following a tone than did subjects who performed alone. Before the tone, muscle tension did not differ for the audience and alone conditions. These findings are clearly difficult to fathom if one considers physiological activity simply as an index of how aroused a person is. However, muscle tension, like the measures we discuss above, undoubtedly reflects task activity as well as arousal. Attempting to inhibit movement may decrease muscle tension. If so, one possible explanation for the Musante and Anker findings may be that *task-related physiological activity* (as well as overt behavior) is accentuated in social conditions. In this case, the decrease in muscle tension caused by the task would be accentuated in the audience condition. Musante and Anker's results are, of course, open to other interpretations. For example, if the task causes subjects to stiffen their bodies, thereby increasing muscle tension, and if the audience distracted subjects from the task, one would expect lower muscle tension in the audience condition. Both explanations, however, illustrate the general point that on this measure, too, differences in task activity, rather than some underlying arousal state, may mediate observed differences in physiological activity.

Vocal Stress

A rather novel technique was used by Brenner (1974) to examine the physiological effects of audience observation. Brenner recorded subjects as they read a poem alone or before an audience. He later analyzed these recordings with the Psychological Stress Evaluator (PSE). The PSE is a machine that responds to inaudible voice signals and which seems to measure muscle tension in the vocal muscles. Brenner's results indicated that subjects in audience conditions exhibited more stress than did those in alone conditions. Interpretation of this finding must be approached with caution, however. Brenner, Branscomb, and Schwartz (1979) note that the PSE must be scored subjectively, and perhaps because of this, the PSE measure shows low reliability. Moreover, the PSE does not correlate highly with other recordings of vocal muscle tension and is subject to a number of recording artifacts. Hence, a simple interpretation of the PSE as a measure of arousal seems inappropriate at this time.

Summary

The research discussed up to this point reveals a complicated and somewhat confusing pattern of findings. Palmar sweating is sometimes greater in audience than alone conditions, whereas skin conductance levels have not been found to differ between alone and audience conditions. Similarly, heart rate does not seem to be elevated by social conditions. In contrast, muscle tension and spontaneous skin resistance responses seem to be elevated in some audience conditions, although the muscle tension effects are suspect due to possible artifacts due to embarrassment, background noise, and so on. In short, there is some marginal support for the notion that social conditions elevate some forms of autonomic (i.e., electrodermal) activity. However, there is no evidence pertaining to the effect of social conditions on electrocortical activity, even though such activity is central to the concept of activation and arousal (Duffy, 1967, 1972; Lacey, 1967). Obviously, the case concerning the crucial mediating role of arousal in social facilitation research is far from closed since, as we have seen in the preceding discussion, there are a number of inconsistent outcomes and several methodological criticisms that seem relevant.

FUTURE DIRECTIONS FOR SOCIAL FACILITATION RESEARCH

At the beginning of this chapter, we indicated that psychophysiological research may provide a key to understanding the underlying causes of social facilitation effects. Even a quick glance at Table 15-1, however, reveals that psychophysiological research to date has not provided conclusive support of any particular theoretical view. Depending on one's perspective, the available data could be interpreted either as evidence for or evidence against a drive or arousal view of social facilitation. Future research hopefully will clarify the complex pattern of findings discussed in the preceding sections. However, to do so may require new paradigms and increased attention to the assumptions and problems underlying physiological measurement. In the present section we outline what we believe to be significant problems and potential prospects for further research concerning the effects of social conditions on physiological activity.

Arousal as a Construct in Social Facilitation

The concept of arousal is a controversial topic in psychophysiology (see Cacioppo & Petty, Chapter 1, and McHugo & Lanzetta, Chapter 23, this volume, for more detailed discussions). Duffy (1962, 1972) assumed that almost any physiological response could be used to index arousal. On the opposite side of the controversy, Lacey (1959, 1967) has shown that this relatively uncomplicated view of arousal severely fails empirical tests. Despite the overwhelming evidence that a unidimensional concept of arousal is inadequate, Duffy (1972) maintains that complete rejection of the concept would be premature at this time. She presents several cogent arguments which suggest that improved measurement techniques and a better understanding of the time course of various physiological reactions will someday provide an index of overall activation. Currently, however, most theorists propose that arousal is a multidimensional concept. Lacey (1967), for example, argues that electrocortical activity, autonomic activity, and behavioral activity are all different forms of psychophysiological activation, while Cacioppo and Petty (1982) argue that subjectively perceived arousal represents yet another manifestation of physiological change. Moreover, these authors argue that at times these various forms of psychophysiological activity may occur simultaneously, while at other times these "arousals" will be poorly correlated. At present, then, it does not seem possible to view these various physiological systems as interchangeable indices of some single underlying arousal state.

In fairness, there is one possible means of integrating the various critiques of the arousal concept with the view that different "arousal" manipulations could have some common effects on behavior and cognition. Most critiques of the arousal construct (e.g., Lacey, 1967) argue that various arousal manipulations affect a variety of physiological systems, and that these effects are manipulation specific and not particularly well correlated across systems (see Chapter 1). This could be correct and still these various manipulations could share some common elements that produce some general effects on task performance, memory, and so on. For example, all these manipulations could cause physiological changes that produce attentional shifts due to attempts of the organism to assess, categorize, and interpret any noticeable physiological change (Schachter & Singer, 1962). Alternatively, the manipulation itself could attract the subject's attention. Responses such as these could absorb attentional capacity, thereby heightening the possibility of attentional overload. Kahneman (1973) and S. Cohen (1978), among others, document a number of task and memory effects that are likely to follow attentional overload which closely parallel many of the effects reported in the social facilitation literature. Indeed, Easterbrook (1959) argued that arousal leads to just the type of restricted cue utilization that Kahneman and Cohen allude to, and Geen (1976) provides data supporting this hypothesis. Since this arousal/overload notion provides an integrated account for a good deal of data, it seems worthy of future research. Figure 15-1C depicts the model described above with one additional feature. Kahneman argues that overload can generate effort/arousal effects. Thus, not only may arousal heighten overload, but the reverse may be true as well, thereby creating a feedback loop. Figure 15-1 contrasts this arousal/overload model to the two other attentional models described earlier, distraction/conflict theory and attentional overload theory.

Note that this arousal/overload notion is distinctly different from the distraction/conflict theory argument that attentional conflict (i.e., overload) leads to elevations in drive. Arousal/overload theory, in contrast, argues that elevations in drive may lead to overload and that it is the latter which is the proximal (i.e., direct) cause of task and memory effects in social facilitation research (see Figure 15-1). Also note that both distraction/conflict theory and arousal/overload theory differ from the nondrive attentional overload theory discussed earlier in the section on theoretical issues. This explanation holds that attentional conflict (due to distraction) causes attentional overload, which, in turn, leads to restricted cue utilization (i.e., a restricted cognitive focus that favors "high-priority" inputs). As noted above, this type of restricted focus is hypothesized to produce just the type of task effects found in social facilitation research. Actually, arousal/overload theory is just an elaboration of attentional overload theory specifying that changes in physiological activity are one class of cues that may contribute to overload. For both views, overload rather than drive is the proximal cause of task effects in the social facilitation literature. Of course, it is conceivable that drive and overload are separate ways of producing social facilitation effects, but given initial indications that drive

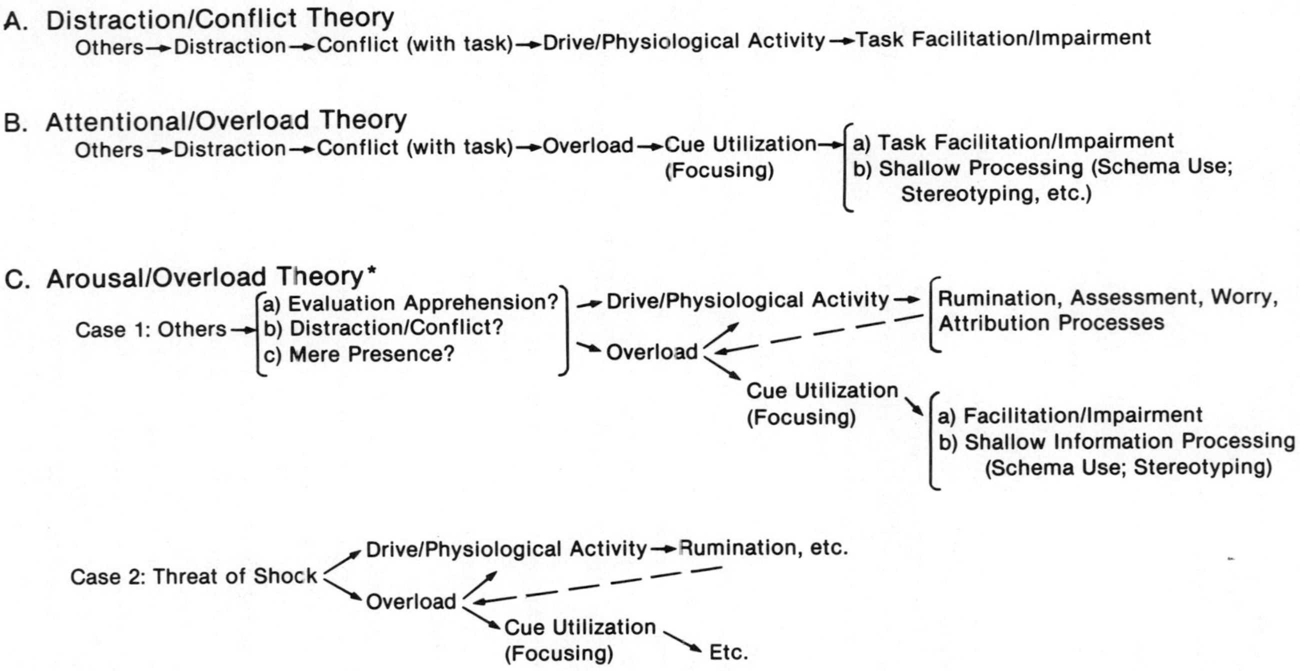

A. Distraction/Conflict Theory

Others→Distraction→Conflict (with task)→Drive/Physiological Activity→Task Facilitation/Impairment

B. Attentional/Overload Theory

Others→Distraction→Conflict (with task)→Overload→Cue Utilization→ a) Task Facilitation/Impairment
(Focusing)   b) Shallow Processing (Schema Use; Stereotyping, etc.)

C. Arousal/Overload Theory*

Case 1: Others → { a) Evaluation Apprehension? b) Distraction/Conflict? c) Mere Presence? } → Drive/Physiological Activity → Rumination, Assessment, Worry, Attribution Processes

Overload → Cue Utilization (Focusing) → a) Facilitation/Impairment b) Shallow Information Processing (Schema Use; Stereotyping)

Case 2: Threat of Shock → Drive/Physiological Activity → Rumination, etc.

Overload → Cue Utilization (Focusing) → Etc.

FIGURE 15-1. Three attentional models of social facilitation. In model C, cases 1 and 2, drive stimuli and consequent rumination are depicted as heightening the probability of overload since both are assumed to absorb and/or shrink cognitive capacity (Easterbrook, 1959). Overload is depicted as heightening drive and/or physiological activity since it is assumed to heighten effort (Kahneman, 1973). This then represents a feedback loop. It is also assumed that frequently the overt manipulation itself will absorb attention, thereby heightening the probability of overload. Thus, in case 2 threat of shock, per se, is depicted as a factor increasing the likelihood of overload.

manipulations do lead to certain forms of cue utilization (Geen, 1976), our prediction is that some form of integrated meta theory will soon emerge. Clearly, some resolution of this type is needed if one wishes to argue that some central construct related to "arousal" manipulations is mediating social facilitation/impairment effects given the complex relationship that exists between physiological and behavioral measures.

New Paradigms and Measurement Strategies

Cardiovascular and Electrodermal Measures

There are recent developments in psychophysiology which suggest that the two most common measures in social facilitation research, heart rate and electrodermal activity, may reflect different aspects of the interaction between the organism and environment. On the one hand, there are some indications that while heart rate increases with behavioral arousal (i.e., activity levels), electrodermal activity does not. Instead, electrodermal activity seems to vary more with nonsomatic, perhaps motivational or attentional factors than it does with motor activity. Miezejeski (1978), for instance, found that heart rate measures increased as finger-tapping rates increased. Skin conductance, however, was not influenced by the rate of finger tapping. These results have been replicated in a number of studies (Carriero, 1975; Epstein, Bourdreau, & Kling, 1975; Roberts, 1974). These data suggest that cardiovascular measures are more likely to reflect changes in motor activity than electrodermal measures. Note, however, that this does not imply that heart rate is not sensitive to motivational stimuli. Indeed, Fowles (1980) proposes that both heart rate and electrodermal measures are sensitive to motivational states. Heart rate, according to Fowles, is linked to somatic activity and incentive effects. Electrodermal measures (e.g., skin conductance) and related indices such as palmar sweat, on the other hand, are hypothesized to respond to punishment or withdrawal of rewards.[14]

If these suggestions are substantiated by future research, this distinction would prove quite useful in assessing more completely those theoretical views which hold that social facilitation is due primarily to anticipation of (or concern with) negative outcomes (e.g., Geen, 1980; Weiss & Miller, 1971). If this is so, Fowles's argument suggests that measures such

---

14. Fowles's assertions are based on an extensive review of the literature and a multicomponent theory of arousal. He contends, as Gray (1975) does, that there are three separate arousal systems: (1) a behavioral activation system (BAS), (2) a behavioral inhibition system (BIS), and (3) a nonspecific arousal system receiving excitatory inputs from both BAS and BIS. Evidence reviewed by Fowles suggests that heart rate is associated with the BAS, which initiates behavior, and that heart rate increases with reward and active avoidance. Electrodermal activity, in contrast, increases with the activity of the BIS, which inputs behavior in response to cues for punishment or frustrative nonreward (extinction).

as skin conductance, spontaneous skin resistance responses, and palmar sweat should be most sensitive to social facilitation manipulations and heart rate should be generally insensitive to these manipulations. Admittedly, the data in Table 15-1 only lend some support to this prediction; palmar sweat and spontaneous skin resistance responses have certainly been sensitive to audience manipulations, while heart rate has not proven sensitive. However, skin conductance has also proven insensitive in social facilitation research. Whether this is due to theoretical inadequacy in one theory or another (e.g., Fowles, 1980; Geen, 1980; Weiss & Miller, 1971) or due to the substantial differences between paradigms used in social psychological research and psychophysiological research remains to be seen. The larger point, however, is that familiarity with psychophysiological developments will frequently aid social psychologists in selecting measures and paradigms to maximize the sensitivity of measurement and minimize the likelihood of irrelevant artifact.

The Parallel Phenomena Strategy

For the most part, social facilitation research has relied on behavioral tasks that have been previously shown to be sensitive to variations in drive (Cottrell, 1972). The goal of this research was to demonstrate that social conditions produced performance effects that resemble the effects of other motivational changes. Thus, the argument that social conditions elevate drive is based on analogy—that is, social conditions have "drive-like" effects on performance. In contrast, psychophysiological measures have been used to look "directly" at psychophysiological symptoms of arousal. This research is weakened by the possibility that observed changes have been artifactually produced and therefore do not actually represent changes in arousal.

One alternative approach is to use the strategy followed with behavioral measures, that is, to assess whether parallel or analogous phenomena result from conceptually related treatments. For example, if a variety of aversive treatments produce a unique pattern of physiological activity and if audience observation produces a similar pattern, one could argue, by analogy, that social conditions are at least aversive. The anticipation paradigm used by Knight and Borden (1979) utilizes this reasoning to demonstrate that anticipating a public speech is like anticipating a threatening event at least in terms of its effect on heart rate, skin conductance, and vasoconstriction.

Note that this use of psychophysiological measures circumvents many of the problems that occur when one tries to argue that a given psychophysiological technique validly measures overall levels of arousal. Instead of agonizing about whether observed psychophysiological change truly represents arousal differences or some irrelevant artifact, one simply examines psychophysiology to see if theoretically meaningful treatments have divergent or parallel effects on physiological behavior. For example, if one had a theory specifying that audience manipulations belonged to a class of manipulations including such treatments as threat, incentive, and hunger, one would have greater confidence in this prediction if all these treatments had similar physiological effects on a variety of indices and these effects were known to be unique to this category of manipulations. How one interpreted this category would depend on one's theoretical orientation, of course, but the parallel pattern would establish some conceptual equivalence between the treatments. This approach requires two cautions. First, this type of data is compelling only when there is a good deal of research demonstrating that a particular pattern of psychophysiological response is *uniquely* associated with a comparison treatment (or treatments) of theoretical interest. Second, a parallel pattern between treatments even on physiological measures does not establish that these treatments are *phenomenologically* equivalent even if they may be functionally equivalent in terms of their effect on behavior. If periodic shock and audience presence during a task both produce similar physiological patterns, we would still expect subjects to be able to discriminate between the two treatments. While phenomenological equivalence may occur on occasion (*threat* of an audience and *threat* of shock may both produce dread and foreboding), observing unique and parallel phenomena between treatments only allows one to infer some conceptual similarity between the treatments in question. In essence, this approach relies on establishing both convergent and divergent validity (cf. Campbell & Fiske, 1959). Although convergent validity is of some interest, the parallel phenomena strategy will only yield definitive data when both convergent *and* divergent validity are established.

Moore (1977), for example, used this approach to see if social conditions could be considered a distracting stimulus (i.e., one that directed attention away from an ongoing task). Moore used a fixed-foreperiod reaction-time (RT) task since distraction produces well-documented behavioral and psychophysiological effects in such tasks (Teece, 1972). In this RT task, subjects must move both hands from base plates on signal in order to depress two response levers. Moore found in audience cells that during the interstimulus interval (ISI) period (i.e., between the warning signal and the response signal), skin conductance was lower and heart rate went down at a slower rate than in an alone control cell. Reaction time was also slower in the audience cell. This was precisely the effect usually found when subjects are distracted during this period. In accord with this, Moore found very similar disruptions in RT and physiological activity when subjects performed the RT task in distracting conditions (i.e., flashing lights). In short, both the audience and distraction conditions were associated with slower RT, lower skin conductance responses, and less cardiac deceleration than an alone control condition. Thus, Moore's study provides psychophysiological evidence that audiences and distracting stimuli produce similar effects during the anticipatory period of a RT task. (See Figure 15-2 for an illustration of this convergent validity.) Moreover, there is evidence that manipulations that should *intensify* attention to the task produce a very different pattern of data, thereby bolstering the divergent validity of this research. Lang, Öhman, and Simons (1978) report that incentives and the interest value of the task primarily affect an acceleratory phase of the cardiac wave form during anticipation periods. Moore's study, in contrast, indicated that the primary effect of audiences and distraction occurred during a deceleratory phase of the cardiac waveform. In this respect,

FIGURE 15-2. Mean skin conductance responses (micromhos) for each condition during successive 2-second intervals of the ISI—first serial position only. Because of complex order effects on some measures, all analyses were based on data from the first block of trials. Data from Moore (1977).

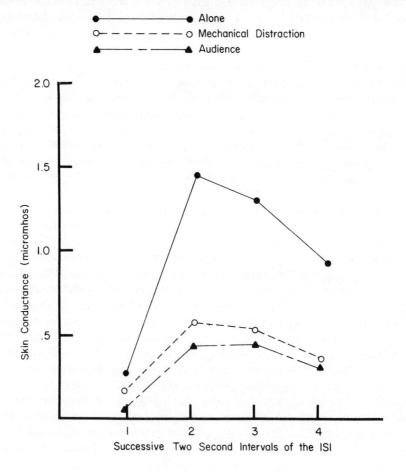

Moore's findings appear to reflect primarily attentional phenomena and not other variables.

Note that data of this type are far superior to the alternative of relying on self-report and recall differences to assess the distracting quality of a stimulus (social presence). Not only is there less possibility of intentional misrepresentation by subjects with psychophysiological measures, but one also gains the ability to ascertain *when* attentional and cognitive processes are affected. In this respect, the strategy used by Moore has much in common with those used by Cacioppo and Petty (1982) to investigate whether cognitive defenses are used by subjects prior to and during the receipt of a persuasive message. First, the researchers establish the *unique* effects that a particular type of verbal processing has on certain psychophysiological indices and then assess whether such a pattern of responding occurs prior to and during various types of messages that differ in their likelihood of eliciting an active cognitive defense. If all links in the nomological net are verified, one has much greater confidence that such cognitive activity frequently occurs in a persuasive context.

Misattribution Strategies

A second alternative to the usual psychophysiological approach in social facilitation research is to adapt some of the strategies used by individuals who study the interaction between cognition and arousal (e.g., Cantor, Zillmann, & Bryant, 1975; Pittman, 1975; Zanna & Cooper, 1974; Zanna, Higgins, & Taves, 1976). If arousal level per se mediates social facilitation effects, heightening irrelevant (i.e., nonsocial) arousal should amplify such effects. This seems the most direct prediction of drive theory, which holds that all sources of drive contribute to energization of behavior (cf. Cantor *et al.*, 1975). It is also possible, however, that the manner in which subjects label the irrelevant arousal will alter its effects. This might occur if performance energization is mediated by some attribution of threat or fear of negative consequences that was contingent on unsuccessful task performance. From a Schachterian viewpoint, this threat would arise from attributing existing arousal to some socially threatening cue. If so, irrelevant drive should heighten social facilitation effects only when subjects can be induced to attribute this irrelevant arousal to the social conditions. This irrelevant arousal could be manipulated via fear (Pittman, 1975), exercise (Cantor *et al.*, 1975), or drug ingestion (Cooper, Zanna, & Taves, 1978), among other manipulations. One would use psychophysiological measures in this paradigm primarily as a manipulation check (cf. Cantor *et al.*, 1975). The advantage of this strategy is that by manipulation arousal, one has a much stronger basis for inferring a causal link between arousal and behavioral effects. The traditional strategy of attempting to document that social conditions produce behavioral changes (e.g., facilitation) as well as some psychophysiological symptom of arousal provides only correlational data on the relationship between arousal and behavior.

A subvariety of the *attributional strategy* is to induce subjects to attribute any arousal they feel to some nonemotional source such as a pill or a noise (e.g., Zanna *et al.*, 1976). Again, a simple drive theory prediction is that such an attribution manipulation should have little effect on social facilitation effects (Cantor *et al.*, 1975). If, however, attributing arousal to a nonemotional source did weaken the behavioral effects caused by social presence, it would suggest some dramatic reformulations in social facilitation theory. Here, psychophysiological measures would be a crucial means of documenting that the attribution manipulations themselves did not actually affect psychophysiological responding in unintended fashion. As an additional feature, one could follow Zanna *et al.*'s procedure of varying whether the pill-produced arousal is described as aversive or not to subjects. If social facilitation is primarily due to subjects' attributing *unpleasant* arousal to the presence of an audience (Geen, 1980), social facilitation effects should be weaker in conditions where subjects are led to attribute *unpleasant* arousal to a pill or a noise instead (cf. Zanna *et al.*, 1976). To our knowledge, there is as yet no research utilizing these research strategies. Undoubtedly, this is due in part to the common acceptance of a simple drive theory explanation of social facilitation effects (Geen & Gange, 1977), which predicts that attributional manipulations would have little impact on social facilitation phenomena. Clearly, this is an area that warrants careful empirical investigation.

Multiple Measurement Strategies

A third alternative to the usual procedure of relying on psychophysiological measures as indices of arousal is to also include self-report and observer ratings of arousal and emotionality. This strategy is already evident in a good deal of clinical research assessing the impact of behavioral treatments for various phobias and fears. For example, Singerman, Borkovec, and Baron (1976) and Cotton, Baron, and Borkovec (1980) used psychophysiological indices, subject self-reports, and Paul's (1966) timed behavior checklist to assess fear among phobics in a public-speaking setting. Paul's timed behavior checklist requires raters to assess overt signs of fear (e.g., poor eye contact, shifting position, nervous use of hands). While observer ratings of anxiety tend to be less sensitive than self-report procedures, when consistent outcomes occur across measures, they substantially raise one's confidence that the psychophysiological measure is reflecting something akin to arousal. Additionally, it may be that perceived arousal and/or observer-rated arousal correlates better with performance differences than does a given psychophysiological measure. If so, one might be wiser to abandon one's view of the psychophysiological measure as an index of arousal than to abandon the hypothesis that arousal affects performance (cf. Cacioppo & Petty, 1982).

SUMMARY AND CONCLUSIONS

Currently, psychophysiological research concerning social facilitation phenomena has failed to provide conclusive support for any particular theoretical perspective; however, there are research strategies emerging that may prove to be more definitive. Whereas the vast majority of the studies reviewed in this chapter were conducted under the assumption that psychophysiological activity provides a straightforward measure of arousal, more promising results may derive from studies that simply look for parallel phenomena in psychophysiological response among various treatments. This research can leave open the question of whether these psychophysiological changes actually represent differences in arousal. The major point is only whether or not parallel and unique phenomena are produced by conceptually related treatments. (*Note.* Strong advantages of this strategy are the ability to pinpoint when various effects take place and to minimize conscious presentational strategies.) The work of Lacey (1959, 1967) and others indicates that physiological measures are complex and by no means straightforward indices of arousal. Rather than being dismayed by this complexity, our suggestion is to utilize it. If a complex response pattern (e.g., long RT, elevated EEG, retarded heart rate deceleration, and low skin conductance) uniquely associated with one treatment (e.g., distraction in a fixed-foreperiod RT task) is also produced by a second treatment (an audience), one has much greater confidence that the two treatments have common elements than if the response pattern is some fairly common and simply one produced by many treatments. Another promising strategy is to utilize manipulations of irrelevant arousal and/or attributional procedures to assess the causal role arousal plays in social facilitation effects. Here psychophysiological measures would primarily be used as manipulation checks. (*Note.* The strong advantage of this strategy is that the causal link between arousal and behavior could be established more convincingly than with other strategies.)

Finally, future work in the social facilitation area would benefit by utilizing multiple measures of physiological activity. As we have noted earlier, different tasks produce different patterns of physiological activity. Hence, it may be more appropriate to think of physiological arousal as a multidimensional state. In this regard, social conditions may affect some dimensions while having little or no effect on other dimensions of arousal. Collecting self-report, behavioral, and physiological data together may further elucidate the dimensions of arousal affected by various social conditions (Cotton *et al.*, 1980; Singerman *et al.*, 1976). Eventually, the accumulation of evidence from studies attacking the social facilitation problem with different measures should enhance our insight regarding the mechanisms responsible for social facilitation effects.

REFERENCES

Allee, W. C., & Masure, R. H.   A comparison of maze behavior in paired and isolated shell-parakeets (*Melopsittacus undulatus shaw*) in a two-alley problem box. *Journal of Comparative Psychology*, 1936, *22*, 131–155.

Bargh, J. A., & Cohen, J. L.   Mediating factors in the arousal–performance relationship. *Motivation and Emotion*, 1978, *2*, 243–257.

Baron, R. S., Moore, D., & Sanders, G. S.   Distraction as a source of drive in social facilitation research. *Journal of Personality and Social Psychology*, 1978, *36*, 816–824.

Borden, R. J., Hendrick, C., & Walker, J. W.   Affective, physiological, and attitudinal consequences of audience presence. *Bulletin of the Psychonomic Society*, 1976, *7*, 33–36.

Bray, R. M., & Sugarman, R.   Social facilitation among interacting groups: Evidence for the evaluation-apprehension hypothesis. *Personality and Social Psychology Bulletin*, 1980, *6*, 137–142.

Brenner, M.   *Stagefright and Stevens' law*. Paper presented at the meeting of the Eastern Psychological Association, 1974.

Brenner, M., Branscomb, H. H., & Schwartz, G. E.   Psychological stress evaluation—two tests of a vocal measure. *Psychophysiology*, 1979, *16*, 351–357.

Brown, J. S., & Farber, I. E.   Emotions conceptualized as intervening variables—with suggestions toward a theory of frustration. *Psychological Bulletin*, 1951, *48*, 465–495.

Bundy, R. S., & Mangan, S. M.   Electrodermal indices of stress and cognition: Possible hydration artifacts. *Psychophysiology*, 1979, *16*, 30–33.

Cacioppo, J. T., & Petty, R. E.   A biosocial model of attitude change. In J. T. Cacioppo & R. E. Petty (Eds.), *Perspectives in cardiovascular psychophysiology*. New York: Guilford, 1982.

Campbell, D. T., & Fiske, D. W.   Convergent and discriminant validation by the multitrait-multimethod matrix. *Psychological Bulletin*, 1959, *56*, 81–105.

Cantor, J. R., Zillmann, D., & Bryant, J.   Enhancement of experienced sexual arousal in response to erotic stimuli through misattribution of unrelated residual excitation. *Journal of Personality and Social Psychology*, 1975, *32*, 69–75.

Carment, D. W.   Rate of simple motor responding as a function of coaction, competition, and sex of the participants. *Psychonomic Science*, 1970, *19*, 340–341. (a)

Carment, D. W.   Rate of simple motor responding as a function of differential outcomes and the actual and implied presence of a coactor. *Psychonomic Science*, 1970, *20*, 115–116. (b)

Carment, D. W., & Latchford, M.   Rate of simple motor responding as a function of coaction, sex of the participants, and the presence or absence of the experimenter. *Psychonomic Science*, 1970, *20*, 253–254.

Carriero, N. J.   The effects of paced tapping on heart rate, skin conductance, and muscle tension. *Psychophysiology*, 1975, *12*, 130–135.

Carver, C. S., & Scheier, M. F.   The self-attention-induced feedback loop and social facilitation. *Journal of Experimental Social Psychology*, 1981, *17*, 545–568.

Catania, J. J., Thompson, L. W., Michalewski, H. A., & Bowman, T. E.   Comparisons of sweat gland counts, electrodermal activity, and habituation behavior in young and old groups of subjects. *Psychophysiology*, 1980, *17*, 146–152.

Chapman, A. J.   An electromyographic study of apprehension about evaluation. *Psychological Reports*, 1973, *33*, 811–814.

Chapman, A. J. An electromyographic study of social facilitation: A test of the "mere presence" hypothesis. *British Journal of Psychology*, 1974, *65*, 123–128.

Chen, S. C. Social modification of the activity of ants in nest-building. *Physiological Zoology*, 1937, *10*, 420–436.

Christie, M. J., & Todd, J. L. Experimenter–subject situational interactions. In P. H. Venables & M. J. Christie (Eds.), *Research in psychophysiology*. London: Wiley, 1975.

Cohen, J. L. Social facilitation increased evaluation apprehension through permanency of record. *Motivation and Emotion*, 1979, *3*, 19–33.

Cohen, J. L. Social facilitation: Audience versus evaluation apprehension effects. *Motivation and Emotion*, 1980, *4*, 21–33.

Cohen, J. L., & Davis, J. H. Effects of audience status, evaluation, and time of action on performance with hidden-word problems. *Journal of Personality and Social Psychology*, 1973, *27*, 74–85.

Cohen, S. Environmental load and the allocation of attention. In A. Baum & S. Valins (Eds.), *Advances in environmental research*. Hillsdale, N.J.: Erlbaum, 1978.

Cooper, J., Zanna, M. P., & Taves, P. A. Arousal as a necessary condition for attitude change following induced compliance. *Journal of Personality and Social Psychology*, 1978, *36*, 1101–1106.

Cotton, J. L., Baron, R. S., & Borkovec, T. D. Caffeine, misattribution, and speech anxiety. *Journal of Research in Personality*, 1980, *14*, 196–206.

Cottrell, N. B. Performance in the presence of other human beings: Mere presence, audience, and affiliation effects. In E. C. Simmel, R. A. Hoppe, & G. A. Milton (Eds.), *Social facilitation and imitative behavior*. Boston: Allyn & Bacon, 1968.

Cottrell, N. B. Social facilitation. In C. G. McClintock (Ed.), *Experimental social psychology*. New York: Holt, Rinehart & Winston, 1972.

Cottrell, N. B., Wack, D. L., Sekerak, G. J., & Rittle, R. H. Social facilitation of dominant responses by the presence of an audience and the mere presence of others. *Journal of Personality and Social Psychology*, 1968, *9*, 245–250.

Crandall, R. Social facilitation: Theories and research. In A. Harrison (Ed.), *Explorations in psychology*. Monterey, Calif.: Brooks/Cole, 1974.

Dabbs, J. M., Johnson, J. E., & Leventhal, H. Palmar sweating: A quick and simple measure. *Journal of Experimental Psychology*, 1968, *78*, 347–350.

Dashiell, J. F. An experimental analysis of some group effects. *Journal of Abnormal and Social Psychology*, 1930, *25*, 190–199.

Davis, C. M., Brickett, P., Stern, R. M., & Kimball, W. H. Tension in the two frontales: Electrode placement and artifact in the recording of forehead EMG. *Psychophysiology*, 1978, *15*, 591–593.

Duffy, E. *Activation and behavior*. New York: Wiley, 1962.

Duffy, E. The nature and development of the concept of activation. In R. N. Haber (Ed.), *Current research in motivation*. New York: Holt, Rinehart & Winston, 1967.

Duffy, E. Activation. In N. S. Greenfield & R. A. Sternbach (Eds.), *Handbook of psychophysiology*. New York: Holt, Rinehart & Winston, 1972.

Easterbrook, J. A. The effect of emotion on cue utilization and the organization of behavior. *Psychological Review*, 1959, *66*, 183–201.

Edelberg, R. Electrodermal recovery rate, goal-orientation and aversion. *Psychophysiology*, 1972, *9*, 512–520.

Edelberg, R. Relation of electrical properties of skin to structure and physiological state. *Journal of Investigative Dermatology*, 1977, *69*, 324–327.

Epstein, S., Bourdreau, L., & Kling, S. Magnitude of the heart rate and electrodermal response as a function of stimulus input, motor output, and their interaction. *Psychophysiology*, 1975, *12*, 15–24.

Fowles, D. C. The three arousal model: Implications of Gray's two-factor learning theory for heart rate, electrodermal activity, and psychopathy. *Psychophysiology*, 1980, *17*, 87–104.

Fowles, D. C., & Schneider, R. E.   Effects of epidermal hydration on skin conductance responses and levels. *Biological Psychology*, 1974, *2*, 67–77.

Fowles, D. C., & Schneider, R. E.   Electrolyte medium effects on measurements of palmar skin potential. *Psychophysiology*, 1978, *15*, 474–482.

Freedman, J., Klevansky, S., & Ehrlich, P.   The effect of crowding on human task performance. *Journal of Applied Social Psychology*, 1971, *1*, 7–25.

Geen, R. G.   The role of the social environment in the induction and reduction of anxiety. In C. D. Spielberger & I. G. Sarason (Eds.), *Stress and anxiety* (Vol. 3). Washington, D.C.: Hemisphere, 1976.

Geen, R. G.   Effects of being observed on learning following success and failure experiences. *Motivation and Emotion*, 1979, *3*, 355–371.

Geen, R. G.   The effects of being observed on performance. In P. B. Paulus (Ed.), *Psychology of group influence*. Hillsdale, N.J.: Erlbaum, 1980.

Geen, R. G.   Evaluation apprehension and social facilitation: A reply to Sanders. *Journal of Experimental Social Psychology*, 1981, *17*, 252–256.

Geen, R. G., & Gange, J. J.   Drive theory of social facilitation: Twelve years of theory and research. *Psychological Bulletin*, 1977, *84*, 1267–1288.

Gray, J. A.   *Elements of a two-process theory of learning*. New York: Academic, 1975.

Haas, J., & Roberts, G. C.   Effect of evaluative others upon learning and performance of a complex motor task. *Journal of Motor Behavior*, 1975, *7*, 81–90.

Hassett, J.   *A primer of psychophysiology*. San Francisco: W. H. Freeman, 1978.

Hebb, D. O.   Drives and C. N. S. (conceptual nervous system). *Psychological Review*, 1955, *62*, 243–254.

Henchy, T., & Glass, D. C.   Evaluation apprehension and the social facilitation of dominant and subordinate responses. *Journal of Personality and Social Psychology*, 1968, *10*, 446–454.

Innes, J. M.   The effect of presence of coworkers and evaluative feedback on performance of a simple reaction time task. *European Journal of Social Psychology*, 1972, *2*, 466–470.

Innes, J. M., & Young, R. F.   The effect of presence of an audience, evaluation apprehension, and objective self-awareness of learning. *Journal of Experimental Social Psychology*, 1975, *11*, 35–42.

Johnson, J. E., & Dabbs, J. M.   Enumeration of active sweat glands: A simple physiological indicator of psychological changes. *Nursing Research*, 1967, *16*, 273–276.

Juniper, K., Blanton, D. E., & Dykman, R. A.   Palmar skin resistance and sweat-gland counts in drug and non-drug states. *Psychophysiology*, 1967, *4*, 231–243.

Kahneman, D.   *Attention and effort*. Englewood Cliffs, N.J.: Prentice-Hall, 1973.

Katkin, E. S.   Relationship between manifest anxiety and two indices of autonomic response to stress. *Journal of Personality and Social Psychology*, 1965, *2*, 324–333.

Kiesler, C. A., & Pallak, M. S.   Arousal properties of dissonance manipulations. *Psychological Bulletin*, 1976, *83*, 1014–1025.

Kilpatrick, D. G.   Differential responsiveness of two electrodermal indices to psychological stress and performance of a complex cognitive task. *Psychophysiology*, 1972, *9*, 218–226.

Kimble, G. A.   *Hilgard and Marquis' conditioning and learning* (2nd ed.). New York: Appleton-Century-Crofts, 1961.

Klinger, E.   Feedback effects and social facilitation of vigilance performance: Mere coaction versus potential evaluation. *Psychonomic Science*, 1969, *14*, 161–162.

Knight, M. L., & Borden, R. J.   Autonomic and affective reactions of high and low socially anxious individuals awaiting public performance. *Psychophysiology*, 1979, *16*, 209–213.

Lacey, J. I.   Psychophysiological approaches to the evaluation of psychotherapeutic process and outcome. In E. A. Rubinstein & M. B. Parloff (Eds.), *Research in psychotherapy*. Washington, D.C.: American Psychological Association, 1959.

Lacey, J. I.   Somatic response patterning and stress: Some revisions of activation theory. In M. H. Appley & R. Trumbull (Eds.), *Psychological stress: Issues in research*. New York: Appleton-Century-Crofts, 1967.

Lang, P. J., Öhman, A., & Simons, R. F.   The psychophysiology of anticipation. In J. Requin (Ed.), *Attention and performance* (Vol. 7). Hillsdale, N.J.: Erlbaum, 1978.

Malmo, R. B.   Activation: A neurophysiological dimension. *Psychological Review*, 1959, *66*, 367–386.

Markus, H.   The effect of mere presence on social facilitation: An unobtrusive test. *Journal of Experimental Social Psychology*, 1979, *37*, 970–988.

Markus, H.   The drive for integration: Some comments. *Journal of Experimental Social Psychology*, 1981, *17*, 257–261.

Martens, R.   Effect of an audience on learning and performance of a complex motor skill. *Journal of Personality and Social Psychology*, 1969, *12*, 252–260. (a)

Martens, R.   Palmar sweating and the presence of an audience. *Journal of Experimental Social Psychology*, 1969, *5*, 371–374. (b)

Martens, R., & Landers, D.   Evaluation potential as a determinant of coaction effects. *Journal of Experimental Social Psychology*, 1972, *8*, 347–359.

Miezejeski, C. M.   Relationships between behavioral arousal and some components of autonomic arousal. *Psychophysiology*, 1978, *15*, 417–421.

Milgram, S.   The experience of living in cities. *Science*, 1970, *13*, 1461–1468.

Moore, D. L.   *Are audiences distracting? Behavioral and physiological data.* Unpublished Master's thesis, University of Iowa, 1977.

Morrison, B. J., & Thatcher, K.   Overpopulation effects on social reduction of emotionality in the albino rat. *Journal of Comparative and Physiological Psychology*, 1969, *69*, 658–662.

Musante, G., & Anker, J. M.   Experimenter's presence: Effect on subject's performance. *Psychological Reports*, 1972, *30*, 903–904.

Obrist, P. A.   The cardiovascular-behavioral interaction—as it appears today. *Psychophysiology*, 1976, *13*, 95–107.

Paul, G. L.   *Insight vs. desensitization in psychotherapy: An experiment in anxiety reduction.* Stanford, Calif.: Stanford University Press, 1966.

Paulus, P. B., Annis, A. B., & Risner, H. T.   An analysis of the mirror-induced objective self-awareness effect. *Bulletin of the Psychonomic Society*, 1978, *12*, 8–10.

Paulus, P. B., & Murdock, P.   Anticipated evaluation and audience presence in the enhancement of dominant responses. *Journal of Experimental Social Psychology*, 1971, *7*, 280–291.

Pittman, T. S.   Attribution of arousal as a mediator in dissonance reduction. *Journal of Experimental Social Psychology*, 1975, *11*, 53–63.

Quarton, R. J.   *Increased dominant responding in the presence of coactors accompanied by cues for rivalry.* Unpublished honors thesis, University of Iowa, 1969.

Rajecki, D. W., Ickes, W., Corcoran, C., & Lenerz, K.   Social facilitation of human performance: Mere presence effects. *Journal of Social Psychology*, 1977, *102*, 297–310.

Rittle, R. H., & Bernard, N.   Enhancement of response rate by the mere physical presence of the experimenter. *Personality and Social Psychology Bulletin*, 1977, *3*, 127–130.

Roberts, L. E.   Comparative psychophysiology of the electrodermal and cardiac control systems. In P. A. Obrist, A. H. Black, J. Brenner, & L. V. DiCara (Eds.), *Cardiovascular psychophysiology—Current issues in response mechanisms, biofeedback, and methodology.* Chicago: Aldine, 1974.

Sanders, G. S.   Driven by distraction: An integrative review of social facilitation theory and research. *Journal of Experimental Social Psychology*, 1981, *17*, 227–251.

Sanders, G. S., Baron, R. S., & Moore, D. L.   Distraction and social comparison as mediators of social facilitation effects. *Journal of Experimental Social Psychology*, 1978, *14*, 291–303.

Sasfy, J., & Okun, M.   Form of evaluation and audience expertness as joint determinants of audience effects. *Journal of Experimental Social Psychology*, 1974, *10*, 461–467.

Schachter, S., & Singer, J. E.   Cognitive, social, and physiological determinants of emotional state. *Psychological Review*, 1962, *69*, 379–399.

Schneider, R. E., & Fowles, D. C.   A convenient non-hydrating electrolyte medium for the measurement of electrodermal activity. *Psychophysiology*, 1978, *15*, 483–486.

Scott, J. P., & McCray, C. Allelomimetic behavior in dogs: Negative effects of competition on social facilitation. *Journal of Comparative and Physiological Psychology*, 1967, *63*, 316–319.

Seta, J. J., Paulus, P. B., & Schkade, J. K. Effects of group size and proximity under cooperative and competitive conditions. *Journal of Personality and Social Psychology*, 1976, *34*, 47–53.

Shapiro, D., & Crider, A. Psychophysiological approaches in social psychology. In G. Lindzey & E. Aronson (Eds.), *The handbook of social psychology* (2nd ed., Vol. 3). Reading, Mass.: Addison-Wesley, 1969.

Singerman, K. J., Borkovec, T. D., & Baron, R. S. Failure of a "misattribution therapy" manipulation with a clinically relevant target behavior. *Behavior Therapy*, 1976, *7*, 306–313.

Spence, K. W. *Behavior therapy and conditioning*. New Haven, Conn.: Yale University Press, 1956.

Strahan, R. F., Todd, J. B., & Inglis, G. B. A palmar sweat measure particularly suited for naturalistic research. *Psychophysiology*, 1974, *11*, 715–720.

Teece, J. J. Contingent negative variation (CNV) and psychological processes in man. *Psychological Bulletin*, 1972, *77*, 73–108.

Thomas, P. E., & Korr, I. M. Relationship between sweat gland activity and electrical resistance of the skin. *Journal of Applied Psychology*, 1957, *10*, 505–510.

Triplett, N. The dynamogenic factors in pacemaking and competition. *American Journal of Psychology*, 1898, *9*, 507–533.

Weiss, R. F., & Miller, F. G. The drive theory of social facilitation. *Psychological Review*, 1971, *78*, 44–57.

Wicklund, R. A. Discrepancy reduction or attempted distraction? A reply to Liebling, Sieler, and Shaver. *Journal of Experimental Social Psychology*, 1975, *11*, 78–81.

Wicklund, R. A., & Duval, S. Opinion change and performance facilitation as a result of objective self-awareness. *Journal of Experimental Social Psychology*, 1971, *7*, 319–342.

Zajonc, R. B. Social facilitation. *Science*, 1965, *149*, 269–274.

Zajonc, R. B. Feeling and thinking: Preferences need no inferences. *American Psychologist*, 1980, *35*, 151–175.

Zajonc, R. B., Heingartner, A., & Herman, E. M. Social enhancement and impairment of performance in the cockroach. *Journal of Personality and Social Psychology*, 1969, *13*, 83–92.

Zajonc, R. B., Wolosin, R. J., Wolosin, M. A., & Loh, W. D. Social facilitation and imitation in group risk-taking. *Journal of Experimental Social Psychology*, 1970, *6*, 26–46.

Zanna, M. P., & Cooper, J. Dissonance and the pill: An attribution approach to studying the arousal properties of dissonance. *Journal of personality and Social Psychology*, 1974, *29*, 703–709.

Zanna, M. P., & Cooper, J. Dissonance and the attribution process. In J. H. Harvey, W. J. Ickes, & R. F. Kidd (Eds.), *New directions in attribution research* (Vol. 1). Hillsdale, N.J.: Erlbaum, 1976.

Zanna, M. P., Higgins, E. T., & Taves, P. A. Is dissonance phenomenologically aversive? *Journal of Experimental Social Psychology*, 1976, *12*, 530–538.

CHAPTER 16

Assessment of Sexual Responding: Arousal, Affect, and Behavior

Kathryn Kelley
State University of New York at Albany
Donn Byrne
State University of New York at Albany

In research conducted over the past two decades, a great deal has been learned about the behavioral effects of erotic stimuli. This knowledge represents a sharp contrast to the relatively recent "dark ages" of sexological practice when, for example, clitoridectomy (surgical removal of the clitoris) was performed in Victorian England to relieve husbands of the threat of their wives' unacceptable sexual insatiability (Barker-Benfield, 1976). Our present understanding of gender differences in responsivity is based on a relatively detailed picture of both subjectively reported and physiologically monitored response patterns. A large portion of the variability in human sexuality can be attributed to learned behavior sequences, not only with respect to gender differences but also for behavior formerly assumed to have exclusively biological antecedents, such as homosexuality.

SEXUAL RESPONDING AS LEARNED BEHAVIOR

In order to interpret the significance and implications of sexual response measurement, we begin with a brief examination of the extensive literature on erotic stimulus effects on subjective sexual and emotional arousal. The stimulus determinants of sexual arousal include internal and external erotic fantasy as well as tactual stimulation, and their effects will therefore be described in general before turning to findings based on physiological measurement in particular. The development of specific measurement techniques has an interesting history which in itself reveals something of the false starts and gradual progress found in the field of psychosexology. The correspondence between subjective sexual arousal and physiological indices indicates its utility in studying the learned behavior patterns on both nomothetic and idiographic levels. Finally, the relation between sexual arousal and several domains of subsequent behavior is described as a consequent of these patterns. We then briefly present a theoretical model that attempts to tie together the various components of sexual stimulation, mediating variables, and sexual behavior.

SUBJECTIVE AROUSAL AND AFFECT IN RESPONSE TO SEXUAL STIMULI

The human attribute of generating sexual fantasy gives us a unique capacity to arouse ourselves independently of situational constraints. The motivational and emotional effects of erotic imagination can influence both the individual who originates it and anyone to whom the fantasy is communicated. Both men and women use internal and external imaginative cues during sexual activity as tools with a variety of functions. We will briefly examine current knowledge about this topic before turning to studies of physiological sexual arousal, *all* of which have used some form of imaginal erotic stimulation to induce excitement.

Functions of Erotic Fantasy

When a person engages in sexual fantasy or processes the fantasies of others, he or she responds to this material subjectively and physiologically as if participating in the imagined activity. There is the experience of sexual arousal and appropriate physiological changes preparatory to engaging in a sexual act. Internally generated fantasies can actually result in higher levels of self-reported arousal than those produced by external stimuli such as erotic photographs or stories (Byrne & Lamberth, 1971). Compared to the effects of reading passages or viewing slides, the erotic value of imagination is considerably enhanced for each individual who is the originator of the scenario rather than the recipient of stimuli created by others. It is possible that external stimuli can sometimes serve to distract the recipients from their own, richer arousal brought about by internal images. That is, the processing of externally supplied erotic information may interfere with autostimulation and thus with arousal, suggesting that with respect to the aphrodisiacal quality of fantasy, homemade is better than store-bought.

Motivational Effects

Behavioral changes occur in response to erotic fantasy, and some of these changes serve to bring potential partners closer together physically and psychologically, thus increasing the probability of sexual behavior. For example, erotically aroused males express more love for female partners than do nonaroused males (Dermer & Pyszczynski, 1978). Such arousal also results in approaching and gazing at opposite-gender strangers (Griffitt, May, & Veitch, 1974). Exposure to erotica also increases the tendency to polarize ratings of the physical attractiveness or unattractiveness of stimulus persons of the other gender. The pretty seem to get prettier and the ugly uglier as a result of fantasy-induced arousal (Weidner, Istvan, & Griffitt, 1979).

The motivational effects of fantasy use during sexual interactions can initiate or heighten sexual interest in a particular partner. If someone experiences good results with a particular kind of fantasy, he or she may repeat its use, perfect it, seek more examples of it, and introduce variations of it in order to increase its value. The sexual content of such an imaginative fantasy can become an "old friend" which Masters and Johnson (1979) describe as having stable, familiar qualities that help the user to become aroused, reach orgasm, and maintain interest in a regular partner. Most sexually active individuals develop a fairly regular pace in predictable circumstances for their erotic behavior, and the ability to rely on a favorite fantasy theme may add variety and enjoyment to pleasant but repetitive sexual experiences (Sue, 1979). The dependable nature of this imagined old friend can be useful in overcoming sexual dysfunctions. For example, sex therapists sometimes instruct clients to develop favorite fantasy themes to utilize in becoming aroused, maintaining arousal, and timing or controlling orgasm.

Emotional and Behavioral Effects

The emotional response to fantasy strongly determines its influence on subsequent sexual activity. A positive affective reaction generally results in activation, pursuance of further stimulation, and approach responses. A negative reaction to fantasy often results in avoidance of additional excitement (Mosher & Cross, 1971). Under some conditions, however, a negative affective response to erotica can be associated with a slight, temporary increase in subsequent sexual behavior, including masturbation among college students (W. A. Fisher & Byrne, 1978a). This negative emotional response has been termed "erotophobia," which, in contrast to its positive counterpart (erotophilia), is characteristic of individuals with a more negative sexual socialization history. Erotophobes report less experience with erotica, which may account for their unexpectedly greater responsiveness to it.

Subjects typically report an increased tendency to engage in sexual behavior during the few hours following exposure to erotic stimuli. Married couples become slightly more likely to engage in heterosexual intercourse (Cattell, Kawash, & DeYoung, 1972; Kutchinsky, 1971), while unmarried individuals are more likely to masturbate (Amoroso, Brown, Pruesse, Ware, & Pilkey, 1971). Even these mild effects decline following continued exposure over several days (Mann, Berkowitz, Sidman, Starr, & West, 1974).

Other than general statements about arousal being elicited by erotic stimuli, along with affective reactions, little evidence has been obtained to indicate precisely how these response systems influence sexuality. For example, do the affective and physiological responses persist over time by means of the reinstatement of internal fantasies about the sexual stimuli until physical gratification occurs? Alternatively, is it possible that attribution processes account for subsequent effects? Cantor, Zillmann, and Bryant (1975) showed that residual physical arousal induced by exercise was misperceived by subjects as attributable to greater sexual excitement and enjoyment in response to an erotic film. It is possible that residual arousal induced by erotica is misperceived by subjects as attributable to greater desire for intercourse or masturbation. See Zillmann (Chapter 8, this volume) for a more detailed discussion of this theoretical approach.

Gender Differences

The question of gender differences in self-reported affective and arousal responses has been the subject of considerable research and controversy. A generation ago, females were compared to males and were described as less interested in and less aroused by sexual stimuli (Kinsey, Pomeroy, Martin, & Gebhard, 1953). Studies since then have corroborated this finding with respect to *affective* responses to erotic depictions of heterosexual activity (W. A. Fisher & Byrne, 1978b) and to written erotic passages (Schmidt & Sigusch, 1970, 1973). Males report more positive feelings than females. With respect to *sexual arousal*, the story is much less consistent. Several recent investigations of subjective arousal to erotica report no gender differences (Byrne & Lamberth, 1971; W. A. Fisher & Byrne, 1978b; Griffitt, 1975; Hatfield, Sprecher, & Traupmann, 1978). In a study of reactions to heterosexual and masturbation slides, Kelley (in press) found more negative and less sexually aroused responses among females than among males on the semantic differential (W. A. Fisher & Byrne, 1978b) and on Griffitt's (1975) scale of self-reported physiological arousal, suggesting that gender similarity in arousal depends on erotic content and possibly on the type of scale used to assess the response.

Increased levels of sexual experience appear to ameliorate the negative emotional responses to erotica observed among females. It appears that the reinforcements associated with sexual activity alter the affective and evaluative responses, as would be expected on the basis of the reinforcement–affect model of evaluative responses (Clore & Byrne, 1974). Griffitt (1975) found heterosexual experience level to be a strong correlate of emotional and arousal responses to heterosexual slide presentations among women. That same experience variable was related to responsiveness to guided erotic imagery in a study of females by Mosher and White (1980). It seems that as female experience level increases, the effects of negative affect and sex guilt are counteracted. For males, it is masturbation experience that more strongly relates to subjective appraisal of erotic stimuli (Griffitt, 1975). Thus, as Kelley (1981b) found in a study of males' and females' affective and arousal responses to heterosexual and masturbatory stimuli, different patterns of reactions to these two topics indicated that in conjunction with sex guilt they assume different roles in sexuality for the genders. Sexually guilty females expressed little sexual arousal and more negative affect in response to both themes, while males and nonguilty females were generally more positive toward and aroused by heterosexual than masturbatory content.

Significance of Fantasizing for Subjective Arousal

These data have demonstrated that a wide range of emotional response to erotic fantasy is measurable within both genders, ranging from intense disgust to great pleasure. Further, gender differences tend to disappear with greater sexual experience. Studies of the subjective experience of orgasm have revealed surprising similarity in the way males and females describe them. Behavioral experts, including psychiatrists and clinical psychologists, could not reliably distinguish men's and women's written descriptions of the orgasmic experience (Vance & Wagner, 1976). An extreme negative response to erotic fantasy may indicate the possibility of sexual dysfunction. Nonorgasmic women, for example, are found to have a disgusted, anxious reaction to their sexual arousal, whereas orgasmic controls react to a state of arousal as pleasant (Heiman, 1977).

With respect to arousal itself, gender differences appear to be minimal. The significance of sexual fantasy for arousal indicates that cognitive and emotional factors contribute to the subjective experiences of sexuality. E. F. Hoon, Hoon, and Wincze (1976) reported the development of a scale of sexual arousability as an indicator of the degree of arousal experienced during a variety of sexual acts. Imagery ability in both genders was related to a higher degree of sexual arousability (Harris, Yulis, & Lacoste, 1980). The cognitive manipulation of erotic stimuli via fantasy thus seems to facilitate arousal as measured on subjective scales. Diminution of cognitive activity and also of sexual activity occurs among males as they age (Giambra & Martin, 1977). That is, the frequency and enjoyment of sexual activity seems to be indicated by erotic imaginal activity levels. Although such correlations leave us with a chicken-and-egg problem, it is at least possible that decreases in fantasy activity are responsible for decreases in orgasm frequency.

The relationship between the content of erotic fantasy and subsequent behavior is less clear. Therapeutic treatments have been devised for the restructuring and/or desensitization of presumably maladaptive fantasy to correct both sexual deviance and dysfunction. Measurement of sexual arousal is commonly used as an adjunct to this therapy to provide information about stimulus content that arouses an individual and to countercondition resultant responses. We know little about the development of arousal responses to inappropriate stimuli. For example, there is little early experience with pornographic material among early sex offenders as retrospectively reported (Goldstein, Kant, & Hartman, 1974). These offenders have typically seen a picture of sexual intercourse for the first time at an age 4 years older than that reported by nonoffenders (Eysenck, 1972). Negative, repressive, and restricted experiences with sexuality have occurred for the eventual offenders, again illustrating the joint roles of cognitive and emotional factors in the subjective arousal responses they report to stimuli of particular content.

In a research area as relatively new as human sexuality, the gaps in psychological knowledge will need to be filled as additional factors are identified. Much of the existing information consists of correlational, nonexperimental data with few of the possible situational parameters manipulated. There are, of course, many obstacles to experimentation in this area ranging from problems of volunteer bias (Kaats & Davis, 1971) to necessary ethical restraints. Nevertheless, the robustness of sexual variables is impressive, and even survey studies performed at the level of dustbowl empiricism can contribute to abstract theorizing. For example, an atheoretical description of the percentage of sexually active teenagers who *fail* to use contraceptives (Alan Guttmacher Institute, 1976) can constitute the baseline starting point for a theoretical approach that pits a reinforcement versus an informational model of social behavior (W. A. Fisher, 1978).

MEASUREMENT OF SEXUAL RESPONDING

This section will examine the psychophysiological techinques used to measure sexual arousal, beginning with psychometric considerations and a brief historical account of laboratory assessment of sexual responses. Several original devices for measuring arousal have been introduced but then faded from the scientific scene as investigators became aware of drawbacks and turned to newer devices. The relationship between objective and subjective physiological assessment will be discussed in some detail, as will the relationship between subjective arousal and physiological processes.

Psychometrics of Assessing Sexual Arousal

Before describing the techniques used to measure sexual arousal, we need first to define the term and to examine some of the psychometric issues raised by attempts to measure this construct.

Arousal

In the most general theoretical sense, sexual arousal refers to a drive state that is based on the need for sexual release. Presumably, this drive leads the organism to engage in consummatory behavior such as sexual intercourse or masturbation. The usual result is orgasm, and the attainment of this goal is drive reducing. As with most human motives, the sex drive is greatly influenced by learning, and human sexual arousal comes to depend not simply on physiological variables but on such factors as conditioned stimuli and cognitive processes (Beach, 1969; Rachman, 1966).

In operationalizing the concept of arousal, psychologists and other researchers interested in human sexuality have not been able to define arousal simply in terms of some stimulus-related experimental manipulation such as deprivation time. Instead, there is reliance on three primary types of response measures.

> 1. There are nonstandardized, relatively simple self-rating scales that range unidimensionally from "not at all aroused" to "highly aroused" (e.g., Levitt & Brady, 1965). These tend to consist of five to seven points along a dimension on which a subject is asked to indicate his or her present subjective state.
> 2. There are equally nonstandardized self-rating scales that ask subjects to make estimates of their physiological responses along dimensions such as "no erection" to "full erection" or "no breast sensations" to "strong breast sensations." See Schmidt, Sigusch, and Schafer (1973) for examples of such measures.
> 3. There are direct physiological measures that are based on the fact that sexual stimulation results in vasocongestion, especially in the genitalia. As will be described in the following section, vasocongestion leads to such measurable bodily changes as penile erection, increased opacity of the vaginal walls, and an increase in genital temperature. For reviews of such devices, see Geer (1975), Hatch (1981), P. W. Hoon (1979), and Zuckerman (1971).

When the term "arousal" is used in the sex research literature, it generally refers to findings based on any and all of these measurement techniques, used interchangeably. This failure to discriminate is probably based on the fact that little is known about the differential predictive qualities of these operations and on the generally positive correlations among them.

Reliability

Most of the familiar concepts of reliability are not really applicable to the devices used to measure sexual arousal. For example, the coefficient of internal consistency has no meaning in the context of single-item measures of self-rated arousal. Further, different levels of arousal on any of the measures in response to different erotic stimuli are assumed to indicate different responses rather than measurement error. Although no one to our knowledge has actually investigated the interjudge consistency that obtains in recording check marks on a rating scale or readings on a vaginal photoplethysmograph, it is generally and probably accurately assumed that with such objective measures any two normal investigators will record the same numerical scores.

At first glance, the coefficient of stability would seem to be an appropriate reliability index for arousal measures. The difficulty here is that repeated exposure to erotic stimuli is found to result in a diminution in arousal that is presumed to reflect decreased drive rather than unreliability of measurement (Kelley, 1981a; Mann *et al.*, 1974).

The only reliability measure that seems at all reasonable to apply here is the coefficient of equivalance. Thus, different self-report rating scales or different measures of penile tumescence should correlate highly. Although such studies have not been done as far as we know, it might be noted that two rating scales could yield spuriously high correlations when used successively because of subjects striving to be consistent and that two physiological measures could yield spuriously low correlations because of diminished arousal with successive stimulation.

Validity

In some respects, the question of validity is as awkward as the question of reliability. At one level, it is like asking about the validity of a thermometer, a clock, a ruler, or of your feelings of hunger. In such instances, what precisely is meant by "validity"?

It seems clear that the current measures of sexual arousal have face validity in that what is generally meant by arousal is a subjective feeling of excitement plus genital changes involving tissue swelling, temperature rise, and erotic sensations. If such bodily changes and self-perceptions constitute the major aspects of sexual arousal, these measures may even be said to have content validity—they represent an adequate sample of the response array.

Construct validity has been established for most of the measuring devices in that they indicate arousal in response to erotic versus nonerotic stimuli (e.g., Abramson, Perry, Seeley, Seeley, & Rothblatt, 1981) and they are appropriately related to subsequent behavior with appropriate sex objects (e.g., Griffitt *et al.*, 1974). Beyond this basic level, however, no one has carried the construct of sexual arousal very far in research linking it to other variables in a theoretical network.

Predictive validity is clearly the most important concept to be examined with respect to measures of arousal. Surprisingly little has been done, however. A few studies have shown that subjects most aroused in one situation were more likely to engage in a sexual act in a subsequent situation than initially unaroused subjects (e.g., Cattell *et al.*, 1972). In addition, the specific stimuli that elicit an individual's arousal (e.g., mutually consenting sex, forced sex, etc.) are found to reflect the specific type of overt behavior in which that individual engages (Abel, Barlow, Blanchard, & Guild, 1977).

As we shall see in the next sections, there are also indications that the various measures of arousal tend to be positively intercorrelated. In other areas of investigation, self-report measures of physiological activity are often found to be unrelated to actual physiological activity (see Pennebaker, Chapter 19, and Blascovich & Katkin, Chapter 17, this volume). Physiological sexual responses, especially for males, represent a marked departure from this generalization.

The intercorrelations of quite different operational measures of arousal could be conceptualized either in terms of concurrent validity or reliability (coefficient of equivalence). The immediate question, though, is how to interpret departures from perfect association. Rather than define one response domain as arousal and a different response domain as only imperfectly predictive of this criterion, it seems more sensible to take the position that different measures constitute partially independent aspects of a higher-order construct. Analogously, a person's height and weight are partially independent indices of size. Let's examine one specific type of measurement discrepancy.

When there are discrepancies between physiological and subjective arousal, the most fruitful question to ask is: "Which measure is a better predictor of subsequent behavior?" Do individual differences in discrepancy (including gender differences) lead to differential sexual behavior, including dysfunctional behavior? Are deviant acts more likely to occur in response to physical or psychological indices of excitement? Does sex therapy result in a decrease in discrepancy? Can biofeedback procedures be designed to bring about congruency between subjective and physiological responses? Conversely, can individuals learn to respond physically only when they simultaneously perceive themselves to be aroused?

As one undergraduate asked when he heard a lecture about the effect of alcohol on physical arousal in contrast to general expectancies about alcohol, "If my girl thinks she's excited, what does it matter?" That is the kind of question to which we will eventually be able to provide answers, using psychophysiological measures of sexual arousal.

Brief History of Laboratory Measurement

Perhaps the first attempt at the scientific measurement of sexual responses came from the laboratory of behaviorist John B. Watson. Watson apparently used a female research assistant as a subject (McConnell, 1980) and promptly encountered a negative evaluation of his work in the form of a divorce instituted by his wife. The data were never published, because Watson was unable to obtain them as part of the divorce settlement.

In the decades that followed, there were very few attempts to study human sexuality experimentally. In the handful of studies that were conducted, the typical subjects were male students who were shown cheesecake photos and asked to give a verbal response such as stories elicited by TAT cards. In the early 1960s Masters and Johnson quietly began the systematic laboratory study of the physical aspects of human sexuality in St. Louis. Their surprisingly popular books, *Human Sexual Response* (1966) and *Human Sexual Inadequacy* (1970), provided descriptive scientific details of the phases of the sexual response cycle.

The Masters and Johnson description of the physiological correlates of human sexual arousal undoubtedly played a pivotal role in encouraging the development of various devices to measure the observed bodily changes. They identified the primary response to effective sexual stimulation as genital and extragenital vasocongestion; the secondary response is an increase in muscle tension, myotonia. The vasocongestive response, reflected in penile erection, breast swelling, nipple erection, sex flush, and clitoral, labial, and vaginal engorgement became the focus of the electronic monitoring and recording of physiological changes during sexual arousal.

Measurement Techniques

Several review articles have provided information about the variety of physiological measures that have been used to measure human sexual responding (Geer, 1975; Jovanovic, 1971; Zuckerman, 1971). For the most part, the measures are confined to specific bodily changes such as genital vasocongestion rather than responses characteristic of general arousal such as heart rate change and pupil dilation.

To induce arousal, experimenters utilize internal fantasies, together with visual and/or auditory erotic stimuli. Such stimulation results in the excitement phase of sexual arousal, which is arbitrarily defined as beginning when a response pattern appears. The genital measurement devices remain at asymptote once maximum vasocongestion is reached at the end of the excitement phase and are thus unable to distinguish the plateau and orgasm phases. Thus, the genital measures will not reflect additional sexual arousal during full penile erection or vaginal vasocongestion. Such limitations of the direct measurement techniques confine their effective use to a relatively narrow range of the sexual response cycle.

Assessing Male Arousal

Both mechanical and chemical indicants of sexual excitement have been employed in measuring the response of males. The two most common chemical approaches consist of determining the levels of secretion of plasma testosterone and urinary acid phosphatase in the blood and urine, respectively. In one experiment, Pirke, Kockott, and Dittmar (1974) found that plasma testosterone levels increased following exposure to an erotic, but not to a nonerotic movie. Subsequent investigations have pointed to the inadequacy of testosterone level as an indicant of sexual activity. For example, Brown, Monti, and Corriveau (1978) observed wide ranges of variability in males in both measured testosterone levels and reported sexual interest and behavior during a week-long period, but there was no covariation between the physiological and subjective measures. Continuing the theme of the relative unimportance of hormonal factors in predicting human sexuality (compared to lower animals), other investigators have found no relationship between testosterone level and male preference for homosexual versus heterosexual partners (Barlow, Abel, Blanchard, & Mavissakalian, 1974). Hormone level is also unrelated to orgasmic dysfunction (Benkert, Witt, & Leitz, 1979).

Secretion of urinary acid phosphatase (UAP) occurs as part of a direct neural influence on the prostate gland during sexual arousal. Such secretion occurs after viewing an erotic film but not films with themes such as anxiety, aggression, or comedy (Barclay & Little, 1972). Males who subjectively reported sexual arousal after viewing erotic pictures showed an increase in UAP (Barclay, 1970). Cognitive factors also contribute to this phenomenon, since a control group who expected to see an erotic movie later increased in UAP levels *before* the external fantasy exposure (Barclay, 1971). Questions still remain as to whether UAP level actually reflects general arousal and/or concomitant sexual arousal under appropriate conditions. The usual overall conclusion of hormonal research on subjective and physiological states of sexual arousal points out the unpredictability of hormone levels and related indicants.

The measurement of penile tumescence has involved a variety of devices to detect volumetric or circumferential variations. For example, a glass cylinder has been used to detect changes in air pressure resulting from tumescence. Since most self-report measures are limited to five to seven points along the arousal dimension, such physical measures involve finer gradations of arousal than subjects are able to verbalize (Abel & Blanchard, 1976). Although this increase in measurement sensitivity would seem to be an obvious methodological advantage, empirical studies that compare the predictive utility of different arousal measures are lacking. There has been considerable use of circumference measures of erection as an approximation of volume changes brought about by blood engorgement. Strain gauges vary in materials and detection methods, and they have been found very useful in the description of the parameters of male sexual responses (Rosen & Keefe, 1978). Because of the nonisotropic characteristics of the penis, penile circumference may not change as length varies, however, so precise measurement would indicate the need for volumetric recording. Also, some investigators have used a thermistor to record penile skin temperature (Jovanovic, 1971) and an anal probe to detect pelvic contractions during orgasm (Bohlen, Held, & Sanderson, 1980).

Assessing Female Arousal

The development of direct genital measures of female sexual arousal has lagged behind that for males. This methodological gap has been attributed to the greater difficulty in observing females' excitement and orgasmic responses relative to males (Masters & Johnson, 1966). Early measurements of female responses included indices of general arousal (S. Fisher & Osofsky, 1968) and vaginal secretions (Shapiro, Cohen, DiBianco, & Rosen, 1968). There were also attempts to measure vaginal contractions with the balloon-like kolpograph (Jovanovic, 1971) and vaginal blood flow with a mechanized diaphragm fitted for each subject (Cohen & Shapiro, 1970). Each of these measures had drawbacks, including reactivity in measuring contractions and complexity in fitting the devices to subjects. Also, the validity of the kolpograph is questionable since it does not show arousal differences between experimental and control sequences of stimulation but does differentiate phases of the menstrual cycle. Some colorful suggestions were made about reactions to it, however. For example, it was suggested that female subjects whose uteruses expelled the water-filled balloon during orgasm must have passive–aggressive personalities (Bardwick & Behrman, 1967). In any event, it was not until plethysmography was introduced that a sensitive measure of female sexual responsivity was available.

Photoplethysmography

Geer (1975) has developed a photoplethysmograph system which reliably measures vaginal vasocongestion during the cycle of sexual arousal. A vaginal probe contains a photoelectric transducer that indirectly measures blood volume by detecting changes in the optical density of the tissue surrounding it (Sintchak & Geer, 1975). Measurement of pressure pulse amplitude, an important indicator of female sexual arousal (Heiman, 1977), reliably discriminated the sequence of changes in arousal during the exposure of females to an erotic versus a nonerotic film (Geer, Morokoff, & Greenwood, 1974) and during masturbation leading to orgasm (Geer & Quartararo, 1976). Resolution as indicated by female photoplethysmography appears to occur relatively slowly, possibly reflecting their physiological capacity for repeated and multiple orgasms.

Thermography

Blood engorgement of tissue produces a temperature rise at that site. Devices to measure temperature change as a result of sexual arousal include the thermistor and heat-screen thermography. The thermistor for women attaches to the labia via a temperature clip and is sensitive to arousal elicited by erotic films (D. Henson, Rubin, Henson, & Williams, 1977), but it is difficult to maintain attachment of the clip to the genital surface (Abel & Blanchard, 1976). Distribution of the temperature changes has been gauged by the use of a thermographic heat screen (Seeley, Abramson, Perry, Rothblatt, & Seeley, 1980). The measure yields a thermogram of temperature distribution which has the advantage of direct comparison between the genders and the possible disadvantage of nonspecific physiological data. Tordjman, Thierree, and Michel (1980) have used the penile thermogram to investigate the possible physiological origin of some erectile dysfunctions. The thermogram method makes it possible to observe a visual pattern of the process of sexual arousal as part of a total interaction, either normal or dysfunctional.

Measurement Problems

Methodological issues in the measurement of human sexual arousal are focused on some problems special to the area. Degree of intrusiveness of the measure can be a problem both psychologically and in the literal sense, and there have been questions raised about the resulting reactivity and nonvalidity of these measures. Bohlen (1980) has called for more sensitive treatment of volunteers who participate in these studies, including more extensive orientation to procedures of anonymity, informed consent, and potential hazards and benefits of the research for the subject. Careful procedures are advised in the orientation process, since in few other psychological research areas must the investigator be concerned about the possibility of acute embarrassment by a stranger mistakenly opening a door to an experimental room, or of the contraction of venereal disease by contaminated devices, or of interference with an unsuspected pregnancy. In order partially to correct the problem of psychological invasiveness of subjective recording procedures, Sarrel, Foddy, and McKinnon (1977) have suggested that arousal be assessed via audiotape rather than on paper-and-pencil scales. Manual activity does not seem to create reactivity difficulties, however, since an experimental study showed that continuous subjective indication of arousal via a lever had no significant influence on physiologically measured arousal (Wincze, Venditti, Barlow, & Mavissakalian, 1980).

Discrepancies in measurement between different types of penile strain gauges have created some concern about artifacts such as subject movement and ease and comfort of handling the devices (Laws, 1977). Masturbation and intercourse as means of experimental arousal would obviously interfere with its measurement by means of strain gauges even though these produce reliable patterns of intense excitement. The most widely used female device, the photoplethysmograph, has two potential sources of artifact: changes in the size of the vaginal barrel which influence the probe's position and distance to the wall, and differences in vaginal lubrication which affect the light reflection's quality or quantity. Also, while masturbation can occur with the probe in place, intercourse cannot. Hatch (1979) has reviewed various methodological issues of the vaginal photo-plethysmograph.

RELATIONSHIPS AMONG MEASURES OF SEXUAL AROUSAL

Variations in the correspondence between physiological measures and the subjects' reported level of arousal have emphasized the need for additional understanding of the psychophysiological aspects of sexual arousal in addition to its basic physiology.

Relationship between Subjective and Objective Measurement

Subjectively reported sexual arousal levels typically correlate in the .40 to .80 range with objective physiological measurement of sexual arousal, although the coefficients drop as low as zero in some dysfunctional groups (Kockott, Feil, Ferstl, Aldenhoff, & Besmyer, 1980). These variables usually reveal higher correspondence for males than for females (Steinman, Wincze, Sakheim, Barlow, & Mavissakalian, 1981). Subjective arousal ratings return to baseline more quickly among females than vasocongestion dissipates (D. Henson & Rubin, 1978). For both genders, the correspondence is highest during plateau and orgasm phases of arousal (Heiman, 1977) suggesting that ascertaining the degree of one's arousal at these higher levels is an easier task than is self-monitoring at the lower levels of the excitement and resolution phases. Figure 16-1 presents a composite picture of the patterns (not absolute levels) of relationships between self-reports and objective measures over the response cycle for both genders. These relationships apparently occur regardless of whether the measurement mode is plethysmography or thermography (Abramson, Perry, Seeley, Seeley, & Rothblatt, 1981; C. Henson, Rubin, & Henson, 1979; Wincze, Hoon, & Hoon, 1977).

The timing of subjective measurement has also been an issue in this research area (Steinman et al., 1981). That is, are subjects asked to report their arousal during or after the erotic stimulation? It is found that males' ratings are highly correlated with physiological arousal regardless of the placement of ratings (continuously during arousal or after stimulation has ceased). The investigators suggested that subjective measurement could yield enough information following arousal and that such a procedure would make the measurement experimentally easier and less potentially reactive. For females, however, maximum level of vasocongestion correlated with self-ratings which were continuous during stimulation or immediately after stimulation; delayed postexperimental ratings were not associated with the physiological measure. The authors suggest that dif-

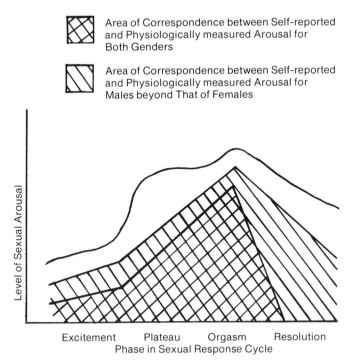

FIGURE 16-1. Self-reported and physiologically measured sexual arousal patterns correspond reasonably well, as shown in this composite comparing the responses of both genders. The correspondence is typically highest at the plateau and orgasm phases and is higher among males than females.

ferential learning of culturally appropriate sexual attributions explains these data, with females trained to be primarily neutral or less attentive to their own physical responses. It should also be noted that obvious anatomical differences between the genders make it easier for males to perceive their genital reactions and hence to make their verbal reports correspond to bodily signals.

Role of Emotions in the Relationship between Subjective and Psychophysiological Responses

Unfortunately, very few data are available with respect to emotional influences on the relationship between subjective and objective measures of sexual arousal. One such study was conducted with female volunteers by Osborn and Pollack (1977). In that experiment, a higher correlation between self-reported and physiological arousal (measured by the plethysmograph) was observed among females who read hard-core erotic stories rather than less arousing erotic ones, perhaps because of a restriction of range in the latter condition. More data are definitely needed to explore this relationship now that valid measures of arousal are available for both genders. We would predict that erotophilic and low-sex-guilt individuals would be more attentive to their physiological reactions than would eroto-phobic and high-sex-guilt ones and hence would yield higher subjective–objective arousal correlations.

Both situational and individual differences in sexual emotionality influence pelvic vasocongestion during sexual arousal. With respect to individual variations, negative attitudes toward masturbation were found to be associated with lower arousal levels measured thermographically among women, but not among men (Abramson, Perry, Rothblatt, Seeley, & Seeley, 1981). Transfer of arousal states was observed among males studied by Wolchik, Beggs, Wincze, Sakheim, Barlow, and Mavissakalian (1980). The males became more highly sexually aroused to an erotic movie following previous exposure to an arousing film involving anger and anxiety.

Influence of Cognitions on the Psychophysiology of Sexual Arousal

Cognitions about the appropriateness of sexual arousal in particular situations undoubtedly influence whether excitement occurs, but little research has been directed to this topic. Contrary to the expectation that the male refractory period inhibits multiple orgasm, some males apparently are able to control the amount of ejaculate consciously in order to be able to continue their sexual activity, but the mechanism and frequency of this phenomenon are unknown (Robbins & Jensen, 1978). According to Hatch (1979), emotions and cognitions modify and enhance the sexual arousal pattern once it has been stimulated. Males are able to inhibit the occurrence of erections in response to an instructional set to do so, even when exposed to an erotic stimulus (Laws & Rubin, 1969). Geer and Fuhr (1976) found that the task of processing increasingly complex cognitive stimuli interfered with penile tumescence compared with subjects not engaged in extraneous cognitive activity; all subjects were exposed to the same erotic auditory stimulus. Once again cognitions can be seen to enhance or to interfere with sexual arousal, suggesting further the importance of cognitive control in human sexuality.

Alcohol Effects on Sexual Responding

There is a great deal of folklore and anecdotal evidence about the role of drugs (including pot and cocaine) in sexual responsivity. Clinical studies show, for example, that dozens of brand name drugs have sexual side effects ranging from impotence to increased libido (Story, 1974). The influence of alcohol on sexual responding illustrates the combinative roles of emotions and cognitions. In our culture, there are clear expectancies as to the effects of alcoholic consumption on sexual responsiveness—"candy is dandy, but liquor is quicker." Despite beliefs about enhanced sexual arousal following alcohol ingestion, both males and females evidence lowered levels of physiological erotic excitement and less intense orgasms at controlled levels of alcohol beyond the relaxation effect (Lang, Searles, Lauerman, & Adesso, 1980; Malatesta, Pollack, Wilbanks, & Adams, 1979; Wilson & Lawson, 1976, 1978). Males more accurately assessed their decreased states of arousal than females, who continued to believe that they were highly aroused.

Gawin (1978) reviewed the possible aphrodisiac effects of pharmacologic agents on the subjective experience of sexual arousal and concluded that more needs to be known about sex and drug interactions. As one example, the combination of an expectancy variable and a dispositional affective variable has been found to influence physiological arousal. Males who *believed* they had consumed alcohol (whether actual alcohol or a placebo) showed an increase in penile tumescence in response to erotic stimuli only if they were high in sex guilt (Lansky & Wilson, 1981). A question yet to be investigated is the relative predictive power of physiological arousal level versus subjective arousal level when the two are discrepant, as in many drug-ingestion situations.

A GENERAL THEORETICAL MODEL

As we have seen in the material presented in the present chapter, an array of stimulus and response variables is involved in the activation of sexual responsivity. A formulation that may be helpful in organizing these variables is the Sexual Behavior Sequence (Byrne, 1977). This is a descriptive model that specifies the constructs of relevance to sexual activation and responsivity and suggests their interactive properties. As outlined in Figure 16-2, sexual behavior is conceptualized as the end point of a sequence that includes a variety of components. The sequence may be initiated by an unconditioned stimulus such as an erogenous caress or by a conditioned erotic stimulus such as an object, an odor, or a musical selection that has been associated with sexual excitement in the past. The role of imaginative responses (both externally and self-generated) has been described in the preceding pages; most of the experimental research in this area uses such fantasies to produce arousal which is assessed on verbal scales (informational responses) or via direct measurement of physiological sexual responses. We have further seen that such arousal leads to preparatory acts such as approach behavior toward attractive members of the opposite sex and to sexual acts such as intercourse and masturbation. Research has also shown the way in which affective and evaluative response tendencies (e.g., anxiety, sex guilt, erotophobia–erotophilia) and

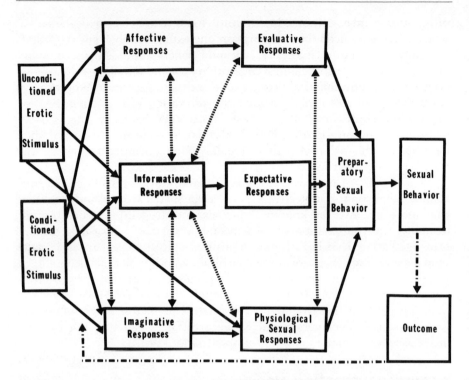

FIGURE 16-2. The model of the sexual behavior sequence describes four interactive response systems evoked by erotic stimuli. The affective–evaluative, informational–expectative, imaginative, and physiological systems mediate the effects of external erotic stimuli on subsequent sexual behavior. The rewarding or punishing outcomes of this behavior provide feedback to the system that influences subsequent behavior. From "Social psychology and the study of sexual behavior" by D. Byrne, **Personality and Social Psychology Bulletin**, 1977, *3*, 3–30. Copyright 1977 by Sage Publications. Reprinted by permission.

expectancies (e.g., alcohol as an aphrodisiac) can affect this process. Finally, though little research has been conducted in this area, the rewarding and punishing outcomes of sexual activity could be expected to affect subsequent interactions when the sexual behavior sequence is activated in the future. This model has recently been shown to be useful in analyzing the determinants of contraceptive behavior among adolescents, identifying its emotional, informational, affective, and imaginal aspects (Byrne & Fisher, 1983).

In a field characterized by atheoretical descriptive approaches, most previous theories have been designed to deal with limited segments of sexuality. Examples include the Freudian description of sexual motivation in terms of libidinal energy, Simon and Gagnon's (1969) role-scripting explanation of gender differences, and Mosher's (1980) analysis of the orgasmic response in terms of depth of involvement. In this burgeoning research area, the need for a more comprehensive model led to the development of the present formulation. It should be noted that Abramson (1983) has also recently proposed a general theory that stresses the importance of the cultural context and norms for sexual behavior. A common theme in each of these relatively new conceptualizations is the recognition that sexuality involves a process of responding simultaneously in one or more of several behavioral realms, including the physiological.

CONCLUSIONS

Although the basic physiological aspects of the human sexual response cycle obviously involve biological processes, the ubiquitous role of psychological variables in initiating, inhibiting, and controlling these responses is unmistakeable. The establishment of such effects inevitably leads us away from a sociobiological explanation of human sexuality and toward an explanation based on sociocultural and learning functions. A concrete example might be helpful. Current evidence suggests that if one wished to predict whether or not married couples would be likely to engage in sexual intercourse on a given evening, psychological variables would be of considerably greater value than physiological variables. That is, we know that exposure to external erotic images such as photographs or films (e.g., Cattell *et al.*, 1972; Mann *et al.*, 1974) or to internal erotic images such as dreams (e.g., Byrne & Lamberth, 1971) is associated with increased probability of intercourse. We also know that neither normal variations in hormone levels (Benkert *et al.*, 1979; Evans & Distiller, 1979; Kraemer, Becker, Brodie, Doering, Moos, & Hambrug, 1976; Raboch & Starka, 1972) nor exposure to sexual pheromones (Morris & Udry, 1978) are related to sexual activity. Beyond existing research on the role of imaginal and affective variables, theoretical models such as the Sexual Behavior Sequence offer guidelines as to other variables that may be identified as mediators of sexual responsiveness, including attitudes, beliefs, and expectancies. In addition, the individual's reinforcement history with respect to sexual acts is hypothesized to be a crucial consideration in attempts to predict sexual behavior.

In the study of other powerful motivations, psychologists have of necessity been forced to approach arousal in an indirect manner. Thus, it has been possible to manipulate deprivation in the study of hunger, to assess generalized physiological activation in the study of anger, to make inferences from overt behavior in the study of attraction, and to fall back on verbal self-reports in the study of almost all motives. Sexuality offers us a unique opportunity. Not only are each of these research techniques applicable to the study of sex, but there is now, in addition, the possibility of direct, specific assessment of physiological erotic excitement. In studying attitudinal responses, social psychologists have developed elaborate deceptions to convince subjects that a machine is a "pipeline to the soul" so that they will respond honestly. Psychosexologists do not have to rely on such a bogus pipeline, they now actually have access to procedures that measure a specific motivational state. Despite the special problems associated with sex research that range from unrepresentative samples to embarrassing psychological and physiological intrusiveness to broad ethnical concerns, the potential payoff in knowledge about a central aspect of human functioning is an important one.

The measurement techniques for reliably assessing sexual arousal are relatively new. It is not surprising that much of the initial work has involved attempts to improve existing devices, to develop more sophisticated ones, and to establish the relationship between these physical measures of arousal and subjective self-reports. What is more exciting, of course, is the fact that the first steps have been taken toward pursuing theoretical questions using these new techniques. Thus, the studies of cognitive processing, emotional influences, gender differences, attitude effects, and the role of drugs all constitute important beginnings in theory-oriented research. It seems likely that theory-oriented research will increasingly characterize the study of human sexuality.

REFERENCES

Abel, G. G., Barlow, D. H., Blanchard, E. B., & Guild, D. The components of rapists' sexual arousal. *Archives of General Psychiatry*, 1977, *34*, 895–906.

Abel, G. G., & Blanchard, E. B. The measurement and generation of sexual arousal in male sexual deviates. In M. Hersen, R. Eisler, & P. Miller (Eds.), *Progress in behavior modification* (Vol. 2). New York: Academic, 1976.

Abramson, P. R. *The sexual system: A theory of human sexual behavior.* New York: Academic, 1983.

Abramson, P. R., Perry, L. B., Rothblatt, A., Seeley, T. T., & Seeley, D. M. Negative attitudes toward masturbation and pelvic vasocongestion: A thermographic analysis. *Journal of Research in Personality*, 1981, *15*, 497–509.

Abramson, P. R., Perry, L. B., Seeley, T. T., Seeley, D. M., & Rothblatt, A. B. Thermographic measurement of sexual arousal: A discriminant validity analysis. *Archives of Sexual Behavior*, 1981, *10*, 171–176.

Alan Guttmacher Institute. *11 million teenagers.* New York: Author, 1976.

Amoroso, D. M., Brown, M., Pruesse, M., Ware, E. E., & Pilkey, D. W. An investigation of behavioral, psychological, and physiological reactions to pornographic stimuli. In *Technical report of the Commission on Obscenity and Pornography* (Vol. 8). Washington, D.C.: U.S. Government Printing Office, 1971.

Barclay, A. M. Urinary acid phosphatase in sexually aroused males. *Journal of Experimental Research in Personality*, 1970, *4*, 233–238.

Barclay, A. M. Information as a defensive control of sexual arousal. *Journal of Personality and Social Psychology*, 1971, *17*, 244–249.

Barclay, A. M., & Little, D. M. Urinary acid phosphatase secretion resulting from different arousals. *Psychophysiology*, 1972, *9*, 69–77.

Bardwick, J. M., & Behrman, S. J. Investigation into the effects of anxiety, sexual arousal, and the menstrual cycle phase in uterine contractions. *Psychosomatic Medicine*, 1967, *29*, 468–482.

Barker-Benfield, G. J. *The horrors of the half-known life.* New York: Harper & Row, 1976.

Barlow, D. H., Abel, G. G., Blanchard, E. B., & Mavissakalian, M. Plasma testosterone levels and male homosexuality: A failure to replicate. *Archives of Sexual Behavior*, 1974, *3*, 571–575.

Beach, F. A. It's all in your mind. *Psychology Today*, 1969, *3*(2), 33–35; 60.

Benkert, O., Witt, W., & Leitz, A. Effects of testosterone undeconoate on sexual potency and the hypothalamic–pituitary–gonadal axis of impotent males. *Archives of Sexual Behavior*, 1979, *8*, 471–479.

Bohlen, J. G. A review of subject orientation in articles on sexual physiology research. *Journal of Sex Research*, 1980, *16*, 43–58.

Bohlen, J. G., Held, J. P., & Sanderson, M. O. The male orgasm: Pelvic contractions measured by anal probe. *Archives of Sexual Behavior*, 1980, *9*, 503 521.

Brown, W. A., Monti, P. M., & Corriveau, D. P. Serum testosterone and sexual activity and interest in men. *Archives of Sexual Behavior*, 1978, *7*, 97–103.

Byrne, D. Social psychology and the study of sexual behavior. *Personality and Social Psychology Bulletin*, 1977, *3*, 3–30.

Byrne, D., & Fisher, W. A. (Eds.). *Adolescents, sex, and contraception.* Hillsdale, N.J.: Erlbaum, 1983.

Byrne, D., & Lamberth, J. The effect of erotic stimuli on sex arousal, evaluative responses, and subsequent behavior. In *Technical report of the Commission on Obscenity and Pornography* (Vol. 8). Washington, D.C: U.S. Government Printing Office, 1971.

Cantor, J. R., Zillmann, D., & Bryant, J. Enhancement of experienced sexual arousal in response to erotic stimuli through misattribution of unrelated residual excitation. *Journal of Personality and Social Psychology*, 1975, *32*, 69–75.

Cattell, R. B., Kawash, G. F., & DeYoung, G. E. Validation of objective measures of ergic tension: Response of the sex erg to visual stimulation. *Journal of Experimental Research in Personality*, 1972, *6*, 76–83.

Clore, G. L., & Byrne, D. A reinforcement-affect model of attraction. In T. L. Huston (Ed.), *Foundations of interpersonal attraction.* New York: Academic, 1974.

Cohen, H. D., & Shapiro, A. A method for measuring sexual arousal in the female. *Psychophysiology*, 1970, *8*, 251.

Dermer, M., & Pyszczynski, T. A. Effects of erotica upon men's loving and liking responses for women they love. *Journal of Personality and Social Psychology*, 1978, *36*, 1302–1309.

Evans, I. M., & Distiller, L. A. Effects of luteinizing hormone-releasing hormone on sexual arousal in normal men. *Archives of Sexual Behavior*, 1979, *8*, 385–395.

Eysenck, H. J. Obscenity—officially speaking. *Penthouse*, 1972, *3*, 95–102.

Fisher, S., & Osofsky, H. Sexual responsiveness in women, physiological correlates. *Psychological Reports*, 1968, *22*, 215–226.

Fisher, W. A. *Affective, attitudinal, and normative determinants of contraceptive behavior among university men.* Unpublished doctoral dissertation, Purdue University, 1978.

Fisher, W. A., & Byrne, D. Individual differences in affective, evaluative, and behavioral responses to an erotic film. *Journal of Applied Social Psychology*, 1978, *8*, 355–365. (a)

Fisher, W. A., & Byrne, D. Sex differences in response to erotica? Love versus lust. *Journal of Personality and Social Psychology*, 1978, *36*, 117–125. (b)

Gawin, F. H. Pharmacologic enhancement of the erotic: Implications of an expanded definition of aphrodisiacs. *Journal of Sex Research*, 1978, *14*, 107–117.

Geer, J. H. Direct measurement of genital responding. *American Psychologist*, March 1975, pp. 415–418.

Geer, J. H., & Fuhr, R. Cognitive factors in sexual arousal: The role of distraction. *Journal of Consulting and Clinical Psychology*, 1976, *44*, 238–243.

Geer, J. H., Morokoff, P., & Greenwood, P. Sexual arousal in women: The development of a measurement device for vaginal blood volume. *Archives of Sexual Behavior*, 1974, *3*, 559–564.

Geer, J. H., & Quartararo, J. D.   Vaginal blood volume responses during masturbation. *Archives of Sexual Behavior*, 1976, 5, 403–413.

Giambra, L. M., & Martin, C. E.   Sexual daydreams and quantitative aspects of sexual activity: Some relations for males across adulthood. *Archives of Sexual Behavior*, 1977, 6, 497–505.

Goldstein, M. J., Kant, H. S., & Hartman, J. J.   *Pornography and sexual deviance*. Berkeley, Calif.: University of California Press, 1974.

Griffitt, W.   Sexual experience and sexual responsiveness: Sex differences. *Archives of Sexual Behavior*, 1975, 4, 529–540.

Griffitt, W., May, J., & Veitch, R.   Sexual stimulation and interpersonal behavior: Heterosexual evaluative responses, visual behavior, and physical proximity. *Journal of Personality and Social Psychology*, 1974, 30, 367–377.

Harris, R., Yulis, S., & Lacoste, D.   Relationships among sexual arousability, imagery ability, and introversion–extraversion. *Journal of Sex Research*, 1980, 16, 72–86.

Hatch, J. P.   Vaginal photoplethysmography: Methodological considerations. *Archives of Sexual Behavior*, 1979, 8, 357–374.

Hatch, J. P.   Psychophysiological aspects of sexual dysfunction. *Archives of Sexual Behavior*, 1981, 10, 49–64.

Hatfield, E., Sprecher, S., & Traupmann, J.   Men's and women's reactions to sexually explicit films: A serendipitous finding. *Archives of Sexual Behavior*, 1978, 7, 583–592.

Heiman, J. R.   A psychophysiological exploration of sexual arousal patterns in females and males. *Psychophysiology*, 1977, 14, 266–274.

Henson, C., Rubin, H. B., & Henson, D. E.   Women's sexual arousal concurrently assessed by three genital measures. *Archives of Sexual Behavior*, 1979, 8, 459–469.

Henson, D., & Rubin, H.   A comparison of two objective measures of sexual arousal of women. *Behaviour Research and Therapy*, 1978, 16, 143–151.

Henson, D., Rubin, H., Henson, C., & Williams, J.   Temperature changes of the labia minora as an objective measure of female eroticism. *Journal of Behavior Therapy and Experimental Psychiatry*, 1977, 8, 401–410.

Hoon, E. F., Hoon, P. W., & Wincze, J. P.   An inventory for the measurement of female sexual arousability: The SAI. *Archives of Sexual Behavior*, 1976, 5, 291–300.

Hoon, P. W.   The assessment of sexual arousal in women. In M. Hersen, P. Eisler, & P. Miller (Eds.), *Progress in behavior modification* (Vol. 7). New York: Academic, 1979.

Jovanovic, U. J.   The recording of physiological evidence of genital arousal in human males and females. *Archives of Sexual Behavior*, 1971, 1, 309–320.

Kaats, G. R., & Davis, K. E.   Effects of volunteer biases in studies of sexual behavior and attitudes. *Journal of Sex Research*, 1971, 7, 26–34.

Kelley, K.   *Familiarity with erotica breeds contempt: Effects of frequency of exposure and novelty of change stimulus*. Unpublished manuscript, SUNY-Albany, 1981. (a)

Kelley, K.   *Heterosexuals' homophobic attitudes and responses to mildly stimulating erotica*. Paper presented at the meeting of the Midwestern Psychological Association, Detroit, May 1981. (b)

Kelley, K.   Gender, sex guilt, and authoritarianism on responses to heterosexual and masturbatory stimuli. *Journal of Sex Research*, in press.

Kinsey, A., Pomeroy, W. B., Martin, C. E., & Gebhard, P. H.   *Sexual behavior in the human female*. Philadelphia: Saunders, 1953.

Kockott, G., Feil, W., Ferstl, R., Aldenhoff, J., & Besmyer, U.   Psychophysiological aspects of male sexual inadequacy: Results of an experimental study. *Archives of Sexual Behavior*, 1980, 9, 477–493.

Kraemer, H. C., Becker, H. B., Brodie, H. X. H., Doering, C. H., Moos, R. H., & Hambrug, D. A.   Orgasmic frequency and plasma testosterone levels in normal human males. *Archives of Sexual Behavior*, 1976, 5, 125–132.

Kutchinsky, B.   The effect of pornography: A pilot experiment on perception, behavior, and attitudes. In *Technical report of the Commission on Obscenity and Pornography* (Vol. 8). Washington, D.C.: U.S. Government Printing Office, 1971.

Lang, A. R., Searles, J., Lauerman, R., & Adesso, V. Expectancy, alcohol, and sex guilt as determinants of interest in and reaction to sexual stimuli. *Journal of Abnormal Psychology*, 1980, *89*, 644-653.

Lansky, D., & Wilson, G. T. Alcohol, expectations, and sexual arousal in males: An information processing analysis. *Journal of Abnormal Psychology*, 1981, *90*, 35-45.

Laws, D. R. A comparison of the measurement characteristics of two circumferential penile transducers. *Archives of Sexual Behavior*, 1977, *6*, 45-51.

Laws, D. R., & Rubin, H. B. Instructional control of an autonomic sexual response. *Journal of Applied Behavior Analysis*, 1969, *2*, 93-99.

Levitt, E. E., & Brady, J. P. Sexual preferences in young adult males and some correlates. *Journal of Clinical Psychology*, 1965, *21*, 347-354.

Malatesta, V. J., Pollack, R. H., Wilbanks, W. A., & Adams, H. E. Alcohol effects on the orgasmic-ejaculatory response in human males. *Journal of Sex Research*, 1979, *15*, 101-107.

Mann, J., Berkowitz, L., Sidman, J., Starr, S., & West, S. Satiation of the transient and stimulating effect of erotic films. *Journal of Personality and Social Psychology*, 1974, *30*, 729-735.

Masters, W. H., & Johnson, V. E. *Human sexual response*. Boston: Little, Brown, 1966.

Masters, W. H., & Johnson, V. E. *Human sexual inadequacy*. Boston: Little, Brown, 1970.

Masters, W. H., & Johnson, V. E. *Homosexuality in perspective*. Boston: Little, Brown, 1979.

McConnell, J. V. *Understanding human behavior* (3rd ed.). New York: Holt, Rinehart & Winston, 1980.

Morris, N. M., & Udry, J. R. Pheromonal influences on human sexual behavior: An experimental search. *Journal of Biosocial Science*, 1978, *10*, 147-157.

Mosher, D. L. Three dimensions of depth of involvement in human sexual response. *Journal of Sex Research*, 1980, *16*, 1-42.

Mosher, D. L., & Cross, H. J. Sex guilt and premarital sexual experiences of college students. *Journal of Consulting and Clinical Psychology*, 1971, *36*, 27-32.

Mosher, D. L., & White, B. B. Effects of committed or casual erotic guided imagery on females' subjective sexual arousal and emotional response. *Journal of Sex Research*, 1980, *16*, 273-299.

Osborn, C. A., & Pollack, R. H. The effects of two types of erotic literature on physiological and verbal measures of female sexual arousal. *Journal of Sex Research*, 1977, *13*, 250-256.

Pirke, K. M., Kockott, G., & Dittmar, G. Psychosexual stimulation and plasma testosterone in man. *Archives of Sexual Behavior*, 1974, *3*, 577-584.

Raboch, J., & Starka, L. Coital activity of men and the levels of plasmatic testosterone. *Journal of Sex Research*, 1972, *8*, 219-224.

Rachman, S. Sexual fetishism: An experimental analogue. *The Psychological Record*, 1966, *16*, 293-296.

Robbins, M. B., & Jensen, G. D. Multiple orgasm in males. *Journal of Sex Research*, 1978, *14*, 21-26.

Rosen, R. C., & Keefe, F. J. The measurement of human penile tumescence. *Psychophysiology*, 1978, *15*, 366-376.

Sarrel, P. M., Foddy, J., & McKinnon, J. B. Investigation of human sexual response using a cassette recorder. *Archives of Sexual Behavior*, 1977, *6*, 341-348.

Schmidt, G., & Sigusch, V. Sex differences in responses to psychosexual stimulation by films and slides. *Journal of Sex Research*, 1970, *6*, 268-283.

Schmidt, G., & Sigusch, V. Women's sexual arousal. In J. Zubin & J. Money (Eds.), *Contemporary sexual behavior: Critical issues in the 1970s*. Baltimore: Johns Hopkins University Press, 1973.

Schmidt, G., Sigusch, V., & Schafer, S. Responses to reading erotic stories: Male-female differences. *Archives of Sexual Behavior*, 1973, *2*, 181-199.

490 BASIC SOCIAL PSYCHOPHYSIOLOGICAL RESEARCH

Seeley, T. T., Abramson, P. R., Perry, L. B., Rothblatt, A. B., & Seeley, D. M. Thermographic measurement of sexual arousal: A methodological note. *Archives of Sexual Behavior*, 1980, 9, 77-85.

Shapiro, A., Cohen, H. D., DiBianco, P., & Rosen, G. Vaginal blood flow changes during sleep and sexual arousal. *Psychophysiology*, 1968, 4, 394.

Simon, W., & Gagnon, J. H. On psychosexual development. In D. A. Goslin (Ed.), *Handbook of socialization theory and research*. Chicago: Rand McNally, 1969.

Sintchak, G., & Geer, J. H. A vaginal plethysmographic system. *Psychophysiology*, 1975, 12, 113-115.

Steinman, D. L., Wincze, J. P., Sakheim, D. K., Barlow, D. H., & Mavissakalian, M. A comparison of male and female patterns of sexual arousal. *Archives of Sexual Behavior*, 1981, 10, 529-547.

Story, N. L. Sexual dysfunction resulting from drug side effects. *Journal of Sex Research*, 1974, 10, 132-149.

Sue, D. Erotic fantasies of college students during intercourse. *Journal of Sex Research*, 1979, 15, 299-305.

Tordjman, G., Thierree, R., & Michel, J. R. Advances in the vascular pathology of male erectile dysfunction. *Archives of Sexual Behavior*, 1980, 9, 391-398.

Vance, E. B., & Wagner, N. N. Written descriptions of orgasm: A study of sex differences. *Archives of Sexual Behavior*, 1976, 5, 87-98.

Weidner, G., Istvan, G., & Griffitt, W. *Beauty in the eyes of the horny beholders.* Paper presented at the meeting of the Midwestern Psychological Association, Chicago, 1979.

Wilson, G. T., & Lawson, D. M. Expectancies, alcohol, and sexual arousal in male social drinkers. *Journal of Abnormal Psychology*, 1976, 85, 587-594.

Wilson, G. T., & Lawson, D. M. Expectancies, alcohol, and sexual arousal in women. *Journal of Abnormal Psychology*, 1978, 87, 358-367.

Wincze, J. P., Hoon, P., & Hoon, E. F. Sexual arousal in women: A comparison of cognitive and physiological responses by continuous measurement. *Archives of Sexual Behavior*, 1977, 6, 121-133.

Wincze, J. P., Venditti, E., Barlow, D., & Mavissakalian, M. The effects of a subjective monitoring task in the physiological measure of genital response to erotic stimulation. *Archives of Sexual Behavior*, 1980, 9, 533-545.

Wolchik, S. A., Beggs, V. E., Wincze, J. P., Sakheim, D. K., Barlow, D. H., & Mavissakalian, M. The effect of emotional arousal on subsequent sexual arousal in men. *Journal of Abnormal Psychology*, 1980, 89, 595-598.

Zuckerman, M. Physiological measures of sexual arousal in the human. *Psychological Bulletin*, 1971, 75, 347-356.

D · CONTRIBUTIONS TO HEALTH

C H A P T E R   1 7

Visceral Perception and Social Behavior

Jim Blascovich
State University of New York at Buffalo
Edward S. Katkin
State University of New York at Buffalo

In this chapter we report the theoretical and methodological background of a line of investigation which we believe has important implications for many theories in psychology, especially in social psychology. By describing a number of empirical studies that we have completed as well as a few that we have planned, we hope to make these implications clear as well as to stimulate interest in visceral perception and social behavior.

Before beginning the actual discussion, a few general points require clarification. First, in this chapter "visceral perception" refers to the self-detection of autonomically controlled responses such as heart beat, gastric motility, bladder distension, and so on. Second, the chapter focuses specifically on the subjective perception of one major visceral response (i.e., heart beat) and its relation to one category of social behavior (i.e., emotional labeling).

THEORETICAL BACKGROUND

William James (1884/1976) theorized that the experience of an emotion consists of the arousal and perception of specific autonomic responses. While there is much empirical evidence supporting the assumption that emotional behavior is associated with autonomic arousal (Plutchik, 1962), there is little *empirical* evidence supporting the assumption that such autonomic activity is accurately perceived. Even in extreme emotional states when a particular emotion is not only clearly identifiable by the individual experiencing that emotion, but also by other observers, it is not clear how accurately the emotional individual is able to perceive the related autonomic activity and/or changes in autonomic activity. For example, a person might "feel" extremely angry and "appear" angry, yet the extent to which that person is aware of autonomic responses which may be related to anger (e.g., vasoconstriction, increases in heart rate and blood pressure) has not been established empirically.

Contemporary modifications of Jamesian theory, such as Schachter and Singer's (1962) cognitive labeling theory of emotion, also emphasize the importance of the perception of autonomic arousal. However, unlike James, Schachter and Singer have argued that there are no unique or specific patterns of autonomic responsivity associated with the phenomenological experience of distinct emotions. Rather, they have postulated that when individuals experience general visceral arousal, they explain it cognitively and label their experience emotionally in the context of available cues. While Schachter and Singer's theory has generated considerable interest and debate concerning the process by which the cognitive labeling of emotion takes place, little attention has been paid to the process by which the individual perceives visceral or autonomic arousal. This absence of empirical research on visceral awareness is particularly striking in view of the common assumption that there is "sufficient evidence of the importance of autonomic feedback to support a cognitive–interpretive, self-attribution theory such as that of Schachter" (Buck, 1980, p. 812).

According to Schachter and Singer the perception of unexplained visceral arousal leads to a relatively neutral and objective search for an explanation. Even critics of Schachter and Singer's theory share their assumption of the importance of visceral perception. For example, Marshall and Zimbardo (1979) and Maslach (1979) disagree with Schachter and Singer and suggest that when an individual experiences unexplained arousal, there is a negative bias, presumably based on past experiences of adrenergic arousal, causing the subject to seek out a negative explanation of the unexplained arousal. Even though Marshall and Zimbardo (1979), Maslach (1979), and Schachter and Singer (1979) have engaged in intense debate concerning the essence of the individual's cognitive response to unexplained arousal, none has questioned the primary assumption that cognitive labeling, and ultimately the experience of emotion, are *secondary to the perception of the visceral arousal.*

Valins (1966) has suggested that individuals merely have to believe that their viscera are aroused in order to begin the cognitive labeling process. This viewpoint, although sometimes interpreted as a derivative of Schachter and Singer's theory, is, in fact, a quite radical departure, since Valins has implied that the accurate perception of visceral arousal is unnecessary for the experience of emotion. However, as Harris and Katkin (1975) have pointed out, there is substantial body of experimental literature which indicates that Valins's data were flawed since his paradigm of providing subjects with misinformation about their visceral activity actually have elicited increased visceral arousal (see Goldstein, Fink, & Mettee, 1972; Hirschman, 1975; Stern, Botto, & Herrick, 1972). Thus, Valins's studies may have been confounded since his cognitive manipulation may also have manipulated visceral responses. Kerber and Coles (1978) have reported that they did not find strong evidence to support Harris and Katkin's (1975) assertion that *actual* physiological changes associated with false physiological feedback were related to affective judgments. Kerber and Coles also noted that the importance of actual physiological changes may depend on the actual level of those changes. However, they failed to discuss the possibility that individual differences in the ability to detect accurately the physiological changes may be important. Since accuracy of visceral detection may be in part a function of physiological activity level, it is possible that the postulated greater weight may actually reflect increased accuracy of visceral self-perception.

While Jamesian and neo-Jamesian theories of emotion have generated numerous experimental studies, there has been no experimental approach addressed directly to the fundamental question of the perception of autonomically controlled visceral arousal. Thus, physiological theories concerning the autonomic basis of emotion place heavy emphasis on the role of visceral self-perception, but sound empirical research has lagged far behind the theories. This has been due in no small part to the lack of technology and methodology for assessing objectively an individual's ability to perceive autonomic activity.

It is clear that objective and quantitative methods for assessing the accuracy of autonomic perception would facilitate empirical study of the relationships among individual differences in the accuracy of visceral perception, induced visceral arousal and the experience and expression of emotion. For instance, in the classic Schachter and Singer (1962) demonstration, it might be predicted that drug-induced arousal would lead to cognitive labeling only for those subjects who accurately perceive the arousal. However, such methods need not be limited to the study of emotion. A similar approach could be used to study the relationships among individual differences in visceral perception, visceral arousal, and other arousal-based theories of social behavior, such as social facilitation, misattribution of arousal, and crowding.

METHODOLOGICAL BACKGROUND

A variety of methods designed specifically for the assessment of visceral perception has emerged from recent research in the field of autonomic self-regulation (Brener, 1977; Brener & Jones, 1974; Katkin, Morell, Goldband, & Bernstein, 1980; McFarland, 1975; Whitehead, Drescher, Heiman, & Blackwell, 1977). The impetus for much of the research has been Brener's "calibration" theory of visceral learning (Brener, 1977; Brener & Jones, 1974), which posits that biofeedback enhances a subject's ability to discriminate visceral responses. The acquisition of such visceral discrimination, according to Brener, facilitates voluntary control over visceral responses. Clearly, the development of valid methods for assessing the accuracy of visceral self-perception is required for experimental testing of Brener's hypothesis. Such methods also have value for investigating the relationship between visceral perception and emotion. Prior to these recent methodological developments, Mandler and his colleagues (Mandler, Mandler, & Uviller, 1958) developed a questionnaire for the subjective assessment of autonomic activity. Thus, previous researchers have attempted to assess visceral self-perception both subjectively and objectively.

Subjective Assessment of Visceral Perception

Mandler et al. (1958) developed the autonomic perception questionnaire (APQ), an extensive list of self-report items. The items on the APQ require respondents to indicate their degree of awareness of autonomically medicated responses such as heart pounding, heart rate, sweating, breathing, and so on. Mandler et al. found that APQ scores correlated positively with scores on anxiety scales containing items requiring the subjective report of physiological events. Furthermore, Mandler et al., reported that persons scoring high on the APQ showed significantly greater autonomic activity (heart rate, electrodermal response, face temperature, and blood volume) than did subjects scoring low on the APQ. Unfortunately, there is no way to indicate the extent to which the APQ or similar instruments reflect accuracy of visceral perception rather than the intensity of visceral arousal.

In addition, subsequent validational research has been disappointing. McFarland (1975) administered the APQ along with his heart activity perception (HAP) test, in which subjects are instructed to press a button in rhythm with their heart beat. McFarland also had subjects increase and decrease their heart rate and provided them with feedback concerning the accuracy of their responses. Although there was no reliable correlation between APQ and HAP scores, subjects who received high scores on the HAP increased their heart rate significantly better than did subjects with low scores on the HAP. McFarland interpreted the low correlation between the APQ and HAP scores as evidence that the two perception tests measured different attributes of the subjects.

Additional failures to confirm the validity of the APQ were reported by Whitehead and his colleagues. In administering the APQ, the rod and frame test, and an objective test of heart beat discrimination (see the following section), Whitehead, Drescher, and Blackwell (1976) discovered the APQ scores did not correlate with heart beat discrimination, and that the APQ items that were specifically related to awareness of heart beat were not correlated with behaviorally assessed measures of heart beat perception. Whitehead et al. concluded that the APQ was not a valid measure of the ability to perceive heart beats. Considering these data, Brener (1977) suggested that *the APQ does not appear to be a reliable measure of autonomic perception*. While he concluded that there is some evidence that individual differences in autonomic perception exist, the extent of that perception cannot be measured reliably by the APQ.

Objective Measures of Visceral Perception

Using laboratory computers, a number of investigators have developed objective techniques for the assessment of accuracy of visceral perception. Because of the simplicity of its measurement, most of this effort has been directed specifically toward the detection of heart beats or heart rate. McFarland (1975), for example, developed the heart activity perception (HAP) test mentioned above as a technique for assessing accuracy of heart rate. Subjects were instructed to press a button in rhythm with their heart beat. The absolute difference between the number of button presses and the number of heart beats occurring during a test interval was divided by the number of heart beats and subtracted from 1 to obtain a measure of heart activity perception. This technique essentially measures the degree to which a subject is aware of his or her heart *rate* over some time interval, and is not particularly sensitive to phasic changes in the heart beats that might occur during the test interval. It is important to note that the perception of heart rate and heart beat are conceptually distinct. Heart rate is inferred from the perception of heart beats *and* time estimation. Heart beat is not inferred in this way and presumably may be perceived directly. Indeed, we maintain that the perception of heart beat is a more fundamental cardiac perceptual process. In order to develop a measure that would more accurately reflect the perceptual sensitivity to phasic changes in heart beats, Brener and Jones (1974) developed their "cardiac activity discrimination" test.

Brener and Jones provided their subjects with brief vibratory stimuli delivered to the wrist. These stimuli were either contingent on the R wave[1] of the electrocardiogram (ECG) or were generated independently of cardiac activity by an external signal generator set to produce a pulse frequency approximately equal to the subject's mean heart rate. After receiving a train of vibratory stimuli for approximately 10 seconds, subjects were asked to judge whether the stimulus train was generated by their R waves or by the external signal generator. A typical experiment would involve 80 or more such discrimination trials. Brener and Jones maintained that the number of trials on which subjects made correct detections is an effective index of cardiac rate discrimination.

1. The "R wave" is the major voltage spike seen on an electrocardiogram. It is an indicator of ventricular contraction.

One deficiency in Brener and Jones's technique was that their subjects could have learned to alter their respiration rate or muscle tension voluntarily, which would have an immediate, profound effect on cardiac rate. By so doing, the subjects would be able to discover a change in the vibratory stimuli that were contingent on their heart beats; similar muscular or respiratory changes would have absolutely no effect on the externally generated noncontingent vibratory stimuli. Although it is not known what percentage of Brener and Jones's subjects were able to use such voluntary manipulations to maximize their correct detections, it is clear that their technique is not foolproof.

Because of this drawback, Whitehead and his collaborators developed a technique in which both contingent and noncontingent signals would be generated continuously by a subject's own ECG. In addition, Whitehead *et al.* (1977) analyzed subjects' responses using the theory of signal detection (TSD; see McNicol, 1972). An important feature of TSD is that it allows the investigator to isolate perceptual sensitivity from response bias components of the subject's response pattern. There is a large literature on the application of TSD to vigilance and perceptual sensitivity for a variety of external perceptual tasks. Whitehead's application of this technique, as well as more recent applications by Ashton, White, and Hodgson (1979), extend the methodological elegance of TSD to the analysis of the perception of internal, viscerally generated signals.

In Whitehead's paradigm, subjects are presented with a train of visual stimuli which are generated by the R waves of the ECGs, and presented after either a 100-msec or a 400-msec delay from the R wave. The subject is asked to discriminate between the signals which are delayed for a "short" or "long" interval after the R wave. Obviously, if a subject tries respiratory or muscular manipulations, both sets of stimuli will be affected equally. Also, if the subjects have no actual perceptual sensitivity of their own heart beats, the two sets of stimuli will be totally indistinguishable. The only way in which subjects can accurately detect the difference between a short delay and a long delay train of stimuli is in reference to their own actual heart beats. Thus, perceptual sensitivity scores greater than chance can be obtained only if the subjects are capable of detecting their own heart beats. Using this paradigm, Whitehead and his collaborators discovered that only a few subjects were able to make the discrimination. Their findings were subsequently confirmed in our laboratory (Katkin *et al.*, 1980). The poor performance of Whitehead's subjects as well as ours led us to conclude that the discrimination task itself was too difficult. Consequently, we set out to devise a task that would preserve the valuable features of Whitehead's paradigm, but would be easier for the subjects to discriminate, assuming that they did indeed have accurate perceptions of their heart beats.

Current Status of Signal Detection Assessment of Visceral Perception

Like Whitehead's, our task is a discrimination task in which subjects are presented with two trains of stimuli generated by their own ECG R waves: stimuli (S+) which have a fixed relationship to the R wave, and stimuli (S−) which have a variable relationship to the R wave. For the S+ stimulus, a subject is presented with a train of 10 tones which occur 100 msec after each of 10 consecutive R waves. For the S− stimulus, the subject is also presented with a train of 10 tones; however, the S− tones have a variable relationship to the R waves.

The logic of the S+ and S− stimuli is presented graphically in Figure 17-1. The two top lines are graphic representations of a hypothetical subject's R waves assumed to occur at equal intervals (1000 msec) for purposes of this illustration. The second line on the left represents a train of S+ tones. Notice that the S+ tones occur precisely at 100 msec after each R wave. The second line on the right represents a train of S− tones. Notice that the tones occur at varying intervals after the R waves. The occurrence of these tones varies from the occurrence of the R waves according to the formula

$$(n + 30\ B_i)\ \text{msec}$$

where n is a random number between 0 and 100 and B_i is the ith R wave. For purposes of this illustration, n is assumed to equal 100. Thus, the first tone in the S− train occurs 130 msec after the first R wave, the second tone in the S− train occurs 160 msec after the second R wave, the third tone 190 msec after the third R wave, and so on, until the tenth tone, which occurs 400 msec after the tenth R wave. The bottom lines on the figure show the intervals between tones. It may be seen clearly that within both the S+ and S− trains of stimuli, the time intervals between tones are constant. As also can be seen in the illustration, the constant interval between S− tones is 30 msec longer than the constant interval between S+ tones. This 30-msec difference is obtained in all cases regardless of the random number n.

We developed this task because we thought that it would be easier for subjects with visceral perceptual sensitivity to discriminate our S+ and S− stimuli than to discriminate Whitehead's S+ and S− stimuli. However, to establish the legitimacy of our task, it was essential to demonstrate that the 30-msec difference between trains of S+ and S− tones was not discriminable.

In order to get an idea of the ease with which the discrimination between S+ and S− tones can be made *with* perception of heart beats, consider what happens (refer to Figure 17-1) if we present subjects with

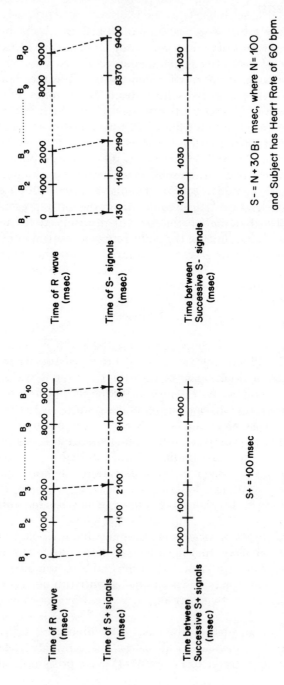

FIGURE 17-1. Logic of discrimination stimuli. From "Empirical assessment of visceral self-perception: Individual and sex differences in the acquisition of heart beat discrimination" by E. S. Katkin, J. Blascovich, & S. Goldband, *Journal of Personality and Social Psychology*, 1981, **40**, 1095–1114. Copyright 1981 by the American Psychological Association. Reprinted by permission.

external signals exactly contingent on their R waves in addition to S+ and S– trains. In the S+ case, subjects would hear each tone precisely 100 msec after the R-wave signal. In the S– case, subjects would hear each tone increasingly delayed from the R-wave signal. To the extent that subjects perceive their heart beats the discrimination between S+ and S– trains becomes a simple task. In our empirical situation, therefore, we can infer the accuracy of the perception of heart beats from the extent to which they can discriminate S+ and S– trains.

The methodological approach to the assessment of visceral self-perception has matured significantly since the early questionnaire studies. McFarland (1975) and Brener and Jones (1974) paved the way for the development of objective assessment of visceral self-perception. Whitehead *et al.* (1977) advanced the technique significantly by introducing signal detection methodology and eliminating the possibility of muscular or respiratory artifacts from the assessment. We believe that we have improved on Whitehead's technique by designing a task which is not so difficult that it precludes assessing a subject's capacity to discriminate.

EMPIRICAL WORK

Completed Studies

Three studies have been run in our laboratory. The purpose of these studies was to assess the reliability of our discrimination paradigm for assessing both the accuracy of an individual's perception of heart beats and the effectiveness of heart beat discrimination training. For purposes of brevity, only the second and third studies will be presented here since they include complete, successful replications of the first study.

Eighteen subjects (9 males and 9 females) were run in two sessions, one week apart. The first session was identical for both experimental and control subjects and constituted a precise replication of an earlier pilot study (Katkin *et al.*, 1980). After arriving at the laboratory the subject was placed in an acoustically controlled, environmental chamber in which temperature and airflow were held constant. Appropriate electrodes were attached to the subject and baseline recordings of heart rate, respiration, and electrodermal activity were made.

Following this, the subject was given tape-recorded instructions appropriate to our visceral discimination task. Briefly, subjects were instructed to discriminate trains of tones which were coincident with their heart from trains of tones which were not. The subjects were then presented with 40 discrimination trials. On each trial they indicated whether the train of 10 tones was coincident or noncoincident with their heart beats, and also indicated the confidence (1 to 4) with which they made the identification. During these first 40 trials, subjects received no feedback about the correctness or incorrectness of their performance. Thus, these trials served as a baseline indicator of their discrimination ability. Following the first 40 trials, subjects were presented with 120 additional trials in which they did receive performance feedback following each trial informing them if their choice was correct or incorrect. In addition, they received a running total following each correctly identified train, indicating the number of correctly identified trains of tones. Both the performance feedback and the running total information were presented to subjects visually via a computer monitor. As mentioned above, both experimental and control subjects were treated identically during the first session. In the second session, one week later, subjects were run in exactly the same manner, except that subjects in the control condition were presented trains of tones driven by a tape recording of their ECG that was made during the first session; they received no feedback about their current, ongoing ECG. In this way we were able to test whether subjects could discriminate the difference in intertone interval (30 msec) between the trains of tones without reference to their actual heart beat.

The results indicated that prior to training (baseline) the *mean* performance of subjects in both the experimental and control groups on the discrimination task was no greater than chance. However, with veridical performance feedback (session 1) regarding the correctness of choices, the mean performance of all subjects in our experiment improved significantly. Overall, both groups in the first session, and the experimental group in the second session, performed better than chance. In the second session, the control group did not perform better than chance (see Figure 17-2). An analysis of variance of the data presented in Figure 17-2 indicated that the groups (experimental–control) $\times$ sessions interaction was statistically significant: $F(1,16) = 6.5$, $p < .025$.

It is important to note that during pretraining in the first session, there were wide variations among individuals in their perceptual sensitivity. Thus, it appears that while some subjects are capable of benefiting from training and others are not, it is also the case that some subjects have already acquired or in some way possess better ability to perceive visceral activity than others. Thus, without performance feedback training, our results parallel Whitehead's. Indeed, our task does not appear to be more sensitive. However, whether or not our task is more sensitive *with* performance feedback training is an open question since Whitehead's task has not been used with such training.

Further analysis of data from the first session revealed a significant and dramatic sex effect.[2] While male subjects improved their discrimination

2. Data were not analyzed for sex differences in session 2 since only half of the subjects (i.e., 9) were actually performing a "live" heart beat discrimination task, whereas in session 1 all 18 subjects (9 males and 9 females) were performing exactly the same task.

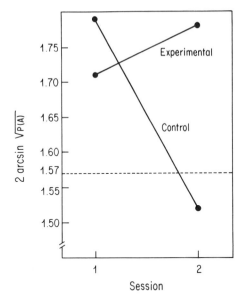

FIGURE 17-2. Mean discrimination performance. From "Empirical assessment of visceral self-perception: Individual and sex differences in the acquisition of heart beat discrimination" by E. S. Katkin, J. Blascovich, & S. Goldband, **Journal of Personality and Social Psychology**, 1981, **40**, 1095–1114. Copyright 1981 by the American Psychological Association. Reprinted by permission.

ability significantly with performance feedback training, females did not. An analysis of variance of the data presented in Figure 17-3 indicated that the sex $\times$ trial blocks interaction was statistically significant: $F(3,48) = 6.22$, $p < .002$. Additional analyses revealed no significant difference in heart rate between males and females or between experimental and control subjects, indicating that cardiac arousal did not underlie either the sex effect or the feedback effect.

An additional study (Koenigsberg, Katkin, & Blascovich, 1981) was conducted with two goals: to replicate the previous findings and to determine if acquired visceral perception would be retained after the cessation of training. This study replicated the first session of the previous study, with an additional period of testing immediately following training. The results confirmed the finding that male subjects acquired visceral discrimination ability more readily than female subjects. The results also demonstrated that there was no decline in discrimination ability after the cessation of training. The implications of this finding are important for future studies in which it would be desirable to train subjects to detect heart beats accurately and then to measure their responses on other tasks after the training period. This is particularly important for studying the relationship between levels of arousal and emotional experience. For example, subjects could be exposed to arousal-inducing situations after being trained to detect visceral activity accurately, and their subsequent emotional behavior could be compared to control subjects who were untrained in visceral detection. Such studies might shed light on the degree to which the

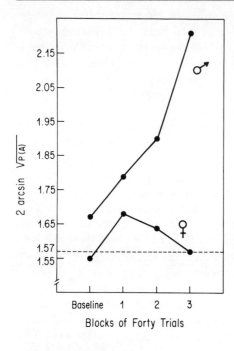

FIGURE 17-3. Mean performance of males and females. From "Empirical assessment of visceral self-perception: Individual and sex differences in the acquisition of heart beat discrimination" by E. S. Katkin, J. Blascovich, & S. Goldband, **Journal of Personality and Social Psychology**, 1981, **40**, 1095–1114. Copyright 1981 by the American Psychological Association. Reprinted by permission.

accurate detection of visceral arousal is a crucial ingredient in emotionally based behavior.

The results of these preliminary studies suggest that our paradigm is a useful one for assessing visceral perception and for training subjects to improve their perception. In addition, the studies suggest that there are sex differences in the ability to learn to perceive heart beats.

Future

Our plans are to conduct additional studies addressed to the following issues: (1) the relationship between various levels of physiological arousal and accuracy of visceral perception; (2) the effects of visceral perceptual accuracy on the attribution of affect in a false physiological feedback paradigm; and (3) the effects of gender and sex-role orientation on visceral perception accuracy.

Our future studies will examine the relationship between arousal and visceral perception. The consensus of most researchers (Adam, 1978; Brener, 1974; Miller, 1978) is that individuals should have little difficulty discriminating visceral activity when they are highly aroused. Recent data reported by Jones and Hollandsworth (1979) confirm this assumption. They reported that sedentary subjects showed poorer heart beat discrimination than moderately or very active subjects. However, after exercise-induced arousal, all subjects showed improved heart beat discrimination. Unfortunately, Jones and Hollandsworth employed the Brener–Jones technique, which may have been confounded by activity level. Thus, there is as yet no unambiguous evidence that visceral arousal per se enhances visceral perception.

Although the relationships among arousal, visceral perception, and emotion are not well documented empirically, it is interesting to note that natural language references to "emotional states" are usually references to states associated with increased physiological arousal. James (1884/1976) himself noted that he did not assume that the perception of *normal* states of physiological activity would define emotion, but only the perception of extreme states of physiological activity. It is possible that the reason that visceral sensations have been implicated so often in "emotions" is that we become aware of those sensations (accurately) only when they are substantially above "normal" baseline levels. Therefore, an empirical investigation of the degree to which level of physiological activity is related to accurate detection of that activity is in the works. We expect that as the strength of ventricular contractions increases, subjects will be better able to perceive their heart beats because the "signal"-to-"noise" ratio is greater. We will test subjects using our signal detection discrimination task with and without training, at rest, at moderate arousal, and at high arousal using physical exercise to induce such arousal.

An additional study will test the notion suggested by Valins that accurate visceral perception is not necessary for the cognitive labeling of emotions. As discussed above, Schachter and Singer theorized that only when individuals experience general visceral arousal do they explain the arousal cognitively and label their experience emotionally in the context of available social cues. Thus, visceral perception is a basic assumption of this theory.

Valins, on the other hand, suggested that visceral perception is unnecessary for such labeling. Rather, he suggested that individuals merely have to believe that their viscera are aroused. Valins (1966) purportedly demonstrated that false heart rate feedback was sufficient to affect the cognitive labeling process. Valins exposed male subjects to 10 seminude female slides. During the presentation of five of the slides, one group of subjects was given auditory heart beat feedback which indicated that their heart rate had sharply increased, and another group received feedback indicating a sharp decrease. Subsequently, both groups rated the attractiveness of the slides which had been presented with false feedback indicating a change (increased or decreased heart rate) higher than the slides presented with feedback indicating no change. The results of the Valins study are equivocal. There is some doubt about the role of actual induced arousal in his subjects (Hirschman, 1975; Stern *et al.*, 1972) and considerable doubt about the equivalence of the concepts of emotion and attribution of arousal (Harris & Katkin, 1975).

Visceral perceptual ability may influence the results of "Valins"-type studies if the typical level of arousal elicited by stimuli is sufficiently great to maximize individual differences in heart beat detection. In this case, good visceral perceivers would not be fooled by false physiological feedback since their own perception may be more veridical. On the other hand, poor visceral perceivers could be expected to be more susceptible to the false feedback manipulation. A second study by Valins (1967) indicates that he was aware of this possibility but was unable to test it directly or appropriately because he lacked a method for assessing and training self-perception of heart beats (Harris & Katkin, 1975; Lykken, 1967). We intend to test this hypothesis by training one group of male subjects to perceive their heart beats accurately while leaving a control group untrained. Subsequently, we will run individuals from both groups in a false physiological feedback experiment.

Finally, we intend to study further the sex × training interaction we have found. Specifically, we will test a *general* sex-role explanation of this previous finding. Neither the male nor female groups in the preliminary studies performed better than chance without training, and the range of performance without training varied from chance to perfect for both sex groups. Nevertheless, the performance of males as a group did improve significantly as a function of the training procedure. It is not likely that visceral perception per se is sex linked, although it does appear that males are more responsive to our training procedures than females. At this point, there is no immediately apparent biological reason for males to be more responsive to these training procedures than females. Assuming that most males are "masculine" and most females are "feminine," several specific sex-role hypotheses could explain the sex effect for visceral perception training found in our pilot work. For example, Deaux (1977) has pointed out performance differences between males and females as a function of task familiarity. Thus, males may perform better than females on our visceral perception discrimination task because of greater socialed familiarity with evaluative and competitive types of tasks. Because of this familiarity, males might experience less confusion and greater motivation to perform. Or, because of familiarity with the task setting involving complex electronic equipment, electrodes, transducers, a computer, and so on, males may simply experience less performance anxiety than females. Other specific sex-role hypotheses can also be generated, for example, sex differences in the need for achievement or field dependence/independence. However, at present such speculation is premature.

In order to pursue any specific sex-role explanation, we must first determine whether sex differences in training are due to sex role in general. We will accomplish this by using sex role and biological gender as independent factors in a future study.

IMPLICATIONS

Theories of the Emotions

The results of our current line of investigation are likely to have substantial implications for most current viscerally based theories of emotion. Such theories assume that the labeling of emotional experience and/or the attribution of affect depend on the perception of internal visceral arousal. Thus, the identification of subjects who differ in the accuracy of such visceral perception should facilitate critical testing of these theories.

Other Social Psychological Theories

Although we have focused on the role of visceral perception in the experience and labeling of emotion, there are many other social psychological theories for which the direct empirical investigation of individual differences in visceral perception is relevant. Implied by these theories is the assumption that some event causes arousal which is consequently perceived and acted upon. Empirical tests of the effects of individual differences in visceral perception on the phenomena which these theories attempt to explain could provide a test of the assumption of visceral perception on which such theories are based. In addition, if such an assumption proved to be tenable, predictions based on such theories could be more precise.

Dissonance theory provides a case in point. Although Festinger (1957) himself never discussed the role of visceral arousal or its perception in his theory, he did assert that dissonance is perceived as an unpleasant state and possesses drive properties. Waterman and Katkin (1967) have demonstrated further that the induction of cognitive dissonance is associated with "drive" and Gleason and Katkin (1979) have shown that dissonance induction is associated with cardiac components of drive. If the experience of cognitive dissonance is related to physiological arousal, individual differences in the perception of such arousal should mediate dissonance-reducing behavior. This is, of course, an empirical question and subject to experimentation using objective indices both of levels of arousal and accuracy of its perception.

Another case is provided by the work of Zillmann and his colleagues on the misattribution of arousal (e.g., Zillmann, 1978; Zillmann, Johnson, & Day, 1974). Zillmann relies heavily on the notion of "residual arousal," which refers to physiological arousal persisting after the decay of the psychological association of that arousal with its cause. It may be that this "psychological" decay is a function of the accuracy with which one continuously perceives the physiological activity. It is possible that if an individual possesses accurate visceral perception he or she will be able to monitor accurately the decline in physiological arousal over time. Thus, for such a person, there should be minimal discrepancy between the physiological and psychological "decay of arousal." Hence, misattribution effects would be more likely for less accurate or poor visceral perceivers. Once again, this is an empirical question that can be examined in the laboratory using objective indices of visceral arousal and perception.

There are many other social psychological theories for which similar applications of visceral perception methodology and training techniques may be generated. A partial list would include cost–arousal models of helping behavior (Piliavin, Piliavin, & Rodin, 1976), drive–arousal theories of social facilitation (Cottrell, 1972; Sanders & Baron, 1975; Zajonc, 1965), and arousal models of interpersonal distance and crowding (Patterson, 1976).

REFERENCES

Adam, G. Visceroception, awareness and behavior. In G. E. Schwartz & D. Shapiro (Eds.), *Consciousness and self-regulation* (Vol. 2). New York: Plenum, 1978.

Ashton, R , White, K. D., & Hodgson, G. Sensitivity to heart rate: A psychophysical study. *Psychophysiology*, 1979, *16*, 463–466.

Brener, J. A general model of voluntary control applied to the phenomenon of learned cardiovascular change. In P. A. Obrist, A. H. Black, J. Brener, & L. V. DiCara (Eds.), *Cardiovascular psychophysiology.* Chicago: Aldine, 1974.

Brener, J. Sensory and perceptual determinants of voluntary visceral control. In G. Schwartz & J. Beatty (Eds.) *Biofeedback: Theory and research.* New York: Academic, 1977.

Brener, J., & Jones, J. M. Interoceptive discrimination in intact humans: Detection of cardiac activity. *Physiology and Behavior*, 1974, *13*, 763–767.

Buck, R. Nonverbal behavior and the theory of emotion: The facial feedback hypothesis. *Journal of Personality and Social Psychology*, 1980, *38*, 811–824.

Cottrell, N. B. Social facilitation. In C. G. McClintock (Ed.), *Experimental social psychology.* New York: Holt, Rinehart & Winston, 1972.

Deaux, K. Sex differences in social behavior. In T. Blass (Ed.), *Personality variables in social behavior.* Hillsdale, N.J.: Erlbaum, 1977.

Egan, J. P. *Signal detection theory and ROC analysis.* New York: Academic, 1975.

Festinger, L. *A theory of cognitive dissonance.* Evanston, Ill.: Row, Peterson, 1957.

Gleason, J. M., & Katkin, E. S. The effects of cognitive dissonance on heart rate and electrodermal response. *Psychophysiology*, 1979, *16*, 180–181. (Abstract)

Goldstein, D., Fink, D., & Mettee, D. R. Cognition of arousal and actual arousal as determinants of emotion. *Journal of Personality and Social Psychology*, 1972, *21*, 41–51.

Harris, V. A., & Katkin, E. S. Primary and secondary emotional behavior: An analysis of the role of autonomic feedback on affect, arousal and attribution. *Psychological Bulletin*, 1975, *82*, 904–916.

Hirschman, R. D. Cross modal effects of anticipatory bogus heart rate feedback in a negative emotional context. *Journal of Personality and Social Psychology*, 1975, *31*, 13–19.

James, W. What is emotion? *Mind*, 1884, *9*, 188–205. Reprinted in S. W. Porges & M. G. H. Coles (Eds.), *Psychophysiology.* Stroudsburg, Pa.: Dowden, Hutchinson & Ross, 1976.

Jones, G. E., & Hollandsworth, J. G. *Heart rate discrimination before and after exercise-induced augmented cardiac activity.* Paper presented at the annual meeting of the Society for Psychophysiological Research, Cincinnati, Ohio, 1979.

Katkin, E. S., Morell, M. A., Goldband, S., & Bernstein, G. L. Individual differences in visceral and external signal discrimination. *Psychophysiology,* 1980, *17,* 322–323. (Abstract)

Kerber, K. W., & Coles, M. G. H. The role of perceived physiological activity in affective judgments. *Journal of Experimental Social Psychology,* 1978, *14,* 419–433.

Koenigsberg, M. R., Katkin, E. S., & Blascovich, J. The affect of pretraining instructional set on the acquisition and maintenance of heartbeat detection in males and females. *Psychophysiology,* 1981, *18,* 196–197. (Abstract)

Lykken, D. T. Valins' "emotionality and autonomic reactivity": An appraisal. *Journal of Experimental Research in Personality,* 1967, *2,* 49–55.

Mandler, G., Mandler, J. M., & Uviller, E. T. Autonomic feedback: The perception of autonomic activity. *Journal of Abnormal and Social Psychology,* 1958, *56,* 367–373.

Marshall, G. D., & Zimbardo, P. G. Affective consequences of inadequately explained physiological arousal. *Journal of Personality and Social Psychology,* 1979, *37,* 953–969.

Maslach, C. Negative emotional biasing of unexplained arousal. *Journal of Personality and Social Psychology,* 1979, *37,* 953–969.

McFarland, R. A. Heart rate perception and heart rate control. *Psychophysiology,* 1975, *12,* 402–405.

McNicol, D. *A primer of signal detection theory.* London: Allen & Unwin, 1972.

Miller, N. E. Biofeedback and visceral learning. In M. R. Rosenweig & L. W. Porter (Eds.), *Annual review of psychology* (Vol. 29). Palo Alto, Calif.: Annual Reviews, 1978.

Patterson, M. L. An arousal model of interpersonal intimacy. *Psychological Bulletin,* 1976, *83,* 235–245.

Piliavin, I. M., Piliavin, J. A., & Rodin, J. Costs, diffusion, and the stigmatized victim. *Journal of Personality and Social Psychology,* 1976, *32,* 429–438.

Plutchik, R. *The emotions: Facts, theories, and a new model.* New York: Random House, 1962.

Sanders, G. S., & Baron, R. S. The motivating effects of distraction on task performance. *Journal of Personality and Social Psychology,* 1975, *32,* 956–963.

Schachter, S., & Singer, J. E. Cognitive, social and physiological determinants of emotional state. *Psychological Review,* 1962, *69,* 379–399.

Schachter, S., & Singer, J. E. Comments on the Maslach and Marshall–Zimbardo experiments. *Journal of Personality and Social Psychology,* 1979, *7,* 989–995.

Stern, R. M., Botto, R. W., & Herrick, C. D. Behavioral and physiological effects of false heartrate feedback: A replication and extension. *Psychophysiology,* 1972, *9,* 21–29.

Valins. S. Cognitive effects of false heartrate feedback. *Journal of Personality and Social Psychology,* 1966, *4,* 400–408.

Valins, S. Emotionality and information concerning internal reactions. *Journal of Personality and Social Psychology,* 1967, *6,* 458–463.

Waterman, C. K., & Katkin, E. S. The energizing (dynamogenic) effect of cognitive dissonance on task performance. *Journal of Personality and Social Psychology,* 1967, *6,* 126–131.

Whitehead, W. E., Drescher, V. M., & Blackwell, B. Lack of relationship between Autonomic Perception Questionnaire scores and actual sensitivity for perceiving one's heart beat. *Psychophysiology,* 1976, *13,* 176.

Whitehead, W. E., Drescher, V. M., Heiman, P., & Blackwell, B. Relation of heart rate control to heart beat perception. *Biofeedback and Self-Regulation,* 1977, *2,* 371–392.

Zajonc, R. B. Social facilitation. *Science,* 1965, *149,* 269–274.

Zillmann, D. Attribution and misattribution of excitatory reactions. In J. Harvey, W. Ickes, & R. Kidd (Eds.), *New directions in attribution research* (Vol. 2). Hillsdale, N.J.: Erlbaum, 1978.

Zillmann, D., Johnson, R. C., & Day, K. D. Attribution of apparent arousal and proficiency at recovery from sympathetic activation affecting excitation transfer to aggressive behavior. *Journal of Experimental Social Psychology,* 1974, *10,* 503–515.

CHAPTER 18

Attentional Factors in the Perception of Bodily States

Michael F. Scheier
Carnegie-Mellon University

Charles S. Carver
University of Miami

Karen A. Matthews
University of Pittsburgh

Pick up virtually any textbook on introductory cognitive psychology and in it you will find some discussion devoted to attentional factors. Clearly, attentional variables are important determinants in the functioning of all information-processing systems. In this chapter we discuss the role played by attentional factors in the perception of bodily states. The discussion begins with a brief but general consideration of attentional processes and how they relate to the self. Also considered here are the various techniques that have been devised to vary self-attention in the laboratory. In the next section we describe more directly the effects that self-attention has on awareness of bodily states, as well as the related effects produced by such awareness on the experience of emotion. Following this and extrapolating from it, we examine how various attentional strategies might get utilized by persons to cope with the bodily changes produced by environmental stressors. The chapter concludes with a general discussion of the ways in which different cognitive representations of a stressful experience can affect reactions to it.

ATTENTION

Attention would seem to be a concept simple enough to make extended discussion of it quite unnecessary. As William James (1890, p. 403) put it, "Everyone knows what attention is." Despite its apparent simplicity, however, the concept, once momentarily grasped, has a decided tendency to become blurred and elusive. As a result, cognitive psychologists have wrestled with the concept for some time now in an attempt to define it (cf. Berlyne, 1974; Posner, 1974).

More recent discussions of attentional phenomena have attempted to avoid this definitional problem entirely. That is, rather than defining attention explicitly, cognitive psychologists have sought to identify the various properties that it exhibits. As an example of this strategy, consider the approach taken by Bourne, Dominowski, and Loftus (1979). They point out that whatever attention *is*, its existence has several discriminable *aspects* (see also Kahneman, 1973). One aspect of attention is its distribution. A person's attention can be diffused (spread over a number of different stimuli) or it can be concentrated. A second aspect of attention concerns the degree of alertness or vigilance that it embodies—in Kahneman's (1973) terms, how much effort is involved. A person may be very alert (attending quickly and easily to even low-intensity stimuli) or very inattentive to even the most salient stimuli.

Yet another property of the attentional process is its selective, or directive nature (see, e.g., Broadbent, 1958; Norman, 1968; Treisman, 1969). That is, persons are capable of isolating specific stimuli—or even specific properties of a given stimulus—for more extensive processing while treating other stimuli or properties of the stimulus in a more cursory fashion. Of course, no single stimulus or stimulus property remains the focus of attention forever. What is focused on can shift rapidly from one moment to the next. A good illustration of this rapid reselection (adapted from Bourne *et al.*, 1979) comes from the behavior of a duck hunter who is watching the skies for incoming birds. At first the hunter searches for the stimulus properties associated with ducks in general—for example, the proper wingbeat or flight formation. Once a flock has been identified as ducks, however, those dimensions are discarded, and attention is shifted to the cues that will enable the hunter to determine whether they are of the type that would make particularly good table fare.

Self-Attention

Of the various properties of attention that have been identified, it is the selective aspect that is most germane to the present discussion. Our usage of the construct, however, will differ somewhat from the way in which it is usually used. Cognitive research on the directional aspect of attention, for example, has generally pursued the selectivity issue with respect to a person's processing of external information. That is, such research typically investigates the attentional and motivational processes within the person that determine how prominent a given environmental stimulus will be compared to other environmental stimuli. Moreover, a similar bias seems to exist within social psychology. Thus, like cognitive research, social psychological research on attention also seems to be generally interested in understanding the differential processing of external information—for example, how one's prior beliefs affect the kind of information that is sought out (e.g., Brock & Balloun, 1967; Kleinhesselink & Edwards, 1975; Mills, 1968). Although such an emphasis is not without merit, it has resulted in at least one unfortunate side effect. Namely, it has caused researchers to ignore another important source of information toward which attention might be directed.

A moment's reflection will reveal that this is indeed the case. Consider, for example, the domain of "all information available for processing." Some of this information originates in the environment, but other information originates from within the person and is related to the self (cf. Bannister & Agnew, 1977; Lewis & Brooks, 1978; Raye, Johnson, & Taylor, 1980). Moreover, just as persons are capable of attending to various aspects of their environments, so, too, do they seem capable of attending to various aspects of themselves. It is this realization that provides the basis for much of the research and theorizing that follows. As will be seen, selectively attending to aspects of oneself has been shown to produce the same effect conceptually as does selectively attending to aspects of one's environment (i.e., a more thorough processing of the information involved). We will review the relevant studies shortly, but a number of remaining issues need to be considered first.

Aspects of Self

One issue that immediately arises concerns our reasons for introducing a concept like self-attention into a chapter on awareness of bodily states. What, if anything, do bodily sensations have to do with the self? While some (perhaps most) readers will not be at all puzzled by couching the present chapter in terms of the self, others certainly will be. The following comments are intended to resolve any ambiguity.

Most persons would agree that the self is not a unitary construct. Rather, it is best viewed as a multifaceted entity, existing at many different levels of complexity. Some aspects of the self are quite conceptual and abstract in nature. For example, the self-concept is a more or less coherent cognitive representation that each person holds of himself or herself (see, e.g., Wylie, 1974). Attitudes are also component aspects of the self, as are one's representation of how one behaves and what one is like. All of these abstract conceptualizations are component parts of what most persons typically think of when they think of the self.

In our view, however, not all aspects of the self are as cognitive and abstract in composition. There are also sensory or perceptual aspects to the self (see, e.g., Buss, 1980). That is, our bodies are equipped with a wide variety of different sensory receptors, whose function it is to pass along to higher processing centers the perceptual input they receive. Some of these receptors—the distance receptors—function primarily to convey information about environmental events and stimuli. But other receptors function to provide us with a continuous flow of information about the status of our own internal bodily states, states typically associated with experiences such as emotions and physical symptoms. Thus, there are internal receptors that alert us to a heavily pounding heart, or a tenseness in our muscles, and there are receptors that enable us to perceive the twinges of pain. The input received from these sensors is no less a perceptual experience than is vision or hearing, but the perceptual experiences all involve some sort of informational input *from within one's own body*. It is this consideration that prompts us to include the information arising from such sources as falling within the domain of self. This also explains why it is that we have introduced a notion like self-attention into our discussion of awareness of bodily states.

We might mention here that our reasoning on this matter is not completely unfounded. The viability of our comments is strengthened by the results of several recent experimental studies, each of which showed that physiological sensations (either perceived or actual) can lead subjects to become more aware of other, nonphysical aspects of the self.

In one of these studies (Fenigstein & Carver, 1978, Experiment 1), subjects were asked to complete a modified version of the Stroop (1938) color-naming task. The Stroop task requires subjects to examine a series of stimuli, each of which is printed in a different color, and to name the color of ink in which each is printed. Subjects in the Fenigstein and Carver study saw a series of words, half of which were self-relevant and half of which were not. In addition to the color-naming task, subjects also completed an attribution task, which required them to assign responsibility for hypothetical outcomes to either themselves or another. While subjects completed the tasks, they were presented with a rhythmic auditory stimulus, which was identified as being either the subject's heartbeat or an irrelevant environmental noise. Results for both dependent measures suggested that identifying the sound as the subject's heartbeat led to enhanced self-focus. That is, latencies for the naming of colors of self-relevant words (but not for self-irrelevant words) were longer in the heartbeat condition than in the noise condition, and greater self-attributions were made in the heartbeat than in the noise condition (see also Fenigstein & Carver, 1978, Experiment 2).

Perhaps even more relevant is a later study conducted by Wegner and Giuliano (1980), which examined the effects of actual physiological arousal. Subjects in their study were asked to lie down on a comfortable lounge chair, to sit in a standard classroom chair, or to run in place for a short time. These manipulations were intended to vary subjects' general arousal in a systematic way, from relatively low arousal to relatively high arousal, respectively. Several minutes later the subjects were given a form containing a series of sentences with words missing. Subjects were to choose a word to go into each blank from three alternatives that were provided. In the target sentences, the three words were personal pronouns. Following the suggestions of Davis and Brock (1975), preferential selection of first-person pronouns was used as the measure of self-focus. As had been predicted, subjects who had relaxed prior to completing this measure made the fewest choices of self-relevant words, subjects who had sat in the chair made an intermediate number of self-relevant choices, and the greatest number were made by subjects who had run in place. Taken together, the results of these various studies strongly suggest that one's bodily sensations do, in fact, comprise important aspects of the self. After all, if bodily sensations were not an integrated part of one's self-structure, it would be exceedingly difficult to explain why it is that making such sensations salient causes a person to reflect in a more intense way about the self more generally.

Self-Focus versus Environment Focus

A second point that needs to be mentioned involves the nature of the attentional model that we will be working with. Specifically, we assume, as do others in the area (e.g., Duval & Wicklund, 1972), that a person only has a limited amount of attention to allocate. Stated more precisely, we assume a *relatively* fixed-capacity model of attention. We say "relatively fixed" because it now seems clear that the absolute amount of attention that one has available can fluctuate somewhat over time. One's momentary level of arousal, the degree of one's tiredness, and the amount of effort one expends in concentrating, for example, can all alter the absolute amount of attention at a person's disposal (see, e.g., Cohen, 1978; Easterbrook, 1959; Kahneman, 1973). Thus, we do not mean to imply that attentional resources can never vary, but only that *at any given moment* a person has only a finite amount of attention with which to work.

This assumption that attentional capacity is relatively fixed has important implications for the distinction that has been made between self-focus and environment focus, in that it suggests that a "mutual antagonism" may exist between focus on the self and focus on the environment. That is, if a person has only a limited amount of attention to allocate, then directing some portion of one's attention to one source of information necessarily means that less attention will be available for processing information coming from other sources. Thus, as attention outward increases, attention to the self is presumed to diminish, and vice versa. We should note, however, that we take no particular stand on whether it is better to conceptualize the direction of attention as rapidly shifting, or as divided among potential objects (cf. Hirst, Spelke, Reaves, Caharach, & Neisser, 1980; Spelke, Hirst, & Neisser, 1976). For present purposes, these two possibilities are equivalent. The fact that we have chosen to phrase the discussion in terms of either shifts or increases and decreases in attentional focus is largely a matter of convenience.

There is a second issue to consider here as well. We have just argued that self-focus and environment focus vary inversely. As more attention is directed inward, less is available to be directed outward. But what is the relationship, if any, between the two states with respect to the type or content of information that is focused on? In contrast to our earlier stand, we suggest that in terms of the type of information that is processed, a high degree of congruence may normally exist between self-focus and environment focus. Here is why.

A person's attention presumably shifts back and forth between self and nonself on a continual basis. But such shifting does not appear to be random. Rather, it seems to be guided in part by the cue implications that are conveyed by the most recent specific object of attention (cf. Hull & Levy, 1979). When we attend to the self, we are often examining an aspect of self that has been suggested by some cue in our environment. And analogously, when we look outward, we are often examining a part of the external world that has been suggested by some cue from within. For example, if the last object of attention has been an environmental event that has been recognized as typically "fear-provoking," an inward focus of attention might be guided specifically to those aspects of self that are presumed to be associated with the experience of anxiety (e.g., a racing heart or queasy stomach). If the most recent self-aspect under scrutiny has been a sense of pain, focus on the environment might be guided by a search for the harm-producing agent (e.g., a piece of broken glass underneath one's beach towel).

The occurrence of this sort of back-and-forth processing makes considerable sense intuitively, in that without it one's experience would become quite disjointed whenever attention fluctuated between environment and self; and this certainly does not seem to be the case. Moreover, it is only by making such an assumption that it is possible to generate precise predictions about the effects that self-focused attention will have.

That is, in most self-awareness research, the attentional manipulations that are utilized are relatively general. They serve to remind persons of themselves, but they do not direct attention toward any specific self-aspect. (There is one very important exception to his assertion which is discussed more fully below.) Rather, researchers simply assume that the subject's attentional focus will naturally drift to the aspect of self that is relevant to the behavioral situation under study. Said differently, it is expected that a particular aspect of the self will be rendered salient by virtue of the situational cues that the particular experimental context contains—an assumption that has now received considerable indirect support from research findings (for details, see Carver & Scheier, 1981).

Thus, it should come as no surprise that a general manipulation of self-attention (e.g., a mirror) can cause attention to be directed to one's emotional experience in some settings, to one's attitudes and values in other settings, and to one's bodily sensations in yet other settings. What is important to understand here, however, is the fundamental assumption on which this experimental approach is based. It is based on the supposition that attentional shifts between environment and self are guided by the cue implications provided by the most recent object of scrutiny (i.e., that there is a back-and-forth processing of self-related and environment-related information).

Varying Self-Attention in the Laboratory

This brings us to the last point that needs to be considered. Specifically, we have argued that the distinction between self-focus and focus on the environment is an important one. We have also suggested that the effect of attending to an aspect of oneself is the same as attending to an aspect of one's environment—a more complete or intensive processing of the information conveyed by the stimulus in question. Without specifying how it is that attentional focus can be varied in the laboratory, however, these assertions would remain idle speculation.

Fortunately, two rather disparate techniques are available for this purpose. One technique involves the use of a self-report instrument to identify and select persons who differ from each other in their chronic tendencies to be self-attentive. The second technique relies on experimental manipulations to alter persons' momentary levels of self-attention. These are discussed, in turn, in the following paragraphs.

It was apparent very early to researchers working in the self-awareness area that people differ in the degree to which they habitually attend to themselves. The disposition to be self-attentive has been labeled self-*consciousness*, to distinguish it from the manipulated state of self-*awareness*, a convention that we will follow throughout this chapter. Self-consciousness is measured by the Self-Consciousness Scale (Fenigstein, Scheier, & Buss, 1975), an instrument that has separate subscales. The *private* self-consciousness subscale, comprised of items such as "I'm generally attentive to my inner feelings" and "I'm constantly examining my motives," was designed to measure the tendency to be aware of the covert and hidden aspects of the self. People who are high on this dimension are presumed to be particularly attentive to their thoughts, feelings, attitudes, and other private self-aspects. In general, the research that has accrued is quite consistent with this conceptualization (for a comprehensive summary of these findings, see Buss, 1980, or Carver & Scheier, 1981).

The *public* self-consciousness subscale, comprised of items such as "I'm concerned about what other people think of me" and "I'm concerned about my style of doing things," was intended to measure the tendency to be aware of the publicly displayed aspects of the self, the self as a social object that has an impact on others. People high on this dimension are thought to be especially cognizant of how they are being viewed by others in their social contexts, and how those others are reacting to them. As with private self-consciousness, the research findings that have accumulated on public self-consciousness are also quite consistent with this conceptualization (again see Buss, 1980, or Carver & Scheier, 1981, for comprehensive reviews).

Both subscales possess adequate reliability (Fenigstein *et al.*, 1975), and a substantial amount of evidence has now been gathered establishing both convergent and discriminant validity (Carver & Glass, 1976; Turner, Scheier, Carver, & Ickes, 1978). Finally, factor analyses have confirmed that the private and public self-consciousness dimensions are factorially sound, and relatively pure and distinct. That is, the correlations between the two subscales, although invariably positive, are generally quite low— typically falling in the high .20s and low .30s (see, e.g., Carver & Glass, 1976; Fenigstein *et al.*, 1975; Turner *et al.*, 1978). Thus, not only are private and public self-consciousness distinct theoretically, they are also relatively independent empirically.

In addition to these biases in the person, there are also situational cues that either raise or lower the level of a person's self-attention. Wicklund and Duval (1971) were the first to attempt to manipulate self-attention in the laboratory. They argued that any stimulus that reminded people of themselves should thereby serve to heighten self-focus. They operationalized this reasoning with manipulations that seemed intuitively to serve as reminders of the self: stimuli such as cameras, mirrors, and tape recordings of subjects' voices.

Later studies provided evidence of the construct validity of such manipulations. For example, Geller and Shaver (1976) obtained indirect support for the position that a camera and a mirror (together) selectively activated subjects' self-relevant memory content. Using a modified version of the Stroop color-naming test, they found that color-naming latencies for self-relevant words were increased by the manipulations, but latencies for other words were not. Additional research has determined that either manipulation by itself resulted in an increased tendency to use self-related language (Carver & Scheier, 1978; Davis & Brock, 1975). There is also evidence that a salient audience increases self-focus (Carver & Scheier, 1978).

When researchers first used these various manipulations, little thought was given to the public–private distinction. The manipulations were used more or less interchangeably. It was implicitly assumed that attention would gravitate toward whatever self-aspect was made salient by the behavioral context. Recent research findings now suggest, however, that these manipulations may differ dramatically from each other in terms of the aspects of the self to which they direct attention. Specifically, this research seems to show that some manipulations (such as cameras and audiences) serve primarily to heighten the subject's cognizance of public self-aspects, whereas other manipulations (such as mirrors) serve mainly to heighten awareness of private self-aspects. For reviews of the relevant findings, see Scheier and Carver (1981) and Buss (1980).

The distinction between private and public self-attention has important implications for understanding the research that has been done on awareness of bodily states. In particular, of the two types of self-attention that have been distinguished, it is private self-attention that is most relevant to persons' cognizance of their bodily states, because such states fall within the domain of the private self. This is not to say that public self-attention is always irrelevant to understanding the research findings that have been obtained (sometimes it is), but only that private self-attention is the variable of primary interest. Thus, in virtually all of the research that is described below, it is private self-attention that was systematically varied, not public. It is to a consideration of this research that we turn next.

CONSEQUENCES OF ATTENDING TO SELF

Self-Focus and Awareness of Bodily States

Casual observation suggests that many persons do not know themselves very well. When asked for a self-description, they provide their questioner with a picture frought with distortions, misperceptions, and inaccuracies. These vagaries in self-report are often unmotivated. That is, the inaccuracies exist simply because people are ignorant of their characteristics, not because of any attempt to deceive. Moreover, they seem to occur regardless of the level of analysis one focuses on. The inaccuracies seem to exist, for example, when the self-reports involve assessments of one's behavioral tendencies (cf. Mischel, 1968). They also seem to exist when the self-reports involve assessments of one's bodily states (cf. Blascovich, 1980).

Part of the problem, at least as it applies to bodily states, is that internal sources of information are not the only determinants of a person's self-reports. To the contrary, many people seem to make extensive use of information from their environments in defining for themselves what their experiences are. For example, people will make use of externally provided information in determining how aroused they are (e.g., Barefoot & Straub, 1971; Valins, 1966). Although the biasing effects of such environmental information does appear to have limits (e.g., Goldstein, Fink,

& Mettee, 1972), the fact remains that people are often led to anticipate internal states before they actually experience them.

Such anticipations no doubt exert a profound influence on the processing of input relevant to the experience (cf. Leventhal, 1980). Indeed, sometimes our expectations may be so powerful that the relevant input information is hardly processed at all. The result is that the expectations do not simply influence our perceptions of our internal states, they dictate them. Stated more directly, we often perceive—even about our own internal states—exactly what we anticipate perceiving. Of course, these expectancy-driven perceptions are not always inaccurate. That is, sometimes our anticipations are congruous with what we are actually experiencing. But at other times they are not, and it is here that the faulty perceptions arise.

The power that such an anticipation can exert is exemplified by the placebo effect. A placebo is an inert substance. After ingesting a placebo, however, people often report experiencing whatever states they have been led to expect to be caused by the placebo (see, e.g., Mechanic, 1968). Apparently, the suggestion provided ahead of time is sufficiently compelling that most people do not direct their attention to a careful examination of the relevant internal cues when reporting on their physical states. Instead, they simply report whatever information had been previously supplied at the verbal or conceptual level. Based on the logic presented earlier, however, one would expect this effect to be minimized, if persons were led to focus more attention on the sensory input—that is, were induced to be privately self-attentive.

Self-Focus and the Placebo Effect

A test of this reasoning was reported recently by Gibbons, Carver, Scheier, and Hormuth (1979). Subjects in this study were given an oral dose of baking soda, which was either identified as baking soda, or misidentified as a drug called Cavanol. Subjects in the latter condition were led to expect the drug to produce changes in heart rate, constriction in the chest, and sweaty palms—in short, symptoms of sympathetic arousal. Subjects for whom the baking soda was correctly labeled were told that they were in the control group, and were not led to expect side effects. After an intervening task, each subject was asked to complete a 16-item symptom checklist, which included the items made salient in the previous stage of the experiment. Half the subjects completed this instrument in front of a mirror, half without the mirror.

The normal placebo effect is to report the symptoms that were ascribed to the drug's action. This, in fact, was what occurred in the absence of the self-attention-enhancing manipulation. Subjects in this group reported experiencing significantly more arousal and more of the specific symptoms ascribed to the drug than did comparable subjects who were not given the anticipation of arousal symptoms. This placebo effect was almost completely eradicated, however, by the presence of the mirror. Apparently, the increase in self-focus led to a more thorough search for evidence of the anticipated symptoms. Indeed, there is evidence that this self-examination was quite specifically for the symptoms that had been mentioned (see Gibbons et al., 1979). This search revealed the absence of the expected symptoms, and this was reflected in the self-reports made by this group of subjects.

Conceptually similar results have since been reported by others (Duncan & Laird, 1980), using a markedly different experimental technique. Specifically, rather than cause subjects to attend to their bodily cues by inducing them to be self-attentive, an expression-manipulation task (Duncan & Laird, 1977; Laird & Crosby, 1974) was utilized to select subjects who evidenced a preference for relying on such self-produced cues or not. The expression-manipulation task requires subjects (without their knowing it) to assume facial positions characteristic of smiles and frowns. They are then asked to rate the amount of subjective affect they are experiencing. Self-produced cue attenders are those who rely heavily on their own facial positions in making their mood judgments. Conversely, situational cue attenders are those who tend not to rely on their own facial cues when inferring their affect state.

In the experiment proper, each group of subjects was asked to perform two further experimental tasks, both of which were expected to produce a moderate amount of fearfulness in them (based on their previous self-reports). One task required them to approach a nonpoisonous snake, until their rising fear prevented them from going further. The second task involved a pain tolerance test. As a prelude to this task, subjects were asked to indicate the maximum level of electric shock that they thought they could tolerate (in fact, no shock was ever given). Prior to completing these tasks, some subjects were given a placebo, which was described as either a relaxer or an arouser. Control subjects received no drug. Following the tasks, all subjects were asked to rate their fear of nonpoisonous snakes and electric shock.

It may be helpful, before describing the results of this study, to consider for a moment what the experiences of the subjects should have been. Situational cue attenders are persons who direct little attention to their own internal states when making judgments about those states. Consequently, when given a relaxer, situational cue attenders should have felt more relaxed, and when given an arouser, they should have felt more aroused. This, in turn, should have caused them to rate both the snake and electric shock as less and more frightening in the relaxer and arouser conditions, respectively.

On the other hand, self-produced cue attenders are persons who do take notice of their own internal states when making judgments about those states. Thus, self-produced cue attenders should have been equally aware of their actual arousal regardless whether they were given a relaxer, an arouser, or neither. This is not to say, however, that the bogus information provided them should have had no effect whatsoever. Subjects given an arouser had at their disposal a viable alternative explanation for the arousal they were experiencing—the pill. The viability of this alternative explanation should have caused arouser subjects to attribute less of their felt arousal to the snake and shock, which in turn should have caused them to rate the snake and shock as being less threatening. In contrast, subjects given the relaxer had no alternative explanation for their arousal. Indeed, these subjects were led to expect that the pill would keep their arousal level relatively low. The effect of this expectancy should have been to cause them to rate the snake and shock as being even more threatening than subjects given no drug, because they were still experiencing considerable arousal in spite of the fact that they had taken a drug that was keeping their arousal artificially low.

In general, the results of the Duncan and Laird study were quite consistent with the reasoning just outlined. Specifically, the results showed that the situational cue group was in fact more responsive to the expected effects of the placebos than was the self-produced cue group. Whereas the situational cue group reported less fear of snakes and electric shock when given a relaxer and more fear when given an arouser, the self-produced cue group reported more fear when given a relaxer and less fear when given an arouser. In brief, consistent with the findings of Gibbons *et al.* (1979), situational cue attenders exhibited positive placebo effects. Self-produced cue attenders, on the other hand, were much less swayed by the information provided them. In fact, their reliance on self-generated cues was so extreme, as the analysis above would suggest, that it actually caused them to show reverse placebo effects—effects that carried over to actual behavior, at least with respect to the shock task (for details, see Duncan & Laird, 1980).

Self-Focus and Other Suggestibility Effects

The placebo effect is one illustration of a broader class of suggestibility phenomena. The reasoning that found support in the Gibbons *et al.* and Duncan and Laird studies (i.e., that attention to internal cues would diminish this sort of suggestibility effect) has also been tested with regard to two other suggestibility phenomena (Scheier, Carver & Gibbons, 1979).

In the first of these studies (Scheier *et al.*, 1979, Experiment 1), male undergraduates were shown a series of slides of nude women. The subjects' task was to rate the amount of arousal produced by each of the stimulus slides. Prior to presenting the slides, the experimenter made an offhand remark that led the subject to expect them to be either extremely attractive and arousing, or extremely unattractive and nonarousing. In reality, all subjects viewed an identical set of slides, each of which had been rated by pilot subjects as being moderately arousing. Self-attention was varied by exposing some subjects to their own mirror images between presentations of the slides (for details, see Scheier et al., 1979, or Neumann, Carver, & Scheier, 1977).

The results of this study indicated a powerful suggestibility main effect: Subjects' ratings were strongly biased by the experimenter's remarks. But this bias was significantly reduced by an experimental manipulation of self-attention, consistent with the findings of Gibbons et al. (1979). Specifically, subjects given the high arousal set tended to report less arousal when self-focus was high than when it was low, and subjects led to anticipate very little arousal tended to report being more aroused when self-focus was high than when it was low.

Although the findings of this study extended the results of Gibbons et al. (1979) in several different ways, there were still some questions that remained unanswered. First was the question of whether the phenomena applied to dispositional self-focus, as well as manipulated self-focus. It was also unclear whether the reasoning was applicable to internal states that were unrelated to arousal (e.g., the perception of taste). Finally, and perhaps most important, there was the question of whether self-focus resulted in more veridical perceptions of the internal state, at the same time that it reduced suggestibility. It was for these reasons that a further study was conducted (Scheier et al., 1979, Experiment 2).

Subjects in this study were persons who were either high or low in dispositional private self-consciousness. They were given experimental instructions that led them to expect to taste a series of solutions of peppermint extract. Their task was to gauge the intensity of each solution (see Scheier et al., 1979, for greater detail). Each subject was first asked to rate the intensity of a standard solution, which served as a baseline. Before giving the subject the second sample solution, the experimenter casually indicated that it should be "a little stronger" or "a little weaker" than the previous one. Independent of this information, the second solution actually was either stronger or weaker than the first one. The subject then tasted and rated the second solution, using the same scale as before. The dependent measure of the study was the degree of change from the first rating to the second rating.

Analysis of subjects' ratings revealed that those who were high in private self-consciousness were significantly less influenced by the experimenter's remarks (when those remarks were incorrect) than were subjects lower in self-consciousness. Moreover, subjects high in self-consciousness tended to be more sensitive to the actual intensity of the second solution. This point is made with greatest clarity by the following analysis. Some subjects who were led to expect weak solutions actually received weak solutions; some subjects led to expect strong solutions did receive strong solutions. For these subjects, there was no conflict between their anticipations and the actual stimulus intensity. Virtually all of these subjects judged the second stimulus in a fashion consistent with their expectations, and this tendency did not differ across levels of self-consciousness. But for other subjects there was a conflict between their anticipations and the stimulus they actually received. Among these subjects, most persons high in private self-consciousness shifted their estimates in the direction *contrary to the anticipation but consistent with the stimulus intensity* (12 did, 5 did not). Among subjects low in private self-consciousness, the pattern was reversed. Most subjects gave reports that were consistent with their anticipations (15) rather than the actual stimulus (5). This difference between self-consciousness groups was highly significant.

These findings are important in that they suggest that self-focus does seem to heighten a person's awareness of actual internal states, in addition to (or rather than) simply making one less susceptible to suggestion. The generality of this conclusion is limited, however, by the fact that the experiment contained an explicit attempt to mislead the subjects. That is, it is impossible to determine from the Scheier *et al.* study alone whether similar effects would be obtained if self-focused subjects were not explicitly primed in such a fashion to focus on their internal states.

Fortunately, data relevant to this issue have been obtained by others. Miller, Murphy, and Buss (1981), for example, have recently conducted a study, the primary purpose of which was to establish the validity of a new scale—the Private Body Consciousness Scale—designed to measure differences among persons in their tendencies to direct attention to internal bodily sensations. All subjects in their study were tested with this new Body Consciousness Scale, but they also completed the more global Self-Consciousness Scale. Several weeks later, the subjects participated in an experiment ostensibly designed to investigate the effects of beverage drinking on subsequent taste perception. All subjects drank a cup of hot chocolate. After a brief delay, they were asked to rate the extent to which they were experiencing various arousal sensations, ostensibly because arousal was known to affect taste perception and it needed to be controlled for. Unknown to the subjects, the chocolate they drank either did or did not contain an additional level of caffeine in the form of No-Doze.

The results offered strong evidence for the validity of the author's new scale. The only subjects to report increased arousal after drinking the caffeine-ladened hot chocolate were those high in private body consciousness. This effect, however, was greatest among persons who were high in private self-consciousness. Thus, private self-attention does seem to be an important determinant of the amount of awareness persons have of their internal states even in contexts in which there is no explicit attempt to mislead them.

Nor is the Miller *et al.* (1981) study the only research that bears on this conclusion. Conceptually consistent results have also been obtained by Pennebaker and Lightner (1980, Experiment 1). In this study, subjects were asked to walk on a treadmill on two separate occasions, spaced one week apart. After each session, subjects were asked to complete a physical sympton checklist, as well as to indicate their level of subjective fatigue. Both assessments dealt with subjects' perceptions of their internal states while they walked. Attentional focus was varied during the second session while subjects walked, by having them don headphones and listen to a series of interesting street noises, or their own amplified breathing, or nothing. Analyses of symptom change scores (from session 1 to session 2) revealed that subjects in the breathing condition reported experiencing significantly more intense physical symptoms than did subjects in either the sound condition or the control condition. The findings also revealed a marginally significant drop in symptom reporting among subjects in the sound condition relative to those in the control condition. The data for subjective fatigue ratings formed a similar pattern. In brief, forcing persons to attend to their own bodies (by reminding them of their breathing) resulted in greater perceptions of physical symptoms and fatigue than if attention was either free or forced to be directed elsewhere.[1]

Conclusions and Limitations

Taken together, the findings generated from the studies reviewed in this section all point to the same conclusion. People seem to be cognizant of their internal bodily sensations only to the extent that their attention is focused inward onto those states. Moreover, this conclusion appears to be valid across a wide variety of different contexts. That is, similar effects are obtained regardless of whether self-attention is varied experimentally by virtue of the presence or absence of a mirror, or is varied dispositionally by virtue of persons' propensities to be high or low in self-consciousness. And similar effects are obtained regardless of whether the internal state in question is associated with feelings of arousal or the experience of taste. In brief, the effects under consideration appear to be quite general and robust.

We would caution people, however, from assuming that the phenomenon has no limits whatsoever. It almost certainly has to. This is the case because there are a number of internal bodily states for which internal cues are either totally lacking or so subtle in form that they go unutilized. For example, there are no known internal cues available for assessing

---

1. An attempt was made in a subsequent study (Pennebaker & Lightner, 1980, Experiment 2) to extend these findings into a more naturalistic domain—specifically, perceptions of symptoms arising from jogging. Although the findings from this study were consistent with the arguments that we have advanced (and with essentially the same set of arguments offered by Pennebaker and Lightner), they are also open to a number of alternative explanations as well, primarily because of the lack of experimental control exerted over the amount of effort subjects expended while running. It is because of this interpretational ambiguity that the study is not more fully described here. Interested readers are referred instead to the original source.

fluctuations in blood pressure (see, e.g., Leventhal, Meyer, & Nerenz, 1980; Leventhal, Nerenz, & Strauss, 1980), and the internal cues produced by one's heart rate appear to be so subtle in form that most people cannot detect them without prior extensive training (see, e.g., Blascovich, 1980; Cacioppo, 1979; Epstein, Cinciripini, McCoy, & Marshall, 1977; Nowlin, Eisdorfer, Whalen, & Troyer, 1971). Given the lack or subtlety of cues associated with such states, there is no reason to expect self-attention to enhance a person's awareness of them. In brief, self-attention should heighten sensitivity to internal states only to the extent that internal cues are readily available that allow one to assess the status of those states.

There is one final issue that needs to be discussed before closing this section. The issue has to do with alternative explanations that might be offered to account for the findings that we have described. Clearly, specific alternative hypotheses can always be invoked to explain the findings of specific studies. Consider, for example, one obvious alternative explanation for the results of the placebo study described earlier, which used a mirror to vary self-focus (Gibbons *et al.*, 1979). We argued that the mirror induced self-attention in that study, thereby making subjects in the placebo condition more aware of the fact that the pill was not having its expected physiological effects. But physiological arousal was not measured in the study. Thus it is impossible to determine for sure whether the pill failed to affect physiology or not. That is, perhaps ingestion of the placebo actually caused subjects to experience the symptoms ascribed to it. If so, perhaps the mirror, rather than enhancing self-attention, simply served to distract subjects from perceiving symptoms that were really there. How do we know that such a process was not in fact occurring in this study?

In answering this question, it is important to bear in mind the parallel that has been established between manipulated self-awareness and dispositional self-consciousness. That is, the parallel findings that have been obtained have important implications for evaluating alternative hypotheses that might arise. How? The mirror and dispositional self-consciousness presumably represent conceptually equivalent ways of varying self-attention. Yet, operationally they are very distinct. By the logic of converging operations (Garner, Hake, & Eriksen, 1956), to the extent that these two methods of varying self-focus produce similar effects on behavior, our faith in the validity of the imputed underlying processes should be thereby bolstered. Stated differently, an attention-based analysis of the findings is enhanced by the fact that it can account for both the effects of a mirror and the conceptually similar effects of dispositional self-consciousness. For an alternative explanation to be equally viable, it must also be able to account equally well for both sets of findings.

Now reconsider for a moment the "distraction" hypothesis that was advanced above. The problem with such an explanation, of course, is that it ignores completely the findings for dispositional self-consciousness.

Thus, while the distraction explanation can provide a reasonable account for the placebo study that used a mirror, it cannot reasonably account for the studies that used dispositional self-consciousness, because subjects in these latter studies were never exposed to a mirror. In brief, the attention-based interpretation is the only explanation of the two that can account for both the effects of a mirror and dispositional self-consciousness. These considerations, in our view, confer a decided advantage on an explanation based on attentional focus. We might add here that similar considerations also apply to the research that has been done examining the effects of manipulated and dispositional self-attention on affective responsivity, research that we turn to next.

Self-Focus, Perception of Internal States, and Emotional Intensity

Over the years, a great many psychologists of widely differing persuasions have shown an interest in the perception of bodily states. This interest has been motivated (at least in part) by the role such internal states are presumed to play in the experience of emotion. That is, following the lead of Schachter and Singer (1962), a number of different personality and social psychologists have come to view the experience of emotion as being strongly influenced by three elements: The existence of some perceptible internal state that differs from one's baseline level; the focusing of sufficient attention on that internal state to result in awareness of its existence; and the use of some knowledge structure to interpret the state.

This is not to suggest that there have been no alterations and changes in the basic analysis over the years. There have been. Leventhal (1980), for example, has recently proposed a model of emotion that differs from the Schachter and Singer analysis in several critical ways. And there has been more than a little disagreement concerning the nature of the specific cues that are utilized in defining emotional experiences—that is, whether the cues are primarily visceral or proprioceptive in nature (e.g., Kleck, Vaughan, Cartwright-Smith, Vaughan, Colby, & Lanzetta, 1976; Lanzetta, Cartwright-Smith, & Kleck, 1976). Moreover, there has even been some disagreement concerning the relative importance of actual physiological change versus perceived physiological change (see, e.g., Valins, 1966).

In spite of these disagreements and alterations, however, belief in the importance of the three factors initially described by Schachter and Singer has not waned. Stated differently, theorists have found it unnecessary to adopt Schachter and Singer's assumptions *in toto* in order to accept the notion that changes in internal states, variations in attention to the state, and interpretive schemas can all have an impact on the nature of a person's subjective emotional experience. Indeed, the same three factors are beginning to crop up in discussions of the multifaceted nature of the experience of symptom states (e.g., Leventhal, 1975; Leventhal & Everhart, 1979; Leventhal et al., 1980; Mechanic, 1972; Pennebaker & Skelton, 1978).

The primary purpose of the present section is to review some recent research bearing on the second of these three influences on emotional state: the direction of attention to the change in state. It has been thought for some time that attentional factors play an important role in emotional experiences (cf. Kanfer & Goldfoot, 1966; Morgan & Pollock, 1977; Walters, 1961), but the role played by such factors has typically been taken for granted rather than studied. That is, it has seemed reasonable that a person will experience emotional states, however the emotion is construed by the person, only to the degree that the emotional cues are attended to. In this regard, the research reviewed in the preceding section suggests that self-focused attention may be a critical determinant of the subjective intensity of the emotional experience, at least in contexts where the emotional state is a salient aspect of the self. Thus, distracting a person who is angry or upset should alleviate the feeling in some measure, whereas inducing the person to focus on it should only make the experience subjectively more intense.

This reasoning has been tested in a recent series of studies. In one experiment, Scheier (1976) exposed half the participants to an anger provocation. He later asked all subjects to report their moods, including a self-rating of anger level. Among subjects in the provocation condition, significantly more intense anger was reported by subjects who had been self-attentive than by those who were less self-attentive (cf. Konecni, 1975). This, in turn, led to significant differences in aggressive behavior.

Scheier and Carver (1977) subsequently pursued this intensification effect further, by testing its generality to a wider variety of emotional states. In one experiment, male subjects were shown a series of slides of nude women, under conditions of experimentally enhanced self-focus or with no manipulation. Subjects were asked to rate the attractiveness of the women in the slides according to the degree of bodily responses that they experienced. Subjects in whom self-focus had been increased made reliably more favorable ratings than did subjects with less self-focus. This finding was subsequently replicated using subjects who varied in their levels of dispositional private self-consciousness (Scheier & Carver, 1977, Experiment 2). In this study the reasoning was extended to the experience of repulsion. That is, some subjects in this experiment viewed slides of mutilated bodies. Among these subjects, significantly greater repulsion was expressed by persons high in private self-consciousness than by those lower in private self-consciousness. A conceptual replication of these effects, concerning the experience of fear, was reported by Carver, Blaney, and Scheier (1979).

Two additional studies extended the reasoning to the experience of elation and depression. Using procedures developed by Velten (1968),

Scheier and Carver (1977, Experiment 3) induced pleasant mood states in some subjects, and depressed moods in others. Then all subjects completed a mood self-report scale, either in the presence of a mirror or with no mirror. Among those given the depression induction, reliably greater depression was reported by self-focused subjects than by those who were less self-attentive. But the comparable tendency among subjects in the elation condition did not attain significance. A final study (Scheier & Carver, 1977, Experiment 4) replicated these effects using individual differences in private self-consciousness.

There is at least one aspect of these findings that deserves further comment. Although it is at least plausible to suggest that the experiences of sexual attraction and repulsion produced mild states of physiological arousal, it seems much less likely that the depression induction produced any arousal change. Depression seems more amenable to the argument that proprioceptive cues help to define the experiential state. We should note, in this regard, that the way in which these various studies were conducted did not preclude the possibility that subjects would gauge their emotional reactions by referring to proprioceptive cues rather than visceral cues. To the contrary, subjects in those experiments received a rather general set of orienting instructions. Their attention may well have gone to proprioceptive cues.

More recent research lends credibility to this speculation. Lanzetta, Biernat, and Kleck (1980) showed subjects attractive and repulsive slides (varied within-subjects), and videotaped subjects' facial expressiveness when viewing each slide. Their data showed that group differences in self-reports of emotional reactions that occurred as a function of self-focus paralleled group differences in facial expressiveness. Unexpectedly, their data failed to replicate the earlier finding that mirror presence caused self-reports of more intense affect. In fact, they found a reversal of that effect, both in self-rated affect and facial expressiveness. Because there were several differences between their research and the Scheier and Carver (1977) studies, the cause of the difference in findings is not clear. One reasonable interpretation, however, stems from the possibility that subjects were aware that they were being videotaped. As Kleck et al. (1976) have noted, people tend to suppress the public expression of their feelings. Enhanced self-focus in a situation in which the display of emotions was public may have led to increased suppression of facial movements. This, in turn, might have resulted in less reported affect. This reasoning is speculative, but it would account for the difference in findings. A more complete answer can only come from further research.

ATTENTIONAL FACTORS IN COPING WITH STRESS

We have seen in previous sections that attention to the self can have important consequences for one's awareness of physical sensations. We have also seen how such heightened awareness can affect the intensity with which emotional states are experienced. Given these potent effects, it seems likely that persons may learn to direct their attention in systematic ways in order to cope with the unpleasant physical sensations produced by life's challenges and dilemmas. In this section we describe the role that attentional processes might play in coping with stress.

Attentional Factors and Type A Behavior

One illustration of the role that attentional factors play comes from research on the Type A behavior pattern, an established risk factor for coronary heart disease. The Type A pattern has been conceptualized as a coping style for dealing with life's challenges and stresses (Glass, 1977). That is, the overt behaviors characteristic of Type A's—competitive achievement-striving, an aggressive hostility, and a sense of time urgency—are thought to reflect the manner in which Type A's stuggle to maintain and to assert control over their environment. Furthermore, it has been observed that Type A's appear extremely alert and hypervigilant (e.g., Bortner & Rosenman, 1967), although they are less able to report task-irrelevant information than are non-Type A's called Type B's. Taking these observations together, it has been suggested that Type A's use a specific attentional strategy for asserting environment control (Matthews & Brunson, 1979). That is, in the face of environmental challenges and stresses, Type A's may focus their attention on doing well on the task at hand and ignore any event that might interfere with their controlling efforts—including physical sensations that, if attended to, would lead to poor performance.

A series of laboratory experiments were conducted to examine these notions (Matthews & Brunson, 1979). The first experiment investigated the performance of healthy Type A's and Type B's on two concurrent tasks, in which one was defined as central or primary, and one was defined as peripheral or secondary. Assumptions of this paradigm are that humans have a limited capacity of attention and that performance on the two tasks varies with the amount of attention allocated to them, provided that the capacity of the individual is fully used. Constriction of attention is said to occur when performance on the secondary task is poor and performance on the central task is the same or better than a specified referent. The primary task was the Stroop color-naming task (described earlier in the chapter), which requires individuals to identify the color of a stimulus word's ink. The task is considered challenging because the stimulus word is the name of a color other than that in which the word is printed (e.g., the word "red" might be printed in blue ink). The secondary task was to depress a response key as soon as a light appeared in the individual's peripheral field of vision. The results revealed that relative to Type B's, Type A's performed more poorly on the secondary task and better on the primary task. Thus, the findings suggest that A's allocate more attention to central tasks and less to peripheral tasks than do B's in relatively unstructured settings.

Because A's attend less than B's to peripheral tasks, it seems reasonable to assume that they might also attend less to *task-irrelevant* peripheral events. If so, the issue then arises of how active a process this inattentiveness of A's might be. That is, the presence or absence of a task-irrelevant peripheral event may simply be inconsequential for A's, who are already attending to central task performance. Alternatively, it may be that A's *actively* inhibit their attention to such peripheral events.

The next two experiments compared these two possibilities. It was assumed that task-irrelevant sounds are peripheral events that can distract from task performance if attention is directed to them. Previous research has shown that the presence of extraneous noise improves performance on the Stroop color-naming task (Hartley & Adams, 1974). Apparently, this occurs because subjects presented with a noise actively inhibit their attention to the noise. In doing so, they also inhibit their attention to other task-irrelevant cues, including the name of the color of the stimulus word (Houston, 1968). Thus, performance is better because subjects are less distracted by the distracting cues inherent in the task. These considerations suggest a way of assessing how active the inattentiveness of Type A's to peripheral events really is. Specifically, if Type A's attend less to task-irrelevant peripheral events than B's do simply because they are attending to the central task, their Stroop performance should not be affected by the presence or absence of a distractor. On the other hand, if Type A's actively inhibit their attention to distractors, the performance of A's should be *facilitated* by the presence of a distractor.

To compare these possibilities, Type A and Type B women and men performed the Stroop color-naming task in the presence or in the absence of a tape of distracting sounds. The results revealed that the performance of Type A's improved in the presence of a distractor, whereas the performance of Type B's deteriorated. Because the latter finding was not expected, the experiment was repeated. The findings again revealed that Type A's performed better in the presence of a distractor than without. This time, however, B's did not show any difference in performance between distractor conditions. Taken together, the results of the two experiments reveal that Type A's tend to actively inhibit their attention to distracting sounds. By doing so, they actively ignore task-irrelevant cues and their performance improves.

Symptom Awareness and Type A

If Type A's do inhibit their attention to distracting, task-irrelevant events (as the relevant research appears to show), it seems likely that they might also ignore any minor internal state that, if attended to, would interfere with performing well. This would be likely to occur even when such information (e.g., a sense of being fatigued) might be useful in regulating one's efforts over the long run. The first systematic study of the reporting of symptom states by Type A's was conducted by Carver, Coleman, and Glass (1976). They used a paradigm designed to produce fatigue in their subjects. Men were required to walk continuously on a motorized treadmill at increasingly sharp angles of incline, while periodically rating their subjective fatigue (cf. Balke, 1954; Balke, Grillo, Konecci, & Luft, 1954). The walking test was to be terminated by the experimenter at a predetermined time unless the subject could not continue. In actuality, the experimenter never signaled the end of the test, and all subjects chose their own stopping points. After a sufficient rest period, each subject completed a running test that enabled assessment of the subject's maximum aerobic capacity (i.e., the person's maximum rate of oxygen absorption). Each subject's walking performance then was scored as a proportion of his maximum oxygen capacity. The results revealed that while Type A's reached a higher proportion of their maximum oxygen absorption rate during the walking test than did B's, they also reported less subjective fatigue. [These findings have been replicated in a similar study of Type A and Type B sixth-grade boys (Matthews & Volkin, 1981).]

Although these results are consistent with the notion that A's ignore internal states during task performance, they are also subject to alternative explanations. For example, the difference in reports of fatigue by A's and B's may have been due to a difference in their subjective standards for evaluating fatigue level. Another possible explanation is that A's in general may be more "macho" than B's. Thus, they may experience as much fatigue as B's, but simply choose not to report it. These ambiguities were subsequently resolved in related research by Weidner and Matthews (1978), using the following reasoning. If either of the foregoing alternative explanations is correct, A's should report little fatigue both during a demanding task, as in Carver *et al.* (1976) study, and at the end of the task. On the other hand, if A's actively ignore fatigue in order to do well on a task, they should fail to report the symptoms during the task, but not at the end of the task, when acknowledgment of symptoms would have no effect on performance.

In the Weidner and Matthews (1978) experiment, Type A's and B's performed a demanding task for 4 minutes and then completed a symptom checklist. Half of each type believed that they were to continue for an additional 4 minutes on the task, half believed they had completed the task. Type A's reported less fatigue as well as less sympathetic arousal symptoms than did B's during the task. However, at the end of the task, A's and B's reported a similar level of symptoms. Taken together with data on the ability of Type A's to ignore distracting events, these data suggest that Type A's ignore internal states when they can interfere with doing well. Thus, they report less intense symptoms during challenging events than do B's. When there is no reason to ignore symptoms, A's and B's report a similar intensity of symptoms.

Additional evidence for these general points is provided by Carver, DeGregorio, and Gillis (1981). In their study, college football players were rated on a number of performance dimensions by their coaches. Among players who were injured by midseason, A's were rated as pushing themselves closer to their limits and performing better than were B's. Of greater relevance is the finding that A's were perceived as having disregarded their injuries during a game to a greater extent than had B's. Stated differently, Type A injured football players were considered likely to ignore their injuries in order to perform well.

In sum, systematic observations and experimentation show that Type A's use a specific attentional strategy for asserting environmental control. They focus their attention on the task at hand and actively ignore information, including physical states, that could interfere with task performance. Consequently, Type A's report less intense symptoms than do Type B's. By so doing, A's might not use information about physical states to regulate their behavior over the long run. They may also ignore the early symptoms of a myocardial infarction, including fatigue, which is a commonly reported prodromal (antecedent) symptom. Consequently, they may delay seeking medical attention. Indeed, this notion is consistent with the observations of Greene, Moss, and Goldstein (1974), who reported that infarction victims, who were predominantly Type A's, delayed seeking medical care (see also Matthews, Siegel, Kuller, Thompson, & Varat, in press).

Sensory versus Evaluative Aspects of the Stress Experience: Some Additional Complexity

Up to this point, we have assumed that a relatively simple relationship exists between attentional factors and coping with stress. On the one hand, ignoring physical states—a style associated with Type A—leads persons to report less intense symptoms. On the other hand, attending to physical states leads persons to report more intense symptoms. It is now time to complicate things somewhat. Specifically, just as individuals can attend to aspects of the self, so, too, do they seem able to attend to various aspects of the symptom experience. In this regard, Leventhal and his colleagues (Leventhal, Brown, Shacham, & Engquist, 1979) suggest that a pain experience consists of stimulus sensations (e.g., aching) and emotional distress components, which under certain circumstances can be separated. Moreover, when separated, allocating different amounts of attention to sensations and to distress should lead to different experiences of pain. In other words, it is important to know what precise aspect of the physical state is being attended to, in order to understand fully the impact that attention has on symptom experience.

These ideas were tested by having subjects immerse their hands in cold water while periodically assessing distress and strength of sensations (Leventhal *et al.*, 1979, Experiment 1). Finger temperature and heart rate were also measured. A third of the subjects were forewarned about the physical sensations they would feel during the experiment (e.g., cold, tingling, numbness); a third were forewarned about the emotional distress they would experience (e.g., apprehension, butterflies, tension, weakness); and a third were forewarned about the specific procedures of the water bath (e.g., bucket size, purpose of the wire screen). Within each of the three groups, half were forewarned that cold water initially causes strong pain; the other half were not forewarned. The results showed that subjects forewarned about the sensation of coldness reported *less* distress and *less* intense sensations during the task than did those subjects forewarned about affective reactions or about specific procedures. Furthermore, among subjects forewarned about the sensation of coldness, those who were *not* also forewarned about the pain from cold water reported less distress and less intense sensations than did those who were forewarned about the pain. The former group, in fact, did experience significantly greater increases in skin temperature than did the other five groups. There were no differences in heart rate among groups.

Leventhal *et al.* interpreted their findings in the following way. When subjects attend to specific sensory features such as "coldness, numbness, pins and needles," these features are encoded prominently in the cognitive representation of the symptom experience. Such a cognitive representation is further thought to facilitate the habituation or reduction of distress, which in turn, is presumed to reduce the sympathetic discharge sustaining peripheral vasoconstriction. On the other hand, when subjects attend to their emotinal reactions, it is the evaluations that are encoded prominently in the cognitive representation of the symptom experience. Consequently, emotional distress reactions continue to be monitored and do not habituate. It can also follow from their work, although they do not say so, that a cognitive representation of a symptom experience that emphasizes the emotional aspects might exacerbate sympathetic discharge. Certainly this possibility is consistent with the previously described work on attention and intensification of emotional states (e.g., Scheier, 1976; Scheier & Carver, 1977).

While the Leventhal *et al.* distress data are by and large consistent with their expectations, the sensation and physiological data are not. The fact that changes in distress and sensation intensity covaried indicate at a minimum that subjects did not completely discriminate between them. Nonetheless, their data do support the notion that attention directed strictly to sensory aspects of the symptom experience has beneficial effects both on intensity of distress and unpleasant sensations.

The finger-temperature data suggest that attention to sensory features of a pain experience can reduce the sympathetic discharge sustaining peripheral vasoconstriction, provided that subjects are *not* forewarned about the strength of pain. If they are forewarned, their finger temperature remains low, suggesting continued sympathetic discharge and sustained vasoconstriction. While it is feasible that the pain warning interfered with the habituation process in the experiment just described, two additional experiments by Leventhal *et al.* (1979, Experiments 2 and 3) utilizing the same cold-pressor test found no differences in finger temperature corresponding to treatment effects. Thus, the role played by sympathetic activation in understanding the impact of attending to and encoding symptom information is unclear from their work.

Pertinent to this issue is other research on the effects of attention on physical states. Bloom, Houston, Holmes, and Burish (1977) studied the impact of coping strategies on sympathetic arousal during a stressful experience. Subjects were administered a sample shock and, thereafter, either were told that they would receive additional painful shocks or told nothing. Some of the subjects were then instructed to read and think about an amusing story (Attentional Diversion Condition), whereas others were instructed to write down reasons why they should not be afraid in this situation (Situation Redefinition). A third group was not given any additional instructions. In fact, no subjects were shocked again. During this time subjects physiological responses were monitored. The results showed that subjects who attended to the story (and consequently not to themselves or to the impending stressor) showed the least sympathetic arousal. Thus, active ignoring was instrumental in reducing sympathetic arousal resulting from the anticipation of shock.

Unfortunately, for our purposes, the Bloom *et al.* (1977) study did not include a condition where attention was directed to physical sensations. Thus, it is not known if attention to the sensations would in fact intensify those sensations. Fortunately, this issue was addressed in a study by Epstein, Rosenthal, and Szpiler (1978). In their experiment, subjects were exposed to six predictable loud noise bursts. Prior to the noise exposure, the subjects were told to attend (1) to their internal reactions, (2) to the noise bursts and other experimental stimuli, or (3) elsewhere. A control group of subjects was given no special instructions. The results showed that those subjects instructed to attend either to their internal sensations or to the noise bursts had greater sympathetic reactions to the bursts than either of the other two groups. Thus, during exposure to noxious stimuli, attention to either the stimuli or to their physical consequences seems to retard habituation. Diverting attention from noxious stimuli does not appear to accelerate the rate of habituation, however.

Taking the findings of Bloom *et al.* (1977) and Epstein *et al.* (1978) together, it appears that attention to the unpleasant sensations produced by a stressor retards habituation to it. Leventhal *et al.* (1979) would suggest that subjects in these studies were attending to the emotional aspects of their physical stress (rather than the purely sensory aspects of it), and thus the emotional distress fails to habituate. Indeed, as noted earlier, attending to emotional states does lead to enhanced reports of emotions.

Self-Focus versus Environment Focus Revisited

We noted earlier that attention to the self and attention to the environment are considered to be inversely related. When more attention is allocated to the self, less is available for processing environmental information. We also noted that in terms of the type of information processed, a high degree of congruence may exist between self-focus and environment focus. Let us now reexamine the implications of this latter assumption for the experience of stress. Consider, for example, the case of listening to aversive noise bursts. If a person attends to the noise bursts themselves, less attention is available for processing the person's own *reactions* to the bursts. If attention should be momentarily directed inward, however, presumably it will be focused selectively on those aspects of the self that are relevant to the person's present situation: specifically, the person's reactions to the noise. Given the natural back-and-forth shifting of attention between environment and self, it is plausible to suggest that instructions to focus on one particular aspect of the environment (the noise) may also serve to make the associated aspect of the self (one's reaction to the noise) more salient whenever focus goes inward.

This process may, in fact, have occurred in the Epstein *et al.* (1978) study. Subjects in that study showed the same failure to habituate to the noise stimuli (i.e., they maintained the same high level of sympathetic arousal), when instructed to attend to either the noise bursts or their reactions to them. Moreover, Epstein and his colleagues are not the only investigators who report that heightened attention to a stressor affects physical states. Matthews, Scheier, Brunson, and Carducci (1980, Experiments 2 and 3) report that subjects instructed to attend to predictable noise bursts rate their symptoms as more intense than subjects not given any special instructions. Thus, it might be the case that attention to a stressor and attention to the sensations produced by that stressor have similar effects on physical well-being.

While these complementary effects can be understood in the context of rapid shifting of attention between the two sources of information (self and environment), they are also consistent with at least one other explanation. It is feasible that a cognitive representation of a stressor might include information about its sensory features, as well as the symptoms experienced as a consequence of the stressor. Similarly, it is feasible that a cognitive representation of symptoms might include the sensory features of their source, *provided that one is identifiable*. The cold-pressor task illustrates this point nicely. When subjects submerge their hand in cold water and are instructed to attend to the water, they probably are aware of the water's coldness in addition to the numbness produced by it. When subjects are instructed to attend to their submerged hand, they are also probably aware of the water's coldness and its resultant physical sensations. In other words, when the stressor is identifiable, subjects may integrate information about the stressor and their reactions to it, either because of an inferred causal link between the two or because the two are phenomenologically integrated.

Two points are noteworthy here. First, we cannot choose between the foregoing two explanations on the basis of available data. In fact, investigators typically do not even discriminate between attention to a stressor and attention to reactions to it in studies of coping strategies during stressful events. For example, in a series of studies by Lazarus and his colleagues, individuals' coping processes were observed as they occurred in stressful events and were categorized on a dimension of extremely vigilant to extremely avoidant. Vigilant strategies are exemplified by excessive monitoring of either or both the stressor and reactions to it, whereas avoidant strategies ignore both. Usually, in these studies, a vigilant strategy led to more difficult and uncomfortable recovery from stressful events than an avoidant strategy (e.g., Cohen & Lazarus, 1973; see also Miller, 1980). Although these studies have made important contributions to the literature, they do little to resolve the issues under consideration here. We simply do not know whether their effects were due to heightened self-focus, environment focus, or both.

The second point of note is that the two explanations offered—shifts in focus of attention and integrated cognitive representations—are not incompatible. That is, early exposure to a stressful event may be characterized by frequent shifts in the processing of self-related and environment-related information. With repeated exposure to the stressor, however, the rapid fluctuation of attention may give rise to an integrated representation of the experience. The particular aspects of the experience that are emphasized presumably determine the effect later attentional focusing has (Leventhal et al., 1979).

Summary and Limitations

In this section we have reviewed data suggesting that ignoring physical sensations—a style associated with Type A—leads persons to report a low intensity of symptoms. In the case of the Type A, ignoring physical sensations appears to occur only when acknowledgment of symptoms could distract from performing well. We have also reviewed data indicating that close monitoring of physical sensations and the stressor that produced them results in perceptions of intense sensations and slowed habituation to the stressor. We have proposed that a cognitive representation of a stress-induced symptom experience may include information about the stressor, if identifiable, as well as information about the physical sensations produced by it. As Leventhal *et al.* (1979) note, unpleasant physical sensations probably include both a sensory feature component that is "objective" and an evaluative–emotional distress component that is not. While the information is integrated into a common experience, emphasis on the emotional aspect of the event might produce further distress or at least delayed habituation of that distress.

It should be noted that we do not believe that attention to one's physical state during stressful events always leads to the perception and experience of intense symptoms. The effects of attention are mediated by the aspects of the symptom experience attended to (e.g., evaluative–sensory features) as well as the characteristics of the stressor (e.g., acute–chronic). An illustration of the latter is the extent of predictability of the stressor. Instructing subjects to attend to an unpredictable event and its consequences is unlikely to enhance symptom intensity because individuals already attend to it at near maximal level (Finkelman & Glass, 1970; Matthews *et al.*, 1980, Experiment 1). In contrast, attention diversion is likely to decrease symptom intensity when the stressor is unpredictable (Bloom *et al.*, 1977; Monat, Averill, & Lazarus, 1972; cf. Houston & Holmes, 1974). On the other hand, diverting attention from a predictable event is unlikely to reduce symptom intensity because individuals should be attending to it at a nearly minimal level, particularly after a substantial period of time has passed. In contrast, increasing attention to a predictable event should enhance symptom intensity (Epstein *et al.*, 1978; Matthews *et al.*, 1980; Monat *et al.*, 1972; Pennebaker, Skelton, Wogalter, & Rodgers, 1978; cf. Leventhal *et al.*, 1979).

CONCLUDING COMMENTS

The primary purpose of the present chapter was to describe the role that attentional factors play in the perception of bodily states. We began with a straightforward hypothesis—attention to a physical state would cause information about that state to be processed more thoroughly. And we presented data consistent with that hypothesis. Self-focused individuals were more aware of their internal experiences than were persons who were less self-focused. The analysis became more complicated, however, when we moved from a discussion of attention to relatively benign sensations (e.g., taste) to a discussion of noxious sensations (e.g., pain). At this point we had to consider not only how attention leads persons to be more aware of their stress reactions, but also how it may retard habituation of those reactions. It also became important to understand how variations in attentional focus can affect the kind of cognitive representation of the symptom experience persons ultimately come to hold. In sum, attentional factors appear to play a critical role in the perception of bodily states and symptom experiences. Although the nature of that role is not simple, we do believe it is systematic.

ACKNOWLEDGMENTS

Preparation of this chapter was facilitated by Grants BNS 80-28159 and BNS 81-07236 awarded by the National Science Foundation to the first and second authors, respectively. It was also facilitated by an American Heart Association (AHA) Established Investigatorship award to the third author with funds contributed by the AHA Pennsylvania Affiliate.

REFERENCES

Balke, B. Optimale koerperliche Leistungsfaehigkeit, ihre Messung und Veraenderung infolge Arbeitsermuedung. *Arbeitsphysiologie*, 1954, *15*, 311.

Balke, B., Grillo, G. P., Konecci, E. B., & Luft, U. C. Work capacity after blood donation. *Journal of Applied Physiology*, 1954, *7*, 231.

Bannister, D., & Agnew, J. The child's construing of self. In J. Cole (Ed.), *Nebraska Symposium on Motivation* (Vol. 24). Lincoln: University of Nebraska Press, 1977.

Barefoot, J. C., & Straub, R. B. Opportunity for information search and the effect of false heart rate feedback. *Journal of Personality and Social Psychology*, 1971, *17*, 154–157.

Berlyne, D. E. Attention. In E. C. Carterette & M. P. Friedman (Eds.), *Handbook on perception.* New York: Academic, 1974.

Blascovich, J. *Visceral perception and social behavior.* Paper presented at the annual meeting of the American Psychological Association, Montreal, 1980. (Available from J. Blascovich, Department of Psychology, State University of New York at Buffalo, Buffalo, N.Y. 14226.)

Bloom, L. J., Houston, B. K., Holmes, D. S., & Burish, T. G. The effectiveness of attentional diversion and situational redefinition for reducing stress due to nonambiguous threat. *Journal of Research in Personality*, 1977, *11*, 83 94.

Bortner, R. W., & Rosenman, R. H. The measurement of pattern A behavior. *Journal of Chronic Diseases*, 1967, *20*, 525–533.

Bourne, L. E., Dominowski, R. L., & Loftus, E. F. *Cognitive processes.* Englewood Cliffs, N.J.: Prentice-Hall, 1979.

Broadbent, D. E. *Perception and communication.* New York: Pergamon, 1958.

Brock, T. C., & Balloun, J. L. Behavioral receptivity to dissonant information. *Journal of Personality and Social Psychology*, 1967, *6*, 413–428.

Buss, A. H. *Self-consciousness and social anxiety.* San Francisco: W. H. Freeman, 1980.

Cacioppo, J. T. Effects of exogenous changes in heart rate on facilitation of thought and resistance to persuasion. *Journal of Personality and Social Psychology*, 1979, *37*, 489–498.

Carver, C. S., Blaney, P. H., & Scheier, M. F. Focus of attention, chronic expectancy, and responses to a feared stimulus. *Journal of Personality and Social Psychology*, 1979, *37*, 1186–1195.

Carver, C. S., Coleman, A. E., & Glass, D. C.   The coronary-prone behavior pattern and the suppression of fatigue on a treadmill test. *Journal of Personality and Social Psychology*, 1976, *33*, 460–466.

Carver, C. S., DeGregorio, E., & Gillis, R.   Challenge and type A behavior among intercollegiate football players. *Journal of Sport Psychology*, 1981, *3*, 140–148.

Carver, C. S., & Glass, D. C.   The self-consciousness scale: A discriminant validity study. *Journal of Personality Assessment*, 1976, *40*, 169–172.

Carver, C. S., & Scheier, M. F.   Self-focusing effects of dispositional self-consciousness, mirror presence, and audience presence. *Journal of Personality and Social Psychology*, 1978, *36*, 324–332.

Carver, C. S., & Scheier, M. F.   *Attention and self-regulation: A control theory approach to human behavior.* New York: Springer-Verlag, 1981.

Cohen, F., & Lazarus, R. S.   Active coping processes, coping dispositions, and recovery from surgery. *Psychosomatic Medicine*, 1973, *35*, 375–389.

Cohen, S.   Environmental load and the allocation of attention. In A. Baum, J. E. Singer, & S. Valins (Eds.), *Advances in environmental research.* Hillsdale, N.J.: Erlbaum, 1978.

Davis, D., & Brock, T. C.   Use of first person pronouns as a function of increased abjective self-awareness and prior feedback. *Journal of Experimental Social Psychology*, 1975, *11*, 381–388.

Duncan, J. W., & Laird, J. D.   Cross-modality consistencies in individual differences in self-attribution. *Journal of Personality*, 1977, *45*, 191–206.

Duncan, J. W., & Laird, J. D.   Positive and reverse placebo effects as a function of differences in cues used in self-perception. *Journal of Personality and Social Psychology*, 1980, *39*, 1024–1036.

Duval, S., & Wicklund, R. A.   *A theory of objective self-awareness.* New York: Academic, 1972.

Easterbrook, J. A.   The effect of emotion on cue utilization and organization of behavior. *Psychological Review*, 1959, *66*, 183–201.

Epstein, L. H., Cinciripini, P. M., McCoy, J. F., & Marshall, W. R.   Heart rate as a discriminative stimulus. *Psychophysiology*, 1977, *14*, 143–149.

Epstein, S., Rosenthal, S., & Szpiler, J.   The influence of attention upon anticipatory arousal, habituation, and reactivity to a noxious stimulus. *Journal of Research in Personality*, 1978, *12*, 30–40.

Fenigstein, A., & Carver, C. S.   Self-focusing effects of false heartbeat feedback. *Journal of Personality and Social Psychology*, 1978, *36*, 1241–1250.

Fenigstein, A., Scheier, M. F., & Buss, A. H.   Public and private self-consciousness: Assessment and theory. *Journal of Consulting and Clinical Psychology*, 1975, *43*, 522–527.

Finkelman, J. M., & Glass, D. C.   Reappraisal of the relationship between noise and human performance by means of subsidiary task measure. *Journal of Applied Psychology*, 1970, *54*, 211–213.

Garner, W. R., Hake, H. W., & Eriksen, C. W.   Operationalism and the concept of perception. *Psychological Review*, 1956, *63*, 149–159.

Geller, V., & Shaver, P.   Cognitive consequences of self-awareness. *Journal of Experimental Social Psychology*, 1976, *12*, 99–108.

Gibbons, F. X., Carver, C. S., Scheier, M. F., & Hormuth, S. E.   Self-focused attention and the placebo effect: Fooling some of the people some of the time. *Journal of Experimental Social Psychology*, 1979, *15*, 263–274.

Glass, D. C.   *Behavior patterns, stress, and coronary disease.* Hillsdale, N.J.: Erlbaum, 1977.

Goldstein, D., Fink, D., & Mettee, D. R.   Cognition of arousal and actual arousal as determinants of emotion. *Journal of Personality and Social Psychology*, 1972, *21*, 41–51.

Greene, W. A., Moss, A. J., & Goldstein, S.   Delay, denial, and death in coronary heart disease. In R. S. Eliot (Ed.), *Stress and the heart.* Mt. Kisco, N.Y.: Futura, 1974.

Hartley, L. R., & Adams, R. G.   Effect of noise on the Stroop test. *Journal of Experimental Psychology*, 1974, *102*, 62–66.

Hirst, W. C., Spelke, E. S., Reaves, C. C., Caharach, G., & Neisser, U.   Dividing attention without alternation or automaticity. *Journal of Experimental Psychology: General*, 1980, *109*, 98–117.

Houston, B. K.   Inhibition and the facilitating effect of noise on interference tasks. *Perceptual and Motor Skills*, 1968, *27*, 947–950.

Houston, B. K., & Holmes, D. S.   Effect of avoidant thinking and reappraisal for coping with threat involving temporal uncertainty. *Journal of Personality and Social Psychology*, 1974, *30*, 382–388.

Hull, J. G., & Levy, A. S.   The organizational functions of the self: An alternative to the Duval and Wicklund model of self-awareness. *Journal of Personality and Social Psychology*, 1979, *37*, 756–768.

James, W.   *The principles of psychology*. New York: Holt, Rinehart & Winston, 1890.

Kahneman, D.   *Attention and effort*. Englewood Cliffs, N.J.: Prentice-Hall, 1973.

Kanfer, F. H., & Goldfoot, D. A.   Self-control and tolerance of noxious stimulation. *Psychological Reports*, 1966, *18*, 79–85.

Kleck, R. E., Vaughan, R. C., Cartwright-Smith, J., Vaughan, K. B., Colby, C. Z., & Lanzetta, J. T.   Effects of being observed on expressive, subjective, and physiological responses to painful stimuli. *Journal of Personality and Social Psychology*, 1976, *34*, 1211–1218.

Kleinhesselink, R. R., & Edwards, R. E.   Seeking and avoiding belief-discrepant information as a function of its perceived refutability. *Journal of Personality and Social Psychology*, 1975, *31*, 787–790.

Konecni, V. J.   Annoyance, type, and duration of postannoyance activity, and aggression: The "cathartic" effect. *Journal of Experimental Psychology: General*, 1975, *104*, 76–102.

Laird, J. D., & Crosby, M.   Individual differences in self-attribution of emotion. In H. London & R. Nisbett (Eds.), *Thinking and feeling: The cognitive alteration of feeling states*. Chicago: Aldine, 1974.

Lanzetta, J. T., Biernat, J. J., & Kleck, R. E.   *Self-focused attention, facial behavior, autonomic arousal, and the emotional experience*. Paper presented at the annual meeting of the American Psychological Association, Montreal, 1980.

Lanzetta, J. T., Cartwright-Smith, J., & Kleck, R. E.   Effects of nonverbal dissimulation on emotional experience and autonomic arousal. *Journal of Personality and Social Psychology*, 1976, *33*, 354–370.

Leventhal, H.   The consequences of depersonalization during illness and treatment. In J. Howard & A. Strauss (Eds.), *Humanizing health care*. New York: Wiley, 1975.

Leventhal, H.   Toward a comprehensive theory of emotion. In L. Berkowitz ((Ed.), *Advances in experimental social psychology* (Vol. 13). New York: Academic, 1980.

Leventhal, H., Brown, D., Shacham, S., & Engquist, G.   Effects of preparatory information about sensations, threat of pain and attention on cold pressor distress. *Journal of Personality and Social Psychology*, 1979, *37*, 688–714.

Leventhal, H., & Everhart, D.   Emotion, pain, and physical illness. In C. E. Izard (Ed.), *Emotions and psychopathology*. New York: Plenum, 1979.

Leventhal, H., Meyer, D., & Nerenz, D.   The common sense representation of illness danger. In S. Rachman (Ed.), *Medical psychology* (Vol. 2). New York: Pergamon, 1980.

Leventhal, H., Nerenz, D., & Strauss, A.   Self-regulation and the mechanisms for symptom appraisal. In D. Mechanic (Ed.), *Psychological epidemiology*. New York: Watson, 1980.

Lewis, M., & Brooks, J.   Self-knowledge and emotional development. In M. Lewis & L. A. Rosenblum (Eds.), *The development of affect*. New York: Plenum, 1978.

Matthews, K. A., & Brunson, B. I.   Allocation of attention and the Type A coronary-prone behavior pattern. *Journal of Personality and Social Psychology*, 1979, *37*, 2081–2090.

Matthews, K. A., Scheier, M. F., Brunson, B. I., & Carducci, B.   Attention, unpredictability, and reports of physical symptoms: Eliminating the benefits of predictability. *Journal of Personality and Social Psychology*, 1980, *38*, 525–537.

Matthews, K. A., Siegel, J. M., Kuller, L. H., Thompson, M., & Varat, M. Determinants of decisions to seek medical treatment by patients with acute myocardial infarction symptoms. *Journal of Personality and Social Psychology*, in press.

Matthews, K. A., & Volkin, J. I. Efforts to excel and the Type A behavior pattern in children. *Child Development*, 1981, *52*, 1283–1289.

Mechanic, D. *Medical sociology: A selective view.* New York: Free Press, 1968.

Mechanic, D. Social psychologic factors affecting the presentation of bodily complaints. *New England Journal of Medicine*, 1972, *286*, 1132–1139.

Miller, L. C., Murphy, R., & Buss, A. H. Consciousness of body: Private and public. *Journal of Personality and Social Psychology*, 1981, *41*, 397–406.

Miller, S. M. When is a little information a dangerous thing? Coping with stressful events by monitoring vs. blunting. In S. Levine & H. Ursin (Eds.), *Coping and health*. New York: Plenum, 1980.

Mills, J. Interest in supporting and discrepant information. In R. Abelson, E. Aronson, W. J. McGuire, J. M. Newcomb, M. J. Rosenberg, & P. H. Tannenbaum (Eds.), *Theories of cognitive consistency: A sourcebook*. Chicago: Rand McNally, 1968.

Mischel, W. *Personality and assessment.* New York: Wiley, 1968.

Monat, A., Averill, J. R., & Lazarus, R. S. Anticipatory stress and coping reactions under various conditions of uncertainty. *Journal of Personality and Social Psychology*, 1972, *24*, 237–253.

Morgan, W. P., & Pollock, M. L. Psychologic characterization of the elite distance runner. In P. Milvy (Ed.), *The marathon: Physiological, medical, epidemiological, and psychological studies*. New York: New York Academy of Sciences, 1977.

Neumann, P. G., Carver, C. S., & Scheier, M. F. An apparatus for varying self-awareness while presenting visual stimuli. *Behavioral Research Methods and Instrumentation*, 1977, *9*, 55.

Norman, D. A. Toward a theory of memory and attention. *Psychological Review*, 1968, *75*, 522–536.

Nowlin, J. B., Eisdorfer, C., Whalen, R., & Troyer, W. G. The effect of exogenous changes in heart rate and rhythm upon reaction time performance. *Psychophysiology*, 1971, *7*, 186–193.

Pennebaker, J. W., & Lightner, J. M. Competition of internal and external information in an exercise setting. *Journal of Personality and Social Psychology*, 1980, *39*, 165–174.

Pennebaker, J. W., & Skelton, J. A. Psychological parameters of physical symptoms. *Personality and Social Psychology Bulletin*, 1978, *4*, 524–530.

Pennebaker, J. W., Skelton, J. A., Wogalter, M., & Rodgers, R. J. *Effects of attention on the experience of physical symptoms*. Paper presented at the meeting of the American Psychological Association, Toronto, August 1978.

Posner, M. I. Psychobiology of attention. In C. Blakemore & M. S. Gazzaniga (Eds.), *The handbook of psychobiology*. New York: Academic, 1974.

Raye, C. L., Johnson, M. K., & Taylor, T. H. Is there something special about memory for internally generated information? *Memory & Cognition*, 1980, *8*, 141–148.

Schachter, S., & Singer, J. E. Cognitive, social, and physiological determinants of emotional state. *Psychological Review*, 1962, *69*, 379–399.

Scheier, M. F. Self-awareness, self-consciousness, and angry aggression. *Journal of Personality*, 1976, *44*, 627–644.

Scheier, M. F., & Carver, C. S. Self-focused attention and the experience of emotion: Attraction, repulsion, elation, and depression. *Journal of Personality and Social Psychology*, 1977, *35*, 625–636.

Scheier, M. F., & Carver, C. S. Private and public aspects of self. In L. Wheeler (Ed.), *Review of personality and social psychology* (Vol. 2). Beverly Hills, Calif.: Sage, 1981.

Scheier, M. F., Carver, C. S., & Gibbons, F. X. Self-directed attention, awareness of bodily states, and suggestibility. *Journal of Personality and Social Psychology*, 1979, *37*, 1576–1588.

Spelke, E., Hirst, W., & Neisser, U. Skills of divided attention. *Cognition*, 1976, *4*, 215–230.

Stroop, J. R.   Factors affecting speed in serial verbal reactions. *Psychological Monographs*, 1938, *50*(5), 38–48.

Treisman, A. M.   Strategies and models of selective attention. *Psychological Review*, 1969, *76*, 282–299.

Turner, R. G., Scheier, M. F., Carver, C. S., & Ickes, W.   Correlates of self-consciousness. *Journal of Personality Assessment*, 1978, *42*, 285–289.

Valins, S.   Cognitive effects of false heart rate feedback. *Journal of Personality and Social Psychology*, 1966, *4*, 400–408.

Velten, E.   A laboratory task for induction of mood states. *Behaviour Research and Therapy*, 1968, *6*, 473–482.

Walters, A.   Psychogenic regional pain alias hysterical pain. *Brain*, 1961, *84*, 1–18.

Wegner, D. M., & Giuliano, T.   Arousal-induced attention to the self. *Journal of Personality and Social Psychology*, 1980, *38*, 719–726.

Weidner, G., & Matthews, K. A.   Reported physical symptoms elicited by unpredictable events and the Type A coronary-prone behavior pattern. *Journal of Personality and Social Psychology*, 1978, *36*, 1213–1220.

Wicklund, R. A., & Duval, S.   Opinion change and performance facilitation as a result of objective self-awareness. *Journal of Experimental Social Psychology*, 1971, *7*, 319–342.

Wylie, R. C.   *The self-concept: A review of methodological considerations and measuring instruments* (rev. ed.). Lincoln: University of Nebraska Press, 1974.

CHAPTER 19

Physical Symptoms and Sensations: Psychological Causes and Correlates

James W. Pennebaker
Southern Methodist University

INTRODUCTION

Historically, the fields of medicine and psychophysiology have been concerned with physiological changes in humans. An implicit assumption of much of this work has been that the person can detect and report these internal changes as specific symptoms or sensations. Unfortunately for the physician, patient, and experimenter, this assumption is not always true. The purpose of this chapter is to acquaint the reader with several factors that can influence the person's perception of internal state. Perceptual, social, developmental, and even cultural factors can radically alter how and when we notice and report symptoms—even when physiological state is comparable between people and settings.

Although we are all familiar with nasal congestion, headaches, pounding hearts, and other sensations, we rarely consider the factors involved in their definition or perception. A sensation is a perception, feeling, or even belief about the state of our body. Although the term "physical symptom" often connotes underlying pathology, we will use the terms sensation and symptom interchangeably. A sensation or symptom is often—but not always—based on actual physiological activity. Above all, a physical symptom represents information about internal state. As such, symptoms are related to virtually all behaviors, whether drinking, sleeping, taking aspirin, or visiting a physician. Symptoms and sensations, then, are both causes and consequences of behavior. They often initiate activity as well as signal that an activity has occurred.

A fundamental assumption of this chapter is that *symptoms are perceived in accordance with the same perceptual processes that have traditionally been implicated in the perception of external stimuli* (see also Brener, 1977; Leventhal, 1975). The awareness of symptoms is dependent on a variety of internal and external cues as well as the sets or schemata that we hold. Because of this, it is critical to note that the awareness of internal sensations does *not* represent a one-to-one correspondence with actual physiological change.

In order to give a flavor of the many directions that symptom research has taken, the present chapter is divided into five sections. The first deals with some of the basic perceptual processes that can influence symptom reporting. This portion of the chapter lays the conceptual groundwork. The following sections deal with developmental, sub- and cross-cultural, and individual difference correlates of the symptom-reporting process. The final section presents a potpourri of related issues, such as emotion, psychosomatics, and physiological bases of symptom perception.

PERCEPTUAL PROCESSES INFLUENCING SYMPTOM REPORTING

Tingling, itching, pain, and specific physical symptoms are perceptions. As with light or sound waves, they are encoded and organized. In order to understand symptom perception, it is instructive to delve briefly into the perception literature. As will be seen, advances in visual and auditory perception are highly relevant to body perception.

Two paradigms have dominated the perception literature for the past 50 years. The first, which assumes a relatively passive perceiver, has been interested in how the individual perceives and reacts to stimuli that are presented. In addition to psychophysical problems (e.g., Stevens, 1975), researchers within this tradition have been interested in orienting responses, color perception, habituation, sensory thresholds, and so on. A more recent paradigm assumes that the perceiver is highly active. Within this approach, researchers are attempting to understand how the organism organizes sensory information as well as seeks out specific types of information so as better to understand the environment. Several highly relevant findings from both approaches are directly related to the symptom-reporting process. (It must be emphasized that the passive–active distinction is not universally accepted. Similarly, researchers within the respective "camps" do not always acknowledge each other's contributions. For more information on these approaches, see Lindsay & Norman, 1977, and Haber & Hershenson, 1973.)

Before discussing the relevant contributions of these literatures to symptom reporting, a real-world example of perception will be helpful. Imagine that you are feverishly writing a paper while sitting alone in your study. All of a sudden, you hear rustling sounds under your desk. You immediately assume that it is a mouse and begin searching for the small, furry creature. As simple as this short vignette may appear, the stages of perception that have occurred are quite complex. First, you must analyze the stimulus characteristics that attracted your attention in the first place (e.g., orienting). Second, we should assess why the perceiver assumed the sound represented the presence of a mouse. Finally, we should examine the implications of the person's selectively looking for the mouse based on the original mouse hypothesis. The processes of orienting, hypothesis formation, and selective search are intimately tied to symptom perception.

Orienting and Competition of Cues

Within the passive school of perception, several researchers have attempted to define which stimuli people are most likely to attend or orient. For example, Berlyne (1960) noted that individuals are more likely to pay attention to visual arrays that are unique, complex, or display motion than arrays that are redundant, simple, or stationary. Similarly, if we assume that a person can process only a finite amount of information at any given time (e.g., Navon & Gopher, 1979), the probability of noticing any given stimulus will be dependent on the number of competing stimuli that are present at the same time. Returning to the mouse example, we will be more likely to notice the initial rustling if the sound is unique *and* if we are not being bombarded by a large number of other types of stimuli at the time.

Our noticing or orienting to physical symptoms can occur in similar ways. If immersed in a task, we will be less likely to notice subtle sensations than if we are in a boring or undemanding environment. In other words, internal sensory and external environmental cues are often in competition for processing. The probability of reporting physical symptoms, then, should be inversely related to the quantity and quality of external information sources. As will be discussed below, a large number of experimental and correlational studies support this reasoning. For example, we have found that people report far fewer physical symptoms during exercise if they are listening to interesting sounds than if hearing their own breathing or nothing at all. Similarly, subjects are less likely to notice signs of fatigue when running on an interesting cross-country course than when jogging on a boring, circular lap course (see Pennebaker & Lightner, 1980).

In a series of studies on coughing in classrooms, we obtained similar results. If one assumes that a cough is an immediate response to the perception of an itching or tickling throat, it would be expected that people would cough at a higher frequency during boring portions of movies or lectures than during interesting portions. In one study, for example, subjects viewed a 17-minute movie that had previously been rated every 30 seconds on its interest value. The movie was then shown to three large introductory psychology courses while experimenters counted the number of coughs during each of the previously rated 30-second segments of the movie. The more interesting the movie segment, the fewer the number of coughs, $r = -.57$, $p < .001$ (from Pennebaker, 1980). These and other studies that we have conducted have consistently shown that self-reported symptoms as well as behavioral measures indicative of symptoms vary as a function of competing stimuli that the person must process (see Pennebaker & Brittingham, 1982, for an extensive review).

Another line of research, dealing with suppression of fatigue, points to a comparable process. Walster and Aronson (1967) required subjects to perform three trials of a fatiguing task. Half of the subjects knew that they would be performing only three trials, whereas the remainder of subjects thought that they would be performing five trials. Self-reports of fatigue were collected after each of the three trials. The authors found that subjects reported feeling less fatigued after three trials if they thought that they still had additional trials to perform. In other words, if they believed that they were still in the midst of the experiment, they were less attentive to fatigue-related sensations (and presumably more oriented to the task at hand). Comparable findings have been reported among Type A coronary-prone college students and children (Carver, Coleman, & Glass, 1976; Matthews, 1979; see also Scheier, Carver, & Matthews, Chapter 18, this volume). Interestingly, we have discovered some analogous findings among residents exposed to ashfalls associated with Mt. St. Helens volcano. Among five of the communities that had received heavy ashfalls, only one was seriously threatened by flooding 6 weeks after the initial eruptions. Although people in this community reported the volcano to be far more dangerous than residents in the other towns, they reported far fewer physical symptoms related to the ash than people in any other area (all p's $< .01$). Residents in the threatened community were preoccupied with the future implications of the volcano and were less attentive to the relatively unimportant ash-related physical symptoms (Pennebaker & Newtson, 1983). The fatigue/symptom suppression idea, then, can be viewed as an extension of competition of cues. If an individual must deal actively with ongoing tasks or crises, he or she would be less likely to notice and report physical symptoms or sensations.

In addition to the experiments noted above, a large number of surveys conducted by the National Center for Health Statistics (NCHS) as well as private investigators have consistently found results that are congruent with the cue competition perspective. For example, individuals who live alone or in social isolation report more physical symptoms (Greenley & Mechanic, 1976; Moos & Van Dort, 1977), report being in worse health (Comstock & Slome, 1973; Wan, 1976), and consume more aspirin and sleeping pills (NCHS, 1979) than do those living with others. Similarly, those people who report that their jobs are boring or undemanding report more symptoms (Coburn, 1975; Weiman, 1977; Wright et al., 1977), depression (Harrison, 1976), and visit health facilities with greater frequency (Moos, 1975) than those who report their jobs to be interesting. Obviously, these studies can be criticized as being correlational rather than causal.

Sickly people may have more trouble making friends, finding spouses, or even holding down interesting jobs. Nevertheless, the findings are consistent with the experimental studies reported above.

Although the competition of cues idea appears to be related to symptom reporting, its use as an explanatory tool is limited. There is far more to perception than orienting toward salient stimuli. Once the person has noticed a given stimulus, he or she must organize the sensory information in order to give it meaning. In addition, it is important to recognize that individuals are usually *searching* for information rather than passively encoding any stimulus that happens to bombard a group of receptors.

Hypothesis Formation and Selective Search

Recall that in the mouse example, our unwitting protagonist assumed that a mouse was present and then selectively looked for a mouse. The formerly passive perceiver is now actively synthesizing and searching for information. Such an active view of perception requires that the organism transform or process available information in order to give it meaning (e.g., Bruner, 1957; Neisser, 1976). This process is necessary since, at any given time, we have access to a tremendous quantity of information. The incoming data, then, must be reduced. This can be accomplished in at least two ways. The first is to restrict which information is encoded in the first place. In other words, information search must be guided. The second way of reducing potential sensory data is by cognitively restructuring, synthesizing, and organizing incoming information. These hypothetical cognitive structures—which are variously called sets, expectancies, templates, tentative or working hypotheses, schemas, scripts—guide our search for information and organize the data gleaned from the search.

Returning to the mouse vignette, the adoption of the mouse hypothesis resulted in the selective search for mouse-relevant information. One can readily see some of the biases and distortions that can occur with such an active perceptual process (Snyder, 1979; Taylor & Crocker, 1981). First, individuals will be more likely to look for hypothesis-relevant than hypothesis-irrelevant information. Consequently, if we hold the mouse hypothesis concerning the rustling sound, we should be less likely to encode information indicating that a loose nail fell on the papers. Second, we will be biased toward confirming our hypothesis. This bias will be positively correlated with the ambiguity of the extant information. Finally, the more potential information that is available in any given setting, the higher the probability that we will be able to confirm any given hypothesis that we adopt.

These principles are directly related to the perception of physical symptoms. In many, if not most cases, we have available to us a large number of internal sensations that are vague, diffuse, and subjective.

Given their ambiguous nature, their perception and interpretation will be greatly influenced by the hypotheses that are adopted. Further, the hypotheses that we have adopted will have a high probability of being confirmed.

An example of this process occurs with "medical students' disease," wherein 70% of first-year medical students adopt the symptoms of one of the diseases that they study (Woods, Natterson, & Silverman, 1966). All the prerequisites for perceptual bias are present. The students are under stress from studying, tests, lack of sleep, and so on. The various stresses undoubtedly result in heightened autonomic activity, thus causing a large number of sensations, such as racing hearts, sweating, fatigue, and so on. In addition, studying about a large number of diseases sets up various disease hypotheses which cause selective search for confirming information. With a large number of potential sensations, the person will have an increased probability of finding sensory information that will verify the hypothesis.

As the example above suggests, illness hypotheses can be set up in a variety of ways. Reading or hearing about a disease or set of symptoms can easily prompt a selective search for verifying information. As most readers can attest, simply seeing someone vomit, faint, or even "look sick" can influence how we perceive internal sensory information. In addition to these relatively transient hypotheses, more longlasting hypotheses concerning body state are often the result of socialization, traumatic experiences (e.g., having a heart attack in years past), or even classical or instrumental conditioning. Some of these factors are discussed in the following sections.

Of particular importance is the fact that the selective monitoring process occurs at several levels of analysis. The hypotheses that we adopt can shape the perception of a single, relatively discrete sensation, a constellation of sensations, or broader categories of sensations, such as perceptions of illness, emotion, hunger, and so on. For example, we recently found that experimentally induced hypotheses could easily change a subject's perception of finger temperature. In the study, subjects were told that a (bogus) ultrasonic noise would have the effect of either increasing or decreasing skin temperature, or would have no effect at all. Finger temperature was continuously monitored while subjects "listened" to the noise. As expected, subjects reported that their finger temperatures had indeed changed in the manded direction. Actual skin temperature, however, did not vary as a function of the manipulation. Of particular interest was the fact that subjects' skin temperatures tended to fluctuate up and down over the course of the study. Within-cell correlations between self-reported skin temperature and actual skin temperature fluctuations indicated that subjects were indeed selectively monitoring their fingers. Those subjects who expected their fingers to become warmer noticed increases in temperature and ignored decreases. Subjects expecting the opposite encoded decreases and overlooked increases (see Pennebaker & Skelton, 1981). Subsequent studies confirmed these findings. That is, when sensory information is ambiguous and/or inconsistent, the person will selectively encode only that information that is congruent with currently held hypotheses.

The perception of broader categories of symptoms can also be the result of hypothesis-guided selective search. A particularly interesting and important example has been reported by Meyer, Leventhal, and Gutman (1980) dealing with hypertensives. In their study, a sample of hypertensive patients were interviewed concerning their beliefs or hypotheses about high blood pressure. All the patients had been told by their physicians that high blood pressure was asymptomatic. Nevertheless, virtually all of the subjects held well-formed hypotheses about specific symptoms that they "knew" covaried with blood pressure elevations. For example, some patients view hypertension as a form of heart disease and thus monitor cardiac sensations. Others believed that hypertension was a vascular disease and were particularly sensitive to vascular symptoms (e.g., headaches, coldness in extremities). The hypotheses held by the subjects influenced how they monitored their bodies and ultimately gauged their need for medical treatment. As an aside, we have recently replicated these findings. In addition, by using within-subject designs we have been able to determine that unique constellations of symptoms covary with fluctuations in blood pressure and blood glucose in insulin-dependent diabetics (Gonder-Frederick, 1981; Pennebaker, 1982; Pennebaker, Cox, Gonder-Frederick, Wunsch, Evans, & Pohl, 1981; Pennebaker, Gonder-Frederick, Stewart, Elfman, & Skelton, 1982). Interestingly, patients' beliefs about covarying symptoms are poorly related to the true covarying symptoms.

Perhaps one of the most important implications of the selective search concept is its relationship to placebo effectiveness (Jospe, 1978; Rickels, 1968). A placebo is an inert substance that is described to the patient as effective. Across hundreds of studies, placebos have been found to reduce symptom reporting, anxiety levels, and other undesirable body states. People typically place great faith in their physicians or healers. Consequently, patients are often willing to adopt their physician-induced hypotheses concerning the effectiveness of a given treatment. The mere fact that the patient visits a doctor in the first place can radically alter the way in which the patient organizes and searches for sensory data. For example, once the sick patient has seen a doctor, he or she may switch from "How sick am I becoming?" to "How well am I becoming?" The very nature of the hypotheses will define the answers (see an extended review of these issues in Skelton & Pennebaker, 1982).

Summary

Individuals perceive physical symptoms and sensations in much the same way as they perceive external environmental events. The probability of noticing a given physical sensation is inversely related to the number of competing stimuli present at any given time. The organization and selective search for symptoms can be highly active. Certain systematic biases may occur in the perception of bodily states for several reasons. First, individuals often have access to a large number of ambiguous sensations that are amenable to a variety of interpretations. Second, the nature of selective search often results in the encoding of hypothesis-relevant or -consistent information at the expense of hypothesis-irrelevant or -inconsistent information.

Although brief, the discussion thus far serves as a conceptual foundation by which to understand much of the symptom-reporting research. As will be seen in the following sections, many of the principles outlined above will be directly relevant to other aspects of the symptom-reporting process.

DEVELOPMENTAL ISSUES IN SYMPTOM REPORTING

The perceptual issues discussed above suggest that the socialization of the child could ultimately influence the ways in which he or she attends to, organizes, and interprets bodily sensations. Within the developmental literature, three recurring themes have been empirically studied. The first assumes that the degree to which the parents are attentive to the child's health will ultimately influence the child's symptom reporting and/or health-seeking responses (e.g., physician visits, absenteeism). A second theme is directly related to the socialization of body-related schemata or hypotheses. Specifically, this approach seeks to learn if the child tends to report the same types of symptoms as the parents. The final approach considers that much of the child's symptom reporting and health problems serve as secondary gains—either to reduce family conflict or to avoid or to be removed from aversive situations. Research findings within each of these categories will be discussed separately.

Attentiveness of Parents

An intuitively appealing idea is that if the parents are overly attentive to the child's health, the child will learn to be overly attentive to his or her bodily sensations, and thus report symptoms to a higher degree. One approach in testing this hypothesis has been to examine the birth order of the child. Presumably, because the firstborn receives more attention from the parents than later borns, he or she should be more attentive to bodily changes. As logical as this reasoning may sound, results from a variety of studies have not provided consistent answers. Of five recent studies examining the relationship between birth order and reported illness (usually by parent), two have found that firstborns are more prone to illness (Franklin, 1973; Sheldrake, Cormack, & McGuire, 1976), two have not found this pattern of results (Friedman, 1975; Gonda, 1962), and one has found a marginally significant trend ($p < .10$) suggesting that firstborn nursery school children are absent due to illness to a greater degree than later borns (Pennebaker, Hendler, Durrett, & Richards, 1981).

Without question, the strongest test of the attentiveness hypothesis has been conducted by David Mechanic (1964, 1979). In his first study, Mechanic interviewed 350 fourth- and eighth-grade children and their mothers concerning perceptions of symptoms by the children, and by the mother for both herself and her child. Correlations were computed between measures of the child's attentiveness to symptoms and the degree of interest in symptoms shown by the mother for both her child and herself. Although the correlations were statistically significant, they accounted for only about 2% of the variance. Mechanic concluded that although weak relationships appear to exist, they were not clinically significant. Interestingly, in a 16-year follow-up with the same subjects, Mechanic (1979) reversed his initial assessment by stating that "factors that focus the child's attention on internal states and that teach a pattern of internal monitoring contribute to a distress syndrome in later life." Note that this syndrome is not exclusively caused by the mother. Rather, the child's attentiveness to internal state may be the result of chronic disease or hospitalization, family distress, and other factors, including parental attentiveness. Whatever the causes may be, this illness syndrome or attentiveness to symptoms persists over an extended period of time.

In sum, the parental attentiveness hypothesis has received weak support. Although a contributing factor to the child's perception of his or her own symptoms, many other variables are undoubtedly influencing this process.

Hypothesis or Schema Socialization

As noted above, the way in which the child organizes and perceives symptoms and sensations may be similar to the parents'. The way that the parent reports symptoms and body-related hypotheses could be adopted by the child. Note that this argument is distinct from the attentiveness issue. A parent, for example, could be oblivious to the child's health but still convey ways by which to define, interpret, and organize sensory experiences.

The research findings to support this hypothesis are again weak. Campbell (1975) found low but positive correlations between the mother's symptom reports and her child's. Mechanic (1964), using a different approach, found that mothers who are under stress report more physical symptoms both for themselves and for their children. As Mechanic notes, this is an important finding in the sense that it is usually the mother's decision (as opposed to the child's) to take the child to a physician, administer medication, and define the child's sick role.

One reason why these results may be so weak is that the respective samples were fairly homogeneous. As will be discussed in the section dealing with cross-cultural differences, general patterns of symptom reporting appear to be roughly similar within but not between cultures. Hence, American mothers and their children may report any of 10 or 12 symptoms (e.g., headaches, tense muscles, stomach pains) whereas a completely different culture may be attentive to a completely different set of symptoms. Statistically, then, analyses on a homogeneous sample will deflate correlations between mother and child symptom patterns.

Secondary Gain in the Symptom-Reporting Process

Perhaps the most consistent developmental pattern is that children in aversive home or school environments report more health problems than do those who are not. One of the most exciting research efforts in this vein has examined the relationship between family dynamics and the child's health. Minuchin and his colleagues (Minuchin, Baker, Rosman, Liebman, Milman, & Todd, 1975) have indicated that family conflict is related to childhood asthma and other disorders. Further, when psychotherapeutic interventions were instituted to reduce family conflict, dramatic improvements were found in the health of the children. This approach assumes that the child's health serves as a homeostatic mechanism in the household. When family conflict increases, the child becomes sick, which, in turn, reduces the conflict. Other studies have indicated that family conflict is related to a child's postoperative reactions (Jessner, Blom, & Waldfogel, 1952), school absenteeism (Boardman, 1975; Pennebaker, Hendler, Durrett, & Richards, 1981), and poor health in general (Mutter & Schleifer, 1966).

Interestingly, these health problems are not limited to family conflict. Two recent studies have found that if the parent and/or teacher view the child as antisocial (e.g., aggressive or shy), increased health problems occur. In one archival study with over 200 nursery school children, the child was more likely to be absent from school due to reported illness (by the parent) if the mother had rated the child as aggressive or shy at the beginning of the school year. This pattern was obtained after controlling for various demographic variables, the child's early health, and measures of family conflict (Pennebaker, Hendler, Durrett, & Richards, 1981). Teacher ratings were similarly related to absenteeism. Finally, in a massive survey of over 1400 parents of children between the ages of 5 and 13, Eisen, Ware, Donald, and Brook (1979) found that parent's perceptions of the child's health and social relations were positively correlated.

It must be noted that these findings may not reflect secondary gains exclusively. It is well known that stress results in massive hormonal and autonomic changes (e.g., Selye, 1976), which, in turn, could make the child more susceptible to disease. At this point it is impossible to disentangle the two explanations. Functionally, the child's getting sick serves as a way of reducing family conflict or avoiding school. Of course, a functional explanation is distinct from a causal one.

Summary

There have been surprisingly few well-controlled and/or longitudinal developmental studies dealing with the development of symptom-reporting patterns in children. At this point we must conclude that parental attentiveness to the child's health and socialization of the child's body schemata are, at the worst, weak, and in the best of all possible worlds, not yet adequately tested. The only consistent finding across all studies is that family or social conflict tends to increase symptom-reporting and illness-related behaviors.

SUBCULTURAL AND CROSS-CULTURAL INFLUENCES

In many cases it is difficult to compare symptom reporting across cultures because of different diets, health practices, and so on. Nevertheless, large and consistent differences typically emerge between disparate cultures that strongly suggest that people vary considerably in terms of the schemata or hypotheses they hold about their bodies and physical sensations. Perhaps some of the most compelling evidence has been found for urban ethnic groups within the United States.

Among American samples, large differences in symptom reporting and responses to pain have been found between subcultures. In a classic study by Zola (1966), it was discovered that Irish-Americans were more likely to seek medical attention for symptoms than Italian-Americans. Further, the symptoms for which they sought medical attention were different. Whereas persons of Irish descent were likely to complain of eye, ear, nose, and throat symptoms, the Italian-Americans typically sought aid for symptoms associated with other parts of the body. Similarly, large differences in response to pain have been found between American-born Jews, Italians, Irish, and Yankees of British descent (e.g., Zborowski, 1969). Not only do these differences emerge for perceptions of aversiveness and overt complaining, but the groups differ in their autonomic responsivity to standardized experimentally induced pain (Sternbach & Tursky, 1965;

Tursky & Sternbach, 1967). The various researchers have attributed these differences to the different meanings each group ascribes to pain. Whereas one group—Jewish—interprets pain as signaling danger with important implications for the future, another group such as the Yankee interprets pain in a more benign, something-to-be-endured fashion.

As might be expected, anthropological studies indicate tremendous variablity in symptom reporting from culture to culture. Margaret Mead (1950) noted that the Arapesh women, when pregnant, did not show signs of morning sickness. According to Mead, this was due to their total denial of pregnancy. Raper (1958) initially assumed that peptic ulcers were a rare occurrence among members of the African tribe he was studying since tribal members never noted or complained of accompanying symptoms. Later autopsies, however, revealed that peptic ulcers were present in virtually the same proportions in the tribe as in England. Apparently, the African tribesmen, not unlike the Arapesh women, were organizing and interpreting their internal sensations in different ways than their Anglo-Saxon counterparts.

Another striking example of cultural differences concerning physical symptoms was conducted among the Panopeans in the Caroline Islands (Fischer, Fischer, & Mahony, 1959). In the culture, the eating of a forbidden, or totem, animal often results in a metaphorical symptom acquisition. For example, a person's ingesting his totem food, such as the turtle "causes him to gasp for air like a turtle . . . or to be subject to a compulsion to flap his arms like a turtle's flippers. An informant, whose sib totem was the eel, reported that his cheeks swelled up like an eel's gills when he violated his taboo."

Finally, cross-cultural and even transhistorical case studies have been amassed examining a phenomenon called mass psychogenic illness (MPI). MPI typically occurs among females in schools or factories, during periods of high stress. In Western cultures, the typical pattern for an MPI outbreak is that one woman will collapse or perhaps vomit. Others soon exhibit similar symptoms in addition to vague complaints of nausea, headache, and dizziness. Interestingly, outbreaks tend to occur along friendship lines (see Colligan, Pennebaker, & Murphy, 1982; Kerckhoff & Back, 1968). In other cultures, such as in Singapore, the patterns and settings of the outbreaks are virtually identical—only the symptoms are different (Phoon, 1982). For example, the Singapore women break into screaming and violent behaviors and report seeing hallucinations that are consistent with their religious beliefs. Even in Western society, the symptoms in MPI cases have changed substantially over the past 500 years. For example, in the Middle Ages it was not uncommon to find outbreaks of dancing or laughing manias, nuns meowing like cats, or even religious visions (Markush, 1973).

The cultural data, then, strongly suggest that people in different cultures at different periods in history do and have perceived their bodies in quite different ways. These differences are quite compatible with the notions of hypothesis formation and selective search. That is, within a given culture, people interpret identical sensory information in ways that are congruent with prevailing medical or religious beliefs. Under appropriate settings, people will selectively attend to internal sensations to verify the hypotheses they hold.

PERSONALITY MEASURES

As might be expected, there are a large number of personality inventories that are related to symptom reporting. In addition, the sheer number of scales that directly measure symptom reporting is expanding rapidly. Within this section of the chapter, we first discuss measures of symptom reporting and then point to several of the psychological constructs that are related. As will be seen, most of the correlates of symptom reporting are related to either attentional focus, competence, or related measures.

Symptom-Report Measures

There are several ways to measure symptom reporting. Perhaps the most standard is to ask subjects the degree to which they typically experience such symptoms as a racing heart, headache, sweating, shortness of breath, and so on. Although some scales will specify a time frame (e.g., within the last year, month), most do not. Scales of this nature include the Cornell Medical Index (Abramson, Terespolsky, Brook, & Kark, 1965), the Hopkins Symptom Checklist (Derogatis, Lipman, Rickels, Uhlenhuth, & Covi, 1974), the MMPI Hypochondriasis Scale (Hathaway & McKinley, 1942), the Somatic Perception Questionnaire (e.g., Shields & Stern, 1979), Langner's (1962) 22-item symptom checklist, Miller, Murphy, and Buss's (1981) body consciousness scale, the Autonomic Perception Questionnaire (Mandler, Mandler, & Uviller, 1958), and our own Pennebaker Inventory of Limbic Languidness or the PILL (Pennebaker, 1982). A particularly interesting quality of each of these scales is that each is internally consistent. This means that a person who reports any one particular symptom is likely to report others. The tendency to report physical symptoms, then, is a stable, unidimensional construct. Although the specific items for each of these scales is relatively similar, it is interesting to note that the researchers who use them often have very different goals in mind.

Some of the scales, for example, have attempted to assess the accuracy by which subjects perceive objectively measured autonomic change (e.g., the Autonomic Perception Questionnaire, the Miller *et al.* body consciousness scale). As a rule, these attempts have produced mixed results (see Pennebaker, 1982, 1983, for an extended discussion of this issue). Other symptom scales are said to measure psychological distress (e.g., the Langner questionnaire), hypochondriasis, or even generalized anxiety (see Spielberger, 1972). Because it is beyond the scope of this chapter to evaluate all the above-mentioned scales, suffice it to say that they are similar in that they tap different aspects of perceived body state.

In addition to the symptom inventories that require subjects to report the frequency and/or occurrence of symptoms in a retrospective manner, many of the studies cited in this chapter simply ask respondents to report the degree to which they are *currently* experiencing selected symptoms. As with the retrospective inventories, such scales are internally consistent and correlate highly with the larger symptom inventories (Pennebaker & Skelton, 1978).

Correlates of Symptom Reporting

Although a large number of individual difference measures correlate with symptom reporting, two general constructs—attentiveness to body and measures of competence or control—have consistently been related to reports of symptoms. Not surprisingly, people who chronically attend to internal states tend to report a large number of symptoms, visit physicians, and take more over-the-counter drugs than do people who are not attentive to their bodies.

For example, Greenley and Mechanic (1976) note that students who identify with introspective others report more symptoms than students who do not. Measures of repression–sensitization correlate with frequency and severity of reported illness and health center utilization (e.g., Byrne, Steinberg, & Schwartz, 1968). Sensitizers process more internal sensory information and more readily perceive the onset of illness. Of particular relevance is the fact that a dispositional measure of self-consciousness (Fenigstein, Scheier, & Buss, 1975) consistently correlates with measures of symptom reporting (Pennebaker & Skelton, 1978). Individuals who are rated as high in private self-consciousness are attentive to their thoughts and moods.

Measures of anxiety level, such as the Manifest Anxiety Scale (Taylor, 1953), are correlated positively with symptom reporting (Lipman, Rickels, Covi, Derogatis, & Uhlenhuth, 1969). In fact, about a quarter of the items on the scale are symptom related (e.g., "I often have butterflies in my stomach"). As an aside, Wine (1971) notes that high-test-anxious subjects perform poorly on exams because they are processing a disproportionate amount of internal sensory information relative to the tests they are taking. This is an intriguing example of the dysfunctional processing of internal cues.

Scales tapping control or competence have also been found to be inversely related to symptom reporting and illness rates. For example, externals on Rotter's I-E scale (Rotter, 1966) report more symptoms than internals (e.g., Kilpatrick, Dubin, & Marcotte, 1974). Measures of self-esteem indicate that the higher the self-esteem, the fewer symptoms reported (e.g., Rosa & Mazur, 1974; Rosenberg, 1965). Helmreich (1972) has noted that the concept of self-esteem implies the ability to control or be competent in dealing with the environment. Manipulated perceived control over the environment also tends to reduce the degree to which subjects report symptoms (e.g., Matthews, Scheier, Brunson, & Carducci, 1980; Pennebaker *et al.*, 1977; Weidner & Matthews, 1978). In each of the examples above, then, individuals who do not perceive themselves as being in control of their environments report more symptoms than do those who feel more in control.

Consistent with these studies, measures of life change and major loss of control events are related to a large number of health-related problems. For example, subjects who report experiencing several major life changes on the Schedule of Recent Experience (Holmes & Rahe, 1967) claim to have more health problems in college (e.g., Marx, Garrity & Bowers, 1975) and in the military (Rahe, Mahan, & Arthur, 1970). The life events scale has also been shown to be related to accidents, heart disease, and cancer, as well as symptom reporting (see Graham, 1972). Other measures of life change (e.g., Jacobs, Spilken, Norman, & Anderson, 1970) report comparable results.

Competence and control measures may be related to symptom reporting for a variety of reasons. One argument is that failure to control the external environment is highly stressful, thus resulting in major physiological upheavals (e.g., Seligman, 1975; Selye, 1976). Another factor may be that loss of control experiences influence the subjects' attention and/or cognitive strategies. For example, Matthews *et al.* (1980) note that unpredictable noise bursts (relative to predictable bursts) cause the person to monitor the external environment more closely. The "psychic cost" of the increased attentional effort is then expressed physiologically. Finally, loss of control experiences may cause the person to adopt symptom-relevant hypotheses and thus selectively search their bodies in greater detail. Several parametric studies must ultimately be conducted to evaluate the loss of control–symptom link.

EMOTIONS, PSYCHOSOMATICS, AND PHYSIOLOGICAL FACTORS

The present chapter has presented several facts and findings concerning physical symptoms in a rather cursory manner. To gain a full understanding of the issues, it would be useful to publish a sequel to *Social Psycho-*

physiology entitled *Physical Symptoms: The True Story.* Because the interested reader may not have the patience to wait for the book (or the movie), this final section will briefly present a few topics that are intimately related to the perception of physical symptoms.

Emotions

For decades, there have been attempts to link emotions, internal sensations, and physiological change. Early research attempted to show that positive emotions were felt in different regions of the body than negative feelings (e.g., Hoisington, 1928; Nafe, 1924). Similarly, specificity theories of emotion that posited a one-to-one correspondence between unique emotions and specific physiological change implicitly assumed that different emotions were characterized by unique sensations (e.g., Cannon, 1931; James, 1890/1950; see also related chapters in this volume). These approaches raise two fundamental questions. First, is there a one-to-one correspondence between perceived emotions and perceived symptoms? If so, what is the causal link between them (i.e., do they occur simultaneously or does one precede the other)?

Over the last few years, we have begun addressing these questions. First, we have found that separate emotions are characterized by unique clusters of reported physical symptoms (Pennebaker, 1982; Skelton, 1981). For example, symptoms of queasy stomach and lump in throat correlate highly with perceptions of guilt; reports of tense muscles, racing heart, and tightness in jaw are related to anger; and so on. By instructing subjects to "feel" each of these unique symptom clusters, they report experiencing the concomitant emotion from which the symptoms were derived. Alternatively, requiring subjects to feel one of several emotions (anger, guilt, joy, fear, embarrassment, sadness) results in the reporting of unique symptom clusters (see Ross, Rodin, & Zimbardo, 1969, for evidence of a comparable process applied to pain reduction).

These findings clearly raise more questions than they answer. Are emotion–symptom clusters the results of culturally defined body hypotheses? Are our beliefs about symptoms congruent with autonomic activity corresponding to the symptoms? If the answer is yes, there are some intriguing—and perhaps frightening—implications for the pharmacological manipulation of even subtle emotions. Finally, the links between emotions and symptoms raise a number of philosophical questions concerning mind and body, specificity, and even linguistic definition of emotion.

Psychosomatics

As noted at the beginning of this chapter, researchers in medicine and psychophysiology have focused almost exclusively on physiological change as opposed to the perception of change. We often tend to overlook the fact that people make health-related decisions based on their perceptions of internal state. Of course, this chapter is not intended to discourage or undermine the physiological approaches. Rather, in conducting psycho-physiological studies, the researchers would be well advised to also collect self-report data concerning the subjects' perceptions. It should be noted that psychophysiological reactions and self-reports of these reactions may, in fact, be relatively independent. For example, one psychological manipulation that may alter autonomic activity may not influence self-reports of that activity, and vice versa. Future research in psychosomatics, then, should attempt to understand the processes affecting both perceived and actual physiological changes, and ultimately, the links between them.

Physiological Influences

There is a certain irony that this chapter, which has dealt with perceptions of internal state, has rarely mentioned the psychophysiological properties inherent in the symptom-reporting process. A harsh critic might suggest that this is analogous to a psychophysicist writing a chapter about judgments of light intensity without ever measuring luminosity. This omission has been intentional. Most studies find very low correlations between self-reports of physiological change and actual change—both between and within subjects (see Blascovich & Katkin, Chapter 17, this volume; Pennebaker, 1982, 1983; Pennebaker *et al.*, 1982; Pennebaker & Skelton, 1978).

In addition, some recent work in our laboratory suggests that we may be approaching the perceived–actual physiological link inappropriately. In recent years, researchers in perception have suggested that individuals encode change information as opposed to static sources of information (e.g., Gibson, 1979; Johansson, vonHofsten, & Jannson, 1980). According to this view, we do not encode absolute levels of visual information or static arrays. For example, if a visual image is projected to a constant area on the retina, the person soon fails to "see" the image (Riggs, Ratliff, Cornsweet, & Cornsweet, 1953). Either the eye must be constantly moving or the environmental stimulus changing in some respect for us to perceive external objects.

Comparable processes may occur in the perception of internal state. That is, we only encode *changes* in autonomic levels. If something such as skin temperature remains constant, we are not able to perceive it. A good example of this may occur among diabetics with fluctuating blood glucose levels. If the patient has an abnormally high but stable blood glucose reading, he or she reports feeling fine. However, if the physician lowers the blood glucose level to a normal (i.e., safe) range, the patient reports symptoms typically associated with very low glucose readings (Pennebaker, Cox, Gonder-Frederick, Wunsch, Evans, & Pohl, 1981).

All of this suggests that symptom researchers have been measuring autonomic activity in a different way than the way in which we perceive the activity. We must ultimately adapt our physiological output to the ways in which individuals encode this information. Our research in this area is in the very early stages. Nevertheless, it may offer new hope to the disappointing results that have traditionally been obtained between perceived and actual physiological activity.

REFERENCES

Abramson, J. H., Terespolsky, L., Brook, J. G., & Kark, S. L.   Cornell Medical Index as a health measure in epidemiological studies. A test of the validity of a health questionnaire. *British Journal of Preventive Medicine*, 1965, *19*, 102–110.

Berlyne, D.   *Conflict, arousal, and curiosity.* New York: McGraw-Hill, 1960.

Boardman, V.   School absences, illness and family competence. In B. Caplan & J. Cassel (Eds.), *Family and health: An epidemiologic approach.* Chapel Hill, N.C.: University of North Carolina, Institute for Research in Social Science, 1975.

Brener, J.   Visceral perception. In J. Beatty & J. Legewie (Eds.), *Biofeedback and behavior.* New York: Plenum, 1977.

Bruner, J. S.   Going beyond the information given. In *Contemporary approaches to cognition: A symposium held at the University of Colorado.* Cambridge, Mass.: Harvard University Press, 1957.

Byrne, D., Steinberg, M., & Schwartz, M.   Relationship between repression–sensitization and physical illness. *Journal of Abnormal Psychology*, 1968, *73*, 154–155.

Campbell, J.   Illness as a point of view: The development of children's concepts of illness. *Child Development*, 1975, *46*, 92–100.

Cannon, W.   Again the James–Lange and the thalamic theories of emotion. *Psychological Review*, 1931, *38*, 281–295.

Carver, C., Coleman, A. E., & Glass, D. C.   The coronary-prone behavior pattern and the suppression of fatigue on a treadmill test. *Journal of Personality and Social Psychology*, 1976, *33*, 460–466.

Coburn, D.   Job-worker incongruence: Consequences for health. *Journal of Health and Social Behavior*, 1975, *16*, 198–212.

Colligan, M. J., Pennebaker, J. W., & Murphy, L. (Eds.).   *Mass psychogenic illness: A social psychological analysis.* Hillsdale, N.J.: Erlbaum, 1982.

Comstock, L., & Slome, C.   A health survey of students: 1. Prevalence of problems. *Journal of the American College Health Association*, 1973, *22*, 150–155.

Derogatis, L. R., Lipman, R. S., Rickels, K., Uhlenhuth, E. H., & Covi, L.   The Hopkins symptom checklist (HSCL): A measure of primary symptom dimensions. *Psychological Measurement in Psychopharmacology*, 1974, *7*, 79–110.

Eisen, M., Ware, J., Donald, C., & Brook, R.   Measuring components of children's health status. *Medical Care*, 1979, *17*, 902–921.

Fenigstein, A., Scheier, M., & Buss, A.   Public and private self-consciousness: Assessment and theory. *Journal of Consulting and Clinical Psychology*, 1975, *43*, 522–527.

Fischer, J., Fischer, A., & Mahony, F.   Totemism and allergy. *International Journal of Social Psychiatry*, 1959, *5*, 33–40.

Franklin, B.   Birth order and tendency to "adopt the sick role." *Psychological Reports*, 1973, *33*, 437–438.

Friedman, R.   Some characteristics of families of children with "psychogenic" pain. *Journal of Clinical Child Psychology*, 1975, *4*, 21–23.

Gibson, J. J.   *The ecological approach to visual perception.* Boston: Houghton-Mifflin, 1979.

Gonda, T. A.   The relation between complaints of persistent pain and family size. *Journal of Neurology, Neurosurgery, and Psychiatry*, 1962, *25*, 277–281.

Gonder-Frederick, L. A.   *Physical symptoms associated with blood pressure and glucose levels in diabetics.* Unpublished master's thesis, The University of Virginia, 1981.

Graham, D.   Psychosomatic medicine. In N. Greenfield & R. Sternbach (Eds.), *Handbook of psychophysiology.* New York: Holt, Rinehart & Winston, 1972.

Greenley, J., & Mechanic, D.   Social selection in seeking help for psychological problems. *Journal of Health and Social Behavior*, 1976, *17*, 249–262.

Haber, R. N., & Hershenson, M.   *The psychology of visual perception.* New York: Holt, Rinehart & Winston, 1973.

Harrison, R.   *Job stress as person-environment fit.* Washington, D.C.: American Psychological Association, 1976.

Hathaway, S. R., & McKinley, J. C.   *Minnesota multiphasic personality inventory.* Minneapolis: University of Minnesota Press, 1942.

Helmreich, R.   Stress, self-esteem and attitudes. In B. King & E. McGinnies (Eds.), *Attitudes, conflict and social change.* New York: Academic, 1972.

Hoisington, L. B.   Pleasantness and unpleasantness as modes of bodily experience. In M. Reymert (Ed.), *Feelings and emotions: The Wittenberg Symposium.* Worcester, Mass.: Clark University Press, 1928.

Holmes, T., & Rahe, R.   The social readjustment rating scale. *Journal of Psychosomatic Research*, 1967, *4*, 213–218.

Jacobs, M., Spilken, A., Norman, M., & Anderson, L.   Life stress and respiratory illness. *Psychosomatic Medicine*, 1970, *32*, 233–242.

James, W.   *The principles of psychology.* New York: Dover, 1950. (Originally published, 1890.)

Jessner, L., Blom, G. E., & Waldfogel, S.   Emotional implications of tonsillectomy and adenoidectomy on children. *Psychoanalytic Study of the Child*, 1952, *7*, 126–169.

Johansson, G., vonHofsten, C., & Jansson, G.   Event perception. *Annual Review of Psychology*, 1980, *31*, 27–63.

Jospe, M.   *The placebo effect in healing.* Lexington, Mass.: Lexington Books, 1978.

Kerckhoff, A., & Back, K.   *The June bug: A study of hysterical contagion.* New York: Appleton-Century-Crofts, 1968.

Kilpatrick, D., Dubin, W., & Marcotte, D.   Personality, stress of the medical education process, and changes in affective mood. *Psychological Reports*, 1974, *34*, 1215–1223.

Langner, T.   A twenty-two item screening score of psychiatric symptoms indicating impairment. *Journal of Health and Human Behavior*, 1962, *3*, 269–276.

Leventhal, H.   The consequences of depersonalization during illness and treatment. In J. Howard & A. Strauss (Eds.), *Humanizing health care.* New York: Wiley, 1975.

Lindsay, P. H., & Norman, D. A.   *Human information processing.* New York: Academic, 1977.

Lipman, R., Rickels, K., Covi, L., Derogatis, L., & Uhlenhuth, E.   Factors of symptom distress. *Archives of General Psychiatry*, 1969, *21*, 328–338.

Mandler, G., Mandler, J. M., & Uviller, E. T.   Autonomic feedback: The perception of autonomic activity. *Journal of Abnormal and Social Psychology*, 1958, *56*, 367–373.

Markush, R. E.   Mental epidemics: A review of the old to prepare for the new. *Public Health Reviews*, 1973, 353–442.

Marx, M., Garrity, T., & Bowers, F.   The influence of recent life experience on the health of college freshmen. *Journal of Psychosomatic Research*, 1975, *19*, 87–98.

Matthews, K. A.   Efforts to control by children and adults with the Type A coronary-prone behavior pattern. *Child Development*, 1979, *50*, 842–847.

Matthews, K., Scheier, M. F., Brunson, B. I., & Carducci, B.   Attention, unpredictability, and reports of physical symptoms. *Journal of Personality and Social Psychology*, 1980, *38*, 525–537.

Mead, M.   *Sex and temperament in three primitive societies.* New York: Mentor, 1950.

Mechanic, D. The influence of mothers on their children's health attitudes and behaviors. *Pediatrics*, 1964, *33*, 444–453.

Mechanic, D. Development of psychological distress among young adults. *Archives of General Psychiatry*, 1979, *36*, 1233–1239.

Meyer, D., Leventhal, H., & Gutman, M. *Symptoms in hypertension*. Unpublished manuscript, Department of Psychology, University of Wisconsin, Madison, 1980.

Miller, L. C., Murphy, R., & Buss, A. H. Consciousness of body: Private and public. *Journal of Personality and Social Psychology*, 1981, *41*, 397–406.

Minuchin, S., Baker, L., Rosman, B., Liebman, R., Milman, L., & Todd, T. A conceptual model of psychosomatic illness in children. *Archives of General Psychiatry*, 1975, *32*, 1031–1038.

Moos, R. *Evaluating correctional and community settings*. New York: Wiley, 1975.

Moos, R., & Van Dort, B. Physical and emotional symptoms and campus health center utilization. *Social Psychiatry*, 1977, *12*, 107–115.

Mutter, A. Z., & Schleifer, M. J. The role of psychological and social factors in the onset of somatic illness in children. *Psychosomatic Medicine*, 1966, *28*, 333–343.

Nafe, J. P. An experimental study of the affective qualities. *American Journal of Psychology*, 1924, *35*, 507–544.

National Center for Health Statistics. *Use habits among adults of cigarettes, coffee, aspirin, and sleeping pills* (Public Health Series 10, No. 131). Washington, D.C.: U.S. Government Printing Office, 1979.

Navon, D., & Gopher, D. On the economy of the human-processing system. *Psychological Review*, 1979, *86*, 214–255.

Neisser, U. *Cognition and reality*. San Francisco: W. H. Freeman, 1976.

Pennebaker, J. W. Perceptual and environmental determinants of coughing. *Basic and Applied Social Psychology*, 1980, *1*, 83–91.

Pennebaker, J. W. Stimulus characteristics influencing estimation of heart rate. *Psychophysiology*, 1981, *18*, 540–548.

Pennebaker, J. W. *The psychology of physical symptoms*. New York: Springer-Verlag, 1982.

Pennebaker, J. W. Accuracy of physical symptoms. In A. Baum, J. E. Singer, & S. E. Taylor (Eds.), *Handbook of psychology and health* (Vol. 4). Hillsdale, N.J.: Erlbaum, 1983.

Pennebaker, J. W., & Brittingham, G. L. Environmental and sensory cues affecting the perception of physical symptoms. In A. Baum & J. E. Singer (Eds.), *Advances in environmental psychology* (Vol. 4). Hillsdale, N.J.: Erlbaum, 1982.

Pennebaker, J. W., Burnam, M. A., Schaeffer, M. A., & Harper, D. Lack of control as a determinant of perceived physical symptoms. *Journal of Personality and Social Psychology*, 1977, *35*, 167–174.

Pennebaker, J. W., Cox, D. J., Gonder-Frederick, L. A., Wunsch, M., Evans, W. S., & Pohl, S. Physical symptoms related to blood glucose in insulin dependent diabetics. *Psychosomatic Medicine*, 1981, *43*, 489–500.

Pennebaker, J. W., Gonder-Frederick, L. A., Stewart, H., Elfman, L., & Skelton, J. A. Physical symptoms associated with blood pressure. *Psychophysiology*, 1982, *19*, 201–210.

Pennebaker, J. W., Hendler, C. S., Durrett, M. E., & Richards, P. Social factors influencing absenteeism due to illness in nursery school children. *Child Development*, 1981, *52*, 692–700.

Pennebaker, J. W., & Lightner, J. M. Competition of internal and external information in an exercise setting. *Journal of Personality and Social Psychology*, 1980, *39*, 165–174.

Pennebaker, J. W., & Newtson, D. Observation of a unique event: Psychological impact of Mt. St. Helens volcano. In H. Reis (Ed.), *Naturalistic approaches to studying social interaction*. San Francisco: Jossey-Bass, 1983.

Pennebaker, J. W., & Skelton, J. A. Psychological parameters of physical symptoms. *Personality and Social Psychology Bulletin*, 1978, *4*, 524–530.

Pennebaker, J. W., & Skelton, J. A. Selective monitoring of bodily sensations. *Journal of Personality and Social Psychology*, 1981, *41*, 213–223.

Phoon, W. H.   Outbreaks of mass hysteria at workplaces in Singapore: Some patterns and modes of presentation. In M. Colligan, J. W. Pennebaker, & L. Murphy (Eds.), *Mass psychogenic illness: A social psychological analysis.* Hillsdale, N.J.: Erlbaum, 1982.

Rahe, R., Mahan, J., & Arthur, R.   Prediction of near-future health change from subjects preceding life changes. *Journal of Psychosomatic Research*, 1970, *14*, 401–406.

Raper, A.   The incidence of peptic ulceration in some African tribal groups. *Transactions of the Royal Society of Tropical Medicine and Hygiene*, 1958, *152*, 535–546.

Rickels, K.   *Non-specific factors in drug therapy.* Springfield, Ill.: Charles C Thomas, 1968.

Riggs, L. A., Ratliff, F., Cornsweet, J. C., & Cornsweet, T. N.   The disappearance of steadily-fixed objects. *Journal of the Optical Society of America*, 1953, *43*, 495–501.

Rosa, E., & Mazur, A.   Validity test of the relation between self-esteem and psychosomatic symptoms. *Humboldt Journal of Social Relations*, 1974, *1*, 144–145.

Rosenberg, M.   *Society and the adolescent self image.* Princeton, N.J.: Princeton University Press, 1965.

Ross, L., Rodin, J., & Zimbardo, P.   Toward an attribution therapy: The reduction of fear through induced cognitive–emotional misattribution. *Journal of Personality and Social Psychology*, 1969, *12*, 279–288.

Rotter, J.   Generalized expectancies for internal versus external control of reinforcement. *Psychological Monographs*, 1966, *80*.

Seligman, M.   *Helplessness.* San Francisco: W. H. Freeman, 1975.

Selye, H.   *The stress of life.* New York: McGraw-Hill, 1976.

Sheldrake, P., Cormack, M., & McGuire, J.   Psychosomatic illness, birth order and intellectual preference: I. Men. *Journal of Psychosomatic Research*, 1976, *20*, 37–44.

Shields, S. A., & Stern, R. M.   Emotion: The perception of bodily change. In P. Pliner, K. R. Blankstein, & I. M. Spigel (Eds.), *Perception of emotion in self and others.* New York: Plenum, 1979.

Skelton, J. A.   *Specificity of bodily information in the self-perception of emotion.* Unpublished doctoral dissertation, The University of Virginia, 1981.

Skelton, J. A., & Pennebaker, J. W.   The psychology of physical symptoms and sensations. In G. Sanders & J. Suls (Eds.), *Social psychology of health and illness.* Hillsdale, N.J.: Erlbaum, 1982.

Snyder, M.   Self-monitoring processes. In L. Berkowitz (Ed.), *Advances in experimental social psychology* (Vol. 12). New York: Academic, 1979.

Spielberger, C. D.   Conceptual and methodological issues in anxiety research. In C. D. Spielberger (Ed.), *Anxiety: Current trends in theory and research.* New York: Academic, 1972.

Sternbach, R., & Tursky, B.   Ethnic differences among housewives in psychophysical and skin potential responses to electric shock. *Psychophysiology*, 1965, *1*, 241–246.

Stevens, S. S.   *Psychophysics: Introduction to its perceptual, neural, and social prospects.* New York: Wiley, 1975.

Taylor, J.   A personality scale of manifest anxiety. *Journal of Abnormal and Social Psychology*, 1953, *48*, 285–290.

Taylor, S. E., & Crocker, J.   Schematic bases of social information processing. In E. T. Higgins et al. (Eds.), *The Ontario Symposium on Personality and Social Psychology.* Hillsdale, N.J.: Erlbaum, 1981.

Tursky, B., & Sternbach, R.   Further physiological correlates of ethnic differences in responses to shock. *Psychophysiology*, 1967, *4*, 67–74.

Walster, B., & Aronson, E.   Effect of expectancy of task duration on the experience of fatigue. *Journal of Experimental Social Psychology*, 1967, *3*, 41–46.

Wan, T.   Predicting self-assessed health status: A multivariate approach. *Health Services Research*, 1976, *11*, 464–477.

Weidner, G., & Matthews, K.   Reported physical symptoms elicited by unpredictable events and the type A coronary-prone behavior pattern. *Journal of Personality and Social Psychology*, 1978, *36*, 1213–1220.

Weiman, C. A study of occupational stressor and the incidence of disease/risk. *Journal of Occupational Medicine*, 1977, *19*, 119–122.

Wine, J. Test anxiety and direction of attention. *Psychological Bulletin*, 1971, *76*, 92–104.

Woods, S., Natterson, J., & Silverman, J. Medical students' disease: Hypochondriasis in medical education. *Journal of Medical Education*, 1966, *41*, 785–790.

Wright, D., Kane, R., Olsen, D., & Smith, T. The effects of selected psychosocial factors on the self-reporting of pulmonary symptoms. *Journal of Chronic Diseases*, 1977, *30*, 195–206.

Zborowski, M. *People in pain*. San Francisco: Jossey-Bass, 1969.

Zola, I. Culture and symptoms: An analysis of patients presenting complaints. *American Sociological Review*, 1966, *31*, 615–630.

CHAPTER 20

Arousal-Induced Eating: Conventional Wisdom or Empirical Finding?

Lynn Spitzer
Yale University

Judith Rodin
Yale University

In recent years, concepts such as "arousal," "activation," and "stress" have been used with increasing frequency in the literature examining human food intake and body weight regulation. Because of numerous clinical reports of stress-induced eating and overeating in the obese (Bruch, 1973; Conrad, 1954; Freed, 1947; Hamburger, 1951; Kaplan & Kaplan, 1957; Leon, 1975; Sjöberg & Persson, 1979), many investigators reasoned that eating or overeating in response to emotional arousal might be a mechanism by which individuals gain weight or maintain an already overweight state. Of special interest was the speculation that some people may eat when emotionally aroused since emotional arousal is often an aversive state and eating is thought to be anxiety reducing (Kaplan & Kaplan, 1957). Bruch (1973) suggested further that emotional arousal is often confused with actual hunger and eating also occurs because of this confusion. These ideas are often referred to as the psychosomatic hypothesis of obesity. There has now been a fair amount of research in this area, which considered experimentally whether the obese did, in fact, eat more in response to emotional arousal as compared to normal-weight individuals and whether eating, in turn, reduced the arousal.

EARLY CONSIDERATIONS
OF THE AROUSAL–EATING RELATIONSHIP

Although most of the studies exploring the notion that anxiety, fear, and other forms of emotional arousal influence eating have employed very similar experimental paradigms, a variety of hypotheses were posed regarding why emotional arousal should be expected to influence eating. For example, in the first experiment to examine the effects of emotional arousal on the eating behavior of both normal-weight and obese individuals, S. Schachter, Goldman, and Gordon (1968) proposed a hypothesis that had very different theoretical roots from the psychosomatic hypothesis discussed above. Specifically, Schachter and his colleagues speculated that overweight individuals were more responsive to food cues in the environment and less responsive to internal physiological signals than were normal-weight individuals (S. Schachter, 1968). Since fear had previously been shown to inhibit gastric motility (Carlson, 1916) and to suppress the release of sugar from the liver into the blood (Cannon, 1915), and since these internal responses were considered to be important physiological correlates of food deprivation, the investigators reasoned that normal-weight individuals should be more responsive to manipulations of fear than overweight persons. More specifically, it was predicted that normal-weight individuals would eat less in response to fear and that the eating behavior of obese individuals would be unaffected by degree of fear.

In order to examine the effects of fear on eating behavior, subjects were threatened with either very painful electrical stimulation (the high-fear condition) or very mild electrical stimulation (the low-fear condition). Then, under the guise of a taste test, they were given the opportunity to eat as much as they liked from a bowl of crackers. Ratings of anxiety were taken before and after eating. Normal-weight subjects in the high-fear condition ate significantly fewer crackers than did their normal-weight counterparts in the low-fear condition. Overweight subjects ate slightly but not significantly more in the high-fear condition than in the low-fear condition. Neither the obese nor normal-weight subjects exhibited significant fear reduction as a consequence of eating. Thus, S. Schachter *et al.* (1968) concluded that their hypothesis was supported by the data and that the psychosomatic hypothesis of obesity, which asserts that the obese confuse hunger with negative affect (Bruch, 1961, 1973) and that overeating reduces states of emotional arousal (Kaplan & Kaplan, 1957), was disconfirmed.

In a subsequent study, McKenna (1972) suggested that the psychosomatic hypothesis would perhaps only be expected to apply when *tasty* food was available. S. Schachter *et al.* (1968) used crackers, and admittedly crackers are a rather neutral food, neither greatly liked nor disliked by most people. McKenna predicted that the replacement of crackers with extremely appetizing and tasty chocolate chip cookies would elicit significant overeating by the obese in an anxious state. In order to produce a state of anxiety in subjects in the experimental condition, McKenna told them that later in the experiment some direct physiological measurements, including a rather extensive blood sample, a urine specimen, and rectal stool sample, would be taken. Subjects in the low-anxiety condition were not led to expect these physiological tests. Using good-tasting cookies, McKenna found a significant interaction between body weight and anxiety.

However, this interaction was accounted for by a reduction in amount eaten by normal-weight subjects under conditions of anxiety as well as an increase in amount eaten by overweight subjects. In addition, there was no evidence of anxiety reduction after eating. McKenna, however, argued that the temporal arrangements of his experiment may have prevented accurate measures of eating-induced anxiety reduction and suggested that anxiety reduction might be an ephemeral effect that had dissipated by the time he was able to assess it.

In a later experiment, Herman and Polivy (1975) incorporated both a good-tasting food (ice cream) and an immediate assessment of anxiety-reduction effects. Unlike previous studies, the investigators were not concerned with obese–normal differences. Instead, they were interested in the effects of emotional arousal on the eating behavior of people who consciously try to control their food intake (i.e., restrained eaters) and those who do not (unrestrained eaters). Emotional arousal was regarded as a disruptor of conscious behavioral regulation, and thus it was predicted that restrained eaters would eat more in response to emotional arousal.

Conducted under the guise of a study on sensory psychology, subjects were threatened with severe electric shock and then given ice cream, presumably to make taste ratings. Actually, the experimenters were interested only in the amount subjects ate. A control group of subjects was offered food in the same way, but was not threatened with severe electric shock. Unrestrained eaters ate significantly less when anxious and restrained eaters ate slightly more, although this increase was not significant. There was no decrease in reported anxiety after subjects had eaten the ice cream.

These three studies essentially produced very similar findings, that is, a small increase in consumption for overweight or restrained eaters experiencing emotional arousal. However, two other studies employing similar experimental paradigms and similar manipulations of emotional arousal have provided no evidence for increased consumption among overweight individuals under conditions of emotional arousal (Abramson & Wunderlich, 1972; Reznick & Balch, 1977).

Another group of studies using different types of procedures designed to increase emotional arousal has found significant effects of emotional arousal on the eating behavior of obese individuals. For example, White (1973) showed subjects films that were meant to arouse distress (Lazarus's subincision film), humor (Charlie Chaplin's *The Tramp*), and sexual feelings (a stag film). Compared to what they ate after viewing a nonarousing film (an India travelogue), overweight subjects ate significantly more after each of the emotional-arousal-inducing films. There were no significant effects of the manipulation of emotional arousal on the food intake of normal-weight subjects. Another study used loud, irregular noise, a flickering light, and an insoluble puzzle as arousal-inducing stimuli (Meyer & Pudel,

1972). Only obese subjects increased their intake in response to these stimuli.

To explain these seemingly disparate effects of different emotion-inducing stimuli on eating behavior of obese individuals, Slochower (1976) noted that the psychosomatic hypothesis implies that the emotional state that triggers eating is diffuse and its source frequently not understood to the individual. If this is the case, it seems plausible that only vague and undefined emotional responses trigger eating in the obese person. The experiments discussed thus far seem likely to differ in the extent to which they encouraged or allowed subjects to label and appropriately interpret their emotional state. Thus, possibly the extent to which subjects found an appropriate explanation or label for their emotional arousal may have influenced its effects on eating behavior. Slochower (1976) tested this hypothesis and found that obese subjects ate more when they could not identify the cause of their emotional arousal than when a clear cause was known. When obese subjects were calm, the presence or absence of a label did not affect their eating.

Finally, it should be noted that subjects not specifically selected or classified according to body weight have also been shown to increase their food intake in response to emotional arousal. For example, a study conducted in a naturalistic, nonlaboratory setting found a significant anxiety-induced increase in amount eaten (Pines & Gal, 1977). They reported that subjects in several classes who were unselected for body weight ate more food during an anxiety-provoking exam than during a nonthreatening lecture. In a laboratory study (Glass, 1967), subjects who, again, were not selected or classified according to body weight, increased their consumption in response to a distressing film.

These data, taken together, suggest that eating induced by emotional arousal sometimes, but not always, increases eating in overweight people and sometimes suppresses eating among their normal-weight counterparts. No single theory advanced thus far is sufficiently parsimonious to explain these findings, and we are led to conclude that they are most likely due to differences in procedure and sampling. As we have said elsewhere (Rodin, 1981b; Spitzer & Rodin, 1981), differences from study to study between overweight and normal-weight subjects appear to depend, for example, on the prior weight history of subjects and whether they are in a static or weight-gaining phase at the time of testing. We have outlined more systematic sampling procedures which should begin to deal with such confounding problems in future research.

The fact that many investigators have used a variety of manipulations to induce emotional arousal and a variety of measures to assess its effects also makes it difficult to integrate and interpret the literature in this area. Throughout this chapter, when possible, we will try to label clearly the type or aspect of arousal that the authors were interested in as well as the type of arousal manipulations and measures that were used.

Recently, the relevant research on arousal and eating in animals has been reviewed by Robbins and Fray (1980). An even more diverse array of putative arousing stimuli has been used in animal research than in human research. For example, electric shock, tail pinch, the presence of complex stimuli, the presence of other animals, and social isolation have all been used as manipulations of arousal. Because of space limitations, it is impossible to review all of these animal studies and the interested reader is referred to Robbins and Fray (1980). Suffice it to say, however, that a variety of putative arousing stimuli do appear to increase amount eaten even in sated animals.

Although the human studies have produced mixed findings on the effects of emotional arousal of amount eaten, most researchers and clinicians, ourselves included, continued to believe that emotional-arousal-induced eating does exist in the real world, at least in some individuals. One reason for this is the consistent and numerous accounts of this phenomenon that are heard routinely in clinical practice and have been regularly reported in the clinical literature (Bruch, 1973; Conrad, 1954; Freed, 1947; Hamburger, 1951; Kaplan & Kaplan, 1957; Leon, 1975; Sjöberg & Persson, 1979). It is important to emphasize, however, that one does not have to hold with an ego-defensive or anxiety-reduction theory in order to explain the relationship between emotional arousal and eating. One alternative is that anxiety and other forms of emotional arousal may be regarded as disruptors of behavior, including self-control, which might then serve to disinhibit hunger-motivated eating behavior. As mentioned earlier, Herman and Polivy (1975) have reported some tendency for normal-weight, chronically self-restrained dieters to overeat when anxious, which may be explained on the basis of a process of disinhibition.

A second alternative is that increased emotional arousal may increase food intake by making an individual more responsive to salient food cues present in the environment (Rodin, 1977). This line of reasoning is supported by the White (1973) study, in which overweight subjects ate significantly more after viewing each of three films intended to arouse very different emotions as compared to viewing a nonarousing film. Importantly, the specific content of the arousing stimulus (i.e., whether the film was distressing, humorous, or sexual) did not affect amount eaten. Thus, pleasant emotional arousal (i.e., humor) as well as unpleasant emotional arousal (i.e., distress) can influence eating in a similar way.

Even though the available clinical and experimental data suggest that emotional arousal does influence food consumption in some individuals, it is clear that the role of arousal in food intake and body weight regulation requires much further clarification.

First, most of the experiments on humans have used manipulations that were intended to produce emotional arousal. When these manipulations were not simply assumed to have their intended effects, manipulation checks generally consisted of some type of self-report of emotional arousal. No measures of actual physiological arousal were taken. Clearly, the subjective feeling that one is emotionally aroused does not *necessarily* mean that an individual will show physiological arousal. Although it seems reasonable to assume that subjective feelings of emotional arousal and actual physiological arousal often occur together, one cannot assume that it is always the case. This is an important point since these two variables may have differential effects on eating behavior. Unfortunately, this distinction has not generally been made by investigators in this area, thus, possibly, leading to such disparate findings as those reported above.

This lack of clarity regarding the distinctions among different types or aspects of arousal is not totally surprising since, at this time, arousal can only be thought of as a working simplification and abstraction of a construct that is not yet well defined. A later section deals explicitly with the concept of arousal as it has been used in the psychological literature.

Aside from the confusion about the meaning of the concept of arousal, another issue that needs to be addressed is the differentiation among eating, overeating, and obesity as responses to any type of arousal. The relationship of arousal to all three of these variables has been imputed, but confused. For example, the data that we have just presented, which suggest that emotional arousal sometimes produces an increase in amount eaten for overweight people, is often cited as evidence that arousal-induced eating causes obesity. This inference, however, is problematic for several reasons.

First, there is no strong evidence at present that an increase in amount eaten, when food intake is induced by arousal, will not be compensated for later in some way, for example, by delaying the next meal or eating less. In addition, even if arousal is shown to lead to overeating, the amount of food one ingests during relatively short time periods cannot be presumed to be the sole determinant of the levels of body weight that are maintained over the long term (cf. Van Itallie, Smith, & Quartermain, 1977). Furthermore, many correlates of obesity have been shown to be consequences of obesity rather than causes (see Rodin, 1977, 1981a, for review). Thus, even if we find a reliable correlation between arousal-induced eating or overeating and obesity, it is imperative to address the possibility that this behavior may be the result of being overweight as well as the possibility that it is a causal factor. In fact, there is also the possibility that the two are related, but both are caused by a third factor.

The present chapter is intended to explore and develop further these and other ideas about the relationship of various types of arousal to eating, overeating, and body weight regulation. In an attempt to do so, we will first discuss the concept of arousal as it has been previously used in the psychological literature. Second, we will discuss arousal theory as it has been applied to the area of human eating behavior. Third, the role of arousal in the conditioning of eating-related responses will be examined in light of recent data. Finally, the implications of this research, in particular, and research in this area, in general, for understanding food intake and weight regulation will be discussed.

THE CONCEPT OF AROUSAL

Arousal as a Nonspecific Energizer

In a number of different versions of what is now commonly referred to as "arousal theory," several investigators proposed similar roles for the concept of arousal (e.g., Duffy, 1957; Hebb, 1955; Lindsley, 1957; Malmo, 1959). An important characteristic of all of these theories is the assumption that the arousal system responds to a variety of stimuli in a nonspecific manner and, in turn, has nonspecific effects on behavior. In other words, they assumed that, although there are different stimuli that influence arousal, the response of the arousal system to each individual stimulus is the same. In terms of its behavioral function, arousal was thought to energize, rather than direct or guide behavior. More specifically, optimal levels of arousal were thought to increase both the strength or intensity of a prepotent response and the probability that the response would be elicited, but not to alter any specific aspects of an individual's motivational state.

Central to arousal theory is the concept of a continuum of arousal, which ranges from a minimum level of deep sleep to a maximum level of extreme effort or intense emotional excitement or disturbance. Generally, the view has been held that there is an inverted-U-shaped relationship between level of arousal and its effect on behavior (Hebb, 1955). Thus, moderate levels of arousal were presumed to have the greatest energizing effect on prepotent behaviors. However, because the parameters of the hypothetical inverted-U curve between level of arousal and its effect on behavior have never been well defined, most researchers in this area have generally assumed that manipulations intended to increase arousal push most subjects toward a more optimal level of arousal. In other words, they are designed to detect only the rising component of the inverted-U-shaped function.

Closely related to the concept of the arousal system as nonspecific, both in terms of its response to precipitating stimuli as well as its behavioral consequences, was the assumption of an identity among psychophysiological measures reflecting autonomic, somatic, and central nervous system activity and measures of behavioral activation. As a consequence, a variety of psychophysiological responses were thought to provide identical and thereby interchangeable measures of arousal.

The view that there is a common nonspecific component of the arousal system that responds to a variety of stimuli in the same manner has led to the premise that the effects of a number of arousal-inducing stimuli are additive. In other words, if two stimuli that have been shown to increase arousal level by 1 unit and 3 units, respectively, are presented serially, they would produce the same level of arousal as another stimulus that has been shown to increase arousal level by 4 units. Theories of generalized arousal have suggested that this should be expected (Berlyne, 1960).

S. Schachter and his colleagues (S. Schachter & Singer, 1962), have presented data suggesting that different emotional states rest on the same pattern of physiological responses and take their form depending on the nature of cognitive labels that are available. This evidence would lend support to the nonspecific arousal hypothesis. However, recently the methodology of this study has been criticized (Marshall & Zimbardo, 1979; Maslach, 1979).

Problems with the Concept of Nonspecificity

Subsequent research has called for a revision of many of these assumptions. First, evidence of disassociation between particular measures of physiological arousal and measures of behavioral arousal (Elliot, 1966; Lacey, 1967a; Mirsky & Cardon, 1962) raised questions about the supposition that any individual measure of physiological arousal could be viewed as a valid index of the degree of activation of the entire arousal system.

Second, empirical evidence relevant to the notion of arousal as a general and nonspecific system has been mixed. Intraindividual correlations among autonomic and electroencephalographic variables and among a variety of autonomic measure themselves were found to be positive, but rather modest in size (Elliot, 1966; Lazarus, Speisman, & Mordkoff, 1963). Further, several investigators have demonstrated distinctive patterns of physiological responses to diverse emotional and other types of stimuli (Ax, 1953; Funkenstein, King, & Drolette, 1956; Mason, 1975; J. Schachter, 1957). These studies suggest that many of the physiological variables that supposedly constitute the arousal system do not respond to stimuli in a totally nonspecific manner.

Third, there is no clear evidence that arousal from different sources is simply additive. Although this assumption is not necessary for a generalized arousal theory to be correct, it has been one component of its principles. One alternative is that there may be enhanced or reduced psychophysiological responding to a second stimulus as a result of exposure to an initial one. In other words, when two arousal-inducing stimuli are presented serially, the increase in arousal produced by the first stimulus may affect the extent of an individual's responsiveness to the second stimulus. This would suggest that the degree to which a specific stimulus arouses an individual will not be the same under all circumstances. For example, stimuli that produce an increase of 1 and 3 units of arousal when presented individually at different times will not necessarily produce a total increase of 4 units when presented serially.

In light of the research discussed thus far, it is not all clear that arousal can be viewed as a general nonspecific system. However, at this time, it would probably be just as inappropriate to assume the opposite point of view—that there is no such phenomenon as general arousal. As Zillmann (1971) has pointed out: "It is sufficient to assume that only the interoceptive feedback of a potentially specific excitatory state is non-specific." In other words, it is not required that the responses of the arousal system to a variety of stimuli be identical but rather that they have something in common.

The low, but positive, correlations generally found among physiological measures thought to be indices of arousal suggest that arousing stimuli affect these responses in somewhat similar, although certainly not identical, ways. Thus, many of the postulates of arousal theory may still be feasible if one assumes that it is the common or nonspecific properties of arousal responses that are the bases for energizing behavior in a general and nonspecific manner. In this model, the specific effects of arousing stimuli may also be seen to influence behavior, but through separate and very different processes. A stimulus may thus be seen as having two effects—a specific one that activates physiological responses involved in eliciting a particular motivational state and a nonspecific one that energizes and thereby allows the relevant responses to occur (cf. Hebb, 1955; Stricker & Zigmond, 1976). In other words, a specific behavior at any given time may be elicited by the currently propotent stimulus. This stimulus, as well as the multiplicity of other stimuli impinging on the individual, tends also to produce nonspecific arousal, and thereby further facilitates responding.

AROUSAL AND EATING BEHAVIOR

Eating as a Prepotent Response

The relevance of arousal theory to research on eating behavior seems relatively clear. An optimal level of arousal is thought to increase the probability that a prepotent response will occur as well as to magnify the strength of the response. If, in a given situation, eating is a prepotent response, an individual should be expected to eat more under an optimal level of arousal than when less aroused.[1] Despite the apparent simplicity of this formulation, however, most of the experiments examining the relationship between arousal and eating behavior have not provided data that can be used to evaluate this hypothesis directly. Since many were designed to test psychodynamic theories of arousal-induced eating, they of course were not likely to assess when and for whom eating is, or is not, a prepotent response.

Even if one is motivated to examine the arousal-induced, prepotent response formulation directly, the methodological demands of doing so are very great because of the difficulty of assessing whether or not eating is a prepotent response. In animal studies, the behavior of an animal in a given setting may be observed over a number of sessions. If the frequency of a variety of behaviors is recorded over these sessions, one may conclude that the most frequent behavior is a prepotent or dominant response, given the same environmental context each time. This procedure has not been widely employed in human experimentation since it would require great effort and the use of sequestered populations.

The absence of such experiments with humans is especially unfortunate since, aside from enabling a specific test of the notion of arousal as an energizer of prepotent responses, the procedure of observing the frequency of behaviors over a number of sessions allows analysis of individual differences. It is very reasonable to suppose that there is a great amount of variation among individuals in terms of whether or not eating is a prepotent response to any given set of circumstances. However, since most research in this area has employed between-subjects designs, individual differences are not explicitly taken into consideration. Rather, they are likely to increase the size of the error term and thus, in some instances, possibly obscure the effects of arousal manipulations. In part, this might account further for some of the contradictory results of the studies on emotional arousal and eating that were discussed earlier.

Much more interesting than the practical problems involved in examining the role of arousal as an energizer of eating when eating is a prepotent response, however, is the theoretical question of how eating comes to be a prepotent response in certain situations. More specifically, what role, if any, does arousal play in this process?

---

1. It should be noted that this idea is similar to Rodin's (1977) hypothesis that arousal increases food intake by making an individual more responsive to salient external stimuli. The distinction between them is that the "prepotent response hypothesis" simply asserts that arousal affects the likelihood of a particular response being elicited, whereas Rodin's 1977 statement was concerned specifically with arousal's effect on the *salience* of the eliciting stimuli. For greater heuristic value, we are here considering the more general statement since even it has not yet been adequately tested.

Conditioning of Prepotent Responses

In trying to answer this question, the first step is to take a closer look at the process by which eating may become a prepotent response to a given situation in the first place. Whether one eats or not, of course, is dependent, at the very least, on various aspects of the individual's physiological state. For example, when individuals have been deprived of food, they are generally more likely to eat than when they just have been fed. However, it has long been recognized that hunger or the desire to eat is not simply a function of a physiological need for food, but rather is partly a learned response to environmental stimuli (Hebb, 1955).

More recently, Rodin (1977, 1978) has suggested that biological responses that promote increased ingestion (e.g., insulin release) can be conditioned to environmental and cognitive cues that have previously been paired with food ingestion. For example, manipulations such as thinking about and looking at food have been shown to affect a variety of physiological responses similar to those produced by the actual ingestion of food (e.g., salivation, insulin secretion, free fatty acid mobilization, gastric secretion, intestinal motility, exocrine pancreatic secretion—Bykov, 1957; Hayashi & Ararei, 1963; Jenkins & Dawes, 1966; Moore & Schenkenberg, 1974; Parra-Covarrubias, Rivera-Rodriguez, & Almaraz-Ugalde, 1971; Penick, Prince, & Hinkle, 1966; Rodin, 1978; Wooley & Wooley, 1973). If, as Powley (1977) has suggested, the augmentation of these responses acts to increase amount ingested, factors that enhance the conditioning process may play a role in determining amount of food consumed subsequently.

We suggest that arousal may affect the magnitude of these conditioned physiological responses in at least two ways. First, given that the association between various physiological responses and environmental or cognitive cues has already been learned, the presence of an optimal level of arousal may serve to energize, and thus intensify, these learned responses. Second, a more subtle role that arousal may play in determining the strength of these learned physiological responses is that it may impact on the conditioning process itself. If optimal levels of arousal enhance and strengthen conditioning of responses to particular environmental stimuli, food consumption in a given situation may be dependent not only on the individual's present level of arousal but also on arousal levels present in similar past situations.

The idea that arousal may facilitate the conditioning of prepotent responses is supported by several studies that have examined the effects of arousal on learning as separate from performance. For example, Rensch and Rahmann (1960) injected hamsters with methamphetamine shortly before discrimination-learning trials. When tested 14 to 94 days later, those animals receiving methamphetamine injections prior to the learning trials performed better than the control animals who were given saline injections prior to the learning trials. This suggests that arousal as manipulated by methamphetamine injection facilitates learning. In human research, Berlyne and his colleagues (Berlyne, Borsa, Craw, Gelman, & Mandell, 1965; Berlyne, Borsa, Hamacher, & Koenig, 1966) studied the effects on recall of another arousal manipulation (the presence or absence of white noise) during paired-associate training. They found that items learned under increased arousal levels were more likely to be recalled 24 hours later. These data clearly challenge the Zajonc (1965) assertion that arousal will always interfere with learning and facilitate performance.

Finally, an interesting animal study has provided evidence for an analogous and conceptually relevant phenomenon. Revusky (1967) showed that the degree of deprivation during prior pairings of a particular food with its ingestion influences the animal's subsequent eating behavior. Specifically, the subsequent preference for, and consumption of, a particular food increases when its ingestion has been previously paired with high level of deprivation. Thus, the degree of deprivation in past experiences evidently influences learning processes that determine, in part, subsequent eating behavior. Since food deprivation has been shown to influence levels of arousal (Campbell & Sheffield, 1953), one possible mechanism for the results of this study is that level of arousal, as opposed to deprivation level per se, may be the critical factor affecting preference. If this is the case, then directly manipulating arousal level during prior pairings of a particular food with its ingestion should influence subsequent eating behavior. The following experiment was intended to test this hypothesis.

EXPERIMENTAL VARIATION OF AROUSAL AND CONDITIONING PROCESSES

To examine systematically the role of arousal in the conditioning of eating-related physiological responses, we decided to employ a conditioning procedure in the laboratory in which the ingestion of a novel food was signaled by the sight and thought of the food. We chose to use a novel stimulus for the obvious reason that if another more familiar food stimulus was used, subjects would bring with them to the laboratory a variety of different, already established learning experiences with the food. As a result, this large variation in individuals would be likely to obscure the effects of the experimental manipulations, which sought to influence de novo a food-relevant experience. In addition, prior experience with a food stimulus would be certain to lessen the impact of the conditioning procedure. An arousal manipulation (caffeine) was introduced during conditioning for half of the subjects to compare reactions to the food stimulus between subjects conditioned under high arousal and those conditioned under low arousal.

Procedure

Subjects were told that the purpose of the study was to examine the effect of a variety of substances on taste and that we were only interested in studying individuals with certain taste preference patterns. With this rationale, we asked subjects to rate a number of foods in terms of both pleasantness and familiarity to see if they had the "taste preference patterns that were needed for the experiment." In this way, subjects who had any prior experience with mangoes were screened out. Subjects also completed personality scales and background measures at this time.

Subjects ($n = 13$) came to the laboratory for two individual sessions at the same time on two separate days. In order to achieve a relatively uniform state of deprivation both between subjects and across sessions, subjects were asked to skip the meal before each of the sessions and to eat and drink nothing but water for at least 12 hours before their scheduled appointment.

In the first session (day 1), the mango sherbet was presented to subjects in a conditioning procedure in which the presentation of the sherbet was paired with its ingestion. An individual conditioning trial consisted of a signal bell a few seconds prior to presentation of a half-teaspoon of mango sherbet. Subjects looked at the sherbet for approximately 10 seconds and then held it in their mouths for approximately 5 seconds to fully experience its taste before swallowing it. The bell in association with the visual presentation of the sherbet was the conditioned stimulus. The sherbet in the mouth represented the unconditioned stimulus. The metabolic responses triggered by the sherbet were the unconditioned responses.

A total of 17 trials was presented.[2] Subjects rated their hunger both before and immediately after the 17 conditioning trials. Immediately after the trials were completed, subjects rated how much they liked the sherbet. This completed the conditioning procedures of the first day. A second session, conducted on a different day, was intended to assess the strength of the conditioning on day 1.

On the second day (day 2), subjects were presented with a bowl of mango sherbet. They rated their hunger both before and after looking at the mango sherbet but before tasting or eating it. Subjects were then given a bowl of lime sherbet together with the bowl of mango sherbet and were allowed to eat as much as they wished of either. Finally, subjects rated how much they liked each of the sherbets.

To this point we have discussed only the conditioning process and the measures used to assess its effect on eating and other related behaviors. To examine the role of arousal in the conditioning process, manipulations

---

2. Presenting 17 trials was a somewhat arbitrary choice that was made on the basis of time constraints.

of arousal were introduced during both sessions. By manipulating arousal on day 1, it was possible to determine if increased levels of arousal during conditioning strengthened the conditioning process. By manipulating arousal during the second session we could determine how arousal level, after some conditioning has occurred, influences eating behavior in response to conditioning cues. In this way we could uncouple and test separately how arousal affects the acquisition of a preference (i.e., conditioning) and/or the intensity of the expression of a preference once conditioning had occurred (the postconditioning phase).

In deciding on the type of arousal-inducing manipulation to use, we looked at the variety of manipulations used in other studies examining the effects of arousal on human behavior. Most eating behavior studies, as we mentioned earlier, used emotion-inducing stimuli such as shock or interpersonal threat to increase arousal. The use of this type of manipulation has several major problems which are especially noteworthy for the area of social psychophysiology.

First, emotional stimuli have been shown to produce distinctive patterns of physiological responses, suggesting that they affect specific physiological parameters as the intended nonspecific influences on arousal level. As a result, behavioral consequences of the physiological responses produced by the stimuli may serve to direct behavior in a specific way as well as to energize it in a general way. Second, emotional stimuli also have distinctive cognitive components. Slochower (1976) has demonstrated that an increase in emotional arousal that has an ambiguous source has a greater effect on eating behavior than an increase in emotional arousal with a known source. Her work implies that when the source of the emotional arousal is easily identified by subjects, it may have a weaker effect on behavior. Finally, as mentioned earlier, one's subjective experience of emotional arousal is not necessarily accompanied by actual physiological arousal.

Ideally, the best of all arousal manipulations is one that has only nonspecific effects and whose source is not obvious to subjects. Unfortunately, until our understanding of the boundaries of the unique and nonspecific characteristics of psychophysiological responding to a variety of supposedly "arousal-inducing" stimuli is better elucidated, we cannot assume that any effects of arousal on eating will not be confounded by other specific influences. But it should be possible to manipulate arousal without revealing its source. Slochower (1976) used slow and fast false feedback of heart rate as an arousal manipulation and subjects were apparently not aware of its putative arousal-inducing role in the experiment. However, evidence regarding whether false feedback induces actual physiological changes is mixed (see the reviews by Liebhart, 1979, or Hirschman & Clark, Chapter 7, this volume). No physiological measures were taken during Slochower's experiment. The only measure of arousal was self-report. Thus, although self-report of emotional arousal was related to the manipulation, it is possible that self-report in this context did not reflect a real change in degree of physiological arousal, but instead was influenced directly by the cognition that one had either a "slow" or "fast" heart rate (cf. Nisbett & Wilson, 1977).

Other studies examining the effects of arousal on human behavior have used small doses of caffeine as an arousal manipulation (Polivy, Herman, & Warsh, 1978; Revelle, Amaral, & Turiff, 1976). Although these studies have not employed any manipulation checks other than self-report scales of mood, caffeine seemed to us a good candidate for an arousal manipulation for several reasons. First, caffeine if disguised on presentation would affect arousal directly through physiological means, and thus there would be no salient emotional source to which subjects might attribute their arousal. Second, caffeine has often been cited as a stimulant, although the evidence is indirect (Gilbert, 1976). In addition, caffeine has been demonstrated to increase subjective feelings of alertness (Regina, Smith, Keiper, & McKelvey, 1974).

In order to eliminate from the study those individuals who were unusually sensitive to caffeine and those who might have, through extensive use, developed a tolerance to caffeine, subjects were carefully questioned prior to participation in the study. Only those volunteers who indicated that they currently consumed fewer than three cups per day of coffee or other beverages containing methylated xanthines such as tea and cola, and never had any adverse reactions to caffeine, were accepted as subjects.

During the first session, subjects were randomly assigned to one of two groups—those who received 200 mg of caffeine and those who received 200 mg of lactose (i.e., placebo). During the second session, these two groups were again randomly divided into those receiving caffeine and lactose. In accord with subjects' knowledge of the purpose of the study (i.e., effects of various substances on taste) and the requirements of informed consent, they were told that, on any day, they would receive one of the following substances—vitamins C, E, or B_{12}; caffeine; or lactose. In this way, subjects were kept blind as to which substance they actually got on any day. The additional substances were included on the list to broaden the subjects' set regarding possible substances, thus helping to control for possible suggestion effects. Experimenters were also blind to the subjects' experimental condition. The measures we used included heart rate, spontaneous and specific skin conductance responses, and verbal report.

Measures of Autonomic Nervous System Activity

Heart rate increases may reflect either more activity in the sympathetic branch or less in the parasympathetic branch of the nervous system. In addition to this autonomic activity, heart rate increases in response to a

host of changes within the circulatory system as well, such as vasoconstriction in certain blood vessels. Situations causing heart rate deceleration
have also been identified in recent years. Lacey and coworkers (1959,
1967a, 1967b) have suggested that cardiac deceleration facilitates sensory
receptivity and thus occurs whenever a person is attending to events in the
external environment. Others have suggested that both the direction and
magnitude of heart rate changes are primarily a function of the overall
state of the musculature in preparation for behavior and are therefore
more a measure of somatic activity than of arousal (Elliot, 1969; Obrist,
Webb, & Sutterer, 1969). However, differences in heart rate can be obscured because sympathetic and parasympathetic actions may be contradictory since heart rate responses are innervated by both parasympathetic and sympathetic branches of the autonomic system.

Skin conductance responses, on the other hand, typically show strong
effects of autonomic activation by external stimuli. These measures are
based on the fact that the elecrical conductance of the skin varies with
activity in the sweat glands, which in turn are innervated by sympathetic
fibers. Some have called them the "most sensitive physiological indicator
of psychological events available" (Montagu & Coles, 1966, p. 261).

Results

Analyses of the data revealed that, surprisingly, the caffeine manipulations had no significant effect on any of the physiological or verbal report
measures. Further, the caffeine manipulation had no systematic effects on
measures of taste preference, hunger, or eating behavior on either the
conditioning (day 1) or postconditioning (day 2) sessions. Either the levels of
caffeine used were not sufficient to arouse subjects or these particular
dependent variables were not the best measures of caffeine's effects on the
arousal system.

It is also possible that other factors present in the experimental context affected arousal, and thus may have obscured or overridden the
effects of the caffeine manipulation. For example, small environmental
changes such as change in noise level in the experimental room greatly
affected many subjects' arousal level as assessed by electrodermal activity
(EDA). Of particular interest was the fact that the bell used to signal the
start of each conditioning trial clearly affected the EDA of all the subjects,
although there were large individual differences in the magnitude of
subjects' responses. Since the bell occurred a few seconds before food
presentation, it seemed reasonable to suggest that subjects who were
more aroused by external stimuli such as the bell might be more aroused
than other subjects during conditioning to the sight of the food. Based on
this line of reasoning, we speculated that if arousal does play a role in the

conditioning of eating-related responses as we originally hypothesized, then individual differences in the extent to which a person's arousal system is activated by specific external stimuli should influence the conditioning process. If the strength of the conditioning is important, it should then influence perceived hunger and eating behavior.

In order to assess individual differences in the extent to which the arousal system responds to specific stimuli, the magnitude of subjects' specific conductance responses to the bell signaling the first conditioning trial was assessed and used as a measure of arousability. (Changes in heart rate were not used since analyses of these data showed that the bell had no significant overall effect on this measure. In other words, changes in heart rate in response to the bell were not reliably different from changes in heart rate in a control period when no stimulus was presented.) We decided that the strongest test of the importance of individual differences would be to use the specific conductance response (SCR) to the bell only on trial 1 as an index of the subjects' arousability. In later trials, arousal might also be increased by the anticipation of the food itself, as classical conditioning theory would suggest. In some ways, although admittedly this is a post hoc consideration, this type of acute punctuated arousal provides an even better test of the present hypothesis than chronically elevated, caffeine-induced arousal, since its discrete occurrence is contiguous with and signals food ingestion.

One might argue that the magnitude of the electrodermal response to the bell may be related to baseline arousal prior to the bell since the law of initial values states that the response of a variable to a stimulus decreases as the prestimulus level increases (i.e., change from baseline is negatively correlated with initial baseline) (Wilder, 1950). However, although the law has been shown to apply to many autonomic responses, Hord, Johnson, and Lubin (1964) found that it did not hold for skin conductance responses. In fact, they point out that, for SCR, the converse of the law of initial values seems to hold—that is, SCR may be positively correlated with prestimulus skin conductance. If this is true, then individual differences in our measure of arousability to external stimuli may correlate positively with chronic level of arousal as assessed by EDA.

Hunger

There were several possible measures of the strength of conditioning that took place. First, we considered increases in subjects' reports of hunger during the first session, from before to after the conditioning trials. A strong correlation with the arousability measure (magnitude of the specific GSR to the first signal) would be impressive since subjects had already been food deprived for at least 12 hours prior to the experiment and had eaten 8½ teaspoons of sherbet by the time the conditioning trials had been completed. The correlation of arousability and the increase in hunger rating was .65 ($p < .01$).[3]

Although there were no direct measures of metabolic activity in this study, ratings of hunger have been considered to be correlates of underlying metabolic activity (Powley, 1977; Wooley & Wooley, 1973). If the conditioning process is influenced by arousal level, the metabolic responses that have been elicited during the conditioning procedure should be larger in those subjects who appear more aroused by the specific stimuli, as the hunger ratings suggest they were. Our additional studies are now assessing this suggestion directly by measuring salivation and endocrine responses.

Even more important than the data presented thus far is the relationship between changes in hunger ratings during the second session, after conditioning had taken place, and arousability during conditioning (session 1). This measure serves to indicate the extent to which the conditioned stimulus (i.e., the presence of the mango sherbet) has now come to influence hunger since hunger ratings were taken before subjects were presented with the mango sherbet and again after the sherbet had been presented but before it was eaten. In fact, arousability on day 1 and an increase in hunger ratings on day 2 were highly correlated ($r = .76, p < .005$). Thus, it appears that arousal during the conditioning processes increases the subsequent expression of hunger-related conditioned responses to the CS (i.e., the visual presentation of the food).

The effect of arousal on the strength of these conditioned hunger-related responses has at least two potential sources. First, level of arousal may enhance the conditioning process itself and thereby create a stronger association between the conditioned stimulus and the conditioned responses. Second, arousal level may influence the magnitude of the response that is being conditioned. This would also lead to stronger expression of the conditioned responses to subsequent presentation of the conditioned stimulus. Although we distinguish between these two processes for conceptual clarity, the present study did not attempt to pull them apart.

Palatability and Consumption

Weaker relationships were obtained between our measure of arousability and perceived pleasantness of the mango sherbet ($r = .37, p < .10$, on both days 1 and 2). Whether or not preference reflects underlying metabolic activity (the CR in the present study) has been the subject of some controversy (Cabanac & Duclaux, 1970; Grinker, Price, & Greenwood, 1976),

---

3. All p values are reported for one-tailed tests since the directions of the correlations are clearly predicted by the hypothesis.

yet the direction of the correlation suggests that it may be influenced by individual differences in arousal during exposure to the food stimulus.

The mango and lime sherbets were available for consumption on day 2. Individual differences in arousability correlated with the amount of mango sherbet eaten ($r = .39$, $p < .10$) but not the amount of lime sherbet eaten ($r = -.27$). Given the very small n, even the marginally significant correlations seem to be extremely suggestive, especially in light of their consistency with the strong and significant relationship between EDA and change in hunger.

Ideally, one would like to use measures of several different physiological responses to assess individual differences in arousability since it has been shown that these are consistent differences in which the effector responds most to external stimulation (Lacey & Lacey, 1958). Thus, one person may respond most in terms of EDA, while another person may show greater changes in blood pressure. As we stated earlier, changes in heart rate were not a good index of arousal induced by the bell since the bell seemed to have very little effect on this measure. However, the fact that there were such strong and consistent data for EDA measures suggests that at least for these data, EDA more closely reflects the variable mediating the extent to which conditioning occurs, and therefore subsequent eating behavior.

The notion that individual differences in EDA response to the bell is an appropriate, if not ideal index of arousability to external stimuli would gain considerable support if it were found to correlate with another potential measure of individual differences in arousability. Geen (Chapter 13, this volume) describes Eysenck's introversion–extraversion concept as a potential measure of individual differences in arousability. In fact, subjects' scores on the Eysenck scale in the present study correlated highly ($r = .59$, $p < .025$) with individual differences in arousability as assessed by the magnitude of the EDA response to the bell.

Finally, since the evidence supporting the hypothesis is based on correlations, the results can obviously be interpreted in alternative ways. One might suggest, for example, that body weight or number of hours of actual food deprivation may be confounded with the arousability measures and, may, in large part, account for the correlations between arousability and the eating-related dependent measures of interest. However, when the effects of these variables were held constant by using partial correlations, the relationship between measures of arousability and the eating-related dependent measures remained essentially unchanged or, in some instances, actually increased in magnitude (see Table 20-1). This suggests, of course, that the relationship between arousability and the eating-related dependent measures are not explained by body weight or hours of food deprivation.

TABLE 20-1. Zero-Order and Partial Correlations of Arousability and Eating-Related Dependent Measures

	ZERO-ORDER CORRELATION	CORRELATION PARTIALING OUT WHETHER SUBJECTS WERE OVERWEIGHT OR NORMAL WEIGHT	CORRELATION PARTIALING OUT NUMBER OF HOURS OF FOOD DEPRIVATION
Arousability and increase in hunger on day 1	.65*	.79**	.64*
Arousability and pleasantness rating of mango sherbet on day 1	.37	.38	.34
Arousability and increase in hunger on day 2	.76**	.78**	.71**
Arousability and pleasantness rating of mango sherbet on day 2	.37	.34	.37
Arousability and amount of mango sherbet eaten on day 2	.39	.41	.31

*$p < .01$.

**$p < .005$.

Individual Differences in Arousability

If there are large individual differences in arousability that relate to differences in conditioning strength and responsiveness to food cues, they can be either inherited or learned. Others have also proposed (notably Maddi, 1968; Thayer, 1967) that there are individual differences in both rate and levels of physiological arousal. Evolutionary pressures may have selected for such characteristics since a strong response when aroused may represent an adaptive strategy for dealing with impending disruption or danger. Thus, the potential for arousability might have an inherited component.

It is also likely that degree of arousability can be modified by learning experiences (e.g., Razran, 1961). One might expect that the more stimuli that have been conditioned to autonomic arousal in the past, the higher that arousal will be, and in turn the more arousable the person will appear to environmental stimuli. Certainly both learned and inherited contributions to differences in arousability are possible.

Clearly, our study was not initially designed to test individual differences in arousability or we would have done it in a different way. Therefore, any conclusions from the data must be seen as suggestive and demanding further research. However, these preliminary data suggest that those individuals who are more arousable may develop more and stronger conditioned responses to a variety of stimuli in the real world than those who are less arousable. Thus, they may show heightened responsiveness on subsequent occasions. Since it is reasonable to assume that food, as compared to other stimuli, is one of the more salient stimuli that people are often exposed to throughout their lifetime, one might expect that those people who are very arousable to environmental stimuli will develop strong conditioned responses to food, thereby showing an arousal-induced prepotent response. In this instance arousal may influence both the acquisition of a conditioned response of a given magnitude and its subsequent expression.

If these individual differences in arousability do affect both the acquisition and expression of conditioned responses to food stimuli, might some people's weight problems be attributed, at least in part, to the mediating processes considered in our experiment? In other words, we might speculate that if arousable individuals experience enhanced conditioning to food quality and stronger expression of these conditioned responses, overeating may be more likely to occur whenever the individual is aroused. Whether this overeating is compensated for under nonarousing circumstances, however, is still an open question. Certainly, obesity is a consequence of more than differences in arousability and arousal-induced eating; it has a large genetic component (Bray, 1982) and is influenced by fat cell morphology (Hirsch & Han, 1969) and different rates of metabolism (Garrow, 1978). But arousability by salient environmental stimuli does indeed appear to be one important potential contributor, and may explain the relationship between arousal-induced eating and obesity without relying on psychodynamic explanations.

ENDOCRINE AND CENTRAL NERVOUS SYSTEM CONTRIBUTIONS TO AROUSAL-INDUCED EATING

Endocrine System

Thus far we have focused our attention on the autonomic nervous system as a measure of arousal's effects on the development and enhancement of the conditioned prepotent response of feeding. Endocrines are also released in response to arousing environmental stimuli, however, including especially the catecholamines (epinephrine and norepinephrine), corticosteroids, insulin, growth hormone, and vasopressin, and could also be seen as measures of arousal. This complicates experimental research into the question of arousal-induced eating since several of these hormones are involved in the metabolizing and digesting of food that is eaten and have been thought to stimulate the onset of feeding as well (Rodin, 1981a). In other words, they are responses both to arousing external stimuli and to the presence of food in the digestive tract. Despite the problems this produces for eating research, in particular, this important link may be one of the underlying mechanisms by which arousal relates to eating.

Recent research has shown that people secrete insulin in response to the sight and smell of palatable foods (Rodin, 1978; Sahakian, Lean, Robbins, & James, 1981; Sjostrom, Garellick, Krotkiewski, & Luyckx, 1980). What has been striking about the data from these experiments is the great variability from person to person in the magnitude of this response. If as we suggested above, insulin is one major nonspecific response to all arousing stimuli, including food, then the more arousable individuals would secrete more insulin (and probably other physiologically significant hormones) in the presence of food cues and other arousing stimuli. Thus we are suggesting that attention to individual differences in arousability could explain why the insulin studies showed such variability from subject to subject in the degree of the insulin response. Arousability would in turn strengthen the conditioning processes and increase the likelihood of food intake on that and subsequent occasions during which the same food cues were present. The probability that individual differences in arousability are linked to different magnitudes and patterns of endocrine responses may be significant for understanding the role of unconditioned as well as conditioned processes in eating behavior.

Brain Neurotransmitters

Work has also been done recently exploring the relationship between arousal, measured at the level of specific central nervous system activity, and eating. By necessity, of course, this has largely been animal work. Recent investigations (Antelman, Rowland, & Fisher, 1976; Wayner, 1974) implicate identifiable catecholamine-containing pathways in the brain as important for the onset of eating, and other activities. Arousal appears preferentially to facilitate brain catecholaminergic function within these pathways and cues in the environment plus the animal's conditioning history determine which responses from the organism's behavioral repertoire are activated by this arousal.

CONCLUSIONS

Historically, the concept of arousal has been of considerable import to social psychologists who have been interested in questions related to the experience and expression of emotions, sexuality and intimacy, and aggression, to cite just a few noteworthy examples. It has also been of considerable interest to investigators considering social and psychological determinants of food intake. However, the concept of arousal itself has never been well defined. Specifically, the boundaries of the unique and general characteristics of different psychophysiological responses to a variety of putative arousal-inducing stimuli are still not clear.

Mason (1975) and Frankenhaueser (1975) have suggested that it is the patterning of different physiological responses rather than the magnitude of any individual responses that will provide a more accurate picture of the effect of an arousal-inducing stimulus because the body's biological systems act in concert with, and affect, one another. For example, Mason (1975) has found that there are a number of distinctive combinations of hormonal responses to different physical stimuli such as heat, cold, heavy exercise, bed rest, and fasting, and psychological events such as grief and depression. Investigators should be aware, therefore, that this is one area in which calculating any group means may be problematic since vast individual differences in patterns of physiological response to the identical stimulus have been identified (Mason, 1975). Presumably, these differences are mediated in part by how individuals appraise the stressor (Lazarus, 1966) as well as by actual differences in the extent of one's physiological responsiveness. Our own future research will examine the patterning of various responses thought to influence eating behavior.

In this chapter we have been especially concerned with the relationship between food intake and arousal. Although the concept of arousal has often been used in research of food intake regulation, investigators in this area have generally focused their attention on the effects of the individual's present state of arousal on amount eaten. In this chapter we have suggested that arousal may also play an important role in the acquisition and conditioning of eating-related responses. More specifically, the presence of increased levels of arousal during the conditioning of hunger-related responses to a particular stimulus were hypothesized to enhance the conditioning process and thus to increase the expression of the conditioned responses to subsequent presentations of the conditioned stimulus. Preferential food intake was shown to be directly affected by this procedure.

Since the experiment suggested that individual differences in arousability affect both the acquisition and expression of conditioned responses to food stimuli, it was questioned whether some weight problems could be attributed, at least in part, to the mediating processes examined in the study. Although this is considered to be a possibility, research addressing whether arousal-induced eating is compensated for over the long term is needed before we can implicate arousal as an important factor in the development or maintenance of obesity.

It was also suggested that arousal-inducing stimuli may play a role in the regulation of food intake through their effects on certain endocrine responses that are involved in the metabolizing and digesting of food that is eaten and that have even been thought to stimulate the onset of feeding. This exciting possibility points to a final common pathway at the physiological level, for the relationship between arousal and food intake.

ACKNOWLEDGMENT

Portions of the research, and the writing of this chapter, were supported by National Science Foundation Grant BNS76-81126 to the second author.

REFERENCES

Abramson, E. D., & Wunderlich, R. A.   Anxiety, fear and eating: A test of the psychosomatic concept of obesity. *Journal of Abnormal Psychology*, 1972, *79*, 317–321.

Antelman, S. M., Rowland, N. E., & Fisher, A. E.   Stimulation-bound ingestive behavior: A view from the tail. *Physiology & Behavior*, 1976, *17*, 743–748.

Ax, A. F.   The physiological differentiation between fear and anger in humans. *Psychosomatic Medicine*, 1953, *15*, 433–442.

Berlyne, D. E.   *Conflict, arousal and curiosity*. New York: McGraw-Hill, 1960.

Berlyne, D. E., Borsa, D. M., Craw, M. A., Gelman, R. S., & Mandell, E. E.   Effects of stimulus complexity and induced arousal on paired-associate learning. *Journal of Verbal Learning and Verbal Behavior*, 1965, *4*, 291–299.

Berlyne, D. E., Borsa, D. M., Hamacher, J. H., & Koenig, I. D. V.   Paired associate learning and the timing of arousal. *Journal of Experimental Psychology*, 1966, *72*, 1–6.

Bray, G.   Role of genetics in determining body weight stability in man. In L. A. Cioffi, W. P. T. James, & T. B. Van Itallie (Eds.), *The body weight regulatory system: Normal and disturbed aspects*. New York: Raven, 1982.

Bruch, H.   Transformation of oral impulses in eating disorders: A conceptual approach. *Psychiatric Quarterly* (New York), 1961, *35*, 458–481.

Bruch, H.   *Eating disorders: Obesity, anorexia nervosa and the person within*. New York: Basic Books, 1973.

Bykov, K. M.   [*The cerebral cortex and the internal organs*] (W. H. Gant, Ed. and trans.). New York: Chemical Publishing Co., 1957.

Cabanac, M., & Duclaux, R.   Specificity of internal signals in producing satiety for taste stimuli. *Nature* (London), 1970, *227*, 966–977.

Campbell, B. A., & Sheffield, F. D.   Relations of random activity to food deprivation. *Journal of Comparative and Physiological Psychology*, 1953, *46*, 320–322.

Cannon, W. B.   *Bodily changes in pain, hunger, fear and rage*. New York: Appleton, 1915.

Carlson, A. J.   *The control of hunger in health and disease*. Chicago: University of Chicago Press, 1916.

Conrad, S. W.   The psychologic implications of overeating. *Psychiatric Quarterly* (New York), 1954, *28*, 211–224.

Duffy, E.   The psychological significance of the concept of "arousal" or "activation." *Psychological Review*, 1957, *64*, 265–275.

Elliot, R.   Effects of uncertainty about the nature and advent of a noxious stimulus (shock) upon heart rate. *Journal of Personality and Social Psychology*, 1966, *3*, 353–356.

Elliot, R.   Tonic heart rate: Experiments on the effects of collative variables lead to a hypothesis about its motivational significance. *Journal of Personality and Social Psychology*, 1969, *12*, 211–228.

Frankenhaeuser, M.   Experimental approaches to the study of catecholamines and emotion. In L. Levi (Ed.). *Emotions: Their parameters and measurement*. New York: Raven, 1975.

Freed, S. C.   Psychic factors in the development and treatment of obesity. *Journal of the American Medical Association*, 1947, *133*, 369.

Funkenstein, D. H., King, S. H., & Drolette, M. E.   *Mastery of stress*. Cambridge, Mass.: Harvard University Press, 1956.

Garrow, J. S. *Energy balance and obesity in man.* New York: Elsevier/North-Holland Biomedical Press, 1978.

Gilbert, R. M. Caffeine as a drug of abuse. In R. E. Gibbins, Y. Israel, H. Kalant, R. E. Popham, W. Schmidt, & R. G. Smart (Eds.), *Research advances in alcohol and drug problems* (Vol. 3). New York: Wiley, 1976.

Glass, L. B. The generality of oral-consummatory behavior of alcoholics under stress. *Dissertation Abstracts International,* 1967, 5205-B.

Grinker, J. A., Price, J. M., & Greenwood, M. R. C. Studies of taste in childhood obesity. In D. Novin, W. Wywricka, & G. Bray (Eds.), *Hunger: Basic mechanisms and clinical implications.* New York: Raven, 1976.

Hamburger, W. W. Emotional aspects of obesity. *Medical Clinics of North America,* 1951, *35,* 483–499.

Hayashi, T., & Ararei, M. Natural conditioned salivary reflex of man alone as well as in a group. In Y. Zotterman (Ed.), *Olfaction and taste* (Vol. 1). Oxford: Pergamon, 1963.

Hebb, D. O. Drives and the CNS (conceptual nervous system). *Psychological Review,* 1955, *62,* 243–254.

Herman, C. P., & Polivy, J. Anxiety, restraint and eating behavior. *Journal of Abnormal Psychology,* 1975, *84,* 666–672.

Hirsch, J., & Han, P. W. Cellularity of rat adipose tissue, effects of growth, starvation, and obesity. *Journal of Lipid Research,* 1969, *10,* 77.

Hord, D. J., Johnson, L. C., & Lubin, A. Differential effect of the law of initial values (LIV) on autonomic variables. *Psychophysiology,* 1964, *1,* 79–87.

Jenkins, G. N., & Dawes, C. The psychic flow of saliva in man. *Archives of Oral Biology,* 1966, *11,* 1203–1204.

Kaplan, H. I., & Kaplan, H. S. The psychosomatic concept of obesity. *Journal of Nervous and Mental Disease,* 1957, *125,* 181–189.

Lacey, J. I. Psychophysiological approaches to the evaluation of psychotherapeutic process and outcome. In E. A. Rubenstein & M. B. Parloff (Eds.), *Research in psychotherapy.* Washington, D.C.: American Psychological Association, 1959.

Lacey, J. I. The evaluation of autonomic responses: Toward a general solution. *Annals of the New York Academy of Sciences,* 1967, *67,* 123–164. (a)

Lacey, J. I. Somatic response patterning and stress: Some revisions of activation theory. In M. H. Appley & R. Trumbull (Eds.), *Psychological stress.* New York: Appleton-Century-Crofts, 1967. (b)

Lacey, J. I., & Lacey, B. C. Verification and extension of the principle of autonomic response stereotypy. *American Journal of Psychology,* 1958, *71,* 50.

Lazarus, R. S. *Psychological stress and the coping process.* New York: McGraw-Hill, 1966.

Lazarus, R. S., Speisman, J. C., & Mordkoff, A. M. The relationship between autonomic indicators of psychological stress: Heart rate and skin conductance. *Psychosomatic Medicine,* 1963, *25,* 19–30.

Leon, G. R. Personality, body image, and eating patterns in overweight persons after weight-loss. In A. Howard (Ed.), *Recent advances in obesity research* (Vol. 1). London: Newman Publishing, 1975.

Liebhart, E. H. Information search and attribution: Cognitive processes mediating the effect of false feedback. *European Journal of Social Psychology,* 1979, *9,* 19-37.

Lindsley, D. B. Psychophysiology and motivation. In M. R. Jones (Ed.), *Nebraska Symposium on Motivation* (Vol. 5). Lincoln: University of Nebraska Press, 1957.

Maddi, S. R. *Personality theories: A comparative analysis.* Homewood, Ill.: Dorsey, 1968.

Malmo, R. B. Activation: A neuropsychological dimension. *Psychological Review,* 1959, *66,* 367–386.

Marshall, G. D., & Zimbardo, P. G. Affective consequences of inadequately explained physiological arousal. *Journal of Personality and Social Psychology,* 1979, *37,* 970–988.

Maslach, C.   Negative emotional biasing of unexplained arousal. *Journal of Personality and Social Psychology*, 1979, *37*, 953–969.

Mason, J. W.   Emotion as reflected in patterns of endocrine regulation. In L. Levi (Ed.), *Emotions: Their parameters and measurement*. New York: Raven, 1975.

McKenna, R. J.   Some effects of anxiety level and food cues on the behavior of obese and normal subjects. *Journal of Personality and Social Psychology*, 1972, *221*, 311–319.

Meyer, J. E., & Pudel, V.   Experimental studies on food intake in obese and normal weight subjects. *Journal of Psychosomatic Research*, 1972, *16*, 305–308.

Mirsky, A. F., & Cardon, P. V.   A comparison of the behavioral and physiological changes accompanying sleep deprivation and chlorpromazine administration in man. *Electroencephalography and Clinical Neurophysiology*, 1962, *14*, 1–10.

Montagu, J. D., & Coles, E. M.   Mechanism and measurement of the galvanic skin response. *Psychological Bulletin*, 1966, *65*, 261–279.

Moore, J. G., & Schenkenberg, T.   Psychic control of gastric acid: Response to anticipated feeding and biofeedback training in man. *Gastroenterology*, 1974, *66*, 954–959.

Nisbett, R. E., & Wilson, T.   Telling more than we can know: Verbal reports on mental processes. *Psychological Review*, 1977, *84*, 231–259.

Obrist, P. A., Webb, R. A., & Sutterer, J. R.   Heart rate and somatic changes during aversive conditioning and a simple reaction-time task. *Psychophysiology*, 1969, *5*, 696–723.

Parra-Covarrubias, A., Rivera-Rodriguez, I., & Almaraz-Ugalde, A.   Cephalic phase of insulin secretion in obese adolescents. *Diabetes*, 1971, *20*, 800–802.

Penick, S. B., Prince, H., & Hinkle, L. E., Jr.   Fall in plasma content of free fatty acids associated with the sight of food. *New England Journal of Medicine*, 1966, *275*, 416–419.

Pines, A., & Gal, R.   The effect of food on test anxiety. *Journal of Applied Social Psychology*, 1977, *4*, 348–358.

Polivy, J., Herman, C. P., & Warsh, S.   Internal and external components of emotionality in restrained and unrestrained eaters. *Journal of Abnormal Psychology*, 1978, *87*, 497–504.

Powley, T.   The ventromedial hypothalamic syndrome, satiety, and a cephalic phase hypothesis. *Psychological Review*, 1977, *84*, 89.

Razran, G.   The observable unconscious and the inferable conscious in current Soviet psychophysiology. *Psychological Review*, 1961, *68*, 81–147.

Regina, E. G., Smith, G. M., Keiper, C. G., & McKelvey, R. K.   Effects of caffeine on alertness in simulated automobile driving. *Journal of Applied Psychology*, 1974, *59*, 483–489.

Rensch, B., & Rahmann, H.   Einfluss des Pervitins auf des Gedachtnis von Goldhamstein. *Pfluegers Archiv fuer die Gesamte Physiologie des Menschen und der Tiere*, 1960, *271*, 693–704.

Revelle, W., Amaral, P., & Turiff, S.   Introversion/extroversion, time stress, and caffeine: Effect on verbal performance. *Science*, 1976, *192*, 149–150.

Revusky, S. H.   Hunger level during food consumption: Effects on subsequent preference. *Psychonomic Science*, 1967, *7*, 109–110.

Reznick, H., & Balch, P.   The effects of anxiety and response cost manipulations on the eating behavior of obese and normal-weight subjects. *Addictive Behaviors*, 1977, *2*, 219–225.

Robbins, T., & Fray, P.   Stress-induced eating: Fact, fiction or misunderstanding. *Appetite*, 1980, *1*, 103–133.

Rodin, J.   Bidirectional influences of emotionality, stimulus responsivity and metabolic events in obesity. In J. Maser & M. E. P. Seligman (Eds.), *Psychopathology: Experimental models*. San Francisco: W. H. Freeman, 1977.

Rodin, J.   Has the distinction between internal versus external control of feeding outlived its usefulness? In G. A. Bray (Ed.), *Recent advances in obesity research* (Vol. 2). London: Newman, 1978.

Rodin, J.   The current status of the internal–external hypothesis of obesity: What went wrong? *American Psychologist*, 1981, *36*, 361–372. (a)

Rodin, J.   Understanding obesity: Defining the samples. *Personality and Social Psychology Bulletin*, 1981, *7*, 147–151. (b)

Sahakian, B. J., Lean, M. E. J., Robbins, T. W., & James, W. P. T.   Salivation and insulin secretion in response to food in non-obese men and women. *Appetite*, 1981, *2*, 209–216.

Schachter, J.   Pain, fear, and anger in hypertension and normotensives. *Psychosomatic Medicine*, 1957, *19*, 17–29.

Schachter, S.   Obesity and eating. *Science*, 1968, *161*, 751–756.

Schachter, S., Goldman, R., & Gordon, A.   Effects of fear, food deprivation and obesity on eating. *Journal of Personality and Social Psychology*, 1968, *10*, 91–98.

Schachter, S., & Singer, J.   Cognitive social, and physiological determinants of emotional state. *Psychological Review*, 1962, *69*, 379–399.

Sjöberg, L., & Persson, L.   A study of attempts by obese patients to regulate eating. *Addictive Behaviors*, 1979, *4*, 349–359.

Sjostrom, L., Garellick, G., Krotkiewski, M., & Luyckx, A.   Peripheral insulin in response to the sight and smell of food. *Metabolism*, 1980, *29*, 901–909.

Slochower, J.   Emotional labeling and overeating in obese and normal weight individuals. *Psychosomatic Medicine*, 1976, *38*, 131–139.

Spitzer, L., & Rodin, J.   Human eating behavior: A critical review of studies in normal weight and overweight individuals. *Appetite*, 1981, *2*, 293–329.

Stricker, E. M., & Zigmond, M.   Brain catecholamines and the lateral hypothalamic syndrome. In D. Novin (Ed.), *Hunger: Basic mechanisms and clinical implications.* New York: Raven, 1976.

Thayer, R. E.   Measurement of activation through self-report. *Psychological Reports*, 1967, *20*, 663–678.

Van Itallie, T. B., Smith, N. S., & Quartermain, D.   Short-term and long-term components in the regulation of food intake: Evidence for a modulatory role of carbohydrate status. *American Journal of Clinical Nutrition*, 1977, *30*, 742–757.

Wayner, M. J.   Specificity of behavioral regulation. *Physiology & Behavior*, 1974, *12*, 851–869.

White, C.   The effects of viewing films of different arousal content on the eating behavior of obese and normal weight subjects. *Dissertation Abstracts International*, November 1973, *34*, (5-B) 2324.

Wilder, J.   The law of initial values. *Psychosomatic Medicine*, 1950, *12*, 392.

Wooley, S. C., & Wooley, O. W.   Salivation to the sight and thought of food: A new measure of appetite. *Psychosomatic Medicine*, 1973, *35*, 136.

Zajonc, R. B.   Social facilitation. *Science*, 1965, *149*, 269–274.

Zillmann, D.   Excitation transfer in communication-mediated aggressive behavior. *Journal of Experimental Social Psychology*, 1971, *7*, 419–434.

CHAPTER 21

Social Psychophysiology and Behavioral Medicine: A Systems Perspective

Gary E. Schwartz
Yale University

INTRODUCTION AND OVERVIEW

The purpose of this chapter is to consider some of the implications of social psychophysiology for the emerging interdisciplinary field of behavioral medicine. It is becoming increasingly clear that an organism's physical health is determined by patterns of processes occurring at biological, psychological, and social/environmental levels (Leigh & Reiser, 1980). This has led some researchers (e.g., Engel, 1977) to propose that the medical model needs to be broadened, if not replaced, by a more comprehensive biopsychosocial model, one that integrates processes occurring at multiple levels. The emergence of behavioral medicine reflects this paradigm shift in thinking regarding a multifactorial approach to understanding the etiology, pathogenesis, diagnosis, treatment, and prevention of illness (Schwartz & Weiss, 1978).

Current theory and research in social psychophysiology, as reviewed in this volume, has important implications for psychology's contribution (i.e., health psychology) to behavioral medicine. Note that implicit in the ordering of its terms, social psychophysiology tends to emphasize the impact of the social environment, as it is interpreted by an organism, on the organism's physiology (see Cacioppo, 1982). Theoretically, in behavioral medicine, too, implicit in the ordering of its terms is a focus on behavioral/social factors as they affect health and illness. It follows that implicit in the ordering of terms in biopsychosocial is a primary focus on biology. For example, the Patient Evaluation Grid (PEG), developed by Leigh and Reiser (1980) to facilitate implementing the biopsychosocial model into clinical practice, begins with the gathering of biological information, moves to the gathering of personal/psychological information, and then moves to the gathering of environmental/social information.

It is understandable why researchers and clinicians coming from a biological tradition tend to approach the problem of health and illness from a biological level first, whereas researchers and clinicians coming from a psychological or social tradition tend to approach the problem of health and illness from a psychological or social level first. However, to reach a comprehensive synthesis will require that the problem be approached from both directions. Historically, more emphasis has been placed on the biological level than on the behavioral or social levels. I believe that social psychophysiology has the potential to bring balance to the emerging field of behavioral medicine by directing its attention to clarifying how social and psychological factors modulate physiological processes in health and illness.

To facilitate the complex task of integrating social, psychological, and physiological variables in health and illness, I will draw on concepts developed in general systems theory (von Bertalanffy, 1968) as they have been applied to living systems theory (Miller, 1978) and cybernetic control theory (Wiener, 1948). For the reader not familiar with systems theory and systems thinking, books by deRosnay (1979) and Weinberg (1975) are excellent introductions to this approach.

The present chapter extends recent writings on the application of systems theory to biofeedback (Schwartz, 1979b), health psychology (Schwartz, 1979a), behavioral medicine (Schwartz, 1980), models of human disease (Schwartz, 1981a), behavior therapy (Schwartz, 1982b), the psychophysiology of emotion (Schwartz, 1982c), and cardiovascular psychophysiology (Schwartz, 1982d).

A SYSTEMS PERSPECTIVE TO SOCIAL PSYCHOPHYSIOLOGY

It is impossible to review the basic tenets of systems theory in a brief chapter and do the theory justice. However, it is essential at the outset that certain key principles be discussed here in order to develop subsequent hypotheses about some of the potential applications of social psychophysiology to behavioral medicine. In particular, in order to appreciate how systems theory can help stimulate theoretical synthesis and interdisciplinary research, it is essential to understand the relationship between (1) interactions of processes, (2) emergent properties in systems, and (3) levels of processes in systems.

According to deRosnay (1979), a system can be defined as a "set of elements in dynamic interaction, organized for a goal" (p. 65). All systems, by definition, are composed of parts (elements), and these elements interact with each other in unique ways, thereby determining the unique behaviors (properties) of the system as a whole. Note that elements do not simply "act" upon one another, they "interact" with each other, and do so dynamically (i.e., the processes are always changing). The parts of a system are, so to speak, social with one another in the sense that they relate with (interact with) each other, forming an organized group of parts that emerge into a whole.

The concept of emergence grows out of the concept of parts interacting with each other. A basic tenet of systems theory is that the behaviors (properties) of a system emerge out of the unique, dynamic interactions of its parts. It follows that if the parts of a system are studied in isolation, it will be impossible theoretically to predict from the properties of parts in isolation what the unique properties of the system as a whole will show when the parts actually interact. The concept that parts must be studied in interaction may at first sound strange, but actually is quite established in psychology. The analysis of variance partitions variance into main effects and interactions. The interactions may be complex, and usually are a source of frustration to researchers interested primarily in simple cause-effect relationships. However, to a systems theorist, the interaction variance is actually the most interesting and important variance, since it is this variance that ultimately reflects the novel interactions among processes and the unique emergent properties of systems.

The phenomenon of emergence is found at every level in nature, from subatomic particles, through atoms and chemicals, to cells, organs and organisms, all the way to groups, organizations, nations, and so on. Although the explanation of emergence is not agreed upon by all theorists, the phenomenon of emergence is well accepted.

The concept of hierarchical levels becomes particularly significant once the ubiquitousness of emergence in nature is appreciated. Table 21-1 (from Schwartz, 1982b) illustrates how levels of systems relate to different scientific disciplines. The table is organized to move from the simple to the more complex, and from the early to the more recent in terms of evolutionary development. Hence, atoms are viewed as composed of subatomic particles, and the discipline of physics has evolved to study the unique properties of different atoms. Subatomic physics studies subatomic particles. The most abstract and basic of physics is called theoretical physics, which integrates mathematics and philosophy of science.

Note that when atoms interact and form more complex molecular systems, a new discipline—chemistry—evolves to study the unique properties of the different chemical systems. The bridge between chemistry and physics (chemicals and atoms) becomes physical chemistry. It makes sense that a good chemist should know physical chemistry and physics, as well as mathematics and philosophy of science.

The emergence of simple living systems (cells) from chemicals is relatively recent in evolutionary time. Cellular biology becomes the new discipline to study the properties of different cells. Note that the jump from chemicals to cells has an intermediate step, called biochemicals, which are very large chemical systems containing carbon, nitrogen, oxygen, and hydrogen. Biochemistry is the field that has emerged to study these

TABLE 21-1. Levels of Complexity in Systems and Associated Academic
Disciplines

According to systems theory, in order to understand the behavior of an open
system at any one level, it is essential to have training in the academic disciplines
below that level, plus have some training at least in the relevant discipline at the
next highest level as well.

LEVEL AND COMPLEXITY OF THE SYSTEM	ACADEMIC FIELD ASSOCIATED WITH THE LEVEL OF THE SYSTEM
Beyond earth	Astronomy
Supranational	Ecology
National	Government, political science, economics
Organizations	Organizational science
Groups	Sociology
Organism	Psychology, ethology, zoology
Organs	Organ physiology (e.g., neurology, cardiology)
Cells	Cellular biology
Biochemicals	Biochemistry
Chemicals	Chemistry, physical chemistry
Atoms	Physics
Subatomic particles	Subatomic physics
Abstract systems	Mathematics, philosophy

Note. From "Integrating psychobiology and behavior therapy: A systems perspective" by G. E. Schwartz, in G. T. Wilson & C. M. Franks (Eds.), *Contemporary
behavior therapy: Conceptual and empirical foundations*, New York: Guilford, 1982.

biochemical systems. A good cellular biochemist should therefore know
biochemistry, chemistry, some physical chemistry and physics, as well as
some mathematics and philosophy of science.

The emergence of more complex, multiorgan organisms is even more
recent in evolutionary time. At the organism level, different disciplines
have emerged to study the organism as a whole. Zoologists classify organisms in terms of structure, whereas integrative biologists, ethologists,
and psychologists study the functioning (behavior) of organisms. Note
that in the same way that the jump from chemicals to cells involved an
intermediate step of biochemistry, the jump from single cells to very
complex multicellular organisms involved an intermediate step of organ
systems. Physiologists study the structure and functioning of organ systems. Different organ systems specialists emerge to study the unique
properties of different organ systems. Hence, neurophysiologists study
the nervous system and cardiovascular physiologists study the cardiovascular system. Theoretically, a good zoologist/ethologist/psychologist
should know some physiology and cellular biology, some biochemistry and

chemistry, some physical chemistry and physics, some mathematics and philosophy of science.

When organisms interact with each other and form groups, the term "social" is typically used to describe these new systems. The discipline of sociology has emerged quite recently to study the structure and functioning of different social groups. The bridge between psychology (which as a discipline typically studies individual organisms) and sociology (which as a discipline typically studies groups of organisms) is called social psychology. Social psychology, therefore, bridges the social/group and psychological/individual levels in the same way that biochemistry bridges the cellular and chemical levels and physical chemistry bridges the chemical and physical levels. According to systems theory, any discipline that cuts across levels comes face to face with studying emergent properties of whole–part interactions. Hence, one discipline's "whole" may be another discipline's "part."

Space does not permit me to further explicate the movement up social/group/organization/nation/ecology levels (see Miller, 1978). However, the principle of emergence and level should now be clear. My purpose in illustrating how systems theory organizes nature and scientific disciplines is to help clarify the unique and difficult challenge facing researchers interested in social psychophysiology. Psychophysiology, by definition, is an interdiscipline—that is, psychophysiology attempts to bridge the individual (psychology) and organ (physiology) levels of structure and functioning. Since psychophysiology is an interdiscipline, and social psychology is also an interdiscipline, it follows that social psychophysiology must bridge three levels of analysis, and therefore three levels of structure and functioning. Theoretically, emergent properties should be evident at both the psychophysiological and social psychological interfaces. Also, it should be impossible theoretically to fully describe the relationship between social variables and physiological processes without considering the interactions emerging at the social psychological and psychophysiological interfaces.

As discussed in Schwartz (1980) regarding the interdisciplinary field of behavioral medicine, it is of fundamental importance not to confuse levels of description and analysis, since each level potentially reflects unique emergent properties. Social psychophysiology bridges three levels, hopefully with the goal of improving our ability to understand and predict how social processes relate to physiological functioning via the mediating level of psychological processing. General systems theory has the potential to provide a common metalanguage that can facilitate the process of translating across these different levels.

DISREGULATION THEORY AND ILLNESS

Social psychophysiology, as conceptualized above, has direct relevance for testing systems theory models of health and illness. Disregulation theory (Schwartz, 1977, 1979a, 1979b, 1982a) is a good example of this approach.

Figure 21-1 is a highly oversimplified but conceptually useful general description of social–psychological–physiological relationships in normal self-regulation and abnormal disregulation. The stages shown in Figure 21-1 can be summarized as follows:

Stage 1: Environmental Stresses/Demands

Stimuli from the external environment impinge on an organism, placing potential strain on the brain (stage 2) and body (stages 3 and 4). Some stimuli (stage 1) can act directly on the body (stage 3) (e.g., physical stimuli such as temperature can produce local vasoconstriction), whereas other stimuli must be processed by the brain in order to influence the body (e.g., social stimuli).

Stage 2: Central Nervous System Information-Processing System

Via sensory receptors and appropriate neural connections to the brain (not displayed in Figure 21-1), the brain registers, recognizes, and interprets the meaning of the environmental stimulation. Psychological processes (or more appropriately, neuropsychological processes) play a major role in determining what pattern of physiological (behavioral) responses will be made in response to the environmental stimuli.

Stage 3: Peripheral Organs

The brain, via neural and humoral connections, regulates patterns of organs coordinated to meet particular needs and reach particular goals. In the same way that "mind" may be thought of as "located" in stage 2, "behavior" may be thought of as "located" in stage 3. All overt behavior, therefore, can be thought of as reflecting organized patterns of peripheral organ functioning. For example, when a subject in a social situation involving personal evaluation (stage 1) interprets the situation as stressful (stage 2) and looks away (stage 3) from the examiner when asked a difficult question (e.g., see Schwartz, Davidson, & Maer, 1975), this eye movement can either be labeled as (1) a behavior (if observed visually by the examiner), (2) a physiological response (if measured using electrodes to directly record the electrooculogram), or (3) a neurophysiological response (if the observer infers, for example, that since the subject's eyes moved to the left, and the subject is right-handed, he probably engaged his right hemisphere in this social stress). Note that the label used (and therefore the selection of the journal in which the data might be published) would depend on the method used to measure the movement and to interpret the movement's significance.

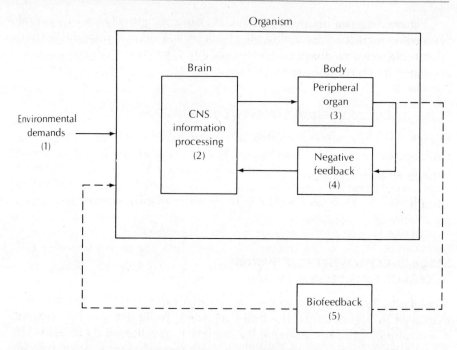

FIGURE 21-1. Simplified block diagram depicting (1) environmental demands influencing (via extero-ceptors, not shown) (2) the brain's regulation of its (3) peripheral organs, and (4) negative feedback from the periphery back to the brain. Disregulation can be initiated at each of these stages. Bio-feedback (stage 5) is a parallel feedback loop to stage 4, detecting the activity of the peripheral organ (stage 3) and converting it into environmental demands (stage 1) that can be used by the brain (stage 2) to increase self-regulation. From Schwartz (1977).

As noted in Schwartz (1978), our tendency to separate behavior, physiology, and neurophysiology as if they each reflected independent processes, when in fact they reflect different levels of one integrated, organized process (at the organism system level), inadvertently discour-ages interdisciplinary theorizing and research. Social psychophysiology should be the field that is explicitly concerned with integrating these different levels of analysis with a special focus on the social level.

Stage 4: Peripheral Negative Feedback

The body contains a very complex array of sensory transducers that measure the dynamic functioning of the body (in terms of physical, chemi-cal, and biochemical processes). This information is fed back to the brain so that the brain can make appropriate adjustments to best achieve certain goals. These adjustment processes are often of the negative feedback variety. That is, as described in cybernetic theory (Wiener, 1948), a subset of general systems theory, negative feedback allows a system to alter its behavior in such a way as to maintain its functioning around a given set point. Negative feedback is the process whereby the brain can counteract changes in the periphery to optimize stability of functioning. Negative feedback is therefore essential for normal, stable movements (i.e., overt behaviors) as well as regulating those physiological processes that comprise and support particular behavioral goals. This is the essence of what Cannon (1932) termed homeostasis.

Stage 5: Biofeedback

It follows that biofeedback is also a negative feedback process (parallel to stage 4), typically using electronic equipment to detect physiological changes and convert the signals into environmental information (stage 1) that can be processed by the brain (stage 2) with the goal of fostering self-regulation. The reader should recognize that the concept of biofeedback as displayed in Figure 21-1 has broad implications for health and illness, including social interactions. Health providers, as well as family and friends, can act as "biofeedback" devices in the sense that people can observe physiological changes (directly or indirectly) and feed this information back to a person. The social environment, therefore, can become an intimate part of the biofeedback (stage 5) loop. Thus, a nurse who takes a patient's pressure and informs the patient that his or her pressure is high is acting as a stage 5 feedback process. Similarly, a person who notices that his or her partner is looking pale may bring this information to his or her partner's attention. The paleness may signify that the partner is coming down with a cold, is tired, is worried about falling in love, and so forth. From a systems perspective, all social interactions can be thought of, therefore, as social psychophysiological interactions.

I believe that it is useful to think of the brain, in collaboration with the body, as acting as a "health care system" (Schwartz, 1979a). That is, one of the brain's primary functions is to detect problems occurring in the body (stage 3, via stage 4 processes), and then to take corrective action to resolve these problems. This self-regulatory process requires that all the components be connected properly, and that the brain has the wisdom, in Cannon's (1932) terms, to pursue the best means of solving the problem.

Self-regulation in systems, therefore, can occur only to the extent that the various components in the system are appropriately connected. If the feedback is interpreted as negative feedback, self-regulation should lead to an ordered set of adjustments. This ordered set of adjustments can be thought of as reflecting the pursuit of health for the system, and, therefore, should lead to "ease" in the system.

It follows that if a person attends to his or her body and interprets this information appropriately, enhanced self-regulation should occur. Altogether, the theory proposes that self-attention (if the information is interpreted in a negative feedback manner) should lead to increased neuropsychological connections, promoting brain–body self-regulation, which in turn should lead to increased order and ease in the system.

Disregulation theory is simply the opposite of self-regulation theory, as briefly summarized above (see Schwartz, 1982a, for a more complete analysis). It follows that if any part of a self-regulating system is, for whatever reason, disconnected (this is an extreme case in a system, but it is a case that well illustrates the general point), self-regulation will be impossible. It follows that in this situation, order in the system will break down. The breakdown in order will be expressed as increased disorder in the behavior of the system. If this disordered functioning reflects certain medical syndromes, the disorder may be labeled as a disease.

One way to promote neuropsychological disconnections, at least theoretically, is to disattend to bodily feedback. If a person does not attend to stage 4 signals reflecting bodily problems, the person will not be able to take appropriate corrective action. Thus, disattention (to essential negative feedback signals) should lead to neuropsychological disconnections, which should produce the process I call disregulation, which will be expressed as increased disorder and potentially be labeled as a disease.

Note that disconnections in complex living systems can be caused by physical, chemical, biochemical, and cellular, as well as psychological and social psychological stimuli. Since this chapter is concerned with social psychophysiology, I will focus on social psychological variables as they can contribute to promoting disregulation. The reader should note, however, that even if the primary disregulation is caused by physical, nutritional, biochemical, or even genetic factors, social psychophysiological processes may play an important contributing role to the diagnosis, treatment, and prevention of such diseases (i.e., disorders of disregulation).

IMPLICATIONS FOR THE SOCIAL PSYCHOPHYSIOLOGY OF DISEASE

There are numerous implications of systems theory for social psychophysiological research concerned with social psychological factors that contribute to the etiology and pathogenesis of disease. Disregulation theory, as a subset of systems theory, becomes especially helpful because it suggests more specific research questions and methodological directions for future research.

For example, a number of studies have recently examined cardiovascular and neuroendocrine responses to various social challenges in Type A and Type B individuals (who are differentially at risk for developing atherosclerotic diseases and myocardial infarction, possibly ending in sudden cardiac death; e.g., Glass *et al.*, 1981). In general, these studies indicate that people classified as Type A, using a standardized interview (assessing verbal and nonverbal reactions in a carefully structured social situation), tend to respond with larger increases in blood pressure and heart rate, as well as measures of plasma epinephrine and norepinephrine, than do Type B subjects. These differences in reactivity are most strongly expressed in situations that require competition and challenge, including time urgency. Typically, Type A and Type B subjects do not differ in resting mean activity in these parameters.

These Type A studies clearly reflect a social psychophysiological paradigm. It appears that in certain social situations, certain individuals show large and potentially maladaptive cardiovascular and neuroendocrine responses that put these individuals at risk for developing serious cardiovascular disease. The next step in such research is to clarify what it is about these social variables, and the mediating psychological variables, that result in such exaggerated and potentially self-destructive physiological reactions.

The approach recommended in this chapter is that appropriate bridges between social psychology and psychophysiology be built, interpreting social psychology and psychophysiology broadly. For example, we can ask the question: Why is it that competition often leads to large increases in multiple cardiovascular responses? A close analysis at the physiological level suggests an answer. The pattern of increases in systolic blood pressure, diastolic blood pressure, and heart rate observed in competitive situations turns out to be a pattern associated more closely with anger and frustration than with fear and anxiety (see Schwartz, Weinberger, & Singer, 1981). Thus, we can speculate that those social situations (stage 1) that trigger anger and frustration at a psychological level (stage 2) should be accompanied by particular patterns of response expressive of these emotions at the behavioral/physiological level (stage 3). Integrating recent research on the psychophysiology of different emotions with recent research on the social psychology of situations that elicit different emotions becomes a potentially fruitful research direction for the future.

Of course, people vary in their reactions to competitive situations. Some of these individual differences probably reflect stage 2 differences (e.g., reflecting stored memories and experiences). Others probably reflect stage 3 differences (e.g., genetic differences in neurochemical sensitivity of particular peripheral organs) and stage 4 differences (e.g., genetic differences in neural sensitivity of particular sensory feedback organs). It follows that if two subjects exposed to the same social situation (stage 1) react with different cardiovascular adjustments (stage 3), these differences can be due to differences at stage 2, 3, or 4, *or any combination of stages 2, 3, and 4.*

This is where a systems perspective becomes particularly useful. By clarifying parts and levels in systems, strategies for becoming more systematic (no pun intended) about uncovering the possible sources of these differences become clearer.

At the present time, the various stage 2, 3, and 4 factors that lead to high cardiovascular reactivity in some subjects and not others in competitive social situations are not well understood. According to systems theory, research strategies that group subjects according to Type A behavior versus grouping subjects according to cardiovascular reactivity will not lead to identical conclusions. This is because not all Type A subjects respond with large cardiovascular responses, and similarly, not all subjects who show large cardiovascular responses turn out to be Type A. Type A is a psychological level (stage 2) category, whereas cardiovascular reactivity per se is, by definition, a measurement occurring at the physiological level (stage 3). Those Type A subjects who actually show *small* cardiovascular responses to competition may differ in family history (possibly genetic predisposition at stage 3) from those Type A subjects who show large cardiovascular adjustments. Or, large cardiovascular responses in subjects who are Type B may be due to differences in genetic predispositions (or other stage 3 and/or stage 4 processes), whereas large cardiovascular responses in subjects who are Type A may reflect an important contribution of stage 2 processes. It follows that subjects who are Type A (stage 2) *and* have a strong genetic predisposition at the periphery (stage 3) should be *most likely* to show large cardiovascular responses and to develop serious cardiovascular diseases.

The systems perspective therefore encourages research that examines *interactions* of social, psychological, and physiological variables, and suggests a systematic framework for interpreting patterns of findings that emerge in terms of different underlying mechanisms. Disregulation theory, as a subset of general systems theory, provides even more specific suggestions within this general framework. For example, another characteristic of Type A subjects is that they tend to push themselves to extremes, and often disattend to their bodies, especially in social situations that they interpret as being competitive. In other words, Type A subjects not only interpret a wide variety of situations as being competitive (with others and/or with self), but in so doing also disattend to bodily cues (since awareness of these cues might serve to discourage them from continuing to compete at such extreme levels). Hence, Glass and colleagues reported, for example, that Type A subjects on an exercise treadmill pushed themselves harder, yet reported less fatigue than Type B subjects.

This suggests the intriguing hypothesis that Type A behavior and its associated cardiovascular reactivity may in part reflect a disregulatory process involving learned disattention to bodily cues in various social situations. The Type A, by being motivated to push him or herself to extremes, may not only place himself or herself at high risk because of the prolonged high stress, but may also promote cardiovascular disorder *as a side effect of the neuropsychological disconnections between brain and body encouraged by the excessive bodily disattention.*

If Type A subjects disattend to their bodies, this disattention should express itself in various ways, as predicted by disregulation theory. For example, even during resting conditions, disregulation theory would predict that homeostatic self-regulatory processes should be less intact in Type A subjects. Heart rate/blood pressure/skeletal muscle relationships should be more disordered (less well regulated in a rhythmic fashion) as a result of the disregulation. Disregulation theory therefore proposes that measures of variance, especially time series and coherence statistics (Porges, Bohrer, Cheung, Drasgow, McCabe, & Keren, 1980) (originally developed in engineering for assessing control processes) should be applied to resting cardiovascular data. Dembroski, MacDougall, and Shields (1977), in their first paper on cardiovascular reactivity in Type A's, noted that Type A subjects did not differ from Type B's in resting heart rate. However, Type A's did show a curious disruption of sinus arrhythmia (which really is not an arrhythmia, but is a true rhythm where heart rate follows breathing regularly in a homeostatically controlled way). Type A's apparently have a breakdown in this normal respiratory–heart rate process. The heart rate of Type A's does not follow breathing in a normal, homeostatic manner. Since Dembroski *et al.* lacked a theoretical framework to interpret these findings, the data were simply mentioned and then disregarded. However, these data become very significant in terms of disregulation theory, especially if future research shows that resting measures of the degree of disorder in this homeostatic self-regulation process is predictive of actual responding to a social challenge.

Another prediction from disregulation theory concerns possible neuropsychological mechanisms (stage 2) that may contribute to this apparent cardiovascular disregulation. As discussed in detail in Schwartz (1982a), it is possible that the denial of pain and other negative emotions may involve a functional disconnection syndrome between the left and right hemispheres. Briefly, our current research suggests the following:

1. A subset of persons, labeled repressors, report very low stress yet score high on defensiveness. These subjects exhibit physiological reactivity which is equal if not greater in magnitude than subjects who report high anxiety (Weinberger, Schwartz, & Davidson, 1979).
2. In right-handed subjects, the left hemisphere is more involved in positive emotions, and the right hemisphere is more involved in negative emotions (Ahern & Schwartz, 1979; Schwartz, Ahern, & Brown, 1979).
3. People who deny negative emotions show greater left–right differences in positive versus negative emotions than do subjects who correctly perceive that they are low anxious (Polonsky & Schwartz, submitted for publication).

4. Extreme left–right hemispheric differences are accompanied by increased cardiovascular disregulation and increased physical illness (Schwartz & Schwaab, in preparation).

Although admittedly preliminary at this time, the available data support the value of linking psychological denial and disattention with functionally produced neuropsychological disconnections that through disregulation may contribute to physiological disorder and thus physical disease. Social situations that encourage disattention should therefore promote neuropsychological disconnections and physiological disorder.

IMPLICATIONS FOR THE SOCIAL PSYCHOPHYSIOLOGY OF HEALTH

Unfortunately, most of the research to date on the psychophysiology of stress has emphasized stimulus conditions that minimize the importance of social factors. These standard paradigms are listed as categories 1 to 3 in Table 21-2. The challenge facing social psychophysiology is to conduct behavioral medicine research that emphasizes categories 4 and 5, and does so in a manner that clarifies the relationships among social, psychological, and physiological levels of interaction.

As implied in Table 21-2, there are numerous paradigms already developed in social psychology that can be potentially integrated with psychophysiology in the study of behavioral medicine. Social psychophysiology may make important contributions not only to the etiology and pathogenesis of disease, but to the treatment and prevention of disease as well.

One area in particular that deserves to be considered in future research concerns the social psychophysiology of healing, broadly defined. By that I mean social psychological variables that, through psychophysiological mechanisms, may facilitate (or counteract) normal healing processes. Variables such as empathy, warmth of the therapist, and even physical contact by a caring professional, spouse, or friend, may have an important impact on healing. Social psychophysiology may provide the tools for better studying the doctor–patient relationship.

In a pioneering book by Lynch (1977) titled *The Broken Heart*, the author reviews epidemiological evidence indicating that enduring human relationships—between children and parents, among friends, and most important, between husbands and wives—are important conditions for emotional and physical health. For example, the data indicate that holding the number of cigarettes smoked constant, those individuals who smoke and have stable family relationships are *less* likely to develop lung cancer than those individuals who smoke but are single, widowed, or divorced. Apparently,

TABLE 21-2. Categories of Stress Paradigms

1. *Simple stresses*
   Deprivation
   Immobilization
   Aversive stimulation
      Noise
      Shock
      Heat/cold
      Electrical stimulation
   Conflict

2. *Mental stresses*
   Vigilance
   Discrimination
   Reaction time
   Mental arithmetic
   Affective imagery

3. *Learning stresses*
   Classical conditioning
      Positive
      Negative
   Operant conditioning
      Reward
      Punishment
      Avoidance

4. *Social stresses*
   Interviews
   Competition/cooperation tasks
   Crowding
   Speech anxiety tasks
   Role-playing tasks
   Social performance/evaluation tasks

5. *Naturalistic stresses*
   Marriage
   Divorce
   Separation
   Death
   Job
   Environmental disaster
   War

stable relationships with animals can have similarly salutary effects on health. One study suggests that the likelihood of recovering from a heart attack is increased if the patient has a stable, caring relationship with a pet.

Lynch proposes that social contact, even in life-threatening environments, can have positive effects on healing and health if the contact reflects genuine concern, caring, and support. In a sample of patients studied in a shock-trauma unit, Lynch and colleagues report that if a patient's hand is held in a caring way, heart rate responses to the stressful environment are attenuated. Furthermore, these salutary effects can occur even if the patient's muscles are paralyzed with curare.

Recently, Drescher, Morrill, Whitehead, and Cataldo (1982) have reported a basic research study on physiological and subjective reactions to being touched. They compared the effects of alpha biofeedback training with human contact on responses to a laboratory stressor. The stressor involved having subjects place one of their hands in ice water. The data indicated that the effects of human contact (touching) occurred most strongly in the cardiovascular system, and that these subjects found being touched both more pleasant and more relaxing than practicing alpha biofeedback. Touching in this study did not reduce the perceived painfulness of ice water but did attenuate the heart rate increase normally produced by pain.

I believe that research paradigms from experimental social psychology can be fruitfully applied to this general area. We can ask questions such as: What kinds of social situations facilitate coping with stress, and thereby facilitate various physiological processes involved in healing? What social factors, including environmental factors and the presence of significant others, can alter the course of illness and healing? Is it possible that caring, supportive relationships act via specific emotional and immune systems to promote well-being? Can other living systems, such as animals and even plants, have health-promoting consequences if they are perceived in a positive, socially caring manner?

Recent research on the psychophysiology of emotion (e.g., Schwartz, Weinberger, & Singer, 1981) support the view that different emotions involve different patterns of central nervous system, neuroendocrine, and physiological responses. It is possible, at least in theory, that certain patterns not only are less stress producing, but specific patterns may actually be physiologically restorative in a health promoting way. It is possible that positive social support may act to reduce disregulation, thereby promoting natural homeostatic self-regulation. This facilitation would be expressed by decreases in disordered physiological variability and by more rapid recovery to physical as well as psychosocial stressors. The challenge of social psychophysiology is not simply to apply current paradigms such as social facilitation, social support, and empathy to fundamental problems in behavioral medicine, but to develop new paradigms that are stimulated by the kinds of questions generated by clinical observations such as those made by Lynch and colleagues in a hospital setting. From a systems perspective, the patient in a hospital is part of a complex social environment. Specifying these social relations may be fundamental to understanding illness and health.

SUMMARY AND CONCLUSIONS

This chapter has, in an abbreviated fashion, attempted to illustrate how social psychophysiology may potentially contribute to behavioral medicine. Social psychophysiology has been interpreted here as reflecting the integration of social, psychological, and physiological levels of analysis and process, emphasizing the emergent interactions that theoretically must occur at both the social psychological and psychophysiological interfaces. Systems theory has been used to help organize and integrate the various methods and findings obtained at these three different levels. Disregulation theory has been used to specify more precisely how social stimuli can potentially disrupt normal homeostatic processes through psychological mechanisms. Disregulation theory stimulates the quantification of patterns of processes in a dynamic manner, with special emphasis on measures of coherence, recovery, and disorder. This chapter is clearly speculative, and only a few examples have been cited to illustrate the general perspective. However, if the general systems perspective set forth in this chapter helps stimulate the reader to consider building new bridges between his or her areas of expertise in experimental social psychology, psychophysiology, and problems in behavioral medicine, it will have achieved its goal.

R E F E R E N C E S

Ahern, G. L., & Schwartz, G. E. Differential lateralization for positive versus negative emotion. *Neuropsychologia*, 1979, *17*, 693–697.

Cacioppo, J. T. Social psychophysiology: A classic and contemporary approach. *Psychophysiology*, 1982, *19*, 241–251.

Cannon, W. B. *The wisdom of the body*. New York: W. W. Norton, 1932.

Dembroski, T. M., MacDougall, J. M., & Shields, J. L. Physiologic reactions to social challenge in persons evidencing the Type A coronary-prone behavior pattern. *Journal of Human Stress*, 1977, *3*, 2–10.

deRosnay, J. *The macroscope*. New York: Harper & Row, 1979.

Drescher, V. M., Morrill, E. D., Whitehead, W. E., & Cataldo, M. F. Physiological and subjective reactions to being touched. *Psychophysiology*, 1982, *19*, 314. (Abstract)

Engel, G. L. The need for a new medical model: A challenge for biomedicine. *Science*, 1977, *196*, 129–136.

Glass, D. C., Krakoff, L. R., Contrada, R., Hilton, W. F., Kehoe, K., Mannucci, E. G., Collins, C., Snow, G., & Elting, E. Effect of harassment and competition upon cardiovascular and plasma catecholamine responses in Type A and Type B individuals. *Psychophysiology*, 1981, *17*, 453–463.

Leigh, H., & Reiser, M. F. *The patient: Biological, psychological and social dimensions of medical practice*. New York: Plenum, 1980.

Lynch, J. J. *The broken heart*. New York: Harper & Row, 1977.

Miller, J. G. *Living systems*. New York: McGraw-Hill, 1978.

Polonsky, W. H., & Schwartz, G. E. *Facial electromyography and the self-deceptive coping style:*

Individual differences in the hemispheric lateralization of affect. Manuscript submitted for publication.

Porges, S. W., Bohrer, R. E., Cheung, M., Drasgow, F., McCabe, P., & Keren, G.   New time-series statistic for detecting rhythmic co-occurrence in the frequency domain: The waited coherence and its application to psychophysiological research. *Psychological Bulletin,* 1980, *88,* 580–587.

Schwartz, G. E.   Psychosomatic disorders and biofeedback: A psychobiological model of disregulation. In J. D. Maser & M. E. P. Seligman (Eds.), *Psychopathology: Experimental models.* San Francisco: W. H. Freeman, 1977.

Schwartz, G. E.   Psychobiological foundations of psychotherapy and behavior change. In S. L. Garfield & A. E. Bergin (Eds.), *Handbook of psychotherapy and behavior change* (2nd ed.). New York: Wiley, 1978.

Schwartz, G. E.   The brain as a health care system. In G. Stone, N. Adler, & F. Cohen (Eds.), *Health psychology.* San Francisco: Jossey-Bass, 1979. (a)

Schwartz, G. E.   Disregulation and systems theory: A biobehavioral framework for biofeedback and behavioral medicine. In N. Birbaumer & H. D. Kimmel (Eds.), *Biofeedback and self-regulation.* Hillsdale, N.J.: Erlbaum, 1979. (b)

Schwartz, G. E. Behavioral medicine and systems theory: A new synthesis. *National Forum,* Winter 1980, pp. 25–30.

Schwartz, G. E.   Disregulation theory and disease: Applications to the repression/cerebral disconnection/cardiovascular disorder hypothesis. In J. Matarazzo, N. Miller, & S. Weiss (Eds.), Special issue on behavioral medicine of *International Review of Applied Psychology,* 1982. (a)

Schwartz, G. E.   Integrating psychobiology and behavior therapy: A systems perspective. In G. T. Wilson & C. M. Franks (Eds.), *Contemporary behavior therapy: Conceptual and experimental foundations.* New York: Guilford, 1982. (b)

Schwartz, G. E.   Psychophysiological patterning and emotion revisited: A systems perspective. In C. Izard (Ed.), *Measuring emotions in infants and children.* Cambridge: Cambridge University Press, 1982. (c)

Schwartz, G. E.   Cardiovascular psychophysiology: A systems perspective. In J. T. Cacioppo & R. E. Petty (Eds.), *Perspectives in cardiovascular psychophysiology.* New York: Guilford, 1982. (d)

Schwartz, G. E., Ahern, G. L., & Brown, S. L.   Lateralized facial muscle response to positive versus negative emotional stimuli. *Psychophysiology,* 1979, *16,* 561–571.

Schwartz, G. E., Davidson, R. J., & Maer, F.   Right hemisphere lateralization for emotion in the human brain: Interaction with cognition. *Science,* 1975, *190,* 286–288.

Schwartz, G. E., & Schwaab, M.   *Repressive coping style, cerebral lateralization and cardiovascular disregulation.* Manuscript in preparation.

Schwartz, G. E., Weinberger, D. A., & Singer, J. A.   Cardiovascular differentiation of happiness, sadness, anger, and fear following imagery and exercise. *Psychosomatic Medicine,* 1981, *43,* 343–364.

Schwartz, C. E., & Weiss, S. M.   Yale Conference on Behavioral Medicine: A proposed definition and statement of goals. *Journal of Behavioral Medicine,* 1978, *1,* 3–12.

von Bertalanffy, L.   *General systems theory.* New York: Braziller, 1968.

Weinberg, G. M.   *An introduction to general systems thinking.* New York: Wiley, 1975.

Weinberger, D. A., Schwartz, G. E., & Davidson, R. J.   Low anxious, high anxious, and repressive coping styles: Psychometric patterns and behavioral and physiological responses to stress. *Journal of Abnormal Psychology,* 1979, *88,* 369–380.

Wiener, N.   *Cybernetics or control and communication in the animal and machine.* Cambridge, Mass.: MIT Press, 1948.

METHODS
OF SOCIAL
PSYCHOPHYSIOLOGY

Fundamentals of Psychophysiological Measurement

F. J. McGuigan
University of Louisville

INTRODUCTION

One of the major aims of social psychology has been to understand readily observable human behavior. Social psychologists have indeed been impressive in their development of methodologies for assessing such overt behaviors (e.g., see Aronson & Carlsmith, 1969). The technology within social psychology for studying small-scale responses such as changes in cardiovascular or covert somatic activity has been available, but it has been widely misunderstood and seldom used for purposes of theory development and testing (cf. Cacioppo, Petty, & Quintanar, 1982). This lack of progress and understanding is due in part to historical trends of social psychology that have dealt largely with such overt social behaviors as interpersonal aggression, attraction, coalition formation, and bargaining. Covert behaviors of social interactions have been essentially ignored.

The classical distinction between overt and covert behavior is not a sharp one. Overt events such as approaching a friend or speaking aloud are readily apparent; but just as clearly, there are events that are hidden from ordinary observation, such as an increase in heart rate or a transient contraction of a small muscle in the tongue. A gray area intervenes between these extremes where we find events that are difficult to classify as being either overt or covert—for example, a slight whisper, a partial blink of the eyes, or a slight behavioral expression of an emotion (e.g., see Hager & Ekman, Chapter 10, this volume).

Whether events are overt, covert, or fall within this transitional area, however, is in principle unimportant to us. The fact that specialized apparatus is required for the observation of small-scale behavior does not mean that covert behavior differs theoretically or in kind from overt behavior. Nor is it theoretically relevant that response events may often be more effectively studied by the methods of psychophysiology than by the classical behavioral methods of observation. The important point is that the reduced motivation or ability of people to control or bias their physiological and psychophysiological reactions make the psychophysiological measurement of the wide range of covert responses underlying overt responses worth the study of social psychologists (see Cacioppo & Petty, 1981; McGuigan, 1978). Let us now briefly consider an overview of the kinds of covert processes with which a social psychophysiologist might deal.

TAXONOMY OF COVERT PROCESSES

In Table 22-1 are a number of the more commonly measured psychophysiological events. We start with the primary division between muscular and glandular responses (I) and neurophysiological processes (II). Muscle responses are best measured through electromyography, whereas brain events are often studied through electroencephalography. This separation of response and central nervous system (CNS) reactions indicates that the two classes of events operate differently and *are* different components of neuromuscular circuits that function during internal information processing. Although we use similar electrical methods for studying these two classes of bodily events, responses obey different laws than do neural events. For an obvious example, muscle fibers move, but neurons do not. It is, then, most efficient to classify systems of responses versus central nervous system reactions separately and to study the interactions of these

TABLE 22-1. Psychophysiologically Measured Covert Processes in Humans

I. Covert responses (which consist of, and only of, muscular and glandular events)
   A. Covert speech responses
      1. Skeletal muscle electromyographic measures, principally from the tongue, lips, chin, laryngeal region, and jaw
      2. Pneumograms
      3. Audio measures of subvocalization ("whispering")
   B. Covert nonoral responses
      1. Skeletal muscle electromyographic measures from the fingers, arm, leg, etc.
      2. Visceral muscle activity (electrogastrogram)
      3. Eye responses, principally the electrooculogram
      4. Cardiovascular measures
         a. Heart rate
         b. Electrocardiogram
         c. Finger pulse volume
         d. Blood pressure
      5. Electrodermal measures (galvanic skin response, skin conductance, etc.)
II. Neurophysiological measures
   In the normal human, electrical activity is studied and recorded through electroencephalography and often further processed to yield evoked potentials, and the contingent negative variation.

events within neuromuscular circuits. Within the first major classification of responses, we focus on skeletal (as contrasted with smooth) muscle responses, eye responses, and respiration. A secondary division then separates responses in the oral (speech) regions of the body (I.A, in Table 22-1) from the nonoral bodily areas (I.B).

Most data on covert speech behavior have been gathered through electromyographic recording (I.A.1). During linguistic processing, the tongue is the most sensitive region; the lips appear to be next most sensitive, and the jaw, chin, and laryngeal regions are relatively insensitive (see, e.g., McGuigan, Culver, & Kendler, 1971; McGuigan & Pinkney, 1973). Pneumograms (I.A.2), potentially important measures of covert oral responses, have not been extensively studied, but we do know that breathing rate increases during such linguistic tasks as silent reading (e.g., McGuigan, Keller, & Stanton, 1964). Breathing amplitude increases during auditory hallucinations (McGuigan, 1966). Audio measures of subvocalization (I.A.3) have been interesting in the study of covert speech behavior, as from highly amplified sounds issuing from the mouth it is possible to understand portions of the prose that children silently read (e.g., McGuigan *et al.*, 1964), or portions of the verbal content of a paranoid schizophrenic's auditory hallucinations (McGuigan, 1966).

Measures of covert nonoral responses (I.B) during cognition also yield valuable information; for example, covert electromyographic finger activity in deaf individuals tells us something about their thought processes (Max, 1937; McGuigan, 1971). The leg is often used as an informative control measure.

Various neurophysiological measures (II) should eventually advance our understanding of the function of the brain during thought, but adequate comprehension of this complex organ will require more advanced techniques of study than we have yet imagined. One major advance within the last several decades has been the development of signal averaging. While the raw electroencephalographic trace tells little of interest, by averaging a number of electroencephalograms during an experimental treatment it has been possible to "tease out" very interesting neural phenomena as in the evoked potential or the so-called "expectancy wave" (the contingent negative variation).

Let us now consider the problem of how to study directly the covert processes specified in Table 22-1. There are relatively minor obstacles to observing overt responses, with most of the difficulties arising only insofar as recording and measurement techniques are concerned. Covert psychophysiological events, on the other hand, can be observed only through the use of equipment that, so to speak, extends the scope of our senses. That magnification is required in order to observe phenomena is not unusual, and we have developed numerous kinds of apparatus that allow us to detect events that could not otherwise be studied. The microscope and the telescope are obvious examples and illustrate the promise of introducing powerful new methods of observation to a field of scientific study. We turn next to a discussion of similarly powerful methods of psychophysiological measurement that may be beneficial for social psychology.

LABORATORY TECHNIQUES FOR MEASURING COVERT PROCESSES

There are four essential features of an electropsychology laboratory for the study of covert processes: (1) *sensors*, which detect the signals of interest; (2) *amplifiers*, which increase the amplitude of the signals sensed; (3) *readout devices*, which display and record the signals; and (4) *quantification systems*, which render the analog signals into numerical values.

In Figure 22-1, we can study the four major components of a relatively advanced psychophysiological laboratory. To the left we can note that the sensors are contained in a specially shielded subject room, and that they enter the amplifiers, located in a second room. Next we note that the amplified signals are recorded on a direct recorder and also on a data tape recorder; the signals are simultaneously monitored on a cathode-ray oscilloscope (CRO) and can be displayed for detailed study on a storage oscilloscope. Finally, the signals enter a quantification system that may be online, or may be employed at a later time, receiving data stored on magnetic tape on a tape recorder or on computer disks (see Cacioppo, Marshall-Goodell, & Gormezano, Chapter 24, and McHugo & Lanzetta, Chapter 23, this volume). We now enlarge on these four laboratory units.

Sensors

The sensor detects the signal of interest. Like a mammalian sense receptor, it is a specialized instrument that is sensitive to a given kind of energy or to a given frequency or amplitude range of a certain kind of energy. Consequently, sensors are designed so that only certain events are detected, while others are rejected. Most sensors in our area of interest are electrodes that sense electrical signals. A pair of electrodes may be fixed on or in the appropriate location of the body, and a difference in electrical potential between the two electrodes may be detected. As we have seen, two principal classes of electrical signals are generated by the muscles and by cerebral neurons. We have also noted that these two classes of events may be studied directly through electronic means, yielding electromyograms and electroencephalograms, respectively.

Surface electrodes, attached on the skin, are more widely used in normal human psychophysiology than are inserted (wire or needle) electrodes. When we attempt to sense subcutaneous potentials with surface

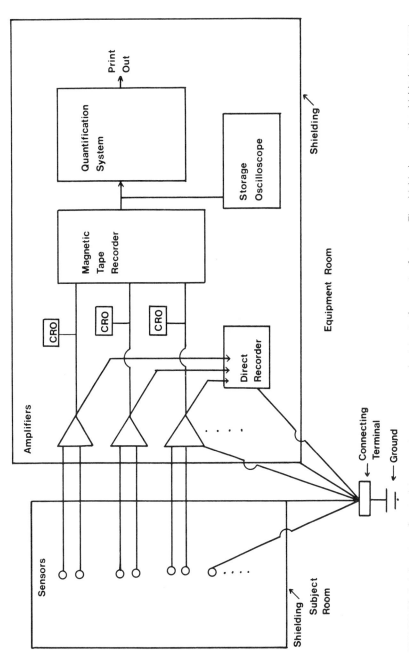

FIGURE 22-1. Laboratory for studying covert processes, emphasizing its four major features. The shielded rooms, the shielded equipment, and the subject are all connected to a common ground.

615

electrodes, cutaneous resistance must be reduced. This can be accomplished by placing a special paste or jelly under the electrode. The jelly forms a metal-electrolyte interface between the skin and the surface electrode which reduces skin resistance, increasing the amplitude of the signal. To reduce cutaneous resistance further, the skin should be rubbed and cleansed with any normal detergent, thus removing oil, salt, and the upper layers of the skin (which consist primarily of dead cells). The electrodes should be attached firmly on the skin so as to prevent movement artifact (movement of an electrode produces a slow signal in the trace that is not part of the bioelectrical signal of interest). This artifact can be eliminated by placing a small adhesive Styrofoam pad over the electrode and perhaps also a piece of tape across the pad onto the skin (elaborations and illustrations of these techniques may be found in McGuigan, 1979, as well as in a number of other laboratory manuals).

More than one pair of electrodes should be attached to the subject so that measurements may be made simultaneously from a number of bodily locations. Single response recording is of limited scientific value. As we shall see shortly, it is important to measure patterns of behavior throughout the body rather than a response in only one region. Another advantage of multiple electrode placement is that suggestion to the subject is prevented or is reduced; if only one set of electrodes is attached in a certain bodily location the subject would expect that something special should occur there. Consider, for instance, how you would feel if electrodes were attached only on your lips—there might be excessive "forced" responding or even inhibition of lip behavior. For an elaboration of this important control procedure, see Chapters 5 through 8 of McGuigan (1978).

There are two general arrangements of electrodes, the bipolar and the monopolar technique. In both techniques the difference in electrical potential between a pair of electrodes is recorded. However, with bipolar recording the two electrodes are placed close together and the leads (wires) from each enter separately into an amplifier. Bipolar techniques are used most commonly in electromyography. With the monopolar technique only one electrode is placed at the bodily region of interest and the second (reference) electrode is placed at a more remote location. Should recording at two bodily locations be desired with the monopolar technique, one electrode would be placed at each location and the potential difference would be recorded between each and the common reference electrode. Monopolar recording is used most prominently in electroencephalography so that several electrodes are placed at selected regions over the brain, with the reference electrode being at the earlobe. The bipolar placement allows more precise recording of activity from a localized region because the potential difference is sensed between two electrodes placed close together. The monopolar arrangement allows the recording of more diffuse electrical activity that is widely spread over larger bodily regions because the distance between the electrodes at the place of interest and the reference electrode is great. Should you use the monopolar technique with electromyography, for instance, you would probably sense other signals thar. those from the skeletal muscle, as, for instance, electrocardiographic ones.

Amplifiers

Once an electrical signal is sensed, it is led from the subject to this second of the four aspects of the laboratory system. In selecting the appropriate amplifiers for the type of biological signals of interest, you might consult a sales representative of selected companies. You can also consult any of several standard laboratory guides.

It is important to employ differential amplifiers, usually solid-state ones using operational amplifiers. Differential amplifiers are especially valuable in rejecting common-mode signals that may interfere with the phenomenon of interest, such as omnipresent 60-cycle current running through your light (and other) circuits (see McGuigan, 1979).

Readout Systems

This third feature of the laboratory system is a unit by which the signal is observed. Readout devices may provide only a momentary signal for study, as in the case of the cathode-ray oscilloscope (CRO), or they may be recording systems that provide a permanent record. A laboratory typically includes both kinds, the CRO for monitoring purposes (to assure that the proper signal is coming through) and the permanent recording system for later study of the signal. An ink-writing polygraph ("electroencephalo-graph") is the most frequently used recording system. Although psychophysiology has made great progress with the ink-writing polygraph, this type of system is not recommended for such covert processes as electromyograms because electromyographic frequencies often range above that for which ink-writing polygraphs provide faithful response recording (i.e., electromyographic frequencies are often too high for a mechanical recording system with the inertia of lag and overshoot to provide a true tracing). High-frequency recorders are preferable. High-frequency recorders typically use an optical system, as when an input signal from the amplifier drives a miniature mirror that reflects ultraviolet light onto photosensitive paper; the signal, recorded on the paper, can then be preserved through chemical fixing processes. Such an optical system can provide a linear response recording as high as 10,000 Hz, although this is not needed for psychophysiology.

When direct tracings are recorded, as with ink-writing or high-frequency recorders, the experimenter's ability to quantify the data is restricted, because the phenomena can only be quantified from the paper records. For this reason, an excellent addition to a laboratory is a multi-channel data tape recorder so that the signals from the amplifiers can be recorded on magnetic tape. Frequency-modulated tape recorders are preferable to direct-recording tape recorders because of less distortion of amplitude and waveform and high repeatability from one playback to the next. The magnetic tape may then be played into a readout device (an ink-writing polygraph, a high-frequency recorder, or a CRO); the signals from the magnetic tape may be "frozen" for study on a storage CRO or photographed with a CRO camera.

The data stored on tape in the original form may also be used for other methods of analysis (such as feeding them into a computer). This added flexibility is important because with it the experimenter can try a variety of techniques of data analysis, some of which may be suggested only after studying the original tracings. It is important that the readout system allow the recording of a number of different channels for simultaneous recordings of different responses.

The mention of different techniques of data analysis brings us to the fourth feature of the laboratory.

Quantification Systems

Investigations conducted in the area of covert processes may be divided into two general classes: (1) those studying a brief, momentary phenomenon, and (2) those studying sustained, long-term processes. The investigator studying a momentary event is probably most interested in an amplitude measure, although other parameters, such as duration and latency, may also be important. The amplitude of the measured event should be compared to some control or baseline value to ascertain whether or not the event occurred reliably. That is, a continuous recording is made when, at some time, the experimental treatment is presented. We would then expect heightened values following the presentation of the treatment. But any bodily region is continuously changing regardless of whether or not the treatment is presented. Hence, the experimenter might measure maximum height of the tracing in a short interval immediately after presentation of the treatment and compare that amplitude with the maximum value in a temporally equal control (baseline) interval sampled some seconds prior to stimulus presentation. A positive effect would be indicated if the treatment values were significantly higher (considering a number of trials) than during the control (baseline) interval.

In the study of longer-term records, signals may be quantified by either amplitude or frequency measures, depending on their characteristics. If the signal is cyclical and repetitive, frequency measures are typically used (although amplitude measures are not thereby precluded). For example, the pneumogram, electrocardiogram, or peripheral pulse are usually quantified by counting the number of cycles per unit time and converting to a rate, such as number of respirations, heart beats, or pulses per minute. Of course, rate is also a primary technique for classifying brain waves.

Where the signal is not cyclical and values are required for relatively longer intervals of time, amplitude measures may be obtained in several different ways. Perhaps the simplest technique is to measure the height of the tracing with a ruler; one would thus compute peak-to-peak amplitude by measuring from the highest point of an event [like an electromyographic (EMG) spike] to the lowest. Amplitude measures are often taken in the case of long-term cyclical signals, as in changes in the amplitude of the pneumogram or of the pulse.

In measuring signals over long intervals of time, data may be sampled by preselecting temporal intervals during which the measure will be taken. More typically, the total tracing may be subdivided into smaller time intervals; in this case, the maximum amplitude of a spike that occurs during each smaller interval (e.g., each 10-second period of a 30-minute record) is measured, and the mean of these maximum amplitude values is computed. The electromyograph is a good example of a record for which this procedure is used, so that changes in maximum amplitude are studied as a function of time and experimental condition.

Hand-measuring techniques are simple, although time consuming, and thus are often replaced by automated procedures. An integration device (which sums the amplitude of the signal from the subject as a function of time) is perhaps the most popular procedure for quantifying sustained records by amplitude measures (integrators are typically included in standard ink-writing polygraphs). Again, the electromyograph is a good example of a measure for which the use of an amplitude integrator is helpful.

In Conclusion

Although complex laboratory equipment is necessary for the study of covert processes, the laboratory system should still be kept as simple as possible. A primary conclusion is that we should have as little apparatus as is reasonably possible and should never develop equipment that is more complicated than necessary to get the job done. One should be wary of the pitfalls that befall researchers who become so enamored with data analysis, equipment construction, and the like, that they needlessly complicate their tasks and sometimes even lose sight of their original research goals. In short, everything else being equal, the simpler the laboratory system, the more efficiently the research can be conducted.

Another general principle of guidance is that it is the psychophysiologist who has to decide how to best accomplish individual purposes in the laboratory. Although it is advisable to study valuable references on psycho-physiological and electronic techniques, and although experts can offer much general advice, such information does not necessarily apply in the unique situation of any individual psychophysiological laboratory. It is advisable to try out different types of supplies and equipment (often manufacturers furnish apparatus on trial) and keep records of perform-ance under a variety of conditions, eventually selecting those that provide relatively good recording under *your* existing laboratory conditions. For example, one might try several different kinds of electrodes, jellies, and pastes and evaluate several different methods of application of these (Styrofoam pads, tape, etc.). Such experiences establish a sound basis for developing standard laboratory procedures.

Relatively simple and inexpensive items often are equal or superior to more expensive and complex ones. For example, over the years we have tried out a large number of different kinds of electrodes and have con-cluded that the relatively inexpensive gold electrodes are completely satis-factory. They can provide excellent recordings and remain usable for years, compared to some that must be discarded almost immediately, or after several months.

SIGNAL-TO-NOISE RATIO

Techniques for reducing electrical noise in the system are important. In this section we consider noise reduction throughout the laboratory system by emphasizing the general principle of maximizing the laboratory's total signal-to-noise ratio. This ratio indicates the degree to which the signal dominates the noise. Everything else being equal, the goal is to develop the largest signal possible and the smallest amount of noise.

The raw signals that the experimenter attempts to record may range below a microvolt. Such signals are extremely weak compared to those that are produced by various human-made devices likely to be present in the laboratory's surroundings. Such unwanted signals can easily obscure the bodily signal of interest. Through specialized techniques it is possible to recover the signal from the noise, but it is much more desirable to prevent noise from entering and developing *within* the recording system.

To maximize the signal-to-noise ratio, there are a number of feasible steps that can either increase the amplitude of the desired signal or reduce the amplitude of noise. Most obviously, the signal-to-noise ratio can be increased by increasing the factor by which the signal of interest is ampli-fied. In principle, the signal may be amplified without limit merely by adding additional amplifiers in series into the circuit. However, there are practical limits to the amount of amplification that can be tolerated. These limits are set by the characteristics of the amplifier and recording systems because, when the signal of interest is further amplified, noise within the system is also amplified. Consequently, mere amplification is seldom productive beyond a certain factor, at which point efforts should be concentrated on noise reduction. Typical amplification factors for such covert responses as EMG range in the neighborhood of 10,000 and 100,000. Active regions, such as the tongue, dictate lower amplification, whereas "control" (inactive) regions, such as the leg, allow high amplification to be used.

Noise Reduction

There are two major sources of noise that are electromagnetically picked up and transmitted within the recording system: (1) signals that are generated within the laboratory itself, and (2) external signals. The former may be subdivided into those that are generated from within and from without the amplifier. Noise within the amplifier may be reduced by quality design and by the use of negative feedback in operational amplifiers (discussed in McGuigan, 1979). Noise generated by laboratory components outside the amplifiers may be reduced by shielding-in all equipment (this is typically already accomplished by the manufacturer); for example, amplifiers are encased in metal, and leads (cables, wires) are shielded within flexible metal conduit. The experimenter then connects the shielding of all equipment together and grounds the equipment so that the major portion of the unwanted signals generated in the equipment is led into the ground (as illustrated in Figure 22-1).

A discussion of reducing noise generated outside the amplifiers is provided by McGuigan (1979) and Cacioppo *et al.* (Chapter 24). We might note that special attention should be paid to shielding the subject, because any noise picked up at the initial electrode stage is amplified. Unlike the signal from the subject, noise that enters the system after the amplifiers is not amplified. Nevertheless, even though it is more important to prevent noise from entering the system prior to the amplifiers, noise picked up by the amplifiers, recorders, and so on, should be minimized by shielding, which should include separate shielding about the apparatus room.

Signal Averaging

Another technique for improving the signal-to-noise ratio is to use signal averagers, now commonly available as separate units or as adjuncts to small digital computers. Signal averaging is appropriate when there is a repetitive signal, but not when the signal is a unique event. Signal-averaging computers average events that are time-locked to a repeated stimulus presentation. After a number of trials, bodily signals that are time-locked to the stimulus are represented as an average output from the computer. Various random fluctuations in each individual signal add and subtract their amplitude values equally (in the long run) at any given time following stimulus presentation; hence, random fluctuations in the bodily (and other) signals over trials average zero amplitude (tend to "cancel each other out"), whereas those events that are regularly locked to the stimulus presentation add or subtract amplitude values consistently. The final summed potential is thus the average of events that are lawfully related to the stimulus. In short, signal averagers present stimulus-related activity that occurs repeatedly over trials and eliminates signals that are out of phase and random with respect to stimulus presentation. For instance, if a light flash is presented on a number of trials, the light stimuli may trigger the signal-averaging computer to analyze the psychophysiological signals immediately following. Brain waves are commonly averaged following a repetitive series of light-flash presentations, and the averaged brain reaction may be quite precisely plotted out (even though the reaction on any of the individual trials is obscured by noise). What is common in the individual sweeps constitutes the average, whereas stray events, tending to be random, are "averaged out." The averager thus produces a single trace that is the average of the inputs of a large number of sweeps. It should now be obvious why signal averaging is not appropriate if there is but one stimulus presentation or if each reaction to the stimuli is different.

The technique of signal averaging is one of the major apparatus advances made in the area of psychophysiology and has produced a large number of valuable findings. Although signal averaging is quite effective in noise reduction, it is still preferable to reduce noise prior to the input of the averager, because the less the noise, the fewer the trials required for a good average trace.

Grounding

The grounding system is so important that if it is defective, all other techniques of noise reduction are relatively trivial. The reason is that if extraneous signals picked up by the shielding and subject are not led off into the earth, or if there is a ground loop in the laboratory grounding system, the extremely small signals generated within the body will be obscured and have little or no chance of being detected.

The primary principle of grounding is that all conducting items in the laboratory should be connected together with a good intralaboratory wiring system; there should then be a single lead from that interconnected system that goes directly into the earth. In this way, electromagnetic transmissions that are picked up by the shielding of the equipment, as well as those that are picked up by the skin of the subject, can be prevented from entering the sensing and recording system by being discharged into the ground.

It is important to emphasize that the grounding wires should be attached to the shielding of each piece of equipment at one and only one point, so that the apparatus, the shielding, and the subject have a single common connection, which should then enter the ground at a single point. For instance, the experimenter would not run a ground wire from the front and another from the back end of the same equipment. It does not help to run multiple grounds from a single item of equipment. In fact, rather than helping, multiple grounds can produce ground loops that may impose a large 60-cycle signal on the psychophysiological signal. In interconnecting the equipment, it is best not to run grounding wires from one item of equipment directly to another; rather, it is preferable for the ground wire from each piece of equipment to go to a common terminal, a terminal that connects with one cable to the earth. Similarly, the subject and the shielding of the rooms have but one ground wire that connects to the common terminal. This principle is illustrated in Figure 22-1, with the exception that we have not indicated separate ground wires to the common terminal for each item of equipment. It is also important that all connections be well made, because loose connections may pick up interference or easily become disconnected and thus disable the laboratory system. The cable that runs from the connection terminal into the ground should provide minimum resistance so that the external signals picked up by the shielding can be effectively conducted into the earth.

GENERALIZING FROM PSYCHOPHYSIOLOGICAL DATA

We have noted that the characteristics of any psychophysiological signal vary with a large number of conditions. For instance, there is constantly changing ambient noise in the environment, and even the most effectively shielded laboratories do not completely exclude all unwanted signals. Another important variable affecting psychophysiological data concerns electrode placement. It is unfortunate that, for both surface and inserted electrodes, precisely constant electrode placements cannot be obtained on successive sessions with the same subject, or among different subjects. For instance, if the experimenter seeks to record chin electromyograms or electroencephalograms, there will be some variation in the placement of the electrodes on repeated measurements of the same subject, or among different subjects. For one thing, the skin resistance will vary somewhat with the particular electrode preparation (e.g., how hard the skin is rubbed) and, for another, the resistance between the electrode and the underlying source of the signal changes somewhat even within an experimental session for a given subject. The precision with which we measure the amplitudes of an alpha wave recorded over a site on the scalp, for instance, is somewhat limited—one cannot guarantee that absolute amplitudes of signals can be confidently measured to the "nth degree" among different subjects, or for a given subject at different times. Approximations to absolute amplitude values are possible when extreme care and experimental techniques have been exercised, but our major sources of inference in psychophysiology rest on relative rather than absolute amplitudes.

In establishing a relative amplitude, an experimenter typically measures a signal under a standard recording condition, such as a baseline value when the subject is at rest. One then compares the amplitude (frequency, etc.) of the signal under some experimental condition with its amplitude under the standard condition. Relative amplitude is thus determined by the change in a subject's behavior during an experimental session from one condition (e.g., rest) to another (e.g., an experimental condition). Typically, a representative value during the resting baseline condition is subtracted from a representative value during the experimental condition to assess the effect of the experimental treatment. Sometimes a ratio (or percentage) increase over baseline is measured instead of a difference. Because of these considerations, most statements about covert psychophysiological processes rest primarily on relative as opposed to absolute values as a function of experimental conditions. These limitations not only apply within each laboratory, but, owing to different techniques and equipment among laboratories, the limitations are even greater when comparing values observed in one laboratory with those observed in another.

The preceding considerations emphasize the importance of establishing a valid baseline. In fact, to ascertain whether or not some experimental treatment produces a response change, it is critical that a low, stable, resting baseline be established for the subject. If the subject is highly aroused prior to engaging in some active thought processes, for instance, the experimenter would have difficulty in ascertaining whether a given covert reaction occurred during those thought processes. It is good practice to produce a state of tranquility in the subject in order to most effectively measure response changes as a function of experimental conditions. A number of procedures can contribute to the establishment of a low-level stable baseline. For one, the concept of a psychophysiological laboratory itself may produce unwanted arousal effects, as in fear. The experimenter should therefore take all possible steps to reassure the subject and to prevent any emotion-arousing terms to be used during the instructions. Further discussion of establishing baselines in psychophysiological research is provided by McHugo and Lanzetta (Chapter 23), and discussion of issues surrounding the psychosocial environment in psychophysiological research is furnished by Cacioppo *et al.* (Chapter 24).

TROUBLESHOOTING

Once the experimenter has developed a stable laboratory, the readout system should be monitored every time some system change is made, such as each time new equipment is brought in. Compulsive checking for the effects of any change will be worth the effort. The purpose is to make sure that the change has not altered normal recording. When checking out the laboratory system, there should be some electrical resistance placed between the electrodes. However, it is not always convenient, nor even desirable, to attach electrodes to a human for the purpose of monitoring signals from them while troubleshooting. A good substitute is a "dummy subject," a 10,000-ohm resistor, which may be placed between the electrodes. With the "dummy" resistance, the experimenter can then monitor a CRO for distorted or unwanted signals without using a live subject.

To locate the source of unwanted signals, one can search throughout the laboratory with the psychophysiologist's "magic wand." A "magic wand" can be easily constructed by placing a 10,000-ohm resistor between the single-ended input to a CRO and the shielding conduit (grounded, of course) of the single-ended cable. By being placed on the end of a long cable connected to an oscilloscope that is set to a low-voltage scale (1 mV per division suffices), the resistor can be moved throughout the lab near pieces of equipment. In this way, stray signals become readily apparent on the CRO and, once detected, their source can be found and properly dealt with. Many strange signals at various frequencies can appear. In addition to those from 60-cycle power lines, interference from other equipment can ride in from other laboratories in the vicinity on ac or dc lines (we once spent 3 days tracing a 2000-Hz signal to the chemistry lab upstairs).

Although one can emphasize the prevention of difficulties, problems still appear when electrodes are being attached to a subject; moment-to-moment monitoring of the signals on a CRO may indicate that the bodily signal is not coming through or that the desired signal is partially attenuated by being superimposed on a 60-cycle signal. At that point, the experimenter needs to discover and correct the problem very rapidly in order to "save the data." If it is a stable, well-constructed laboratory, broken connections are an unlikely source of the problem, so attention can be turned to higher probability sources. There might be poor contact between the electrode and the skin surface; a break in the electrode lead itself is not frequent. One might diagnose such problems by placing each lead of an ohmmeter on the surface of each of the two electrodes respectively in order to measure interelectrode resistance. The rule of thumb is that resistance in excess of 10,000 ohms may prevent the desired bodily signals from adequately entering the amplifiers. The experimenter could then use the ohmmeter to run a continuity check to ensure that there is no break in the electrode leads. If the electrodes are in satisfactory condition, they may be removed and then replaced after further massaging of the skin to reduce cutaneous resistance. Incidentally, although it is typical to measure resistance with an ohmmeter, a measure of impedance (with an Electrode Impedance Tester) is actually preferable for biphasic signals like EMGs and electroencephalograms, whereas resistance is the measure appropriate for dc signals. Furthermore, measuring resistance with an ohmmeter might produce a slight, but harmless, shock for the subject, whereas shocks are not possible with the impedance tester.

Another possible problem that can appear while preparing the subject is that there are conductive paths of detergent, water, or electrode paste between two placements on the skin; these could virtually eliminate useful EMG signals from the subject.

Problems like these with electrodes would appear in only one channel, whereas trouble in all channels would indicate a more general problem (poor subject ground, extraneous noise, etc.). Extraneous noise may come from a piece of equipment that has been overloaded or perhaps from some change in the environment, such as a new TV station in the vicinity. [A TV station emits a high-frequency signal that can penetrate inexpensive shielding like copper mesh; in this case, the signal would wax and wane at 60 cycles per second (a "sync signal"), appearing in the records as 60 Hz, yet not emanating from a power line.]

LABORATORY SAFETY

Shock hazard to subjects and experimenters, the primary laboratory danger, is a function of the amount of current that flows through the body. To gain some perspective, a current less than 1 mA is readily perceptible, whereas 10 to 100 mA can cause pain, burns, and tetanus of the involved musculature. Currents in excess of 100 mA are likely to cause cardiac and respiratory arrest. Shock hazards exist to the subject because the subject is grounded by a special electrode; hence, just as when one is in the bathtub, any contact with a power line could cause electrical current to be conducted through the body with potentially fatal consequences.

The best protection is never to bring 110- or 220-V ac power lines into the subject room and never to use any equipment in the subject room that requires such a power source. (As noted earlier, another argument against bringing electrical equipment into the subject room is that the equipment is a source of electromagnetic transmission that produces undesired noise.) If, however, it is necessary to bring ac-operated equipment into the subject room, it is critical that a grounded subject not be allowed to touch that equipment, as it may be conducting leakage currents from the lower line that activates it. Leakage currents are typically small, and their presence is not commonly recognized. Such currents can range from well below threshold to fatal levels, depending on various conditions.

In the case of electrodes inserted beneath the skin, the danger is easily fatal. When using surface electrodes, the danger of shock to the subject is less, but still present. With inserted electrodes, a safety standard is to assure that there is less than 5 one-millionths of an ampere flow through the subject. There have been reports of patients in hospital beds with implanted electrodes being electrocuted by turning on their bedside lamp—the leakage current on the lamp was sufficient to be fatal.

Methods of eliminating shock hazards include use of only battery-operated equipment in the vicinity of the subject and careful grounding of any necessary line-operated equipment that the subject could conceivably touch. Each piece of apparatus should be grounded separately to the common point at which the subject's ground wire connects (see Figure 22-1). This common point should be connected to the primary laboratory ground cable. Whenever possible, avoid using a grounded outlet like a water pipe for the ground system, because these may become unsafe with age and corrosion. Similarly, avoid having two separate ground systems within the reach of the subject, for there can exist considerable differences in voltages and currents between the two ground systems. With proper grounding in the subject's vicinity, safety even in the event of equipment malfunction can be assured.

Small shocks can occur in the laboratory through a variety of unusual circumstances. We have mentioned one, merely testing electrode resistance with an ohmmeter. Even such small shocks are undesirable, because they can provide a bad experimental set for the subject. To keep subjects' expectations positive, it is advisable never to use intentional shock in a psychophysiological lab; this precaution could help prevent the arousal of gruesome rumors about the lab that can make it difficult to attract subjects, who already have a tendency to think that all the electrical equipment means that shock is in store for them. Although we have concentrated on shock hazards to the subject, the principles apply equally to the experimenter; the difference is that we *know* the subject is grounded. But if the experimenter should become momentarily grounded by accidentally touching a grounding cable, there are many ways in which the experimenter, too, can be shocked (e.g., coming into contact with excessive leakage current on an oscilloscope, or with an instrument that has an electrical short).

CONCLUSION

Although it is advisable to study the many valuable references on psychophysiological and electronic techniques, and although experts can offer much general advice, such information does not necessarily apply in the unique situation of any individual psychophysiological laboratory. A general procedure for the psychophysiologist is to try out a number of different types of supplies and equipment (remember, you might obtain apparatus on trial) and keep records of performance under a variety of conditions, eventually selecting those that provide relatively good recording under the existing laboratory conditions. For example, one should try several different kinds of electrodes, jellies, and pastes and evaluate several different methods of application of these (Styrofoam pads, tape, etc.). Such experiences establish a sound basis for future standard laboratory procedures.

In this chapter we have reviewed various technical considerations for studying psychophysiological processes. More advanced and detailed sources of information about equipment and methodology may be found in two issues of the *American Psychologist* (March 1969 and March 1975) that have been devoted to instrumentation in psychology. Articles in the 1969 issue that are of direct interest for the study of covert processes are those by White on evoked cortical responses, by Vladimirov and Homskaya on eye recording, by Ax and by Johnson and Naitoh on general instrumentation, and by Mackay on telemetry; also, an article by Haith gives an application of infrared television to the study of ocular behavior in the human infant.

In the 1975 issue, the psychophysiologist might pay attention to the use of biomedical telemetry (Sandler, McCutcheon, Fryer, Rositano, Westbrook, and Haro), cardiovascular psychophysiology (Obrist, Gaebelein, and Langer), blood pressure monitoring (Krausman), eye-movement recording (Monty; Young and Sheena), "alpha machines" (Schwitzgebel and Rugh), biofeedback instrumentation (Paskewitz), microwaves (Justesen), and the measurement of genital responses (Geer). Both issues also consider the general use of computers, the 1975 issue giving the greater coverage because of the sizable advances in computer technology (especially solid-state electronics and packaging) that have allowed the development of the small, inexpensive computer. Computers have numerous, extremely valuable applications in the social psychophysiology laboratory, particularly for data reduction and stimulus control. Social psychophysiological data probably pose the most difficult analysis problems of any that psychologists face. It is not unusual for many miles of "squiggles" to be recorded in a day's work, making it difficult and time consuming to define a response. However, computers can perform this task. For example, McGuigan and Pavek (1972) programmed a computer to search for response outputs from the various electrode placements on their subjects. The computer continuously computed the mean and standard deviation of the analog signals; when an amplitude was identified that exceeded a certain number of standard deviations from the mean, a response was defined, and the latency, duration, and amplitude of the response were printed out. With this method they found a most interesting eye response that would not have been detected by visual means alone.

ACKNOWLEDGMENT

Much of this information was adopted from McGuigan (1979) with the kind permission of Lawrence Erlbaum, the publisher. For elaboration of some of the topics presented here, kindly consult that source.

REFERENCES

Aronson, E., & Carlsmith, J. M.   Experimentation in social psychology. In G. Lindzey & E. Aronson (Eds.), *The handbook of social psychology* (Vol. 2). Reading, Mass.: Addison-Wesley, 1969.

Cacioppo, J. T., & Petty, R. E.   Electromyograms as measures of the extent of affectivity of information processing. *American Psychologist*, 1981, *36*, 441–456.

Cacioppo, J. T., Petty, R. E., & Quintanar, L. R.   Individual differences in relative hemispheric alpha abundance and cognitive responses to persuasive communications. *Journal of Personality and Social Psychology*, 1982, *43*, 623–636.

Max, L. W.   An experimental study of the motor theory of consciousness: IV. Action-current responses in the deaf during awakening, kinaesthetic imagery and abstract thinking. *Journal of Comparative Psychology*, 1937, *24*, 301–344.

McGuigan, F. J.   Covert oral behavior and auditory hallucinations. *Psychophysiology*, 1966, *3*, 73–80.

McGuigan, F. J.   Covert linguistic behavior in deaf subjects during thinking. *Journal of Comparative and Physiological Psychology*, 1971, *75*, 417–420.

McGuigan, F. J.   *Cognitive psychophysiology—principles of covert behavior*. Englewood Cliffs, N.J.: Prentice-Hall, 1978.

McGuigan, F. J.   *Psychophysiological measurement of covert behavior: A guide for the laboratory*. Hillsdale, N.J.: Erlbaum, 1979.

McGuigan, F. J., Culver, V. I., & Kendler, T. S.   Covert behavior as a direct electromyographic measure of mediating responses. *Conditional Reflex*, 1971, *6*, 145–152.

McGuigan, F. J., Keller, B., & Stanton, E.   Covert language responses during silent reading. *Journal of Educational Psychology*, 1964, *55*, 339–343.

McGuigan, F. J., & Pavek, G. V.   On the psychophysiological identification of covert nonoral language processes. *Journal of Experimental Psychology*, 1972, *92*, 237–245.

McGuigan, F. J., & Pinkney, K. B.   Effects of increased reading rate on covert processes. *Interamerican Journal of Psychology*, 1973, *7*, 223–231.

CHAPTER 23

Methodological Decisions in Social Psychophysiology

Gregory J. McHugo
Dartmouth College

John T. Lanzetta
Dartmouth College

INTRODUCTION

Methodological issues in social psychophysiology are essentially the same as those in psychophysiology. The purposes of research in the related fields may differ, but methods of recording and quantifying the data, and the interpretations of the bioelectric signals, are based primarily on the research of psychophysiologists. Over the past several decades the latter group has explored a wide range of substantive and measurement problems; has developed, or has encouraged equipment manufacturers to develop, improved methods for detecting, recording, and analyzing bioelectric signals; and has been active in adapting computer technology to the laboratory. The accumulating literature on these topics is an invaluable source of information for social psychologists venturing into this field. At the same time, the volume of literature, the lack of consensus on central issues, the esoteric and unfamiliar language, the technical complexity of the procedures, and the dynamic nature of the field are troublesome.

Most social psychologists are interested in using physiological measures to index the strength of an "emotional" or "arousal" state or a covert "cognitive" process that is hypothesized to mediate social behavior. The major concern is with finding a valid, reliable, and sensitive measure of the implicated state or covert process. Rarely is the bioelectric signal of interest either in its own right or because of its relationship to other bioelectric signals. Thus, many substantive issues in psychophysiology are of concern only to the extent that they influence the interpretation of data or that they point to methodological problems. For example, individual response stereotypy (discussed below; see also Cacioppo & Petty, Chapter 1, this volume) was an exciting finding in psychophysiology, but is of significance to the social psychophysiologist because it contributes to inflated error variance. Similarly, the research of several investigators (e.g., Lacey, 1967; Lacey & Lacey, 1970; Obrist, Gaebelein, Shanks, Langer, & Botticelli, 1976; Obrist, Webb, & Sutterer, 1969) on the variables influencing heart rate is significant for social psychologists because it questions the use of heart rate as a simple index of arousal.

From the point of view of the social psychologist the ideal state of the art in psychophysiology would be a data base in which measures were linked to underlying states unambiguously, and procedures for recording, scoring, and analysis were specified for each measure. Unfortunately, the knowledge base is not so far advanced, and, of necessity, social psychologists interested in using physiological measures must acquire familiarity with some basic methodological issues and must face numerous choices.

In this chapter we identify the major issues and choice points that have to be confronted. At times we may suggest possible ways to handle specific problems, but more often we will point to sources of information bearing on a decision, either because the number of options at a choice point are too extensive to describe or because there is no consensus about an approach or procedure. For us this is an opportunity to reflect on our recent experience in expanding our research capabilities in social psychophysiology. Our intention is to review the issues and decisions that we have faced and to indicate which resources have been most useful in the process. The first section of this chapter raises some general questions concerning the use of physiological measures and experimental design. Later sections explore issues of recording, measurement, and analysis of bioelectric signals. A final section concerns the use of computers in psychophysiological laboratories.

CHOICE OF PHYSIOLOGICAL MEASURES

Compared to subjective reports or overt behavioral indicators, physiological measures are difficult to obtain, to process, and to analyze. Why, then, would an investigator want to use such measures? To a psychophysiologist the answer is self-evident; the bioelectric signals reflect the action of particular structures and processes in the human body and thus are as worthy of study as any other responses. But to a social psychologist interested in an index of an emotional state or a covert process, the justification must lie elsewhere. We might summarize the reasons that most investigators turn to physiological measures as follows:

1. They provide a reliable and valid index of a hypothetical construct.
2. They enhance the convergent validity of constructs that are measured imperfectly by verbal or behavioral measures.

3. They provide a continuous rather than a discrete measure of a process or state.

4. They are more "sensitive" to subtle changes in underlying states.

5. They sometimes provide the only direct measure of a process or state.

6. They are often less subject to voluntary control and thus less vulnerable to "demand characteristics."

7. They are less "reactive," because the purpose of the measure can be better disguised.

Offsetting these potential advantages are a number of disadvantages that must be considered in making a choice. Physiological recording procedures are obtrusive; they typically require constraining the activity of subjects; and they are time consuming. The "psychological" impact of these procedural requirements has not been established, but may include increases in anxiety, irritability, boredom, and fatigue. The recording procedures may also foster "self-focusing," which, in turn, can modify the processes being measured. On the other hand, these procedures may create a "bogus pipeline," thereby increasing the validity of subjective measures. Although physiological recording procedures may be no more obtrusive than other social psychological procedures (e.g., videotaping or self-reports), researchers should be aware of these possible psychological effects.

In addition to possible adverse effects on subjects, the primary disadvantages of physiological measurement are the expense and technical expertise required. There are costs associated with the time needed for subject preparation and adaptation to the laboratory setting and for ensuring recording precision and safety. Furthermore, the time spent in data reduction and analysis, the modification of the data base to correct for artifact, and the loss of data due to subject idiosyncrasies or equipment malfunction are additional expenditures. There are also significant costs involved in obtaining the necessary technical expertise to use the equipment properly and to analyze the data appropriately. Finally, there is the large expense of purchasing and maintaining the equipment.

Given the costs and difficulties of obtaining physiological measures, the social psychologist should examine carefully the assumptions underlying the choice of such measures and balance the presumed advantages against the offsetting disadvantages. In general, the requirements of a single study rarely justify the setting up of a psychophysiological laboratory; typically, such laboratories are created in support of a program of research in which physiological measurement plays a central role. As an alternative to setting up a laboratory, an investigator could explore the possibility of short-term access to a laboratory and to the measurement expertise required for the period necessary to complete a study. If the value of physiological measures for understanding social behavior is established by further research, we may witness the growth of collaborative research between social psychologists and psychophysiologists, resulting perhaps in the emergence of shared, regional laboratories for physiological measurement.

If, upon weighing the relative advantages and disadvantages of physiological measures, the decision is made to employ them, the investigator must select a specific measure(s). As noted above, social psychologists often use physiological measures to index "states" while exploring the effects of various experimental manipulations. Historically, the primary objective has been to assess arousal or emotional response. Organs and processes controlled by the autonomic nervous system (ANS), and more especially by the sympathetic branch of the ANS, were usually the focus of attention. Even with this limited objective investigators had a wide choice of measures, such as heart rate, skin resistance, blood pressure, and pupil diameter. As interest has expanded to include assessment of cortical states, expressive behavior, and covert muscle patterning, the list of possible physiological systems to be monitored has also expanded. The choice has been complicated further by the growing sophistication in recording and data analysis, which has encouraged the examination of various parameters of particular measures and the use of multiple measures.

Whatever the organ or process recorded, the social psychologist is more interested in the construct validity of the measure than in the physiological process underlying its behavior. How, then, is one to assess the relative construct validity of the alternative measures? Typically, prior research provides the best initial guidance, but often tradition within an area may suggest one measure, say skin resistance level, while the specialists advocate another, say skin conductance level, and innovators clamor for yet another, say skin potential. Review chapters in respected handbooks (e.g., Venables & Christie, 1980) and reports of parametric research, when available, are useful in guiding the decision. As an example of the latter, Boucsein and Hoffmann (1979) compared skin resistance and skin conductance levels within subjects and found few differences in results.

In addition to construct validity, reliability, sensitivity, ease of recording, and other such issues should all be weighed in making the choice. For example, it may be wrong to assume that reliability is assured because a physiological measure is involved. The reliability, that is, the repeatability, of electromyographic (EMG) measurement has been argued (e.g., Grossman & Weiner, 1966) and since found to vary with such factors as recording technique and task (Gans & Gorniak, 1980; Graham, 1979) and scoring procedure (L. H. Epstein & Webster, 1975).

The number of measures to use is another difficult decision. A single index is often of limited validity, because most physiological states and processes are multivariate. Multiple measures may improve the specification of the underlying process. In addition, multiple measures allow convergence on the hypothetical construct, thereby improving validity. How-

634 METHODS OF SOCIAL PSYCHOPHYSIOLOGY

ever, as more measures are added, the problems compound at each level of recording, measurement, and analysis. The data, and hence conclusions, are richer and more informative, but the complexity may be overwhelming and communicability may suffer.

The use of arousal as a hypothetical construct and its attendant measurement serves to exemplify the issues of which and how many measures to employ in psychophysiological research (see also Chapter 1). Based on Cannon's (1915) notion of integrated responses by the body in preparation for fight or flight, Duffy (1957) proposed a unidimensional bodily response of activation that reflected the intensity of the preparatory reaction. Malmo (1959), in a series of studies, supported the notion of a unidimensional activation (arousal) continuum, and later research on the reticular activating system suggested an underlying mechanism that could be responsible for this unidimensional arousal. A number of investigators have strongly challenged the theory, at least at an operational level. Lacey (1967) was especially critical, pointing to a variety of ways in which the assumption did not accord with data:

> 1. Some arousing situations invoke both the parasympathetic and the sympathetic system and thus are associated with changes in only certain indices and not others, for example, sexual arousal.
> 2. Specific stimulus situations appear to be associated with particular patterns of responding, not with simple increases or decreases in uni-dimensional arousal. This has been called the principle of *stimulus response specificity* (see Chapter 1).
> 3. As a corollary to the above, some situations appear to be associated with *directional fractionation* of response. That is, one finds an increase in one index of arousal (e.g., skin conductance) and a decrease in another (e.g., heart rate).

The implication of the critiques of a unidimensional arousal continuum appear obvious, at least at the operational level: no single measure can provide unequivocal evidence of different levels of arousal. Yet at the theoretical level the concept of unidimensional arousal is alive and healthy (Schachter, 1964; Zillmann, 1978), and for many social psychologists the primary utility of physiological measures resides in their potential for providing a measure of this hypothesized underlying state.

There are no satisfactory solutions to the dilemma posed by the conflicting views short of abandoning the concept of unidimensional arousal. Since at the theoretical (hypothetical construct) level the concept appears viable and useful, compromises must be made. An investigator could use multiple measures and derive an index of arousal based on a summation (of standard scores) across measures, or use an index for each individual based on the maximum response on any of the measured dimensions. These procedures have not been widely employed, and they clearly rest on untested assumptions. More typically, an investigator attempts to establish beforehand that a particular measure covaries with the intensity of the stimulus to be used, and then operationally defines arousal in terms of this measure. No assumptions are made about the generality of the measure across situations or the effects of the situational manipulation across measures.

If, for example, one wants to measure the magnitude of arousal produced by dissonance, one could find a physiological measure that co-varies with decision latency or decision conflict, because both are pre-sumed to produce differences in dissonance. As such, this measure would operationally define arousal for this set of eliciting stimuli. No assump-tions could be made that other dissonance-producing situations would necessarily covary with this measure or that other potential measures of arousal would covary with the stimuli employed.

This widely employed "solution" may, in part, be responsible for many of the failures to replicate studies in which arousal states are assessed. Often experimenters testing related hypotheses involving arousal as a mediating variable have employed different evoking stimuli and used dif-ferent measures of arousal. Ambiguity in interpretation presumably will continue until some consensus is achieved regarding the theoretical and operational status of the concept of unidimensional arousal.

DESIGN AND PROCEDURE CONSIDERATIONS

The time-dependent growth and decay of bioelectric signals, the potential influence of habituation and sensitization, the prevalence of high individual variability in physiological response, and the possible influence of baseline response levels on the magnitude of phasic responses all create problems for the design of an experiment and constrain the procedures employed. Measures such as phasic skin resistance lag the onset of a stimulus by 2 to 4 seconds and take a minimum of 6 to 10 seconds to decay, whereas others, such as heart rate or muscle action potential, have rapid onset and decay. Clearly, the experimental procedure should reflect the *time-dependent characteristics* of the particular measures taken. Thus, in repeated-measures designs, intertrial intervals should be long enough to permit decay of the response to baseline levels before initiation of a new trial or closed-loop procedures (discussed below) can be used to ensure return to baseline between trials.

Habituation (see Chapter 1) is a well-established phenomenon with respect to skeletal muscle responses, but less well established for many autonomic indices. For skin conductance (SC) repeated presentation of a conditioning stimulus results in decreasing frequency and/or amplitude of the SC response, but this is often presumed to be a measure of the change in the orienting response (see below and Chapter 1) to the stimulus. When SC reflects an emotional response (UCR) to an aversive stimulus, it is less clear that gradual decrements will occur upon repeated presentations of the stimulus. Such variables as surprisingness, uncertainty, and novelty appear to mediate the effect, and, under some circumstances, evidence of *sensitization* (see Chapter 1) may be obtained.

The problems raised by habituation and sensitization have mainly to do with repeated-measures designs. If the design includes repeated measurement within subjects, counterbalancing can control for some of the effects due to order or repetition, but cannot eliminate such confounds as floor effects, reduction in sensitivity, or carryover between trials. When the design is repeated measures between subjects, additional problems are posed, because experimental conditions may differ in terms of novelty, surprisingness, potency, and so forth. Differences between groups in SC response could thus result from different rates of habituation in the experimental conditions because of this variability in novelty or surprisingness.

There are no ready solutions to the measurement confounds that can be produced by habituation and sensitization. Awareness of the variables that influence these effects should facilitate attempts to equate stimuli across experimental conditions, but this is easier stated as a goal than accomplished in practice. Often, pretesting of the stimuli can alert one to potential problems in between-subjects designs. For within-subject designs, habituation trials are typically introduced prior to experimental trials on the assumption that habituation effects will have dissipated after a few exposures to the stimulus.

Malmo and Shagass (1949) were among the earliest investigators to demonstrate that individuals may differ consistently in their patterns of response to various stressors, which has been labeled *individual response stereotypy* (see Chapter 1). In their study some patients characteristically responded to stress with increases in muscle tension, whereas others responded with changes in heart rate. Lacey and Lacey (1958) later showed that nonpatient samples also responded to various stressors differentially.

It is difficult to decide what to do about this phenomenon. One could pretest subjects using multiple measures and pick that measure for each subject which covaries best with variation in the intensity of some stressor, but this is a cumbersome procedure and not free of criticism. The problem with any proposed solution is that individual differences in response on any one measure may be due to a variety of factors, such as constitutional differences that modulate response to a stressor, differential experience with the stressor, and differences in magnitudes of orienting response or in rate of habituation to the stressor stimulus. To assume that individual response stereotypy is responsible for all the variance in level of response is unwarranted. In practice, most investigators ignore the problem and treat individual differences as "error," whatever the source.

As noted above, an interrelated response pattern, called the *orienting response*, is typically evoked by a change in stimulation. Included as part of this response pattern are increases in SC, vasoconstriction in the periphery, vasodilation in the head, and decrease in heart rate. The use of any of these measures as an index of an emotional or arousal state is thus subject to ambiguity of interpretation, because the response may be composed of an orienting reaction to the stimulus per se, as well as an emotional reaction to the content (meaning) of the stimulus. Because the orienting response typically habituates rapidly, the problem can be handled by using a series of habituation trials or by ignoring the data obtained in the first few trials of a repeated-measures design.

Several other issues pertaining to physiological measures create design and analysis problems. They are the law of initial values, range corrections, missing and aberrant data, and inflated error variance due to experimental procedures.

In 1950 Wilder called attention to the fact that the larger the ANS response in a prestimulus phase, the smaller is the response to stimulation. He named this phenomenon the *law of initial values* (LIV; see Chapter 1). Later work suggests that labeling the observation as a law overstates the generality and reliability of the relationship; it is not obtained for all ANS measures, or for all prestimulus levels, but it is sufficiently pervasive to create interpretation problems. If the magnitude of the subject's response to a stimulus is inversely related to the level of response in a baseline or prestimulus period, and if this effect is due to an internal mechanism controlling the response (e.g., homeostasis), then the change (phasic response) might not reflect accurately the magnitude of the underlying emotional response. Most suggestions for handling this problem rest on the assumption that the phenomenon does reflect the operation of a homeostatic (negative feedback) mechanism that modulates the amount of change as a function of level of initial response.

Statistical corrections for the LIV have been proposed by Lacey (1956), who derives an *Autonomic Lability Score,* and by Benjamin (1967), who suggests the use of covariance analysis. The former is a special case of the latter, and both permit comparisons between the poststimulus scores of two individuals or groups corrected for differences in prestimulus response levels. Before use of either of these statistical corrections, investigators should determine whether their data need to be adjusted by computing the correlation between prestimulus levels and the magnitude of the phasic response to stimulation. In a between-subjects design one could also reduce the confounding effects of LIV by employing a matching procedure. Subjects showing similar prestimulus levels could be randomly assigned to each of the experimental groups. This is more difficult to accomplish with physiological measures than with test scores or demographic characteristics, and it has rarely been employed.

Lykken, Rose, Luther, and Maley (1966) suggested *correcting the range* of electrodermal responses as a means of enhancing intersubject comparisons and reducing error variance due to individual physiological differences.

This requires the addition of standardized procedures within an experimental session in order to determine each subject's response range; these values are then used during quantification to correct response amplitudes for differences in range among subjects. Lykken and Venables (1971) and Lykken (1972) have discussed range correction procedures for electrodermal and heart rate responses and should be consulted if such a correction is deemed appropriate.

Because psychophysiological research is highly technical, *missing data* are often present in the final data matrix due to equipment failures or other factors. Often one or several trials may be lost for a given subject, or one of several measures will be missing for a given trial. The data analyst thus must decide whether to drop that subject (trial) entirely, or to replace the missing data with values based on that subject's performance, or on the performance of all other subjects. The problem is pervasive, but the resolution will depend on the proportion of missing data points for a given trial, subject, or group. One defense is to anticipate an analysis strategy that does not require equal cell sizes everywhere. Another strategy may be to run enough subjects so that one can randomly select subjects to provide equal cell sizes for each analysis. Repeated measurement that permits aggregation of the data may also circumvent the problems of missing trials or repetitions.

It may also happen that some subjects are aberrant in their responding in the laboratory, and hence become *outliers* in final distributions. This is particularly a problem in social psychophysiology, where the stimulus material is often distal and cognitively mediated. Hence, the independent variable(s) will have less impact than desired and dependent variable distributions will be skewed. Subjects may be ill, medicated, anxious, bored, or nonresponsive, and the researcher must decide whether or not to include their data in the statistical analyses. A standardized screening procedure can reduce the number of outliers. Researchers should give thought to this problem in advance and devise pretests that include physiological measures, so that aberrant subjects can be detected at the outset. If they go undetected until the final analysis, they still may be dropped from the study, but the consequences may be more severe for analysis and interpretation. Basic sources on statistics such as Winer (1971) and more specialized treatments for psychophysiologists such as Levey (1980) contain discussions of procedures for handling missing data and outliers.

Finally, the complexity of a *social* psychophysiological experiment contributes to inflated error variance. The recording procedures are obtrusive and possibly stressful, the laboratory environment is novel, and experimental procedures may range from complex and demanding to ambiguous and confusing. These and other *psychosocial* factors contribute to inflated error variance, as do individual differences in physiological responding. Researchers thus must be mindful of one fundamental reality. We can structure experimental settings as rigorously as possible, we can stand-ardize our procedures, and we can control virtually all of the *exteroceptive* experience of our subjects, but we cannot directly control the subject's *interoceptive* experience. Experimental control affords precise specification of the stimuli that impinge on the subject from the external environment, whether as setting variables (e.g., temperature, humidity, illumination) or as experimental variables (e.g., instructions, task stimuli, trial cues). How-ever, the subject's internal physiological processes are continuous and dynamic. They are the background over which the experimental manipula-tions are laid and from which discrete time series are extracted so that responses can be measured. In other areas of psychological research, the experimenter controls the information impinging on the subject and pre-sumably most influencing the response, which itself is often overt. In the psychophysiological laboratory, we attempt to control the relevant ex-ternal information, but we record from ongoing internal processes, which may be influenced by a variety of external and internal (linguistic and imaginal) stimuli that are independent of manipulated variables.

This lack of specification of interoceptive experience, together with variation in the numerous external realms, physical and psychological, cumulate to produce wide variation among subjects in response to labora-tory treatments. The more that researchers can do to reduce these sources of variation, the more likely are statistically significant effects to emerge. This is where *closed-loop* experimental procedures, in which feedback from the subject during the session determines the scheduling of experimental events, can be used to reduce error variance. In closed-loop procedures onset conditions for each trial are preselected based on the response of one or more measures. That is, at the beginning of the session, extensive baseline data are collected. This may involve periods of relaxation, minimal stimulation, or "neutral" stimulation. From this period, a baseline is com-puted that must be maintained for a predetermined period of time before any trial may begin.

Most classically trained experimentalists are accustomed to fixed pro-cedures, that is, *open-loop* programming, where trials occur as prepro-grammed. With the real-time computational ability of the laboratory com-puter, open-loop programming can be replaced with procedures that ensure greater standardization and therefore less error variance associated with the procedures themselves. It is a simple matter for the closed-loop program to account for trend over the session within a measure such as skin resistance level, so that the return to baseline before a trial can be monitored intelligently. Simple feedback to the subject could be provided between trials to facilitate the return to baseline. In addition, a subject's motivation and ability to return to baseline could be pretested, lest, for example, the failure to do so becomes an avoidance response in face of aversive stimuli.

RECORDING BIOELECTRIC SIGNALS

Equipment

The easy availability of sophisticated hardware can deceive the researcher, who has the capital to invest in the equipment, into believing that all one has to do is purchase and install the equipment in order to start doing psychophysiological research. In fact, the problems only begin once the hardware is in place and are only compounded by bad decisions at the hardware stage. Expert advice should guide the selection and installation of the necessary hardware. In the long run an established company with available expertise and reputable service is often the better bargain. Equipment with inherent flexibility of application should be purchased when possible, so that future configurations can be accommodated without additional purchases. Mixing manufacturers can cause problems also, because their equipment often operates at different voltage and current levels and therefore may be incompatible. This chapter assumes that a laboratory computer is involved in the research, so it is crucial to ensure that the peripheral equipment used to detect, amplify, process, and store the analog signals is compatible with the computer, whether through the analog-to-digital (A/D) converter or through a digital input/output (I/O) device. Also, provided that the expertise and facilities are available, reliable, high-quality equipment can be constructed locally at great savings. Several journals, such as *Psychophysiology* and *Behavior Research Methods and Instrumentation*, publish technical reports that contain sufficient detail for local adaptation.

Installation

Some of the most difficult and frustrating problems in psychophysiological research occur before the first subject enters the laboratory. Ensuring the proper *grounding* of all equipment and of the subject is essential for safe operation, and adequate *shielding* of the laboratory and the data transmission lines is necessary to ensure proper signal processing. Local expertise, from engineers, physicists, or trained colleagues, should be sought to ensure the success of this preliminary phase. The published literature, such as McGuigan (1979) and Gale and Smith (1980), is useful in establishing a laboratory, but cannot substitute for on-site, expert consultation.

Expert advice will be needed further in the *calibration* of the equipment prior to actual use in an experiment. Improper calibration at the outset can render data useless, as can the failure to ensure that the calibration is maintained throughout the experiment. Frequent systematic checks are essential and are easily accommodated through use of the local computer. For the most part, calibration requires the input of a standard signal (which should also be calibrated) that is then processed through the recording system. The output signal will depend on amplification ratios, but this can be calculated and the output values should agree with calculated values within a specified accuracy level. The outputs, of course, should not vary over time. The laboratory should be prepared for an experiment so that little adjustment of the equipment is required during the experimental phase itself. Adjustments during an experiment are risky, unless the quantification procedures take them into account, which can be tedious and error-prone.

Electrode Technique

Once the equipment is installed, calibrated, and working with minimal electrostatic interference, the laboratory is ready for an experimental subject. The first decisions in psychophysiological recording concern electrode technique (see McGuigan, Chapter 22, this volume). *Electrode location* is one concern, and, where possible, adherence to standards is advisable. For example, Jasper (1958) informed electroencephalographic (EEG) researchers of standard locations for scalp electrodes, Lykken and Venables (1971) suggested standard electrode locations for recording electrodermal activity, and Davis (1959) proposed standard surface EMG electrode placements. Individual differences in physiognomy are inevitable, so investigators should standardize procedures by employing reference points to minimize variation among subjects in electrode placement.

Depending on the research problem at hand, *laterality differences* may be a concern. Electrodes may be placed bilaterally, but if not, unilateral placements should be made with laterality differences in mind. The past decade spawned numerous studies of hemispheric EEG asymmetry beginning with Galin and Ornstein (1972), and more recently laterality differences have been found in electromyographic (Schwartz, Ahern, & Brown, 1979) and electrodermal (Lacroix & Comper, 1979) research. Where these differences are important to current research, subjects may be screened preexperimentally for indicators of laterality such as handedness from which eligibility can be determined. Electrode placement could then reflect the assessment of each subject's laterality.

Additional decisions concern *electrode procedures*, such as type and size of electrode, type of placement (e.g., bipolar vs. monopolar), type of conducting medium used between the electrode and the skin, and the techniques used to prepare the skin surface for electrode placement. Investigators can find assistance in reports of parametric research particular to a given measure. As examples, Williamson, Epstein, and Lombardo (1980) compared horizontal and vertical bipolar EMG electrode placements in the context of frontalis biofeedback training; Mitchell and Venables (1980) examined the relationship of electrodermal activity to electrode size; and

Schneider and Fowles (1978) compared several electrolyte media for electrodermal recording.

The researcher should consult the experts to ensure proper electrode technique for each measure. In addition, the target literature for the anticipated research should be consulted so that procedures conform to those used previously in a specific area of research. Unfortunately, discrepancies sometimes exist between what the specialists advise and what colleagues in a given research area have done. On the one hand are pressures to conform to the standards of the psychophysiologists to ensure the scientific rigor and validity of the results, but on the other hand are the pressures of tradition in each separate subdiscipline, which may determine acceptance of the results within their intended domain.

The recent provision of publication guidelines for electrodermal (Fowles, Christie, Edelberg, Grings, Lykken, & Venables, 1981) and for heart rate (Jennings, Berg, Hutcheson, Obrist, Porges, & Turpin, 1981) research is welcome and should aid decision making as it pertains to the collection, analysis, and reporting of such data.

Analog Signal Processing

Once proper electrode technique has ensured adequate sensing of the physiological response, the remaining stages of recording are those of electronically processing an analog signal. *Amplification* of one sort or another is required, because most physiological signals are very small in amplitude. Often, *filtering* is necessary or desirable. The researcher may know the frequency range of interest, so that low-pass and high-pass filters can be used to reject unwanted information from the analog signal. For example, an EMG researcher may discard all frequencies below 100 Hz and above 500 Hz, because the activity of interest lies within this 400-Hz band or because the activity within this band is sufficiently representative of all activity that filtering is justified to ease further processing. However warranted, filtering is irreversible, and researchers must be cautious about such modification of the raw waveform.

In some applications, early stages of signal processing involve the use of a notch filter to remove electrostatic interference at a specific frequency due to standard electrical transmission lines (e.g., 60 Hz in the United States and 50 Hz in Europe). This is to be avoided if possible by techniques such as shielding, because electronic filtering is imprecise. In actuality, a normal distribution of frequencies with a mean of 60 Hz will be eliminated, thus distorting the analog input in what may be an undesirable fashion.

Subsequent to amplification and filtering, the usual requirements of analog signal processing are for *display* and *storage*. Display is most often by means of an ink-writing oscillograph or a cathode-ray oscilloscope. The former produces hard copy that can serve archival purposes, and facilitates visual analysis and artifact detection. Most oscillographs are restricted mechanically to display frequencies less than about 100 Hz. As a result, if the user wishes to score the data from the oscillograph record, the raw waveforms with high-frequency components must be modified by such procedures as integration prior to hard-copy display. The oscilloscope, unless photographed, does not provide a permanent record, but it is useful for calibration and for continuous monitoring of incoming analog signals during a session to ensure proper equipment functioning. Its frequency and amplitude display capabilities greatly exceed those of an ink-writing device.

In addition to choosing the types of display, it is necessary to decide when to display the signal; should the raw signal or some processed version of it be shown? Such decisions dovetail with the decision of how and what to store. In the past, the raw signal and processed versions of it were recorded on paper and analyzed as such. With the advent of FM tape recorders, raw data were often displayed on paper in real time, but stored on tape for further processing by computers. Today, with the availability of computers that are dedicated to single laboratories, these procedures are often altered. In our laboratory, an ink-writing oscillograph records the raw EMG signals, whereas the computer stores digitized versions of the integrated EMG on floppy disk. This allows us to monitor the lower frequencies of the raw EMG signals in real time both to ensure proper equipment functioning and to detect the occurrence of artifact, but scoring and manipulation of the integrated EMG waveforms are performed by the computer. Such factors as analysis requirements, individual preferences, and available hardware will determine the specific forms of display and storage of the data.

Unfortunately, because of the facility of computers for rapid reduction and analysis, raw data are sometimes not stored and are thereby irretrievable for future analysis. We know of no formal guidelines, but our experience would suggest that some record of the raw analog signals be retained. As noted above, a paper record is one option for complex analog signals (e.g., EMG), because they make heavy demands on computer memory and processing capacity, but less complex waveforms [e.g., galvanic skin responses (GSRs)] can be efficiently stored by the computer.

We have assumed that this chain of procedures, from sensing through amplification and filtering to display and storage, occurs prior to A/D conversion by the computer. Although it is possible to accomplish all of these tasks beyond sensing with the computer, such use is inefficient. Hardware processing of analog signals is preferred as far down the chain as possible. Once the analog signal is passed to a computer for digitization, programming problems are introduced due to hardware constraints, often related to processing speed and memory capacity. The operation of the computer will be greatly restricted if it performs real-time analog signal processing at too early a stage.

MEASUREMENT ISSUES IN ANALOG SIGNAL PROCESSING

There are two aspects of measurement in psychophysiological research: modification and quantification. Modification means changing such characteristics of the analog signal as polarity, shape, and component frequencies. These changes usually occur in hardware before quantification. Quantification refers to the process of converting the raw or modified digitized waveform into the desired units of analysis.

Modification

An initial division is made into those procedures that modify *frequency* characteristics versus those that modify *amplitude* characteristics. This division depends on the signal being processed, the stage of processing, and the specific application. For example, EEG data may be frequency-analyzed initially by extracting only a band of frequencies from the complex input wave, and then amplitude may be modified through suitable integration. In EMG research, integrated amplitude is used often to index muscle tension, but in some settings frequency characteristics are studied as signs of muscle pathology.

Each researcher must be clear about the interaction of the frequency and amplitude characteristics of a given analog waveform and then decide what information is relevant. In many cases, tradition and convention may dictate a modification, but new and useful information may be available in other characteristics of a waveform. Earlier we mentioned the dilemma concerning what form of signal to store as the permanent record of the research. This bears directly on the issues of signal modification. How much modification should be performed on the raw analog signal prior to permanent storage? Should one filter and integrate an EMG signal prior to storage, because this is the waveform of eventual interest, or should one preserve the raw signal and perform the modifications in poststorage analyses? These are questions that each researcher will answer based on practical and professional considerations, such as computer memory and storage capacity or the necessity for raw data archives.

There are numerous signal modification procedures; all may be performed on the digitized waveform by computer or on the analog waveform by peripheral hardware. The reason for performing signal modification prior to the computer interface relates to the sampling rate (also known as the Nyquist rate) and hence the amount of computation required by the computer to process unmodified analog signals. The sampling theorem states that in order to recover the analog function exactly, it is necessary to sample the signal at a rate greater than twice the highest frequency (known as the Nyquist frequency) (Stearns, 1975). Therefore, to sample a raw EMG waveform, where the highest frequency may approach 2 kHz, and to perform A/D conversion, the computer must sample more than 4000 points per second from the analog waveform. In addition, averaging the raw waveform requires taking the absolute value of each point (rectification) and then entering each new value into a running average that is then stored at preselected intervals (e.g., 4 points per second) to represent the integrated EMG waveform. This amount of processing by the computer is demanding, especially with multiple analog channels and other experimental procedures that require simultaneous computer control. In this case, it is much simpler to perform the averaging in peripheral hardware and then to sample the modified waveform at the desired rate for storage and further analysis (i.e., 4 points per second).

Each research program will dictate the type of analog signal modifications required. Raw EEG and EMG signals often are *integrated* prior to quantification. This involves rectifying the input and then either cumulating it with a voltage-based or time-based reset or averaging it and retaining a "smoothed" version of the input. These forms of modification have been discussed by Shaw (1967); several types of integration are compared in Figure 23-1.

Heart rate may be derived from the raw waveform in several ways. It may be necessary to detect only peaks (i.e., heart beats), in which case a cardiotachometer can be used to provide an analog signal in beats per minute, or the time between adjacent peaks may be computed to produce an analog signal known as heart period in milliseconds (interbeat interval). Other forms of analysis of heart rate involve the complete electrocardiogram, where certain pathologies are in question or specific responses of the heart are being studied.

EEG processing often involves the isolation of specific frequency bands for analysis. The alpha band (8 to 13 Hz) is often extracted from the input waveform and then integrated and analyzed for relative amplitude at various sites. Signal averaging of the EEG waveform is another form of modification that is often used in evoked potential research. In this case, multiple instances of a time-locked analog waveform are superimposed so that the signal (i.e., the evoked response) emerges from the noise within the individual trials.

The purpose of modification is to produce a new waveform that is appropriate for the analyses required by an experiment. Some modifications will be dictated directly by the nature of the research, whereas others will be selected by the researcher as convenient to the specific purposes. It is from this modified signal that quantification and final scoring will take

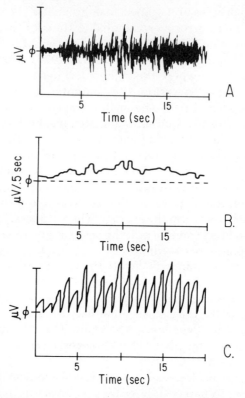

FIGURE 23-1. Schematic illustration showing two forms of integration of a raw EMG signal (A). The first (B) shows full-wave voltage averaging (also known as smoothing or as contour-following integration) with a time constant of .5 second. The second (C) shows time-based resetting cumulative integration with a 1-second reset.

place. Often, it is this waveform that will be passed to the local computer for quantification and analysis.

One possible strategy is to save the modified signal as the basic data for all subsequent analyses. Compared to a raw waveform, the computer can sample the modified signal at a much lower rate in real time and still provide adequate precision. These data can then be stored on floppy disk or another computer-addressable medium for later processing. This allows great flexibility in analysis, because most of the information in the raw data is preserved. Alternatively, where discrete trials are recorded, the computer may reduce the input analog waveform to a summary statistic, such as the mean amplitude over each specified interval, and save only these few values. If no further analyses are required or of interest, such a strategy is highly efficient, because few data are stored. We prefer the former strategy, because it preserves temporal information and allows for subsequent exploratory analyses and computer-generated graphical displays, but the data storage requirements are greater.

Storing the modified analog signal also allows for an important step in processing, namely, the *removal of artifact*. In many applications, subject movement, speech, or other activity may cause artifactual responses to appear in certain input signals. Removal of such inappropriate responses from these data arrays is a tedious, but often essential task. Although perhaps true, it is unwise to assume that such occurrences are randomly distributed and will not affect statistical analyses. The means for removing artifact will vary. In our laboratory, the paper record of the raw EMG data will often reveal artifact. These instances can be checked against a record of the experimental session, perhaps on videotape or as noted by the experimenter during the session. Computer programs then remove those responses that are known to be artifactual and substitute values for those points that will not bias subsequent analyses, such as a mean derived from adjacent time periods.

Quantification

Strictly speaking, the data have been quantified throughout processing, but for our purposes quantification begins with the computation of units of analysis. The steps in the quantification process are shown in Figure 23-2. At the computer interface the input analog signal is transformed into arbitrary units through *analog-to-digital* conversion. As the voltage of the input signal varies, the values read from the A/D converter vary, but the units are now arbitrary. Converting the digitized waveform, now a data array, to *real-world units* is a simple programming matter, requiring constants such as the gain and sensitivity of the amplifier, the A/D value for zero volts, and so forth. It is important to realize that the conversion of the digitized waveform to real units, however noble, is bound to be inaccurate. Recall the number of steps that have occurred from the point of electrode contact with the subject's skin to the modified signal that is passed to the computer. There are signal-to-noise problems at each juncture, as well as hardware error, and as a result, the final waveform, while perhaps a reliable variant of the initial signal, is appropriate only for relational analysis and not for absolute comparisons. In other words, measurement error and bias can intercede at numerous points, and conversion back to real-world units can only approximate the amplitudes of the original signal.

Further quantification may be called for after computation of meaningful units. *Mathematical conversions* are used sometimes to rescale the data point for point. Linear transformations such as computing deviation scores or z scores are familiar to most psychologists and are not specific to a given psychophysiological measure. Other mathematical conversions are specific

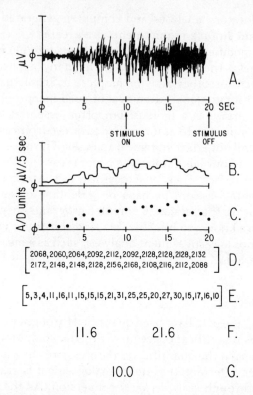

FIGURE 23-2. Schematic illustration showing the stages in the scoring process for an EMG signal from a 20-second trial in which a stimulus was present for the latter 10 seconds. The raw EMG (A) is passed through a full-wave voltage averager (B) with a time constant of .5 second and then sampled at 1 Hz (i.e., 1 point per second) through the analog-to-digital converter (C) to produce a data array with 20 values (D), now in A/D units. This array is converted back to EMG units (E) with a mathematical conversion $[(x - 2048)/4]$, and then the converted array is collapsed over time by computing the mean amplitude prior to and during stimulus presentation (F). Finally, a phasic score for this trial is computed by subtracting the baseline (prestimulus) mean from the response mean (G).

to the variable of interest and the arguments for and against the conversion should be consulted. These conversions are often nonlinear and hence change the characteristics of the distribution, making these procedures both conversions of units and transformations of scale. For example, skin resistance level in ohms is frequently converted to skin conductance level in micromhos, and heart rate in beats per minute may be converted to heart period in interbeat interval (milliseconds). Both conversions involve a reciprocal transformation and a constant term to rescale the units. Such conversions are done because of convention, for convenience of interpretation, to modify the distributions to permit or to improve statistical analysis, or to minimize the influence of an inherent characteristic of the data, such as nonindependence or susceptibility to the law of initial values. Caution is urged, because these conversions can be misleading. Some researchers measure skin conductance level or interbeat interval directly using different peripheral hardware, and the directly measured and the mathematically converted variables may not be the same, although they are indistinguishable in print (see Lykken & Venables, 1971; Venables & Christie, 1980). Figure 23-3 demonstrates the differences in an analog waveform that result from various conversions.

In other instances researchers compute more *complex indices*, combining either the information from several similar channels or from different measures. For example, laterality scores are prevalent in EEG research, where the activity of one cerebral hemisphere is represented as a proportion of the other hemisphere's activity or of the activity of both hemispheres (e.g., Galin & Ornstein, 1972; Morgan, McDonald, & MacDonald, 1971). Such a summary index increases efficiency of analysis by summarizing information from both cerebral hemispheres in a single index. Other researchers have proposed the use of composite indices for summarizing autonomic activity (e.g., Wenger & Cullen, 1972).

After each data array has been converted to the appropriate units of analysis or after multiple arrays have been combined into composite units, further quantification involves *reduction over time*. All the processing to this point has preserved the point-for-point characteristics of the waveform or has computed a new waveform without altering temporal characteristics. This is essential if the data array is to be analyzed by time-series procedures, but often in social psychology the activity during discrete blocks of time is reduced to a summary statistic and then aggregated over repetitions, trials, subjects, and groups in conventional analysis of variance. As such, the *epoch* becomes the building block in the data analysis, where an epoch is defined as an instance of behavior that emerges distinctly from surrounding time periods.

For example, the researcher often averages data (as amplitudes) over time within each epoch to summarize the activity during that time period. Such analyses deal with *level* of responding, as summarized usually by the mean, but also may use other measures of central tendency, such as the median or the mode. Other statistics also may be used to summarize an epoch, such as the peak amplitude, peak–trough difference, number of peaks, latency of peak response (rise time), or latency of recovery. Each researcher should select thoughtfully the appropriate summary statistic when collapsing over time within each epoch. This decision may be guided by research traditions or may be based on hypothesized response patterning. The overriding goal is to best summarize the activity of each measure during a specific period of time, usually as some measure of amplitude.

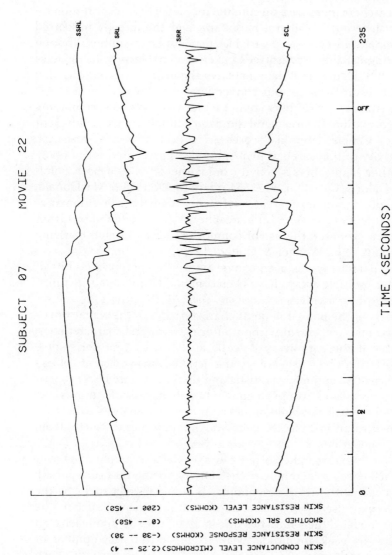

FIGURE 23-3. Computer-generated plots showing one subject's electrodermal response to an impactful film segment. Note the differences in ordinate range for each plotted array. The actual recorded and stored data array was skin resistance level (SRL) ($\bar{X}$ = 385.95, **SD** = 10.85, **n** = 235, skewness = .202); the other three plotted arrays are mathematical conversions of these data. Smoothed skin resistance level (SSRL) was computed by averaging over 3-second intervals ($\bar{X}$ = 385.92, **SD** = 10.74, **n** = 79, skewness = .25). Skin resistance response (SRR), also known as phasic skin resistance, is the first differenced version of SRL, which is computed by differencing successive adjacent pairs of data points ($\bar{X}$ = .032, **SD** = 2.10, **n** = 234, skewness = −3.22). Skin conductance level (SCL) is a reciprocal transform

In some applications, measures of *variability* over time are of interest. Research hypotheses may predict changes in the variability of response amplitudes as a function of experimental conditions, and hence a summary statistic is needed to capture this information for further analysis. The range of amplitudes or the variance (also, log variance, standard deviation) during the epoch are often appropriate measures of variability. Other, less well-known statistics are available for summarizing variability and may have desirable properties; their use depends on the measure being analyzed, its behavior during the imposed experimental conditions, and the intended statistical procedure. For example, the successive difference mean square (SDMS) and the number of reversals (NREV) have been suggested as appropriate measures of variability in heart rate, where the presence of linear trends complicates the use of conventional variance statistics (Heslegrave, Ogilvie, & Furedy, 1979; Luczak & Laurig, 1973; Wastell, 1981). An important point for those steeped in the traditions of social psychology is that experimental effects in psychophysiology are often in variability rather than level, and new perspectives on what constitutes a "response" are required. Furthermore, the choice of statistic to summarize the activity of a given psychophysiological measure within each epoch should be based on a comprehensive review of prior research and thorough understanding of the data at hand.

Once the data for each epoch have been reduced over time, most research in social psychophysiology involves the computation of a *phasic score* (change score, difference score) to represent the subject's response. This is done by subtracting the activity during a *baseline period* from a *response period*. That is, response magnitude is described in relative terms: stimulus on versus stimulus off, task present versus no task, condition A versus condition B, condition A versus no condition, or condition A versus neutral condition. Summarizing the response during the stimulus interval is accomplished easily, because the experimenter (and presumably the computer) knows exactly when the trial began and ended, when the stimulus appeared and disappeared, and so on. The only choice is which summary statistic(s) to extract from the epoch, as discussed above.

The problem for the computation of a phasic score is determining what to use as the appropriate baseline from which to measure the response. Conventionally, one uses the time period immediately preceding stimulus onset as the baseline for the response period. As such, the baseline value may vary from trial to trial, but each response is relative to what occurred immediately prior to the cue that began the response interval or the stimulus that evoked the response. Although conceptually straightforward, this approach may harbor difficulties. What if the subject anticipates on some trials and not on others? What happened *after* the response interval? Does the postresponse baseline period look like the preresponse baseline period? Rote approaches to computing phasic scores may overlook or obscure interesting data. Again, awareness of the time-series context of psychophysiological responses suggests care in specifying baseline conditions from which to measure phasic change.

There is a disturbing tendency among researchers to use a different-length time period for the baseline computation than for the response computation. Because the baseline period serves as a "control" for the response period, similarity along as many dimensions as possible, including duration, is desirable. In many instances, analysis of the baseline periods alone should precede analysis of phasic responses. Baselines within an experiment may be compared for trends over time or for differences in level or variability between groups or conditions. These cautions under-score the need for the experimenter to consider various procedures for collecting appropriate baseline data to be used in the computation of phasic scores. Closed-loop experimental procedures, which were discussed above, offer an alternative to extensive baseline collection and reliance on phasic scores, because the subject returns to the predetermined baseline levels before each trial, which makes response amplitudes relative to a single baseline.

STATISTICAL ANALYSIS OF SOCIAL PSYCHOPHYSIOLOGICAL DATA

Analysis strategy often will be predetermined by experimental design. Most social psychophysiologists come to their research with the biases of traditional experimental psychology, that is, for fixed-effects between-subjects analysis of variance. In some applications, this strategy is appropriate, but with increasing frequency alternative approaches to statistical analysis may be necessary and desirable.

One reason for the failure of psychophysiological data to meet the assumptions of traditional analysis of variance stems from the use of phasic scores, which often produce *skewed distributions*. There are procedures to correct skewness, such as removing outliers or mathematically trans-forming the scores (e.g., square root, logarithms), but these procedures may be problematic. In the former case, one is throwing out data from subjects who may have overresponded in the hypothesized direction, whereas in the latter case, one's statistical results are based on trans-formed data and interpretive difficulties may arise.

Where there is a theoretical justification for a *mathematical transforma-tion*, such as is the case in psychophysics, the central issue is which trans-formation to apply to the raw data. On the other hand, if the purpose is solely to draw in outlying data points so that parametric statistical tech-niques may be employed, the use of transformations is questionable. Here we reiterate the problem for social psychophysiology: Variability of re-sponses may be due both to physiological differences among subjects and to differences in the psychological impact of the experimental stimuli and setting. When a nonnormal distribution results due to the latter cause, mathematical transformations may increase the probability of inferential error. Disentangling the components of overall variation due to either physiological or psychological differences among subjects becomes an important, albeit difficult task for the researcher.

Social psychophysiologists might consider adding *standardized procedures* to all experimental sessions, such as those employed when range corrections are anticipated. The idea here is to assess independently subject lability using standardized, impactful stimuli so that variations in response to the experimental stimuli can be judged as due to intersubject physiological differences or to differential psychological responsivity. Where responsivity to the standardized stimuli covaries strongly with that to the experimental stimuli, the "take" of the independent variable may be judged as strong and mathematical transformation of the skewed raw data distribution is appropriate. Where responsivity is less clearly related between the standardized and experimental conditions, mathematical transformations to correct skewness may be inappropriate.

Furthermore, it will often be the case with phasic scores that the assumption of *homogeneity of variance* will be violated. There may be more variation among experimental subjects than among control subjects, or there may be more variation in one experimental condition than in another. That is, a strong correlation may exist among means and their associated measures of dispersion. Seldom are tests for homogeneity of variance/covariance reported in the research literature; instead, casual reference is given to the robustness of analysis of variance in face of these violations. Some researchers, who are mindful of such problems for traditional analysis of variance, use appropriate nonparametric tests to analyze psychophysiological data (e.g., Cacioppo & Petty, 1979a, 1979b; Schwartz, Fair, Salt, Mandel, & Klerman, 1976). As such, problems in the data for parametric analysis are made explicit, and less restrictive techniques are used to test experimental hypotheses. Guidelines are needed to assist researchers in choosing among analytic techniques when the data fall within the fuzzy region between clearly meeting or not meeting the assumptions of parametric tests.

More detailed discussions of the analysis problems related to mathematical transformations, nonnormality of distributions, and heterogeneity of variance and covariance can be found in most source books on psychophysiological methods, such as Levey (1980) and Johnson and Lubin (1972), and in review articles, such as that of Richards (1980).

Another problem for analysis in social psychophysiology is the *repeated-measures* nature of much of the research. Often, the most logical and practical experimental design includes within-subjects factors and hence involves repeated exposure to experimental conditions. The amount of time devoted to preparing for physiological recording and to adapting the subject to the laboratory setting often motivates the collection of extensive data from each participant. There are two forms of repeated-measures design. The first is the repetition of similar trials so that more stable indices of behavior can be obtained through aggregation or so that changes over time can be observed (e.g., learning, habituation, or extinction). The other is the exposure of single subjects to multiple experimental conditions so that the same subjects appear in both control and treatment cells. Both strategies should reduce error variance, which is a primary consideration when designing social psychophysiological experiments. S. Epstein (1980) has argued for increased aggregation over stimuli/situations and over trials/occasions, in a manner akin to the prevalent practice of aggregation over individuals, in order to enhance generalizability and to increase replicability. These arguments are particularly apt for social psychophysiologists, where such procedures will help reduce incidental variance, that is, variance due to factors other than the independent variables.

The analysis of repeated-measures designs has been discussed for many years, but the advice is often contradictory. In addition, the procedures are time consuming and often opaque to users. Homogeneity of variance/covariance must be assured, which is a stringent criterion. The persistent problem in psychophysiological research is the nonindependence of repeated measurements. That is, adjacent data points are correlated more strongly than nonadjacent points, thus violating the circularity assumption (autocorrelation) for analysis-of-variance models. Corrections have been suggested for traditional analysis of variance such as that of Greenhouse and Geisser (1959), but these strategies are conservative. Multivariate analysis of variance is often preferred (e.g., Davidson, 1972), but it is foreign to many researchers, and with multiple dependent variables, its use is complicated. Richards (1980) has reviewed many of these issues, and Keselman and Rogan (1980) have described procedures for avoiding positive bias in repeated-measures F tests.

Analysis problems are complicated further when there are *multiple dependent variables*. Many traditional multivariate strategies, usually based on the linear (regression) model, are appropriate. Social psychophysiological research normally involves multiple dependent variables, so multivariate analysis strategies are necessary for a fuller understanding of the *patterns* in the data. There is a distinction between analyzing differences among patterns within response systems and analyzing multiple dependent variables from more than one response system. In the former case, the response of a single system, such as the face or the sympathetic nervous system, is modeled as a patterned response. Each psychophysiological measure is viewed as a component of an integrated response. For example, Fridlund and Izard (Chapter 10, this volume) discuss the analysis of patterned EMG data from multiple sites on the face as an index of facial expressive behavior. When multiple dependent variables are obtained from more than one response system, the analyst may use multivariate techniques to test hypotheses concerning covariation among these systems or to avoid Type I errors due to conducting multiple univariate tests where the dependent variables are not orthogonal (e.g., Englis, Vaughan, & Lanzetta, 1982).

A general strategy for multivariate analysis is to explore first the relationships among the dependent variables used in a study, eliminating redundancy through the guidance provided by such techniques as factor analysis, cluster analysis, canonical correlation, and the various forms of linear and nonlinear regression. Once the relationships among the measures are understood, differences among groups of subjects or among conditions within subjects can be examined. For example, linear discriminant analysis is a powerful tool for analyzing group differences. The same statistical procedures are available for repeated-measures discriminant analysis, where one wishes to discriminate among conditions or occasions within groups. Here researchers must beware of heterogeneity of variance/covariance, because discriminant procedures are extensions of multivariate analysis of variance. Ray and Kimmel (1979) have provided an overview of these multivariate options for psychophysiological research.

Ray (1980) has also proposed the use of path analysis to model relationships among multiple dependent measures in psychophysiological research. Although path analysis may be appropriate statistically and conceptually, *structural equation modeling* is a superior technique (Bentler, 1980; Jöreskog, 1977; Jöreskog & Sörbom, 1979). These latter techniques are mathematically complex, but are explicit and powerful conceptually (see recent applications by Zajonc, 1980, and Bentler & Speckart, 1981). Structural equation models allow for such options as multiple dependent measures, multiple occasions (repeated measures), corrections for measurement error, and fixed and free coefficients. Structural relationships among *latent* variables are described by a *causal model,* which is parameterized from a *measurement model* that is based on the *observed* variables. For example, arousal is a latent variable (i.e., a hypothesized state) that may be estimated from such measures as skin conductance response, systolic blood pressure, and self-report. As such, a causal model can test the impact of arousal on other latent variables, such as attitudes and behaviors, which themselves may be variously measured at one or more points in time. These techniques are the most sophisticated multivariate hypothesis-testing strategies available today, integrating and superseding such techniques as path analysis, covariance analysis, and factor analysis.

Two further developments in statistical analysis that have been made available by high-speed digital computers are appropriate for psychophysiological data, but they are relatively untried. Both are time-series techniques and reflect our belief that investigators will profit from awareness of analytic strategies that are natural for some social psychophysiological data structures.

The first is based on the work of Box and Jenkins (1970), who integrated autoregressive and moving-average techniques into ARIMA modeling. With these procedures the stochastic component of a time series is modeled by weighting past values and past shock terms (error terms). One advantage of time-series procedures is that tests of the statistical significance of model parameters are not biased as they are in ordinary least-squares regression approaches (e.g., ANOVA), where autocorrelation among error terms is likely. Once the parameters of an ARIMA model have been identified and estimated, complex intervention hypotheses may be tested. If this time-series hypothesis, called a transfer function, increases the model's predictability, the parameters of this intervention component (transfer function) will be statistically significant. Because transfer functions can test variously shaped intervention hypotheses, these procedures may be more appropriate in social psychophysiological research than the hypotheses in traditional analysis of variance, which are typically step functions (i.e., tests of differences among means). Figure 23-4 illustrates the difference between these two forms of hypotheses. In addition, ARIMA modeling has grown in sophistication to the point where the simultaneous analysis of multiple time series is possible. Glass, Wilson, and Gottman (1975) have described time series methods for experimental research in psychology; McCain and McCleary (1979) and McCleary and Hay (1980) provide a basic introduction to ARIMA modeling. The task for the experimenter becomes one of building a theoretical model and structuring an experiment to accommodate this type of statistical analysis.

The second development is *spectral analysis*, that is, the analysis of analog (continuous, time-series) data in the frequency domain. EEG researchers are sophisticated in these procedures, but other psychophysiologists have lagged in the application of these techniques to their data. These procedures are well suited to the analysis of rhythmic processes such as heart rate or respiration rate, where an understanding of the constituent sinusoidal functions is of interest. Brillinger (1975) has presented the mechanics of spectral analysis.

More relevant to social psychophysiology are spectral analytic techniques that involve relationships between time series. For example, Porges, Bohrer, Cheung, Drasgow, McCabe, and Keren (1980) described a new statistic, the weighted coherence, which is analogous to R-squared in general linear model (regression) applications or omega-squared in ANOVA. That is, weighted coherence summarizes the degree of redundancy between two physiological functions within a frequency band of interest, whereas R-squared is the proportion of shared variance between those two functions over time in the amplitude domain. These authors have used the weighted coherence between respiration rate and heart period as

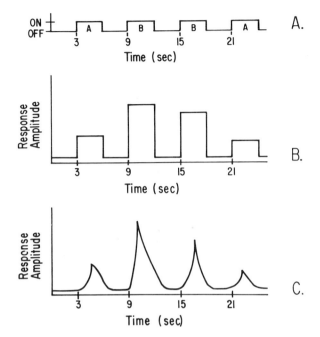

FIGURE 23-4. Graphical comparison of two possible statistical models of a hypothesized experiment in which two stimuli are presented twice (A). An analysis-of-variance model (B) hypothesizes differences in mean amplitude between conditions and habituation within conditions. A time-series model (C) (an ARIMA transfer function) hypothesizes differences in response latency, peak amplitude, and recovery time between conditions, as well as habituation within conditions.

a measure of respiratory–cardiac coupling in a study of the effects of methylphenidate on hyperactive children (Porges, Bohrer, Keren, Cheung, Franks, & Drasgow, 1981). Such statistics as the weighted coherence have many potential uses in psychophysiological research. It could be computed for all pairs of dependent measures as an index of similarity or coupling, and then the resultant matrix could be analyzed by cluster analysis procedures to study patterning in the frequency domain. Both frequency-based (spectral analysis) and time-based (ARIMA modeling) time-series techniques hold great promise as they evolve and become more widely used in the analysis of psychophysiological data.

COMPUTERS IN SOCIAL PSYCHOPHYSIOLOGY

The use of computers has been discussed throughout the preceding sections, but further comments are offered concerning some issues and possibilities associated with laboratory computers and their relationships with larger institutional computers (see also Cacioppo, Marshall-Goodell, & Gormezano, Chapter 24, this volume).

There are multiple information sources available to aid prospective users. Manufacturers of computer equipment provide detailed literature and on-site consultation as required. They will tell you what a particular machine can and cannot do. Processing speeds, programming languages, facility of adaptation to laboratory use, communications facilities, and hardware and software support are all important issues to be discussed with competing vendors. Computer manufacturers usually do not know about specific applications; they probably do not have peripheral hardware for the specialized recording done in a psychophysiological laboratory. However, given the specifications of the peripheral hardware, the computer expert can advise on compatibility. Similarly, manufacturers of peripheral recording, storage, and display equipment can advise on compatibility if given the specifications for a particular computer. For some psychophysiological measures, there are specialized monographs or articles on computer implementation and utilization. For example, Basmajian, Clifford, McLeod, and Nunnally (1975) authored a monograph for EMG applications. Other resources, both primary (e.g., *Behavior Research Methods and Instrumentation*) and secondary (Mayzner & Dolan, 1978; Uttal, 1968), can familiarize the user with the potential uses of the laboratory computer in a given application.

There are several components that are desirable for most laboratory computers. These include a central processor and core memory, an A/D converter, a D/A converter, a scientific timer, a hardware multiply/divide unit (floating-point processor), a digital interface (parallel I/O) unit, a storage medium (e.g., floppy disk or cassette tape), a display medium (e.g., incremental plotter or graphics terminal), and a serial interface unit for control terminals and line printers.

Computers are categorized by word size, that is, the number of bits per word in memory. Common sizes for smaller laboratory computers are 8-, 16-, and 32-bit words. The word size directly affects the size of the numbers that can be stored and manipulated by the machine. A scientific computer should be able to handle floating-point numbers (i.e., decimals), as well as the more easily handled fixed-point numbers (i.e., integers). In some applications, a storage medium may not be necessary, because the data for a single experimental session can be stored in core memory and then passed through a communications link to a mainframe computer for further processing. As such, local utility is limited, but many functions can still be performed. The decision about local storage depends on the availability, cost, and reliability of the institution's mainframe computer, as well as ease of intercommunication.

Several of the primary functions of the laboratory computer are analog signal processing, experimental control procedures, and data analysis. Analog signal processing was discussed above. The laboratory computer can be interposed at various points in the stream of events from sensing to quantification. Analog signal recording and modification are done better in peripheral hardware, but graphical display, data storage, quantification, and analysis may be handled by the local computer.

The second function of the local computer is the control of events during an experimental session. This process is aided greatly by providing convenient connections between the parallel and serial I/O units of the computer and peripheral devices. In our laboratory, each computer's parallel I/O unit connects to an interface panel that contains ports for power drivers at several voltages (5, 12, and 28 V), a bank of relays for computer-controlled switch closures, and a bank of connectors for input from peripheral devices to the computer. The computer thus operates peripheral devices such as slide projectors, video cameras, and feedback devices. The scientific timer, in conjunction with the interface panel, provides the programmer with all the necessary control of events. The digital inputs from the environment to the computer include experimenter-triggered switches and subject-controlled reaction time and rating scale devices. The programming of an experiment is done in software, which greatly increases speed of preparation and flexibility. A computer with a high-level language that is accustomed to laboratory applications and that has such features as parallel processing with interrupts is desirable to accommodate the programming of experiments that include control of peripheral devices, A/D conversion of input signals, and digital inputs.

Another use of the computer for real-time experimental control is closed-loop programming, as discussed earlier. Events can be scheduled during the session according to contingencies set by the computer using information from the subject and the experimenter. Baselines can be monitored continuously and the experimenter can be informed throughout the session of the "behavior" of the subject. Experimental events can be timed in accordance with overt or covert subject responding, as the situation demands. As an example of closed-loop programming, Pope and Gersten (1977) have described a computer-automated shaping procedure for EMG biofeedback-assisted relaxation training.

The third use of the computer at the local level is for analysis of the data. Artifact can be removed through procedures designed to scan data arrays and replace specified segments with appropriate values. Making this a first step ensures that artifact does not persist to the final stages of statistical analysis. Then data can be quantified (i.e., converted to appropriate units) and aggregated for further statistical analysis. The rapidly developing area of computer graphics should be exploited fully to allow for the visual analysis of computer-generated graphical data displays. Coupland, Taylor, and Koopman (1980) demonstrated the utility of three-dimensional cartographic plots of EEG data. The power of human visual information processing is utilized more fully when experimental data are displayed graphically, and researchers will better understand the time-series context of psychophysiological research. Statistical analysis can then be performed, providing that such use is appropriate for the laboratory computer.

As a final section, appropriate use considerations will be discussed briefly, because computer uses and misuses are increasingly important issues. The basic question here is how much processing is done with the laboratory computer before (if ever) passing the data to a larger computer for further analysis. The answer to this question is complex, but awareness of some important considerations is helpful. The bottom line is to do those things locally that the small computer does best and then pass the data to the next larger computer for the things that it does best, and so on. As computers become more prevalent and communications links become faster and more reliable, appropriate use considerations will become more and more relevant.

Most laboratory computers have limited memory capacity and smaller word size than those of a larger mainframe computer. Statistical procedures that require matrix manipulations and that generate large or very small numbers may be impossible or imprecise on smaller computers; they are certainly less efficient. Most small computers, even if capable of floating-point processing, do not come with guaranteed statistical software. Writing complex programs may be possible at the local level, but is time consuming and error prone. Also, many small computers come with programming languages that are not meant for large-scale floating-point processing, although they may be highly efficient at collecting data and controlling peripheral events.

The practice in our laboratory has been to pass data arrays to the institutional computer for all large-scale statistical analyses. Sophisticated software is available, reliable, maintained regularly, and very efficient. It is a simple matter to assemble the appropriate data array in the laboratory computer, perhaps score it and reduce it somewhat, and then pass it to the larger computer. This allows us to collect, quantify, and analyze our data from the laboratory, using the local computer as a communications device with a more powerful computer when appropriate.

Each experimenter's blend of local and remote processing will vary with the trade-offs involved. If the remote computer is expensive to use, if the queues are long and the mode of operation inefficient (i.e., batch vs. time-shared), and if the software is not supported or powerful, then local processing will prevail. It is up to each researcher to judge the appropriateness of the locale for each computer use. In the final resolution, software considerations should outweigh hardware considerations. Just because the local computer can do the job does not necessarily mean that software development will be easy, that precision will be adequate, or that speed will be sufficient.

SUMMARY AND CONCLUSIONS

Social psychophysiological research is complex because the special problems of obtaining physiological data combine with those already present in social psychological research. Advantages arise primarily because the physiological variables permit additional constructs to enter statistical models. The choice of how many and which physiological measures to obtain will be influenced by prior research, present expertise, and the hypotheses to be tested. As in all areas of research in psychology, the psychometric properties of each measure must be considered foremost, but physiological measures require additional attention to numerous practical details.

In addition to those psychosocial factors that add incidental variance to experiments in social psychology, there are a host of sources of further variation inherent in the use of physiological measures. Experimenters must be especially attuned to these abundant sources of unwanted variance, so that experimental design reflects an attempt to minimize their influence. Extensive pretesting of stimuli, procedures, and even subjects may be required before adequate tests of experimental hypotheses are possible. Furthermore, awareness of the dynamic time-series context from which physiological measures are derived will aid in the design and execution of experiments in social psychophysiology.

Psychophysiological recording is sophisticated, and it involves the fusion of diverse expertise. Technical engineering problems abound, as do numerous choice points where the investigator(s) will be influenced by research traditions and up-to-date parametric data.

The length and varied content of the section on measurement attest to the possible pitfalls and the large number of decisions facing a social psychologist who uses psychophysiological measures. The form of analog signal modification often will be preselected by the measures chosen, as time has nurtured conventions for each. There will still be decisions to make, because one needs to determine just what form the final analog signal will take prior to quantification. Decisions will also be influenced by the nature and point of the computer interface with the peripheral recording hardware.

The problems of quantification are more varied and less bound by tradition. The removal of artifact is frequently an essential requirement. Computing units of analysis is functionally simple, but often conceptually difficult. The decision as to which measures to extract from each epoch is also difficult and is surely a point for creative exploration and reasoned alternatives. Finally, the reduction of the data from each epoch to a phasic score is complicated by the need for a representative baseline.

The statistical analysis of data from social psychophysiological experiments is a complex endeavor. Tests of hypotheses within traditional approaches based on the general linear model may be biased for several reasons, and thus researchers must be wary of their application. Tests to ensure compliance with the assumptions of conventional tests and explicit acknowledgment of the shortcomings are recommended. With increasing frequency, multivariate data structures are emerging from psychophysiological laboratories, and hence multivariate statistical procedures are appropriate. Nonparametric techniques and structural equation models or time-series approaches are suggested as alternatives to conventional analyses; the former maintain the conceptual structure of the research hypotheses, whereas the latter may require a restatement of the problem. In social psychophysiology, where experimental conditions may extend over time and where stimuli may be complex, time-series approaches may be especially valuable in testing experimental hypotheses.

The increasing availability of small, dedicated laboratory computers requires additional expertise and decisions. The specific configuration will vary across laboratories, but the importance of decisions concerning appropriate use, maintainability and flexibility, software development, and communications facilities are invariant. The enhanced data collection, storage, manipulation, display, and analysis capabilities afforded by the local computer, and its links to other computers, will allow researchers to test more complex theoretical (and hence statistical) models and thereby understand the underlying processes more fully.

ACKNOWLEDGMENTS

The preparation of this chapter was supported by National Science Foundation Grant 77-08926 and by funds from the Lincoln Filene endowment to Dartmouth College. The authors thank Craig A. Smith for his comments on earlier versions of this chapter.

REFERENCES

Basmajian, J. V., Clifford, H. C., McLeod, W. D., & Nunnally, H. N.   *Computers in electromyography.* London: Butterworths, 1975.

Benjamin, L. S.   Facts and artifacts in using analysis of covariance to "undo" the law of initial values. *Psychophysiology,* 1967, *4,* 186–201.

Bentler, P. M.   Multivariate analysis with latent variables. *Annual Review of Psychology,* 1980, *31,* 419–456.

Bentler, P. M., & Speckart, G.   Attitudes "cause" behaviors: A structural equation analysis. *Journal of Personality and Social Psychology,* 1981, *40,* 226–238.

Boucsein, W., & Hoffmann, G.   A direct comparison of skin conductance and skin resistance methods. *Psychophysiology,* 1979, *16,* 66–70.

Box, G. E. P., & Jenkins, G. M.   *Time series analysis, forecasting and control.* San Francisco: Holden-Day, 1970.

Brillinger, D. R. *Time series: Data analysis and theory.* New York: Holt, Rinehart & Winston, 1975.

Cacioppo, J. T., & Petty, R. E. Attitudes and cognitive response: An electrophysiological approach. *Journal of Personality and Social Psychology,* 1979, *37,* 2181–2199. (a)

Cacioppo, J. T., & Petty, R. E. Lip and nonpreferred forearm EMG activity as a function of orienting task. *Biological Psychology,* 1979, *9,* 103–113. (b)

Cannon, W. B. *Bodily changes in pain, hunger, fear, and rage.* New York: Appleton, 1915.

Coupland, S. G., Taylor, M. J., & Koopman, R. F. EEG landscapes: An application of computer cartography. *Psychophysiology,* 1980, *17,* 413–417.

Davidson, M. I. Univariate versus multivariate tests in repeated-measures experiments. *Psychological Bulletin,* 1972, *77,* 446–452.

Davis, J. F. *A manual of surface electromyography.* Montreal: Allan Memorial Institute of Psychiatry, McGill University. (Republished as WADC Tech. Rep. 59-184. Wright-Patterson Air Force Base, Ohio: U.S. Air Force, 1959.)

Duffy, E. The psychological significance of the concept of "arousal" or "activation." *Psychological Review,* 1957, *64,* 265–275.

Englis, B. G., Vaughan, K. B., & Lanzetta, J. T. Conditioning of counter-empathetic emotional responses. *Journal of Experimental Social Psychology,* 1982, *18,* 375–391.

Epstein, L. H., & Webster, J. S. Reliability of various estimates of electromyogram activity: Within and between subject analyses. *Psychophysiology,* 1975, *12,* 468–470.

Epstein, S. The stability of behavior: II. Implications for psychological research. *American Psychologist,* 1980, *35,* 790–806.

Fowles, D. C., Christie, M. J., Edelberg, R., Grings, W. W., Lykken, D. T., & Venables, P. H. Publication recommendations for electrodermal research. *Psychophysiology,* 1981, *18,* 232–239.

Gale, A., & Smith, D. On setting up a psychophysiological laboratory. In I. Martin & P. H. Venables (Eds.), *Techniques in psychophysiology.* Chichester: Wiley, 1980.

Galin, D., & Ornstein, R. Lateral specialization of cognitive mode: An EEG study. *Psychophysiology,* 1972, *9,* 412–418.

Gans, C., & Gorniak, G. C. Electromyograms are repeatable: Precautions and limitations. *Science,* 1980, *210,* 795–797.

Glass, G. V., Wilson, V. L., & Gottman, J. M. *Design and analysis of time-series experiments.* Boulder: Colorado Associated University Press, 1975.

Graham, G. P. Reliability of EMG after electrode removal and replacement. *Perceptual and Motor Skills,* 1979, *49,* 215–218.

Greenhouse, S. W., & Geisser, S. On methods in the analysis of profile data. *Psychometrica,* 1959, *24,* 95–112.

Grossman, W. I., & Weiner, H. Some factors affecting the reliability of surface electromyography. *Psychosomatic Medicine,* 1966, *28,* 78–83.

Heslegrave, R. J., Ogilvie, J. C., & Furedy, J. J. Measuring baseline-treatment differences in heart rate variability: Variance versus successive difference mean square and beats per minute versus interbeat intervals. *Psychophysiology,* 1979, *16,* 151–157.

Jasper, H. H. The ten twenty electrode system of the International Federation. *Electroencephalography and Clinical Neurophysiology,* 1958, *10,* 371–375.

Jennings, J. R., Berg, W. K., Hutcheson, J. S., Obrist, P., Porges, S., & Turpin, G. Publication guidelines for heart rate studies in man. *Psychophysiology,* 1981, *18,* 226–231.

Johnson, L. C., & Lubin, A. On planning psychophysiological experiments. In N. S. Greenfield & R. A. Sternbach (Eds.), *Handbook of psychophysiology.* New York: Holt, Rinehart & Winston, 1972.

Jöreskog, K. G. Structural equation models in the social sciences. In P. R. Krishnaian (Ed.), *Application of statistics.* Amsterdam: North-Holland, 1977.

Jöreskog, K. G., & Sorböm, D. *Advances in factor analysis and structural equation models.* Cambridge, Mass.: Abt Books, 1979.

Keselman, H. J., & Rogan, J. C.   Repeated measures F tests and psychophysiological research: Controlling the number of false positives. *Psychophysiology*, 1980, *17*, 499–503.

Lacey, J. I.   The evaluation of autonomic responses: Toward a general solution. *Annals of the New York Academy of Sciences*, 1956, *67*, 123–164.

Lacey, J. I.   Somatic response patterning and stress: Some revisions of activation theory. In M. H. Appley & R. Trumbull (Eds.), *Psychological stress: Issues in research*. New York: Appleton-Century-Crofts, 1967.

Lacey, J. I., & Lacey, B. C.   Verification and extension of the principle of autonomic response-stereotypy. *American Journal of Psychology*, 1958, *71*, 50–73.

Lacey, J. I., & Lacey, B. C.   Some autonomic-central nervous system interrelationships. In P. Black (Ed.), *Physiological correlates of emotion*. New York: Academic, 1970.

Lacroix, J. M., & Comper, P.   Lateralization in the electrodermal system as a function of cognitive/hemispheric manipulations. *Psychophysiology*, 1979, *16*, 116–129.

Levey, A. B.   Measurement units in psychophysiology. In I. Martin & P. H. Venables (Eds.), *Techniques in psychophysiology*. Chichester: Wiley, 1980.

Luczak, H., & Laurig, W.   An analysis of heart rate variability. *Ergonomics*, 1973, *16*, 85–98.

Lykken, D. T.   Range correction applied to heart rate and to GSR data. *Psychophysiology*, 1972, *9*, 373–379.

Lykken, D. T., Rose, R., Luther, B., & Maley, M.   Correcting psychophysiological measures for individual differences in range. *Psychological Bulletin*, 1966, *66*, 481–484.

Lykken, D. T., & Venables, P. H.   Direct measurement of skin conductance: A proposal for standardization. *Psychophysiology*, 1971, *8*, 656–672.

Malmo, R. B.   Activation: A neurophysiological dimension. *Psychological Review*, 1959, *66*, 367–386.

Malmo, R. B., & Shagass, C.   Physiological studies of reaction to stress in anxiety and early schizophrenia. *Psychosomatic Medicine*, 1949, *11*, 9–24.

Mayzner, M. S., & Dolan, T. R. (Eds.).   *Minicomputers in sensory and information-processing research*. Hillsdale, N.J.: Erlbaum, 1978.

McCain, L. J., & McCleary, R.   The statistical analysis of the simple interrupted time-series quasi-experiment. In T. D. Cook & D. T. Campbell (Eds.), *Quasi-experimentation: Design and analysis issues for field setting*. Chicago: Rand McNally, 1979.

McCleary, R., & Hay, R. A., Jr.   *Applied time series analysis for the social sciences*. Beverly Hills, Calif.: Sage, 1980.

McGuigan, F. J.   *Psychophysiological measurement of covert behavior: A guide for the laboratory*. Hillsdale, N.J.: Erlbaum, 1979.

Mitchell, D. A., & Venables, P. H.   The relationship of EDA to electrode size. *Psychophysiology*, 1980, *17*, 408–412.

Morgan, A. H., McDonald, P. J., & MacDonald, H.   Differences in bilateral alpha activity as a function of experimental task, with a note on lateral eye movements and hypnotizability. *Neuropsychologia*, 1971, *9*, 459–469.

Obrist, P. A., Gaebelein, C. J., Shanks, E. M., Langer, A. W., & Botticelli, L. J.   Cardiovascular behavioral interactions. In D. I. Mostofsky (Ed.), *Behavior control and modification of physiological activity*. Englewood Cliffs, N.J.: Prentice-Hall, 1976.

Obrist, P. A., Webb, R. A., & Sutterer, J. R.   Heart rate and somatic changes during aversive conditioning and a simple reaction time task. *Psychophysiology*, 1969, *5*, 696–723.

Pope, A. T., & Gersten, C. D.   Computer automation of biofeedback training. *Behavior Research Methods and Instrumentation*, 1977, *9*, 164–168.

Porges, S. W., Bohrer, R. E., Cheung, M., Drasgow, F., McCabe, P. M., & Keren, G.   New time-series statistic for detecting rhythmic co-occurrence in the frequency domain: The weighted coherence and its application to psychophysiological research. *Psychological Bulletin*, 1980, *88*, 580–587.

Porges, S. W., Bohrer, R. E., Keren, G., Cheung, M. N., Franks, G. J., & Drasgow, F.   The influence of methylphenidate on spontaneous autonomic activity and behavior in children diagnosed as hyperactive. *Psychophysiology*, 1981, *18*, 42–48.

Ray, R. L.   Path analysis of psychophysiological data. *Psychophysiology*, 1980, *17*, 401–407.

Ray, R. L., & Kimmel, H. D.   Utilization of psychophysiological indices in behavioral assessment: Some methodological issues. *Journal of Behavioral Assessment*, 1979, *1*, 107–122.

Richards, J. E.   The statistical analysis of heart rate: A review emphasizing infancy data. *Psychophysiology*, 1980, *17*, 153–166.

Schachter, S.   The interaction of cognitive and physiological determinants of emotional state. In L. Berkowitz (Ed.), *Advances in experimental social psychology* (Vol. 1). New York: Academic, 1964.

Schneider, R. E., & Fowles, D. C.   A convenient, non-hydrating electrolyte medium for the measurement of electrodermal activity. *Psychophysiology*, 1978, *15*, 483–486.

Schwartz, G. E., Ahern, G. L., & Brown, S.   Lateralized facial muscle response to positive and negative emotional stimuli. *Psychophysiology*, 1979, *16*, 561–571.

Schwartz, G. E., Fair, P. L., Salt, P., Mandel, M. R., & Klerman, G. L.   Facial muscle patterning to affective imagery in depressed and nondepressed subjects. *Science*, 1976, *192*, 489–491.

Shaw, J. C.   Quantification of biological signals using integration techniques. In P. H. Venables & I. Martin (Eds.), *A manual of psychophysiological methods*. New York: Wiley, 1967.

Stearns, S. D.   *Digital signal analysis*. Rochelle Park, N.J.: Hayden, 1975.

Uttal, W. R.   *Real-time computers: Technique and applications in the psychological sciences*. New York: Harper & Row, 1968.

Venables, P. H., & Christie, M. J.   Electrodermal activity. In I. Martin & P. H. Venables (Eds.), *Techniques in psychophysiology*. Chichester: Wiley, 1980.

Wastell, D. G.   Measuring heart rate variability: Some comments on the successive difference mean square statistic. *Psychophysiology*, 1981, *18*, 88–90.

Wenger, M. A., & Cullen, T. D.   Studies of autonomic balance in children and adults. In N. S. Greenfield & R. A. Sternbach (Eds.), *Handbook of psychophysiology*. New York: Holt, Rinehart & Winston, 1972.

Wilder, J.   The law of initial values. *Psychosomatic Medicine*, 1950, *12*, 392–401.

Williamson, D. A., Epstein, L. H., & Lombardo, T. W.   EMG measurement as a function of electrode placement and level of EMG. *Psychophysiology*, 1980, *17*, 279–282.

Winer, B. J.   *Statistical principles in experimental design*. New York: McGraw-Hill, 1971.

Zajonc, R. B.   Feeling and thinking: Preferences need no inferences. *American Psychologist*, 1980, *35*, 151–175.

Zillmann, D.   Attribution and misattribution of excitatory reactions. In J. H. Harvey, W. Ickes, & R. F. Kidd (Eds.), *New directions in attribution research* (Vol. 2). Hillsdale, N.J.: Erlbaum, 1978.

CHAPTER 24

Social Psychophysiology: Bioelectrical Measurement, Experimental Control, and Analog-to-Digital Data Acquisition

John T. Cacioppo
University of Iowa

Beverly S. Marshall-Goodell
University of Iowa

Isidore Gormezano
University of Iowa

INTRODUCTION

Social psychophysiological research is distinguished by its integrative analysis of physiological and social factors and systems (cf. Cacioppo, 1982; Cacioppo & Petty, 1981a; Schwartz & Shapiro, 1973; Shapiro & Schwartz, 1970). Contributions to this book attest to the advances that have been made in understanding how physiological mechanisms are affected by social factors, explaining complex social behaviors that are affected by both situational and internal (e.g., detected physiological) events, and constructing testable and more precise social psychological predictions. This approach also promises to lead to the development of more realistic social psychological theories resulting from investigators considering the physiological substrates of overt behavior and the biological limitations to which their abstract theories must ultimately adhere.

Electrophysiological measures can be expected to yield unambiguous information, however, only if recorded properly and obtained within an experimental design that exposes the contingencies between the bioelectrical events and social psychological constructs. Obtaining valid and reproducible bioelectrical measurements is a small technical wonder in itself. "You've got to pull out a low-level voltage from high-level noise, build or employ equipment to survive anything from liquid spills to high-voltage pulses and—most important—make sure the patient is protected from electrical hazard while you're about it" (Svetz & Duane, 1975, p. 68). In the first portion of this chapter, we elaborate on some of the basics of electro-physiological measurement that were broached in preceding chapters. Next, we outline issues regarding the experimental context and survey potentially confounding variables. Afterward, we describe a flexible yet relatively inexpensive laboratory for social psychophysiological research that we have developed at the University of Iowa, and the procedures for experimental control and analog-to-digital data acquisition that we have adopted are explained. The description of the Iowa laboratory is used to illustrate in concrete terms some of the issues and decisions that are raised in this and the preceding two chapters. We end the chapter by discussing a few nonelectrophysiological procedures for social psychophysiological research.

BIOELECTRICAL MEASUREMENT

Bioelectrical signals generally range in magnitude from a millivolt (mV), such as might result from the ventricular contraction of the heart, to a few microvolts (μV), such as might result from the muscle action potentials of a small skeletal muscle. Extracting these signals can be difficult because the person in a laboratory is basked in about 10 V of electrical "noise," which arises from surrounding electrical sources (e.g., lighting, power lines, motors, transformers) and from the similar coupling of the body and apparatus to powerline grounds (Svetz & Duane, 1975).

Bioelectrical signals can be classified as spontaneous or event-related, and as tonic or phasic. *Spontaneous or nonspecific activity* refers to bioelectrical events that occur in the absence of a designated or identified stimulus. For instance, subjects may vary in their responding to the experimenter or laboratory. Unless attributes of the experimenter or laboratory are manipulated or assessed in some manner (e.g., Rankin & Campbell, 1955), the physiological responses to these stimuli would be included in the category called spontaneous or nonspecific, since these would be among the physiological responses that appeared "unrelated" to specific stimuli or experimental events. The opposite of a spontaneous physiological response is an *event-related response*, which can be characterized by a stable temporal relationship to an actual or anticipated stimulus. An event-related physiological response is sometimes said to be "evoked" or "elicited."

Orthogonal to the classification of a response as spontaneous or event-related is the categorization of a physiological response as phasic or tonic. *Phasic physiological responses* refer to short-term bioelectrical events that return to their prior level of activity. When a bioelectrical event persists and appears not as a transient shift, but rather as an adjustment in the level of activity, the change in activity would indicate a change in *tonic physiological response*. A sudden quickening of the heart beat when concentrating on a difficult task would clearly classify as a phasic change as long as heart rate returned to its normal (i.e., prestimulus) level within a matter of seconds. The distinctions between tonic and phasic physiological responses can at times be difficult to determine in practice, and interested readers might wish to consult the discussion of phasic responses by McHugo and Lanzetta (Chapter 23, this volume) and texts on techniques in psychophysiology for the details of these distinctions for any given system of response (e.g., Brown, 1967; Greenfield & Sternbach, 1972; Martin & Venables, 1980; Stern, Ray, & Davis, 1980; Venables & Martin, 1967).

But how are bioelectrical signals recorded in the first place? We turn to this question next.

The Laboratory Context

In many pioneering and some contemporary studies in social psychophysiology, little attention has been given to the laboratory context. A polygraph has been wheeled into a room accommodating a subject, electrodes or transducers were applied to the subject, and bioelectrical recordings were obtained from the subject. This procedure may seem expedient, particularly if a sound experimental design is employed, but at a minimum extraneous sources of electrical and auditory noises threaten the sensitivity and validity of the psychophysiological measures obtained. In this section we briefly summarize the major considerations that should be given when developing a laboratory for social psychophysiological research. Although there are a few sources of helpful information that readers may wish to consult (e.g., manufacturers' literature), we found Gale and Smith's (1980) compilation of the suggestions of a large sample of the members of the Society for Psychophysiological Research and of the Psychophysiological Group of Great Britain to be a particularly valuable resource.

According to Gale and Smith (1980), there are five areas of concern: extraneous auditory noise, extraneous electrical noise, extraneous psychosocial noise, computer installation, and technical assistance.

Extraneous Auditory Noise

As Gale and Smith (1980) note, the principal sources of disturbing auditory noise are (1) traffic outside the building (e.g., automobiles, airplanes, students passing between bars), (2) traffic inside the building (e.g., students passing between classes; sounds from adjacent animal, children, or group processes labs), (3) machinery (e.g., elevators, typewriters, telephones, workshops), (4) the building (e.g., water running through pipes, rain or winds striking the exterior of the building), and (5) the control room of the laboratory (e.g., experimenters, slide projectors, relays, computer printers). The decision regarding the location of the laboratory can minimize the problems arising from the first four sources of noise. In addition, with the advent of closed-circuit television, the control room and subject's chamber can be separated by a wall and sound-attenuating material rather than by large observation windows. Apparatus, such as the polygraph, computer, slide projector, and tape deck, can be placed in the control room to minimize the sounds that they might produce while in use. For instance, we found that the sound made by a slide projector was disturbing to (i.e., elicited autonomic responses from) subjects sitting in an otherwise quiet environment. At present, our subject's chamber and control room are located adjacently at the end of a hallway of social psychological laboratories, and we use a small projection window to present visual stimuli from the control room to subjects in their quarters. All the cables that pass between the rooms do so through conduits that are stuffed with foam. These arrangements have been the most important and effective of those available to attenuate distracting and extraneous sounds in the subject's room.

The control and subject's rooms can be constructed to attenuate the remaining noise. Gale and Smith (1980) indicate that soundproofing tiles and other fabric inside the subject's chamber are ineffective in attenuating sounds coming from outside the chamber and suggest that soft lining (e.g., thick curtains) be installed around the source of the noise (e.g., in the control room) to reduce echo and transmissions to the subject's room.

Achieving reasonable sound attenuation is not difficult or expensive, particularly if the laboratory can be located in a quiet part of the building. Complete sound attentuation, however, is not only very expensive, but can be dissettling to subjects. Hence, a careful decision about where to locate the laboratory, a modest investment to insulate the equipment in the control room, and a limited investment to insulate the subject's chamber from other intrusive noises are probably best for most purposes.

Extraneous Electrical Noise

The need to reduce or eliminate external electrical interference is another consideration when selecting the location of the laboratory. Major sources of electrical interference include elevators, workshops (e.g., arc welding), flickering neon lamps, motor relays, fluorescent lights and dimmers, and ventilation control systems (Gale & Smith, 1980). To some extent, the differential amplifiers used commonly in electrophysiological recording serve to attenuate these confounding electrical signals. Differential amplifiers are so named because they take the difference between the two input signals obtained from the electrodes or transducer and magnify this difference. Theoretically, the electrical signals ("noise") that appear at both inputs simultaneously have no effect on the output of the amplifier. In practice, unfortunately, differential amplifiers are imperfect in function, and low-level bioelectrical events can be lost in the sea of electrostatic noise that emanates from external electrical sources (for more details on amplifiers, see McGuigan, Chapter 22, this volume). Accordingly, locating the laboratory away from major sources of external electrical interference can reduce the problem as well as minimize the need for expensive apparatus, such as shielding around the subject's room (see McGuigan, Chapter 22).

Ideally, lighting and equipment should be powered by a dc rather than an ac supply; at a minimum, incandescent rather than fluorescent room lighting should be employed, as these procedures will aid in minimizing extraneous electrical interference in psychophysiological recordings. Carpeting in and around the laboratory should be the electrically groundable type, as electrostatic discharges can be detrimental to microcomputer and control-logic equipment. Finally, and importantly, proper grounding procedures, which are discussed in detail in Chapter 22 (see also Gale & Smith, 1980; Stern et al., 1980), are necessary to attenuate extraneous electrical interference and to ensure the safety of the subject and experimenter.

Extraneous Psychosocial Noise

The laboratory artifacts that plague social psychologists in studies of overt behavior (e.g., demand characteristics, evaluation apprehension, experimenter bias) are no less a problem in social psychophysiological research, since reliable and valid measures of social psychological constructs are the object of study in both settings. The presence of electrical instrumentation, cables, and bioelectrical sensors can exacerbate the investigator's problem of involving the subject in the experimental task per se, for although psychophysiological measures are noninvasive, they can most certainly be obtrusive. Social psychologists, who have nearly perfected the instructional manipulation (cf. Aronson & Carlsmith, 1969), are quick to appreciate the care with which the experimental instructions and task must be prepared. Less obvious, perhaps, is the importance of the experimenters being skilled technicians in the laboratory. The behavior of the experimenters in a social psychophysiological study can be a major determinant of the ease with which subjects can adapt to the sensors that are attached and the electrical equipment they know stands nearby. Subjects generally find the sensors, electroconductive gels, adhesives, and so forth, to be novel. If the experimenters appear unknowledgeable about procedures or apparatus, or incompetent in performing their task, the subjects may become anxious about their own safety and, consequently, become less attentive to the various experimental stimuli. Thus, the sensitivity and reliability of the electrophysiological responses to the experimental treatments can be enhanced greatly by training experimenters in the technical aspects of psychophysiological recording and the social aspects of establishing rapport with the subject while remaining objective and detached. Finally, double-blind procedures can be used to minimize experimenter bias and are feasible to employ if the critical experimental instructions can be automated or delivered from the control room following the preparation of the subject.

Ideally, the preparation of the subject for electrophysiological recordings is done in a separate room that is carpeted (to help minimize noise and echos), painting in a soothing (e.g., pastel) color, and furnished in a comfortable style (e.g., minimal electrical wiring in view, paintings on the walls) to attenuate any anxieties he or she may have about participating in the study. Although some equipment is unavoidable in this room, the less intimidating or unusual the room appears to the subject, the more quickly he or she will adapt to the setting and respond solely to the experimental treatments. Of course, when the subject is ultimately led to the testing room, another period of adaptation will be required. Again, the less intimidating or unusual the room appears to the subject, the more quickly he or she will adapt to the extraneous environmental factors.

Computer Installation

The large quantities of data involved and the need for precise, flexible, and sophisticated manipulations of experimental treatments have made the use of computers in social psychophysiological research particularly attractive. There are, however, several issues that might be considered when selecting and interfacing a computer to the polygraph. Obvious concerns such as space, adequate power, air conditioning and humidifying equipment, and cables and conduits for interfacing the computer to the other equipment in the laboratory can create major problems for installation if overlooked (Gale & Smith, 1980). Additional issues that we faced while developing a microcomputer-based laboratory for social psychophysiological research are detailed in the following major section of this chapter.

Technical Assistance

Many researchers who wish to employ electrophysiological equipment have extensive expertise that do not intersect with electronics. For this reason, technical assistance in developing and maintaining a laboratory is common. However, the need for technical assistance can be reduced substantially by investing 6 months in the intensive study of electronics and computer systems (Gale & Smith, 1980). Although one is unlikely to learn enough in 6 months to do without technical assistance, the selection of, and communication with, those providing the technical support can be greatly improved by such study. Of course, consulting with knowledgeable colleagues can also be helpful. Moreover, outline what skills you need, or what technical tasks are at hand, *before* seeking technical support. The technician is likely to know less about the requirements and limitations of your particular research objective than you know about (or are willing to learn about) electronics.

There also appears to be a strong lure of hardware and fancy equipment, particularly (though not exclusively) to those providing technical support:

> Psychophysiology does have its own brand of sophisticated alchemy, of course; there are now several manuals of a very technical nature, which discuss (in what may appear to the outsider as obsessional and excruciating detail) problems of electronic circuitry, electrode preparation and placement, waveform analysis, computer storage of data, and so on. My view is that this sophistication has been misplaced, since technical aspects have often been overemphasized at the expense of the art of *experimentation*. (Gale, 1973; italics added)

It is expedient, therefore, to inform the technicians that modifications in an operating system (e.g., replacing floppy disks with a hard disk storage system) must be accomplished in a manner that minimizes the disruptions of ongoing research so that you are able to maintain, for the most part, an uninterrupted program of research on social variables. (We have found that the projected "downtime" for design modifications is generally badly underestimated.)

Psychophysiological Data Collection

Overview
As outlined in Chapter 22, collecting physiological measures can be examined in four major stages: (1) sensing, (2) amplifying, (3) recording, and (4) quantifying. To review briefly, *sensing* involves the selection and application of the appropriate electrodes or transducers required to detect the desired bioelectrical signal while attenuating background electrical noise. Once a signal has been detected, enhancement of the signal and attenuation of the background noise is accomplished during the *amplification* stage using, for example, differential amplifiers. In the *recording* stage, the physiological analog signals are stored using chart-and-pen recorder and/or FM tape recorders. Laboratory computers are increasingly employed to digitize analog signals and record these values as the ultimate object of statistical analyses (Law, Levey, & Martin, 1980).

Representative Problems and Sources of Artifacts
One complication in the interpretation of physiological measures is that large differences exist among individuals in the stability and reactivity of their physiological responses. This idiosyncratic source of variance can be diminished by collecting and correcting for prestimulus differences in responding and/or by treating your major independent variables as within-subject factors in mixed-factor experimental designs. In between-subjects designs, of course, a physiological response is measured as a function of

factors that are varied between subjects. In within-subject designs, the baseline physiological level is established prior to each trial or block of trials, physiological changes are measured relative to the pretrial baseline level, and treatments are varied within or between blocks of trials. We have attempted to blend the best of each in mixed-factor designs wherein we conduct two versions or "replications" of each experiment, with replications treated as a between-subjects factor and differing primarily in the ordering of the experimental stimuli (e.g., Cacioppo & Petty, 1981b).[1] Each replication includes multiple practice and experimental trials, which, in turn, consist of epochs such as a variable-length intertrial interval (the last several seconds of which serve as the baseline interval for that trial), the pretaped announcement of a question or forewarning, a postwarning/ prestimulus (wait) interval, the presentation of the test stimulus for the primary task (e.g., a decisional problem, a controversial editorial), and a brief post- (overt) response interval. The partitioning of a trial is not invariant, but rather can be accomplished in whatever manner best suits an investigator's goals.

A second methodological procedure useful in social psychophysiological research is the paced or time-locked procedure (Kahneman, Tursky, Shapiro, & Crider, 1969; see Shapiro & Schwartz, 1970). In the time-locked procedure, the subject is given information and responds at specified moments during a recording trial (e.g., at a slide change). Moment-by-moment physiological responses throughout the trial are recorded. Subsequently, average physiological response profiles are determined for each subject and condition. The averaging procedure can actually serve to magnify small but consistently positive or negative bioelectrical events that are masked in a random distribution of "noise" (e.g., the averaged electrocortical potential or contingent negative variation—see Chapter 22). In other instances, the time-locked procedure simply aids discriminating between tonic and phasic activity, differentiating the experiment's event-related responses from spontaneous responses, and assessing the covariation among responses obtained from several modalities (e.g., physiological, verbal, motoric) by providing a clearer picture of the form and time course of the physiological responses.

Third, there are generally low intercorrelations among physiological responses (Lacey, 1959, 1967) except following particularly novel or intense stimuli (e.g., a gun shot—Darrow, 1929; see Lang, 1971; Lazarus,

---

1. Inclusion of "Replications" as a factor allows one to generalize more confidently from findings that emerge across the replications to other sequences of treatments. Generalization is limited only if the Replication factor interacts with a within-subject factor. This mixed design also allows investigators to standardize the psychophysiological data within subjects, for although this standardization procedure may eliminate a main effect attributable to the Replication factor, it does not eliminate interactions involving the Replication and within-subject factors.

1966; Mewborn & Rogers, 1979). One implication of this dispersion of physiological activity is that a multivariate analysis of a profile of physiological responses may yield information about patterns of physiological responses that is not apparent in univariate analyses (see Fridlund & Izard, Chapter 9, this volume; Schwartz, 1982). McHugo and Lanzetta (Chapter 23, this volume) provide a summary of the various multivariate procedures currently employed in psychophysiological research.

Fourth, potentially confounding influences are inherent when comparing two distinct populations, such as people who differ in public self-consciousness (see Scheier, Carver, & Matthews, Chapter 18) or extraversion (see Geen, Chapter 13). In all likelihood, there are differences between the two populations other than the variable of interest, and these differences may be capable of influencing psychological and physiological responses (Pollin, 1962). There theoretically will always be differences between groups unless the groups are constituted randomly, and ultimately, the only means of increasing the reasonableness of the argument that a dispositional or group characteristic is responsible for a particular manner of physiological responding is to manipulate this characteristic.

Finally, social-developmental or longitudinal studies employing electrophysiological measures are complicated by the effects of seasonal environmental variables on physiological responses.[2] Lengthier periods of acclimatization than might normally precede an experimental session, range corrections (Lykken, Rose, Luther, & Maley, 1966), transformations to normalize the data (see Levey, 1980), and within-subject comparisons for longitudinal studies can be utilized to minimize the variance in physiological responding that is attributable to seasonal or irrelevant environmental factors.

EXPERIMENTAL CONTROL AND ANALOG-TO-DIGITAL DATA ACQUISITION: AN ILLUSTRATION OF A MICROCOMPUTER-BASED LABORATORY

As the instrumentation and recording procedures in psychophysiology become more standardized, and the experimental control of potent factors in the setting becomes more complete, reproducible chart-and-pen (analog) records of subtle physiological responses to a stimulus are increasingly attainable. *The acquisition of comparable analog records of physiological responding is*

---

2. Wegner (1962), for instance, reported that these factors almost ended his psychophysiological research:

> The school-age subjects of the Fels Research Institute came for biannual testing. My first two sets of data showed little correspondence, even though an air-conditioned laboratory has been employed during the summer. Fortunately, I continued work in the second winter and found winter-to-winter consistencies that were not reflected in the summer data. (p. 106)

not sufficient, however, for achieving psychophysiological results that are comparable across laboratories or studies. Psychophysiological data are not analyzed in their analog form, but rather they are digitized and summarized using descriptive statistics. The manner (e.g., sampling rate) in which the analog data are digitized, the nature of the parameters (e.g., amplitude, magnitude, variance) extracted from the digital representation of the analog signal, the manner in which a given set of parameters is extracted (e.g., using reciprocals, range corrections, transformations), and the nature of the inferential statistics employed when analyzing the extracted parameters can *each* affect the final results obtained and the conclusions drawn.

A simple example should illustrate. The integrity of an analog waveform can be retained in a digital array only if the rate of analog-to-digital (A/D) conversion is at least twice as fast as the fastest frequency in the analog signal (see Figure 24-1). Obviously, the array of digital values needed to represent transient physiological responses can become large quickly, and human errors, either in the A/D calculations or in the transcriptions, can become quite likely.

Computers in psychophysiological research have proven to be a powerful tool, for several reasons. First, the experimental control and timing of events can be very specific, simplifying the process of signal averaging and the detection of event-related physiological responses. Second, the A/D conversions can be programmed to occur tirelessly and reliably at high speeds if necessary. Third, response detection and parameter extraction through the use of computers require a formal explication of procedures, rendering these procedures (in the form of computer programs) open for public scrutiny and replication. Fourth, as evidenced in several of the preceding chapters (e.g., see Chapters 13 through 15), whether physiological activity is thought to vary as a function of social factors depends in part on what physiological effector is monitored and what parameters are extracted. For instance, Moore and Baron (Chapter 15) report that the mere presence of others typically has no effect on heart rate, but, occasionally at least, it has an excitatory effect on skin conductance responses. The overall physiological effects of the mere presence of others is difficult to determine from these data, since seldom is more than one parameter examined in any given study. However, the processing speed of computers has substantially reduced the cost of recording multiple measures simultaneously and extracting several parameters from each (e.g., skin conductance level, skin conductance response amplitude), so that the effects of social factors on physiological systems can be more accurately determined. Moreover, the study of the reciprocal influence of social and physiological systems is aided by the simultaneous recording of people's reportable, behavioral, and physiological responses. Again, laboratory computers are proving to be of assistance, as they can often provide the needed speed, reliability, and storage capacity for the volumes of data obtained.

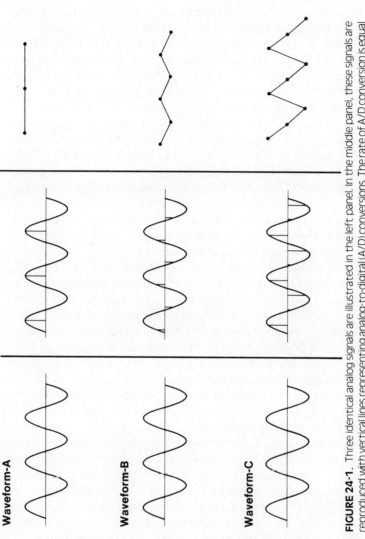

FIGURE 24-1. Three identical analog signals are illustrated in the left panel. In the middle panel, these signals are reproduced with vertical lines representing analog-to-digital (A/D) conversions. The rate of A/D conversion is equal to the frequency of the fastest component of the analog signal in waveform A in the middle panel, twice the frequency of the fastest component of the analog signal in waveform B of the middle panel, and three times the frequency of the fastest component of the analog signal in waveform C. In the right panel, the analog signals are reproduced from the digital arrays obtained from the A/D conversions depicted in the middle panel. The waveforms reproduced in the right panel, rather than the original waveforms in the left panel, form the basis for data processing and analysis, thereby illustrating that the rate of A/D conversion is one of several technical factors independent of bioelectrical measurement that govern the comparability of results across psychophysiological studies.

In this section of the chapter we describe a relatively inexpensive and flexible microcomputing system developed specifically to control social psychophysiological experiments, collect analog and digital data, and extract dependent variable measures for the reportable, physiological, and motoric states. Readers not interested in using computers in psychophysiological research may wish to forgo this discussion and proceed directly to the following section, "Nonelectrophysiological Procedures."

Hardware Configuration

The hardware configuration of the Iowa Social Psychophysiological Laboratory is displayed in Figure 24-2. Although the microcomputers employed in this laboratory are typically marketed as personal (hobby) computers, their design allows their conversion to a powerful laboratory computer. Specifically, we employ the general hardware configuration of the Apple II/FIRST system developed and described by Scandrett and Gormezano (1980). Our system consists of two 16-sector Apple II Plus microcomputers, each augmented by an AM9511 floating-point processor and 8253 programmable counter/timer configured to provide a real-time clock. Each microcomputer is equipped with 48K of memory, a random access memory card that provides up to an additional 16K of memory, two 5¼-inch minifloppy disk drives, and a 9-inch video monitor. The primary microcomputer (see Figure 24-2) is additionally equipped with a 16-channel 8-bit A/D converter, a 16-channel 8-bit D/A converter, and two 8255 programmable peripheral interface (PPI) chips providing a pair of 24-bit digital input/output (I/O) buffers, which are used for experimental control and digital data acquisition. At present, up to eight physiological (analog) responses may be sensed and recorded simultaneously from a human subject.[3] The channels in the system include one dc channel for electrodermal (EDA) input, six ac channels for EMG or EEG inputs, and one channel for moment-by-moment heart rate input. Other input devices include a hand-held potentiometer for subjects to indicate their moment-by-moment subjective state, up to 11 reaction-time keys for discrete behavioral responses, and a panel of 10 switches for entry of judgments, ratings of attitudes, and decisions in choice situations. Output devices that can be switched on or off include a slide projector, the paper drive on the polygraph, a display panel containing a row of five lights, a large-dial galvanometer for use in providing veridical or bogus feedback, two tone generators, and a tape deck. In addition, a probe stimulus may be presented

3. The typical sampling rate employed is 100 observations per channel per second, which can quickly yield more data than can be stored internally in the computer. Hence, data must be transferred periodically from the computer to the hard disk. By using "virtual arrays" during data collection, this transfer of data from the primary microcomputer to the hard disk essentially becomes invisible to the subject and user.

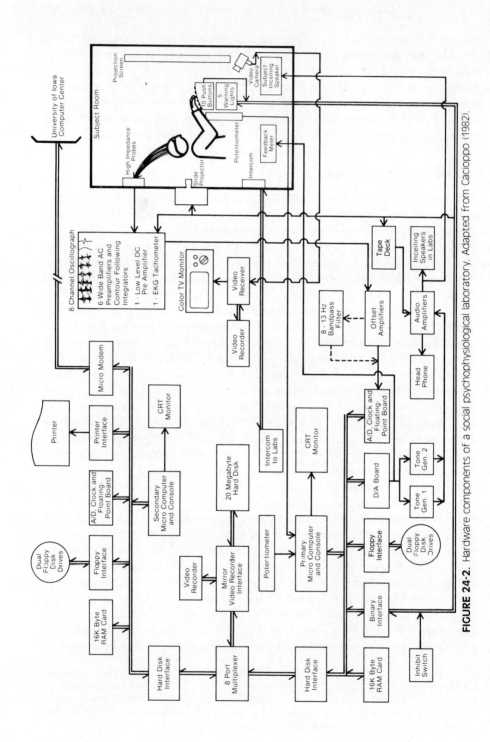

FIGURE 24-2. Hardware components of a social psychophysiological laboratory. Adapted from Cacioppo (1982).

during the task epoch on some trials. The probe stimulus (e.g., a brief tone) initiates a secondary task that subjects perform by pressing a reaction-time key as quickly as possible whenever the stimulus is presented. Subjects' reaction time to the probe stimulus is used as an independent measure of the proportion of the individual's total available processing capacity that he or she utilizes while performing the primary task (e.g., see Tyler, Hertel, McCallum, & Ellis, 1979). The primary microcomputer serves to time the presentation of the stimuli and demarcate the epochs while also identifying and recording physiological, attitudinal, and behavioral responses obtained during or following a trial. The secondary microcomputer, which can serve as a backup for the primary microcomputer, is typically dedicated to data processing and analysis. The secondary microcomputer is specially equipped with a printer/plotter and a micromodem that provides an interface to the university mainframe computer system (see Figure 24-2).

Despite the availability of 64K of memory in each microcomputer, memory limitations have proven to be a problem. Hence, we acquired a 20-megabyte hard disk, which can be accessed concurrently by users at both the primary and secondary microcomputers. The 20-megabyte hard disk has removed any serious restrictions on the size of the experimental programs or arrays of data employed during an experimental session. The 20-megabyte disk can eventually become cluttered with programs and data from previous sessions unless provisions are made for transferring files from the hard disk to a long-term storage medium. As depicted in Figure 24-2, we have interfaced a videorecorder to a hard disk, which allows us to store and retrieve volumes of information using compact video-cassettes.

Software System

The software system that we employ is called FIRST and is an adaptation by Scandrett (Scandrett & Gormezano, 1980) of FORTH (Moore, 1974), which is an interactive, high-level language developed for use on computers with severely limited memory size (e.g., 8K words). Like FORTH, FIRST is a dictionary-based language, but FIRST is specifically tailored for the most efficient laboratory use of the modified microcomputers that we employ.

The basic FIRST language consists of a dictionary of about 450 words which can be executed by entry on the keyboard. The available functions support a monitor, a disk operating system, an efficient compiler, a macro assembler, a well-developed text editor, high-resolution graphic capabilities, keyboard input and video output facilities for numerical and character string data, and routines for line printer operations and hard-copy graphics.

FIRST provides for hardware multiplication and division of 16- and 32-bit integers as well as 32-bit floating-point operations. These include a full selection of transcendental functions (direct trigonometric, inverse trigonometric, log, exponent, square root). Numerical calculations are particularly rapid due to the use of the AM9511.[4] Compiling time in FIRST is short, which expedites debugging a program (the full language can be reassembled in a matter of seconds), and the modular nature of programming in FIRST allows small portions of a program to be written and tested with much greater ease than in BASIC or from an EDITOR/ASSEMBLER. Once written and tested, a set of FIRST instructions can be represented by a single word, which acts much like a call for a machine-language subroutine in BASIC.

FIRST, therefore, provides the ability to define new functional words as combinations of previously defined words. After a new word has been added to the dictionary, it can be used as a component of still newer words. A FIRST program is thus developed in a hierarchical manner, starting with the 450 words in the FIRST language and building new intermediate words. For example, the word SLDCH, which stands for slide change, advances the slide projector carousel one time, and is one of many specially designed words that links the primary microcomputer to the peripheral equipment. These intermediate words are combined into still more comprehensive words, which define the sequence of operations to be performed. For instance, the word TRIALA, which represents one of several different types of trials to which a subject might be exposed, is comprised of a series of words (or subroutines) defined previously in the program that deals with specific and distinct aspects of this particular type of trial (e.g., timing of slide changes, inclusion of probe stimulus, A/D recording). Entering the most comprehensive word (e.g., RUN) executes the series of subroutines that constitute a complete session.

No formal distinction is made between the operating system, the compiler, and the program. Every program is essentially a new language designed to be the most suitable for the control and computational demands of a particular experiment. Each program need not be built from scratch, however, but rather a new program typically requires changes only at the upper levels of the language (e.g., definition of Trial words). The intermediate words that control output devices such as the tape recorder and slide projector and sample input devices such as the polygraph channels and subject's keyboard, once written, can be used in any

---

4. All numerical calculations are done in R.P.N. (reverse Polish notation) on a 4-byte-wide, 256-byte-deep software stack. Entering a numerical value pushes that number on to the top of the arithmetic stack, and arithmetic operators operate on the stacked values. Because of easy, compiled-in-stack manipulations, large stack scratch space, and extensive use of the floating-point processor hardware, FIRST completely supersedes the functions usually provided by the Applesoft (floating-point) BASIC or integer BASIC by both its very high processing speed and its flexibility.

program. Similarly, the intermediate words written to sample A/D input from EDA, EMG, EEG, HR, potentiometers, and so forth, can be reused, much as one reuses subroutines in other programming languages. In addition, the intermediate words that control timing are written as variables so that changes in the duration of epochs and stimuli within epochs may be accomplished by simple editing of experimental parameters.

Applications: An Illustration

Prior to an experimental session, the experimenter loads a test program, which is used to calibrate the polygraph, A/D chip, and so forth. Following calibration and checks of input and output devices, the experimenter loads an interactive program that displays the current experimental setup (e.g., A/D sampling rate, instruction and stimulus epochs in milliseconds, number of practice and experimental trials, and filtering characteristics for each of the eight physiological channels) and permits changes to be entered on the keyboard. These values are stored for later use in parameter extraction and analysis programs, executed from the secondary microcomputer. The program pauses at various points to permit the experimenter to provide preexperimental instructions, obtain preexperimental response (e.g., questionnaire) measures, and apply physiological sensors, and await the subject's adaptation to the laboratory. When all is ready for the experiment to begin, the experimenter enables the program that controls the presentation of specific, prerecorded instructions to the subject, followed by a pretreatment baseline and a series of practice and experimental trials. The A/D counts from each channel are sampled every 10 msec, and these digitized values are recorded on disk. If instructional manipulations or the presence of others are involved, these procedures can be either automated using audio- or videorecording equipment or performed "live" as part of the programmed sequence of events.

Following an experimental session, a separate program is employed using the secondary microcomputer to extract the appropriate parameters from the signals recorded on each channel. For example, the extracted measures for channels with integrated EMG input include the number and amplitude of the peak responses emitted during each epoch (e.g., prestimulus, stimulus), the magnitude of the integrated EMG activity in microvolts per second evinced during each epoch, the variability of the integrated EMG activity, and so forth. The data obtained from the parameter extraction program can then be summarized across trials by another program and input into classification (data processing and analysis) programs.

We are now in the process of developing a library of generalized programs for experimental control/data acquisitions, parameter extraction, signal analysis, statistical analysis, and data plotting. An example of a signal analysis algorithm that has been programmed in FIRST is a fast Fourier transform routine, whereas an example of a statistical routine program is FANOVA, a mixed design analysis of variance program.[5] When especially complex or unusual analyses are desired, we transfer the data at 300 baud over a standard telephone line (via a micromodem) to the university mainframe computer.

A considerable setup time for a computerized laboratory for social psychophysiological research can probably be expected. Acquisition and construction of the hardware configuration can often be slowed by the need for components not available locally. Development of the interfaces, subroutines, and prototype programs for experimental control/data acquisition and data analysis can be particularly time consuming, but can be facilitated by perusing similar programs developed in other laboratories. Fortunately, you can expect the daily operation and modification of established prototype programs to require less time and expertise than does the initial programming.

The few problems we have encountered following the establishment of the Iowa laboratory are relatively minor. Although the small size of the microcomputers make them easily portable, movement exacerbates the tendency for the component chips to loosen from their sockets. Particular care might also be taken when moving or handling the hard disk, floppy disks, and/or floppy disk drives, since dust or movement *can* result in a partial or complete loss of the stored data. Investigators should plan on keeping duplicate copies of all program and summary data files, for instance, on floppy disks or videocassettes.

NONELECTROPHYSIOLOGICAL PROCEDURES

The preceding description of a microcomputer-based laboratory for experimental control, A/D data acquisition, and data processing illustrates the kinds of options that might be considered and decisions that must be made when using bioelectrical measures in social psychophysiological research. There are, however, alternative, nonelectrophysiological procedures that are useful in social psychophysiological research. In this section we survey three nonelectrophysiological methods that have shown

5. Since the data array is virtually paged from disk into computer memory, thousands of input values are permitted. Although the number of levels within each factor, including the Subject factor, is essentially unlimited, the total number of different factors permitted by the current version of FANOVA in any mixture of within- and between-subject factors is nine when our high-resolution graphical plotting facilities are simultaneously present in computer memory. (Deletion of the graphics vocabulary permits a modest extension of the number of factors handled by FANOVA.)

particular promise: verbal measures of physiological activity, the misattribution procedure, and exogenous agents that alter physiological activity
(e.g., drugs, pacemakers).

Verbal Measures of Physiological Activity

Perhaps the oldest and most straightforward procedure is to ask the
subject to describe his or her bodily sensations (cf. Hassett & Danforth,
1982). The James–Lange theory of emotions, for instance, assumed that
people could, at a minimum, distinguish the idiosyncratic bodily reactions
that accompanied divergent emotional reactions. Studies of the relationship between the electrophysiological and verbal covariants of emotion
indicated large discrepancies existed, and the accuracy and validity of
verbal reports were implicated (e.g., Syz, 1926; see Blascovich & Katkin,
Chapter 17, this volume).

Nisbett and Wilson (1977) have argued more recently that people
cannot accurately report the causes (antecedents) of their behavior or
emotions. Their critique of verbal reports as data about psychological
processes applies to stimuli arising from within an individual's body as well
as to those emanating from the external environment. Although the
experiments and interpretations offered by Nisbett and Wilson (1977)
have been criticized on a number of grounds (see Ericsson & Simon, 1980;
Sabini & Silver, 1981; Smith & Miller, 1978; White, 1980), their caveat
regarding the interpretation of verbal reports nevertheless warrants commentary. Verbal reports concerning an individual's bodily sensations or
states can be viewed as symptomatology data whose accuracy is open to
empirical study. As detailed in the chapter by Blascovich and Katkin
(Chapter 17), verbal reports of *specific* bodily states (e.g., resting heart rate)
and reactions (e.g., increase in heart rate) have proven to be fairly inaccurate. Similarly, the causes of bodily reactions are typically reported
inaccurately by people (see Pennebaker, 1982). Nevertheless, the verbal
reports of physiological activity can constitute an informative set of data in
social psychophysiology as long as they are used to complement rather
than replace actual physiological data (e.g., see Pennebaker, Chapter 19,
and Scheier *et al.*, Chapter 18).

Although the apparent dissociation between specific verbal and electrophysiological measures of ongoing physiological activity quelled research
in this area, investigations of the operant conditioning of visceral activity
has led to a renewed interest in proprioception and interoception (Brener,
1977). From the point of view of operant conditioning theorists, an individual's detection of a physiological change need not be accurate as long
as it is a perceptible event that is correlated with the physiological change.
For instance, individuals may not be able to discriminate between large

changes in heart rate and skin conductance, but nevertheless reliably report being more "aroused" when one or both of these responses occur than when they do not (see Thayer, 1970).

More recently, Mackay (1980) has contended that adjective checklists (e.g., the stress-arousal checklist) provide an integrative measure more representative of general physiological arousal than any single psychophysiological variable. In a review of verbal measures of physiological activity, Mackay (1980) cites two lines of evidence for this proposition. The first derives from research that indicates verbal reports of arousal (e.g., as assessed using adjective checklists) correlate more highly with physiological composites (e.g., heart rate and skin conductance) than do pairs of physiological variables (e.g., Thayer, 1967, 1970). The second line of evidence comes from a deductive rather than inductive research strategy: Subjects are exposed to discernable external stimuli (e.g., noise) that are hypothesized to alter physiological arousal, and verbal measures of physiological arousal are administered. Generally, self-reports of arousal have covaried with the expected effects of the independent variables on physiological activation (see Mackay, 1980). The validity of verbal measures of general physiological arousal, however, is still questionable, for two reasons. First, self-report measures of arousal may be more highly correlated with the average of several physiological measures of arousal than with any single physiological measure (or than are any two physiological measures) of arousal because of the reduction in measurement error that is achieved by using multiple measures to gauge a common construct. Second, Zillmann (see Chapter 8, this volume) has clearly demonstrated that following exercise reportable arousal subsides more quickly than does changes in blood pressure. Hence, independent variables that excite specific effector systems may also alter verbal reports of arousal, but this convergence is apparently lost soon afterward (see also Lang, 1971).

At this point, the validity of verbal measures of actual physiological activity cannot be accepted without strong reservations. Nevertheless, the basic independence among the physiological, reportable, and behavioral responses to experimental treatments provides a wealth of information that can be tied empirically and theoretically to social behaviors (e.g., see Fazio & Cooper, Chapter 5).[6] Thus, verbal measures of physiological activity (or activation) should not be taken as an index of physiological activity per se, but rather as an index of a reportable state that may or may not be related highly to the targeted physiological process.

6. Although the change in reportable states is assumed to be based in a physiological change, it is an error to equate the two since (1) numerous physiological changes go unnoticed (e.g., Cacioppo & Petty, 1982; see Cacioppo & Petty, Chapter 1), (2) situational factors can alter the bodily sensations that are perceived (see Pennebaker, 1982; Scheier *et al.*, Chapter 19), and (3) the same reportable state may be accomplished by a variety of physiological mechanisms (Schwartz, 1982).

The Misattribution Paradigm

A second procedure that has been effective in social psychophysiological research is misattribution. The most common sequence of events involves the subject ingesting a placebo that he or she believes has specific (experimenter-specified) side effects. This misattribution procedure is based on the principle that people search for causes of an unexplained internal state, such as a sudden feeling of tension or arousal (see Chapters 5 through 8). In their search, people consider external as well as internal causes and sometimes misattribute the true cause of a felt bodily state (e.g., increased sympathetic activity, epinephrine in the bloodstream), to something that *seems* to be a reasonable cause at the time (e.g., a pill they recently ingested). Of course, only when a stimulus can have the same effects on a person as he or she is experiencing at the moment will misattribution be likely to occur (see Zillmann, Chapter 8). The nature of the internal state that the people are experiencing, therefore, can be inferred indirectly by determining the type of "side effect" that elicits misattribution. Thus, in the misattribution paradigm, subjects are either exposed or not to treatments that are believed to affect physiological responding and are either exposed or not to a possible external cause for the consequent bodily sensations.

Several studies in the area of cognitive dissonance, for instance, used misattribution procedures to investigate the sensations associated with the state of cognitive dissonance (see Fazio & Cooper, Chapter 5). A study by Higgins, Rhodewalt, and Zanna (1979) nicely illustrates the procedure. Subjects were told that they were to ingest a pill (a placebo) as part of a study on visual acuity. Subjects were told that the pill might cause them to feel "unpleasantly sedated" (unaroused–unpleasant), "relaxed" (unaroused–pleasant), "tense" (aroused–unpleasant), "pleasantly excited" (aroused–pleasant), or nothing in particular (no-side-effects control group). These subjects voluntarily wrote a persuasive message advocating a position with which they initially disagreed while they believed they were waiting for the pill to take full effect. Higgins *et al.* (1979) found the placebo with the possible side effect of making the person feel "tense" lessened attitude change. More important, however, they found that a pill described as possibly causing a feeling of unpleasant sedation blocked attitude change even more completely. Overall, the characteristic of felt unpleasantness (or stress) was more effective in eliciting the misattribution of dissonance to the pill (and the consequent reduction of pressures to change one's attitude) than was the characteristic of felt arousal (cf. Fazio & Cooper, Chapter 5). Of course, there may be large discrepancies between the nature of and the sensations from one's bodily responses. Cognitive dissonance may have sympathetic-like physiological effects, but feel most like a state of unpleasant tension. Hence, the nonelectrophysiological and electrophysiological procedures that we have discussed thus far can provide complementing rather than redundant information (Cacioppo & Petty, 1982b).

Exogenous Agents That Alter Physiological Activity

A third procedure that has occasionally been employed in social psychology involves utilizing exogenous agents that alter physiological activity in well-defined ways (e.g., Cacioppo, 1979; Schachter, 1971). For example, drugs might be administered to enhance or attenuate a physiological reaction that presumably mediates a socially significant behavior (e.g., helping, attitude change). One of the best known studies of this type is Schachter and Wheeler's (1962) study of emotional plasticity. Subjects were told that they were in a study of the effects of vitamins on vision. Subjects were injected with either epinephrine, a saline solution (placebo), or chlorpromazine (a peripherally active agent that diminishes the activation of sympathetically innervated structures). Subjects were misinformed about the nature of the injection, however; all were told that, following the prick of the injection, they would feel no side effects from the drug. Subjects were exposed to a comedy film shortly thereafter. (The exact time period between injection and film presentation was adjusted so that the effects of the drug would occur shortly after the start of the film.) Schachter and Wheeler (1962) found that subjects injected with epinephrine or the placebo tended to act more amused during the film than did subjects injected with chlorpromazine. Although the theoretical support this study provided for Schachter and Singer's (1962) theory of emotional plasticity has been questioned (e.g., see Zillmann, 1978), the merits of this innovative *methodology* persist (e.g., Cooper, Zanna, & Taves, 1978).

CONCLUSION

This chapter has focused on the nature and measurement of bioelectrical activity, and on computer control and A/D data acquisition. The discussion was designed to provide a basic understanding of the general issues involved in and instrumentation available for electrophysiological recording. Discussion was not focused on any one physiological recording procedure [e.g., average evoked potential (AEP) recording], although sources for this information were suggested. Discussion of the nature of bioelectrical activity stressed the importance of laboratory construction, sound and electrical insulation, psychosocial considerations, laboratory safety, and experimental design. It was noted that an important and physiologically significant event could be masked by electrical artifacts. Sources of electrical artifacts and potentially confounding variables were, therefore, described, and a few procedures for their elimination were indicated.

Bioelectrical measurement was segmented for purposes of exposition into four stages: sensing, amplifying, recording, and quantifying (see also

McGuigan, Chapter 22, and McHugo & Lanzetta, Chapter 23). Sensing was used to refer to the transformation of a physiological event to a valid, electrical representation that could be transmitted to amplification equipment. Since the electrical signals of interest to most investigators are extremely small (e.g., 1 mV), a magnification of the signal is required. This step was referred to as amplification. The third stage, recording, referred to the attainment of a permanent record of the detected stream of physiological events. The final stage discussed was quantification (signal processing and analysis). Issues considered during the quantification of bioelectrical signals include transformations of the data, utilization of procedures to check and correct for preexisting differences in physiological responses across groups, and selection of appropriate statistical procedures for deriving or testing hypotheses.

A specific microcomputer-based laboratory for social psychophysiological research was described to illustrate the kinds of options available and the kinds of decisions that might be made to obtain electrophysiological recordings. This system was established specifically to control social psychophysiological experiments, collect analog and digital data, and extract dependent variable measures for the monitored physiological, reportable, and motoric responses. The inexpensive laboratory microcomputer employed has been augmented by a hardware floating-point processor, additional memory, and an A/D converter chip. In addition, a software system (FIRST) was developed specifically for psychological experimentation and A/D data acquisition was described. FIRST is an interactive, high-level, structured programming language that, thus far, has been sufficiently fast that repeated tedious machine-language programming has seldom been needed for stimulus control and data acquisition.

The final section surveyed nonelectrophysiological procedures that have been used in social psychophysiological research. Three procedures were surveyed: verbal reports of bodily state, misattributional procedures, and exogenous agents that alter an individual's physiological state. The survey of these procedures indicated that each complements rather than replaces electrophysiological procedures, as the electrophysiological and nonelectrophysiological procedures appeared to provide only partially redundant information about the role of physiological and situational factors in social behavior.

ACKNOWLEDGMENTS

The authors would like to thank David Shapiro for helpful comments on an earlier draft of this chapter and Gertrude Nath for assistance in the preparation of this chapter. The laboratory for social psychophysiological research described in this chapter was developed with the support of NSF Grants BNS-7818667 and 8023589, NIH Biomedical Research Support Grant, and a University Faculty Scholar Award to the first author. The original development of the FIRST hardware and software was facilitated by NSF Grants BNS 7684561 and 8005907, NIMH Grant MN 16841, and NIDA Grant DA 01759 to I.G., and by NIMH Grant MH 15773 to B.M.-G. Correspondence should be addressed to John T. Cacioppo, Department of Psychology, University of Iowa, Iowa City, Iowa 52242.

REFERENCES

Aronson, E., & Carlsmith, J. M.   Experimentation in social psychology. In G. Lindzey & E. Aronson (Eds.), *The handbook of social psychology* (2nd ed., Vol. 2). Reading, Mass.: Addison-Wesley, 1969.

Brener, J.   Visceral perception. In J. Beatty & J. Legewie (Eds.), *Biofeedback and behavior*. New York: Plenum, 1977.

Brown, C. C.   *Methods in psychophysiology*. Baltimore: Williams & Wilkins, 1967.

Cacioppo, J. T.   The effects of exogenous changes in heart rate on facilitation of thought and resistance to persuasion. *Journal of Personality and Social Psychology*, 1979, *37*, 487–496.

Cacioppo, J. T.   Social psychophysiology: A classic perspective and contemporary approach. *Psychophysiology*, 1982, *19*, 241–251.

Cacioppo, J. T., & Petty, R. E.   Electromyograms as measures of extent and affectivity of information processing. *American Psychologist*, 1981, *36*, 441–456. (a)

Cacioppo, J. T., & Petty, R. E.   Electromyographic specificity during covert information processing. *Psychophysiology*, 1981, *18*, 518–523. (b)

Cacioppo, J. T., & Petty, R. E.   A biosocial model of attitude change. In J. T. Cacioppo & R. E. Petty (Eds.), *Perspectives in cardiovascular psychophysiology*. New York: Guilford, 1982. (a)

Cacioppo, J. T., & Petty, R. E. (Eds.).   *Perspectives in cardiovascular psychophysiology*. New York: Guilford, 1982. (b)

Cooper, J., Zanna, M. P., & Taves, P. A.   Arousal as a necessary conditon for attitude change following induced compliance. *Journal of Personality and Social Psychology*, 1978, *36*, 1101–1106.

Darrow, C. W.   Electrical and circulatory responses to brief sensory and ideational stimuli. *Journal of Experimental Psychology*, 1929, *12*, 267–300.

Ericsson, K. A., & Simon, H. A.   Verbal reports as data. *Psychological Review*, 1980, *87*, 215–251.

Gale, A.   The psychophysiology of individual differences: Studies of extraversion and EEG. In P. Kline (Ed.), *New approaches in psychological measurements*. London: Wiley, 1973.

Gale, A., & Smith, D.   On setting up a psychophysiological laboratory. In I. Martin & P. H. Venables (Eds.), *Techniques in psychophysiology*. Chichester: Wiley, 1980.

Greenfield, N. S., & Sternbach, R. A.   *Handbook of psychophysiology*. New York: Holt, Rinehart & Winston, 1972.

Hassett, J., & Danforth, D.   An introduction to the cardiovascular system. In J. T. Cacioppo & R. E. Petty (Eds.), *Perspectives in cardiovascular psychophysiology*. New York: Guilford, 1982.

Higgins, E. T., Rhodewalt, F., & Zanna, M. P.   Dissonance motivation: Its nature, persistence, and reinstatement. *Journal of Abnormal and Social Psychology*, 1979, *15*, 16–34.

Kahneman, D., Tursky, B., Shapiro, D., & Crider, A.   Pupillary, heart rate, and skin resistance changes during a mental task. *Journal of Experimental Psychology*, 1969, *79*, 164–167.

Lacey, J. I.   Psychophysiological approaches to the evaluation of psychotherapeutic process and outcome. In E. A. Rubinstein & M. B. Parloff (Eds.), *Research in psychotherapy*. Washington, D.C.: American Psychological Association, 1959.

Lacey, J. I.   Somatic response patterning and stress: Some revisions of activation theory. In M. H. Appley & R. Trumbull (Eds.), *Psychological stress: Issues in research*. New York: Appleton-Century-Crofts, 1967.

Lang, P. J.   The application of psychophysiological methods to the study of psychotherapy and behavior modification. In A. E. Bergin & S. L. Garfield (Eds.), *Handbook of psychotherapy and behavior change: An empirical analysis.* New York: Wiley, 1971.

Law, L. N., Levey, A. B., & Martin, I.   Response detection and measurement. In I. Martin & P. H. Venables (Eds.), *Techniques in psychophysiology.* Chichester: Wiley, 1980.

Lazarus, R. S.   *Psychological stress and the coping process.* New York: McGraw-Hill, 1966.

Levey, A. B.   Measurement units in psychophysiology. In I. Martin & P. H. Venables (Eds.), *Techniques in psychophysiology.* Chichester: Wiley, 1980.

Lykken, D. T., Rose, R., Luther, B., & Maley, M.   Correcting psychophysiological measures for individual differences in range. *Psychological Bulletin,* 1966, *66,* 481–484.

Mackay, C. J.   The measurement of mood and psychophysiological activity using self-report techniques. In I. Martin & P. H. Venables (Eds.), *Techniques in psychophysiology.* Chichester: Wiley, 1980.

Martin, I., & Venables, P. H. (Eds.).   *Techniques in psychophysiology.* Chichester: Wiley, 1980.

Mewborn, C. R., & Rogers, R. W.   Affects of threatening and reassuring components of fear appeals and physiological and verbal measures of emotion and attitudes. *Journal of Experimental Social Psychology,* 1979, *15,* 242–253.

Moore, C. H.   FORTH: A new way to program a minicomputer. *Journal of Astronomy and Astrophysics Supplement,* 1974, *15,* 497–511.

Nisbett, R. E., & Wilson, T. D.   Telling more than we can know: Verbal reports on mental processes. *Psychological Review,* 1977, *84,* 231–259.

Pennebaker, J. W.   Accuracy of symptom perception. In A. Baum, J. E. Singer, & S. E. Taylor (Eds.), *Handbook of psychology and health* (Vol. 4). Hillsdale, N.J.: Erlbaum, 1982.

Pollin, W.   Control and artifact in psychophysiological research. In R. Roessler & N. Greenfield (Eds.), *Physiological correlates of psychological disorders.* Madison: University of Wisconsin Press, 1962.

Rankin, R. E., & Campbell, D. T.   Galvanic skin response to Negro and white experimenters. *Journal of Abnormal and Social Psychology,* 1955, *51,* 30–33.

Sabini, J., & Silver, M.   Introspection and causal accounts. *Journal of Personality and Social Psychology,* 1981, *40,* 171–179.

Scandrett, J., & Gormezano, I.   Microprocessor control and data acquisition in classical conditioning. *Behavior Research Methods and Instrumentation,* 1980, *12,* 120–125.

Schachter, S.   *Emotion, obesity, and crime.* New York: Academic, 1971.

Schachter, S., & Singer, J. E.   Cognitive, social, and physiological determinants of emotional state. *Psychological Review,* 1962, *69,* 379–399.

Schachter, S., & Wheeler, L.   Epinephrine, chlorpromazine, and amusement. *Journal of Abnormal and Social Psychology,* 1962, *65,* 121–128.

Schwartz, G. E.   Cardiovascular psychophysiology: A systems perspective. In J. T. Cacioppo & R. E. Petty (Eds.), *Perspectives in cardiovascular psychophysiology.* New York: Guilford, 1982.

Schwartz, G. E., & Shapiro, D.   Social psychophysiology. In W. F. Prokasy & D. C. Raskin (Eds.), *Electrodermal activity in psychological research.* New York: Academic, 1973.

Shapiro, D., & Schwartz, G. E.   Psychophysiological contributions to social psychology. *Annual Review of Psychology,* 1970, *21,* 87–112.

Smith, E. R., & Miller, F. D.   Limits on perception of cognitive processes: A reply to Nisbett and Wilson. *Psychological Review,* 1978, *85,* 355–362.

Stern, R. M., Ray, W. J., & Davis, C. M.   *Psychophysiological recording.* New York: Oxford University Press, 1980.

Svetz, P., & Duane, N.   The ABCs of bioelectric measurements. *Electronic Design,* 1975, *16,* 68–72.

Syz, H. C.   Observations on the unreliability of subjective reports of emotional reactions. *British Journal of Psychology,* 1926, *17,* 119–126.

Thayer, R. E.   Measurement of activation through self-report. *Psychological Reports,* 1967, *20,* 663–678.

Thayer, R. E.   Activation states as assessed by verbal reports and four psychophysiological variables. *Psychophysiology*, 1970, 7, 86–94.

Tyler, S. W., Hertel, P. T., McCallum, M. C., & Ellis, H. C.   Cognitive effort and memory. *Journal of Experimental Psychology: Human Learning and Memory*, 1979, 5, 607–617.

Venables, P. H., & Martin, I.   *A manual of psychophysiological methods*. Amsterdam: North-Holland, 1967.

Wegner, N. A.   Some problems in psychophysiological research. In R. Roessler & N. Greenfield (Eds.), *Physiological correlates of psychological disorders*. Madison: University of Wisconsin Press, 1962.

White, P.   Limitations on verbal reports of internal events: A refutation of Nisbett and Wilson and of Bem. *Psychological Review*, 1980, 87, 105–112.

Zillmann, D.   Attribution and misattribution of excitatory reactions. In J. H. Harvey, W. J. Ickes, & R. F. Kidd (Eds.), *New directions in attribution research* (Vol. 2). Hillsdale, N.J.: Erlbaum, 1978.

SECTION IV
EPILOGUE

A Contrasting Frame of Reference: Soviet Contributions to Social Psychophysiology

John T. Cacioppo
University of Iowa

Richard E. Petty
University of Missouri–Columbia

INTRODUCTION

> Reactions are a *biosociological* conception, under which it is possible to group all the phenomena of the living organism, from the simplest to the more complicated forms of human behavior in the conditions of social life. The reactions of man in connection with his social relations acquire a social significance. In this we observe the main distinction between psychology and physiology. The latter also studies the reactions of man, but studies them without any reference to his social relations, while in psychology these relations constitute the principal content of the reactions studied. (Kornilov, 1930, p. 268)

Scientific study progresses as models are developed to describe a certain set of phenomena closely. The models may be rudimentary or overly simplified at first, but refinements or replacements follow as more knowledge about the area becomes available. In principle, a model is retained as long as it fits the observations in a simple, economical, and testable fashion. The more untestable assumptions or propositions required to bridge the gap between the model and the data, the less attractive, more cumbersome, and vulnerable the model.

In the preceding chapters we have seen a variety of models bearing on social processes. Each has expanded the set of phenomena typically addressed to include hypotheses, mediations, or observations at the physiological as well as at the social level. Many of the models that have been described may have initially appeared familiar, but most harbor significant refinements and extensions deemed necessary by the broader context of data about which the authors wrote. Less obvious to most readers of this collection of works are several distinctive features of these models that are so common to Western psychology that they form a transparent frame of reference. These features include (1) the strong emphasis on experimentation as a means of identifying the phenomena to be explained, (2) the focus on the individual (e.g., his or her qualities, dispositions, attitudes) as the unit of analysis and the object of environmental (e.g., social) influences, (3) the utilization of a potpourri of methods and theoretical doctrines in an effort to someday build a general theory supported by the accumulated experimental observations, and (4) the rejection of a priori philosophical assumptions about the nature of humankind. Although there are sound arguments for these features (cf. Boring, 1950; Brown, 1961), one contribution gained from a survey of Soviet psychology is obtaining an appreciation for the benefits and limitations of our particular frame of reference as Western psychologists. There are, of course, alternative windows through which these same phenomena may be viewed. The frame of reference of Soviet psychology, for instance, suggests alternative models for some of the social psychophysiological data reviewed in the preceding chapters and has resulted in novel paradigms and databases that must ultimately be accommodated by Western psychological models.

Before proceeding to the general Soviet perspective on psychological processes, we should note that *social* psychology in the USSR is a relatively new field of inquiry and is more similar to what we term industrial/organizational than experimental social psychology (Cole & Maltzman, 1969; Lomov, 1978–1979; Strickland, 1979). This applied brand of social psychology is now in sharp demand in the USSR because of its practical significance, but its theoretical integration with general Soviet psychology is still under way (Krauss, 1976; Petrovskiy, 1971; Strickland, 1980). The major contributions of Soviet psychology to social psychophysiology, therefore, derive not from their work in social psychology but rather from their advanced work in psychophysiology (e.g., Sokolov, 1972) and their general systems approach to thought and action within a sociohistorical context (e.g., Anokhin, 1969; Wertsch, 1981).

As in Western psychology, Soviet psychology is focused on measurable quantities and is inquisitive about all levels and aspects of human reactions (physiological, verbal, behavioral, social, political). In Soviet psychology, however, there are stronger emphases on avoiding eclectic approaches that imply assumptions about humankind that are incompatible with those of Marx, and on devising comprehensive analyses of human reactions that integrate physiological, verbal, behavioral, social, and political levels of phenomena into a single, coherent system. Although behavior is an object of Soviet psychological inquiry, the varieties of behaviorism that flourished in America in the early 1900s were rejected in Soviet psychology as providing too limited a view of human reactions (an error termed "mechanical materialism"). Thus, while Western behaviorists in the earlier part of this century asserted that consciousness was outside the purview of a scientific psychology, Soviet psychologists embraced the study of consciousness in line with their endorsement of "dialectical materialism."

Dialectical materialism refers to the notion that all events are interconnected and in a constant state of flux. The dialectic, or what Marxism holds to be "the universal law of nature, history, and thought" (Cropsey, 1972, p. 765), refers to the sequence of affirmation ("thesis"), negation ("antithesis") and negation of the negation ("synthesis"). Human reactions in society can be viewed in terms of spiritual or psychical events, as they commonly were several hundred years ago, but this perspective (thesis) is antagonistic to scientific inquiry. Human reactions can, alternatively, be viewed in terms of matter, but this perspective (antithesis) can be antagonistic to the concept of consciousness:

> Mechanical materialism makes an initial assumption that thought, consciousness, and sensation have merely a subjective, or even a fictitious, existence. It divests matter of all those qualities which have some subjective or mental content. As a result, it lands itself in a contradiction. It creates the necessity for a realm of nonmental reality. (McLeish, 1975, p. 139)

The Soviet synthesis of this thesis and antithesis was to view consciousness as "a property which emerges historically at the point where matter has reached a certain level of complexity" (McLeish, 1975, p. 86). The effects of these different traditions can be seen in that Western psychologists might observe the "products" of consciousness and emphasize the inferential nature of the models of consciousness that are thereby derived, whereas Soviet psychologists, who are much more likely to be studying consciousness, tend to view the multitude of factors and events (e.g., physiological, social) leading to a conscious act as *components* of consciousness, and derive models based on their observations of the "process" of consciousness.

As implied by the concept of dialectical materialism, everything is affected by change and relation. The species is evolving, while individual members of the species are born, grow, and die. An organism is defined within its species by its relation among others (i.e., social context) and in time (i.e., historical context). When compared with members of the species in the past, the organism may be said to represent the spearhead of the species, whereas it may represent the opposite when compared with future generations. This relatively obtuse point, which is rarely seen in Western psychological literature (cf. Gergen, 1973), is much more common in the Soviet psychological literature because of their strong convictions that people's reactions to any single stimulus varies as a function of factors at other levels (e.g., social, developmental), and interpretations vary with the context.

A simplified example of the type of theorizing might be helpful. In Soviet psychology, sociohistorical processes are thought to influence communicative processes such as speech. Speech (and other symbolic processes), in turn, is viewed as intimately tied to thought and to the development and activity of the nervous system. For instance, the states of excitation and inhibition within the organism are conceived as influencing the perceptions of, reflections of (i.e., thoughts about), and responses to signs and symbols in the environment. Since the human environment is a social environment, an individual's activity constitutes actions within a society that, in turn, molds the everchanging sociohistorical context influencing speech and thought.

As might be expected, the abstract experimental approach characterizing many Western psychological inquiries of individual human properties is criticized in the Soviet literature for failing to consider properly the impact of human history, society, and relations on thought and action (Shikhirev, 1980). Similarly, attempts to reduce psychological processes to the level of physiological or biological events are criticized for failing to consider the effects that emerge as the complexity of the organism increases (see Schwartz, Chapter 21, this volume).

> Dialectic psychology concedes willingly enough that man's biology and physiology provide the springboard for his psychical development and that they most certainly participate in its progress. However, this participation does not proceed in any mechanical or invariable manner. (London, 1950, pp. 84–85)

Thus, there is a tendency for contemporary Soviet researchers to employ psychophysiological methods, include developmental and sociocultural factors, and collect observations in naturalistic settings. Social and physiological processes are theoretically viewed as constituting not so much different areas of inquiry as different levels of inquiry about the same general process or system.

We should emphasize that the results reported in the Soviet literature, at least those that are easily accessible to Western psychologists (e.g., in English translation), have in many cases been unreplicable in Western laboratories. Several factors may be responsible for this state of affairs. Soviet psychologists view the operation of many psychological processes as contingent on the particular sociocultural environment from which the subjects were drawn (Shikhirev, 1980), a view that is similar to a position occasionally voiced by Western social psychologists (cf. Gergen, 1973). Hence, it might be argued that difficulty by Western psychologists in replicating results reported in the Soviet literature are due more to the sociocultural and historical differences between the East and West than to any other factor. Although possible, several other factors are noteworthy. Typically, we have found fairly sparse reports in the literature regarding the exact methods, instrumentation, material, and data reduction procedures used in Soviet experiments. Moreover, we have found a general tendency by Soviet psychologists to interpret data based on few, if any, inferential statistical analyses. Hence, generalizations drawn from the observations of a few individuals may represent unreliable differences between these individuals. Finally, the predilection for Soviet psychologists to collect data in less than perfectly controlled (e.g., educational) settings may contribute as well to the difficulty Western researchers have encountered in replicating Soviet findings, since Western researchers tend to attempt the replications in more carefully controlled laboratory studies. There is also some pressure to construct interpretations that are in accord with the Marxist conception of man, although this pressure does not appear to exert a substantial bias in the research literature (cf. McLeish, 1975). In any case, findings reported in the Soviet literature might best be viewed as being of questionable generalizability until successful replications are available in Western psychological laboratories.

BRIEF HISTORY OF SOVIET PSYCHOLOGY

Soviet psychology developed in the context of scores of years of socio-political crises, and the essential nature of Soviet psychology (and its contributions to social psychophysiology) may not be fully appreciated without some rudimentary knowledge about its history. In addition, a basic understanding of the environment out of which Soviet psychology grew might aid readers who wish to keep somewhat abreast of the Soviet psychological literature. We therefore sketch the history of Soviet psychology in this section. The interested reader may wish to consult McLeish (1975), Lomov (1978–1979), Corson and Corson (1976), or Rahmani (1973) for more detailed discussions of the history of Soviet psychology, or *Soviet Psychology*, English summaries in *Voprosy Psikhologii*, various government documents, and occasional edited works and books of Soviet psychological research that appear in English translation (e.g., Cole, John-Steiner, Scribner, & Souberman, 1981; Cole & Maltzman, 1969; Sokolov, 1972).

Science in general and psychology in particular were slow to develop in Tsarist Russia due to several sociocultural factors (McLeish, 1975; Rahmani, 1973):

> 1. Tsarist Russia was characterized by an isolationism from other societies.
> 2. A Christian Orthodox religion presupposing the dualistic nature of humankind was accepted by or imposed on all citizens and served to maintain the autocracy (even though Peter the Great, a Russian Tsar, established the Soviet Academy of Sciences).
> 3. Serfdom and illiteracy characterized the vast majority of citizens.

4. Families were patriarchal and extended.
5. The governmental bureaucracy greeted opposition or the expression of dissent with censorship, intimidation, and elimination.

Russian intellectuals in this environment were exposed to severe surveillance and restriction, but a minority emerged who resisted the ruling pressures and who tended to develop their ideas to their logical extreme. Since the number of such intellectuals was too small at any one time to bring about a direct change in the sociopolitical climate of Russia, the intellectuals realized a need to recruit the understanding and support of the masses to bring about a sociopolitical change (McLeish, 1975). Apparently, one means of doing this pursued by the intellectuals was to undermine the need for the dominant sociocultural (e.g., religious) beliefs by developing materialistic explanations for practical human social behavior (i.e., behavioral phenomena observable to the masses of illiterate peasants). The Orthodox Church in Russia, which supported the autocracy by persecuting intellectual dissenters, provided psychical explanations for such pervasive events as consciousness. Thus, a natural objective for the early intellectuals was to develop a materialistic account of consciousness as it manifests in normal, daily activities. It was in part for this reason that one of the most distinctive characteristics of Soviet psychology is the total rejection of dualistic theories of any kind (e.g., mind–body, spiritual–material, ideal–actual) as the basis for explaining human thought and behavior and their focus on the natural, physiological substrates of thought and actions observed in a social context. Although we cannot hope to provide a comprehensive summary of the history of Russian psychology here, it is possible to sketch the development of Soviet psychology by summarizing the contributions of a few prominent Soviet intellectuals.

Lomonosov (1711–1765) is credited by McLeish (1975) with laying the groundwork for contemporary Soviet psychology. Lomonosov, who was one of the founders of Moscow University, appealed to empiricism as the arbiter of philosophical arguments, explanations of social phenomena based on natural and lawful forces rather than arbitrary decisions of Tsars or divine interventions, and the search for the interconnectedness of forces, objects, and events. Radishchev (1749–1802) and Belinsky (1811–1848) advanced the position of dialectical materialism by advocating notions of evolution wherein humans were viewed as "kin—born of the same womb—to everything that lives on the earth; not only beast and bird but also plant, fungus, metal, stone, earth" (Radishchev, 1907, p. 149, cited in McLeish, 1975). Belinsky went on to assert the basic unity of the human organism, setting the stage for contemporary Soviet psychological inquiries. He argued that psychology must be practical while based on physiology:

> Pure thought, mind without flesh, is a logical dream, a lifeless abstraction. But this does not imply that mental activity can be explained solely in terms of physiological laws—on the contrary. Mental activity has its own specific features which can only be studied in the activities of the mind itself. Nevertheless, [Belinsky] maintained, "Psychology which is not based on physiology is as unsubstantial as a physiology that knows not of the existence of anatomy." (McLeish, 1975, p. 42)

Chernyshevsky (1828–1889) spent the last 27 years of his life as an exile in Siberia for expressing his ideas, which included: "materialistic monism, demand of the objective method, the principle of determinism, [and] the affirmation that psychics reflecting the reality appears in the activity of man" (Budilova, 1978, p. 30). Chernyshevsky is considered a Russian pioneer of the concept of humans as social organisms. He postulated that people's actions were motivated by self-interest (or needs) rather than abstract principles, but argued that it is the social organization rather than the individual that is responsible for the form and morality of an individual's deeds.

Sechenov (1829–1905), who was influenced significantly by Chernyshevsky, helped establish both the Russian fields of physiology and psychology. Sechenov (1973) employed the notion of materialistic monism as the basis for a program of physiological research, which he set forth in his book, *Reflexes of the Brain*. Interestingly, Sechenov began as an idealist (i.e., he believed that mental activities derived from spiritual sources), but while working in the laboratories of Helmholtz in Germany and Claude Bernard in France, he adopted materialism as his basic premise. In his doctoral dissertation ("Data for the Future Physiology of Alcoholic Intoxication," 1860), Sechenov advanced the notions that there was a unity between the organism and the conditions of their existence, the forces governing organic and inorganic nature were the same, and the mysteries of consciousness could be unraveled using the objective methods of physiology (premises still apparent in Soviety psychological research). Following Sechenov's discovery of the process of "central inhibition" in the nervous system,[1] he proposed that mentation manifested externally in muscular movement (i.e., action), and that instances of mentation separated from action resulted from the central suppression of a reflexive muscular response (Sechenov, 1973). Unlike Watson, Sechenov viewed the external muscular movements as a component rather than the essence of thought. Sechenov

---

1. Central inhibition in the nervous system can be illustrated by placing salt on the lesioned end of a decapitated frog's spinal cord; spinal reflexes, such as the movement of a frog's leg following pinching, are completely inhibited by this application of salt. This demonstrates that the overt response normally elicited by an external stimulus can be attenuated or inhibited by neural factors within the central nervous system.

also posited that activity of behavior has different levels. The lowest level pertains to the physiological processes underlying the behavior, whereas the highest level "involves a special subsystem of personality designated as 'self' and appearing in the process of interpersonal communication" (Yaroshevskiy, 1979, p. 107). Thus, Sechenov more than anyone was responsible for outlining the premises and methods of contemporary Soviet psychology.

Pavlov (1849–1936), a Russian physiologist who studied the digestive system and, later, the conditioned response, succeeded Sechenov as the major force in Soviet psychology. Pavlov's research on the classical conditioning of salivary responses in dogs is well known to Western psychologists. Less well known to some, however, is Pavlov's influential theoretical transition in interpreting his data (Corson & Corson, 1976; McLeish, 1975). Pavlov began by explaining his data in terms of the subjective state of the dog, basing his explanations on the analogy to human experience. His attempts to develop a predictive rather than a descriptive model of the dog's behavior using the anthropomorphic concepts he thereby derived ultimately proved frustrating. The physiological concepts of excitation and inhibition of nerve centers proved to be far less frustrating ingredients for Pavlov's model of the conditioning of an organism's behavior using "distant" external events. Pavlov dropped all subjective and dualistic explanations in his model of the dog's behavior in favor of developing a model based on physiological (particularly cortical) functioning. This move, and Pavlov's expositions on its merits, had a dramatic influence on the development of Soviet psychology (e.g., see Kurtsin, 1976).

In the next section we sample aspects of contemporary Soviet psychological research that bear more directly on the social psychophysiological issues broached in preceding chapters. Recall that reports of Soviet psychological research available in English translation typically contain sparse information about the exact methods employed, involve naturalistic rather than strictly controlled laboratory observations, and are based on nonstatistical analyses of data. Thus, while the following reports may prove useful in generating hypotheses, alternative viewpoints on existing data, or new phenomena that may ultimately need to be explained by existing Western psychological theories, replications and extensions of this work are needed before the actual value of the research can be determined.

CONTEMPORARY SOVIET WORK

Arousal and Wakefulness

As we noted in Chapter 1 of this volume, physiological arousal has been used to refer to the nonspecific, energizing aspect of behavior. This concept has played and continues to play an important role in organizing social psychophysiological data (e.g., see Batson & Coke, Chapter 14; Fazio & Cooper, Chapter 5; Geen, Chapter 13; Moore & Baron, Chapter 15; Spitzer & Rodin, Chapter 20; Zillmann, Chapter 8). As has been noted by these and other contributors to this volume, however, the concept of arousal has been difficult to operationalize and, hence, meaningful theoretical work has been impeded.

Several solutions to this problem have been suggested, such as using an aggregate physiological index (see McHugo & Lanzetta, Chapter 23) or self-report responses to an adjective checklist (Mackay, 1980; cf. Cacioppo, Marshall-Goodell, & Gormezano, Chapter 24). A unique procedure that might prove informative in understanding at least one aspect of the concept of "arousal" is outlined by Luria (1973) in an article entitled "The Quantitative Assessment of Levels of Wakefulness."

You may recall from preceding chapters that the problems with present social psychophysiological procedures for assessing a person's "arousal" include:

1. The various physiological responses to an "arousing" stimulus are sometimes poorly correlated.
2. The physiological responses to different but purportedly equally arousing stimuli are inconsistently correlated.
3. Reportable and physiological measures of arousal are not consistently correlated and, indeed, appear to change across time in a different fashion.

These specific problems are circumvented by the procedures outlined by Luria (1973) and demonstrated in Luria and Vinogradova (1959). Luria (1973) (1) conceptualizes the nonspecific, energizing aspects of the central nervous system as varying with the person's "wakefulness" and enabling the person's system of selective associations; (2) apparently does not find any single measure of physiological activity, such as EEG activity, to be monotonically related to the person's state of wakefulness; and (3) argues instead that the existence and intensity of the orienting response (i.e., a pattern of physiological responses—see Chapter 1) to semantic associations reflect the organism's underlying state of "wakefulness." Since consciousness, or the stream of reportable states, is such a pervasive issue in Soviet psychology, it should not be too surprising that the concept of "wakefulness" rather than "arousal" has been a focus of the study of the nonspecific actions of central nervous system (CNS) activity in Russia, and that wakefulness is defined in terms of people's ability to respond discriminately to human signals, such as words.

In the early part of this century, a number of Soviet psychologists were investigating the structural organization of the brain and localization of functional systems in the cerebral cortex. Following the report by Moruzzi and Magoun (1949) of nonspecific actions emanating from the reticular formation, Soviet psychologists "began to examine the *nonspecific functions of the brain*—the processes of waking, levels of consciousness, and general levels of activation" (Luria, 1973, p. 74). In their investigations, Soviet psychologists took as their starting point Pavlov's "law of strength," which holds that significant stimuli evoke strong physiological responses, whereas insignificant stimuli evoke weak physiological responses. This organization of the CNS, according to Luria (1973), ensured the clear, selective functioning of the cerebral cortex, which is to say that the stream of reportable states would be coherent and highly discriminating of external stimuli. Interestingly, Pavlov's "law of strength" holds for a person who is awake and alert, but exceptions to it are observed as the person passes from wakefulness to deep sleep (Luria, 1973). As the person begins this transition, EEG activity slows and becomes more synchronous, and what previously had been classified as "significant" and "insignificant" stimuli begin to elicit the same type of response. (Although the nature of this "response" was not specified explicitly by Luria, it appears from the report that some measure of cortical activity or orienting response was employed.) This epoch of the transition is called the "equalizing phase." As the person continues through this transition from wakefulness to sleep, a "paradoxical phase" is encountered where "insignificant" stimuli actually elicit stronger responses than do "significant" stimuli. Finally, in what Luria (1973) describes as the "ultraparadoxical phase," significant stimuli fail to elicit any response, whereas responses continue to be seen following the presentation of insignificant stimuli. In Luria's words:

> In the normal (optimal) state of the cortex, important (significant) stimuli easily become dominant, and weak (insignificant) stimuli are forced into the background; and the course of conscious processes assumes an organized character. However, as the cortex passes into the "phasic" state and cortical tone is reduced, this selective functioning of mental processes is inevitably disturbed. Important (significant) stimuli are reduced to the same level of importance as weak (insignificant) stimuli, and they lose their dominant character; they cease to act as determinant factors, and the train of thought no longer gives the appearance of organization; well-ordered associations directed toward a particular goal give way to incidental, uncontrolled associations; haphazard images begin to rise to the surface of consciousness, and the organized flow of consciousness is disrupted. (pp. 75–76)

As noted, and consistent with the Soviet focus on verbal thought, the psychophysiological index of wakefulness is keyed to changes in the pattern of physiological responses that follow the spoken word. The reasoning is that as wakefulness recedes, the nonspecific actions of the brain stem that energize the various specific functional systems involving higher cortical processes are reduced, and the selective nature of the word meanings becomes increasingly disrupted:

Incidental and insignificant associations that are elicited by a word, but that are normally ignored, begin to assume the same importance as significant, dominant, semantic associations; and as a result, the train of thought loses all semblance of organization. . . . Might not this fact serve as a starting point for evaluating the level of reduction of cortical tone, for providing an objective description of the operating potentialities of the cortex, and, in the final analysis, for quantitatively assessing wakefulness. (Luria, 1973, pp. 76–77)

Luria's assessment procedure was as straightforward as his rationale (Luria, 1973; Luria & Vinogradova, 1959). As we noted in Chapter 1, the presentation of a novel or significant stimulus (e.g., word) can elicit an orienting response. (Recall from our discussion in Chapter 1 that Pavlov, 1927, was the first to document the orienting response.) The orienting response habituates when the stimulus is presented repeatedly, but re-appears when the stimulus is changed. The orienting response intensifies when the physical presentation of the stimulus is intensified (up to a point, after which a defense rather than an orienting response is elicited); it diminishes as the intensity of the stimulus decreases; and paradoxically, it is strengthened again as the stimulus approaches the sensory threshold level. If the stimulus is initially irrelevant to the subject (i.e., it possesses no particular significance to the person), extinction of the orienting re-sponse (i.e., habituation) proceeds quickly. Luria and Vinogradova (1959) note that the orienting response to a stimulus can be made more stable and durable with the help of a verbal instruction (e.g., having the subject press a button on hearing a particular stimulus) or a UCS (e.g., a painful stimu-lus accompanying the stimulus).

In the Soviet studies, only "neutral" words (i.e., words that possessed no special emotional or symbolic significance to the subjects) were em-ployed. During the study, a subject hears a list of words and is instructed to press a button with the right hand every time a particular test word is announced. Thus, one word out of the list of words (i.e., the test word) is selected to serve as the "significant" stimulus, and this word attains sig-nificance through its function as the signal for an overt response. The words in the list are pronounced, each separated by a brief (15- to 30-second) delay. The subject initially displays an orienting response (as assessed by vasoconstriction in the left hand and vasodilation in the temporal artery) to each presentation, but at some point during this reading of words (typically after 15 to 20 words have been announced), the subject habitu-ates to the reading of the words and ceases to evince an orienting response to each word as it is announced. In normal, waking subjects, the announce-ment of the test word at this point elicits the button press and an orienting response. The announcement of words that are semantically related to the test word does not elicit the voluntary button press that the test word elicits, but it is accompanied by an orienting response. The more semantically similar the word is to the test word, the more pronounced is the orienting response. No orienting response is observed following the announcement of unrelated words or words that are related *phonetically* to the test word (Luria & Vinogradova, 1959).

In another study using the same procedure, two groups of mentally retarded children who differed in the severity of their disability served as subjects (see Luria, 1973). The children with the milder form of retardation displayed the orienting response to the test word, words that were semantically related to the test word, and words that were phonetically related to the test word (even though only the test word elicited the overt button-press response). The remaining words did not elicit an orienting response. Children with a severe disability, and those children with the milder form of disability but who were younger, displayed the orienting response to the test word and to words similar in sound to the test word, whereas words semantically related to the test word and words totally unrelated to the test word did not elicit the orienting response.

If the older children with the milder form of retardation were tested when they were not fatigued (e.g., early in the schoolday), orienting responses were observed primarily in response to words similar in meaning (rather than in sound) to the test word. When the same experiment was conducted later in the schoolday (e.g., after 5 hours of classes), this finding had reversed: Words similar in meaning to the test word generally failed to elicit the orienting response, whereas words similar in sound did elicit an orienting response. This was interpreted as evidence that reduced wakefulness due to fatigue led to the expected quantitative differences in autonomic response patterning (Luria, 1973).

One implication of Luria's reasoning and data worth noting at this point is that as wakefulness decreases, the likelihood of semantic processing decreases at a faster rate, and to a lower point, than do shallow (e.g., phonetic, orthographic) levels of stimulus processing.

Luria (1973; Luria & Vinogradova, 1959) describes a second procedure similar to the first except that, following habituation to the word list, the test word is accompanied by a painful stimulus (i.e., a UCS such as an electric shock) rather than an instruction to press a button. After 18 to 25 repetitions of this pairing, the presentation of the test word was found to elicit a defense rather than an orienting response (as indicated by vasoconstriction in the hand and temporal artery of the head—see Cacioppo & Petty, Chapter 1). At this point, Luria (1973) suggests, wakefulness could be measured by examining the subject's autonomic response patterning (e.g., orienting vs. defense response) elicited by neutral words that are semantically related, phonetically related, and unrelated to the test word. The results of such a study using normal subjects, reported in Luria and Vinogradova (1959), indicated that words similar in meaning evoked a defense response. Words that were not precisely related in meaning but nevertheless were related semantically, and words related phonetically to the test word, evoked an orienting rather than defense response, whereas unrelated words did not evoke a consistent autonomic pattern.

Luria and Vinogradova (1959) assessed what in essence were the experimental demands of their studies. They reported that the subjects *"were unable either exactly to formulate the aims of the experiment, or to designate exactly that group of words evoking definite vascular reactions"* (p. 103; italics theirs). It is also worth emphasizing that "neutral" words were employed in all these studies. This may be an especially important facet of their procedure if wakefulness is to be assessed. For instance, Oswald (1966) reports that sleeping people display a phasic EDA response and a large-amplitude burst of asynchronous EEG activity (the "K complex") when their own or be-loved's name is announced, but not when a name of an unfamiliar person is announced. Similarly, a mother may sleep through an alarm clock but awaken to a less intense cry or unusual sound coming from her child. Hence, the reasoning developed by Luria for quantifying wakefulness may hinge on the use of words that initially possessed no particular significance or emotional value and that still have not attained a particularly high level of importance to the subjects.

These procedures for assessing the nonspecific actions of the brain, what Luria (1973) terms "wakefulness," provide an interesting contrast to the procedures outlined elsewhere in this book for assessing nonspecific bodily reactions, or what social psychologists have occasionally referred to as a person's physiological arousal. Interestingly, Luria's procedures could easily be adapted to the experimental designs commonly employed in social psychophysiological research. For instance, subjects could be randomly assigned to alone or group conditions to determine whether or not mere presence (see Moore & Baron, Chapter 15) results in between-group differences in the nature and intensity of the autonomic response pattern elicited by semantically, in contrast to phonetically, related and unrelated words; the nature and intensity of the autonomic response patterns displayed by introverts and extraverts exposed to these procedures, and differences in fatigue using a modified version of these procedures, might be examined and explained (see Geen, Chapter 13); one or both of the assessment procedures outlined above might be employed following the presentation of a counterattitudinal essay under high- and low-choice conditions to determine the effect of cognitive dissonance (see Fazio & Cooper, Chapter 5); and so on.

Finally, an opinion voiced by a number of contributors to the present volume is that the concept of "arousal" in social psychology needs to be refined or partitioned into its various functional components. Even though there are some similarities between the Soviet concept of wakeful-ness and the concept of arousal in social psychology in the West, we believe it best to retain Luria's term "wakefulness" to refer to the phenomenon assessed using the procedures outlined above rather than adding yet another operationalization to the list presently included under the term "arousal."

Attitudes

Western psychologists have long sought psychophysiological indices of attitudes (see Cacioppo & Petty, 1981a; Cacioppo & Sandman, 1981; Petty & Cacioppo, Chapter 3; Tursky & Jamner, Chapter 4) and, more recently, the mechanisms by which bodily processes and attitude change are related (Cacioppo & Petty, 1982; Fazio & Cooper, Chapter 5; Hirschman & Clark, Chapter 7; Petty & Cacioppo, Chapter 3; Rogers, Chapter 6). In the Soviet psychological literature, we found a number of interesting references to or brief reports of related work. The most detailed reports pertained to what has been termed the "classical conditioning" or "indirect attitude response" approach (Cacioppo & Sandman, 1981; Petty & Cacioppo, Chapter 3), and we discuss this work first. We also found a few intriguing passages in contemporary work that pertained to what we have termed the "emotional response" or "direct attitude response" approach to attitude assessment using physiological measures. Although we had not found definitive evidence in the Western psychological literature that autonomic activity reflected the polarity and intensity of affective responses (see Chapter 3), we did find several passages in the contemporary Soviet psychological literature suggesting that phasic EDA and heart rate responses could be used to index these parameters. The paradigm used in the Soviet research is slightly different than any employed previously by Western social psychologists and may merit investigation. Hence, even though most of the original reports of this Soviet research were not accessible to us, we have summarized what we could obtain in the section "Emotional and Cognitive Response Approaches." Afterwards, a section summarizes reports in the Soviet literature that imply that, with properly prepared and delivered materials, people's attitudes are especially susceptible to change during the transition from normal levels of wakefulness to sleep.

Classical Conditioning Approach

This approach involves monitoring an induced (i.e., classically conditioned) physiological response rather than a naturally occurring physiological response to an attitude object or issue. Accordingly, the conditioning of the response is a necessary antecedent to attitude assessment. The details of the classical conditioning approach are outlined in Petty and Cacioppo (Chapter 3) and Tursky and Jamner (Chapter 4). The basis of this approach grew out of the work of the Soviet laboratories of Kragnogorsky and

Ivanov-Smolensky in the late 1920s and early 1930s, when, according to Razran (1961), it was observed that a conditioned response elicited by the sound of a metronome was also evoked by the announcement of the word "metronome," and vice versa. Razran (1961) also summarizes an early Russian study wherein semantic conditioning was adapted for gauging an individual's attitudes toward sociopolitical slogans. According to Razran, a 13-year-old boy was conditioned to salivate to the word *khorosho* (well, good) and to differentiate this word and response from the word *plokho* (poorly, badly, bad). To validate the conditioning procedure, the boy's secretion of saliva was monitored for the 30 seconds beginning with the spoken sentence *Khorosho uchenik otvechayet* ("Well the student answers") and similarly for the spoken sentence *Plokho vorobey poyot* ("Poorly the sparrow sings"). The boy was found to secrete 14 and 3 drops of saliva, respectively, providing support for the efficacy of the semantic conditioning. Over the course of the next several days, the boy's salivary responses to socio-political slogans and sentences were assessed. The data reported by Razran (1961) are summarized in Table 25-1. The secretion of saliva during the 30-second epoch beginning with the announcement of the statements with which the boy was likely to approve averaged 18.8 drops of saliva; beginning with the announcement of the word *plokho* averaged 1.5 drops; and beginning with the announcement of statements with which the boy was likely to disapprove averaged 1.5 drops of saliva (see Table 25-1).

The classical conditioning approach to the study of attitudes is cumbersome in regard to the equipment involved and the initial conditioning that must be done (see Cacioppo & Sandman, 1981; Petty & Cacioppo, Chapter 3). Nevertheless, as Tursky and Jamner (Chapter 4) have delineated, this methodological cost may well be worth it in some instances to obtain a more accurate and complete mapping of a person's attitude domains and to study the discrepancies that are sometimes observed across levels of analysis (e.g., psychophysiological, psychophysical, verbal, behavioral).

Emotional and Cognitive Response Approaches

One of the more surprising statements we encountered while surveying contemporary Soviet research was the assertion that the direction and intensity of a person's emotional response to an object or issue are reflected in autonomic changes. Western research using autonomic responses to gauge attitudes has confounded the emotionality and the novelty/signal value of the attitude objects. Hence, it was unclear whether the observed autonomic changes (typically, skin conductance responses) reflected an orienting response or the emotionality of the stimulus (Cacioppo & Sandman, 1981). Putlyaeva (1980), in an article entitled "The Function of Emotions in the Thought Process," indicated that the same problem

TABLE 25-1. Salivation to Statements following Conditioning

TEST STATEMENT*	DROPS OF SALIVA
Negative statements	
The pupil was fresh to the teacher	0
Brother is insulting sister	1
The pupil failed to take the examination	2
The Fascists destroyed many cities	2
The pupil broke the glass	2
My friend is seriously ill	2
Intermediate statement	
The pupil passed the examination with a mediocre grade	10
Positive statements	
The pupil studies excellently	14
Leningrad is a wonderful city	15
The Soviet Constitution is the most democratic	17
The Soviet people love their Motherland	17
The fisherman caught many fish	18
The children are playing well	19
The Soviet Army was victorious	23
The pioneer helps his comrades	23
The enemy army was defeated and annihilated	24

Note. Adapted from Razran (1961).
*In addition to these statements, the word *khorosho* was announced seven times and elicited an average of 14.7 drops of saliva, whereas the word *plokha* was announced two times and elicited an average of 1.5 drops during the 30-second recording interval.

had been recognized in Soviet psychology and, more interestingly, that a resolution using a distinctively Soviet paradigm had been reached:

> Some investigators considered the GSR to be an index solely of an orienting response, whereas others regarded it as an indicator of emotional states. These two points of view were in each case demonstrated with empirical data by their adherents. It was especially designed studies by V. S. Merlin (1960), and A. E. Ol'shannikova (1969) that not only confirmed the presence of GSRs in both cases but also made it possible to distinguish between these cases on the basis of the pattern of development and extinction of a GSR. Thus, these two viewpoints complemented, rather than contradicted, one another. (p. 24)

The Soviet resolution to the problem was apparently based on the fact that the orienting components of an autonomic response to an attitude stimulus should habituate with repeated presentations, whereas the components of the autonomic response pattern attributable to the emotional nature of the stimulus should not (at least, not as quickly). Putlyaeva (1980) goes on to summarize the nature of the autonomic pattern reflecting a person's positive or negative reaction to a stimulus (presumably following habituation):

1. Phasic increases in EDA are noted regardless of the individual or the polarity of the individual's emotional response to the stimulus.
2. Consistent directional changes in heart rate are observed *within individuals* in response to a positive or negative stimulus.
3. Averaging heart rate responses across individuals leads to an "apparent" dissociation between EDA and heart rate responses to the stimulus, with the former showing increases and the latter exhibiting no consistent overall change. This "apparent dissociation" of heart rate and affective response is avoided by obtaining background data from each subject to take into account that for some subjects "positive emotions caused a slowing of the pulse rate, whereas in others, the pulse rate speeded up" (Putlyaeva, 1980, p. 26).

Hypnopaedia and Persuasion

Hypnopaedia stems from the Greek words *hypno* meaning sleep and *paidea* meaning education or tuition and refers to instruction during sleep and low levels of wakefulness. Incidental or spontaneous learning during what behaviorally appears to be sleep states was first documented by Sviadoshch while he observed neuropsychiatric patients under his care (Rubin, 1971; Sviadoshch, 1968). Although most of the studies stimulated by Sviadoshch's observations and accessible to Western psychologists have dealt with the learning of foreign languages (particularly English), a few studies have examined attitude change. We begin by summarizing the "principles" of successful hypnopaedia as gleaned from studies of learning (cf. Rubin, 1968, 1971), and then survey the few studies pertaining most to attitude change (cf. Budzynski, 1976; Sviadoshch, 1968).

The acquisition of information through hypnopaedic training appears primarily during hypnagogic reverie and light sleep rather than during EEG slow-wave sleep (Levy, 1969; Simon & Emmons, 1955). When information is presented during EEG slow-wave sleep, learning is poor and then only when the presentation of the information also evokes desynchronized EEG activity ("K complexes"), REM (paradoxical) sleep, or lighter sleep (Cooper & Hoskovec, 1967). Rubin (1971), after reviewing the literature on hypnopaedia, concludes that "sleep-learning" is actually a misnomer, that "familiarizing and learning verbal material at the beginning of bedtime behaviour lapsing into drowsiness and light sleep is analogous with hypnopaedia" (p. 42), that complex material cannot be learned by hypnopaedic procedures alone, but that hypnopaedic procedures can substantially augment the learning of simple and complex materials.

The effectiveness of hypnopaedia as a supplementary teaching method for complex material is believed to be the result of the enhancing effect of low levels of wakefulness on a person's unquestioning acceptance of (e.g., reduced counterargumentation to) the material being presented: "Speech assimilated during sleep, in contrast to that assimilated during waking state is not subjected during assimilation to the critical processing, and is experienced on awakening as a thought of which the source remained outside consciousness" (Sviadoshch, 1968). This observation, when applied to the area of persuasion, has potentially far-reaching implications. Consider Bliznitchenko's (1968) report of a study in which there was a radio instruction of the English language by means of the hypnopaedic method. The radio broadcasts were aired daily (except Saturday and Sunday) from December 21, 1965, to February 16, 1966, and "embraced some 2000 residents of Dubna, a town not far from Moscow known as a centre of nuclear physicists" (Bliznitchenko, 1968, p. 202). Bliznitchenko's study, which apparently did not examine the utility of the hypnopaedic method for persuasion, was reportedly successful: hypnopaedic instruction facilitated the acquisition of English by many of the residents of Dubna. There were no control comparisons, however, and the significance of the hypnopaedic training per se is difficult to assess. Nevertheless, the fact that the method can apparently be used on large masses of people suggests the potential social impact of the procedure should hypnopaedic instruction and persuasion prove to be effective.

Rubin (1971) argues that the format of hypnopaedic tutorials is particularly important. He suggests that a hypnopaedic tutorial possess the following characteristics:

1. It should begin with a positive suggestion to listen and remember the story.
2. The duration of sounds is increased by 10 to 15%.
3. The range of frequency is restricted to 120 to 200 Hz.
4. The timbre of the speaker's voice is designed to be pleasant to the listener(s).
5. There is an equal emphasis on all components of a sentence.
6. There are no abrupt changes in tempo or intonation.
7. There is a frequent repetition of the information presented with no changes in sequence
8. With each repetition the speed of speech quickens and volume decreases to a whisper.

But the recipient apparently need bear no responsibility for preparing these materials, nor does he or she necessarily have to voluntarily approve of the entire training program (e.g., by being privy to the persuasive intent of a communicator) for hypnopaedia to be a theoretically effective procedure for undermining the person's critical evaluation of a persuasive appeal (see Budzynski, 1976).

We might note in this regard that research on hypnopaedic instruction and persuasion may have much in common with the area of distraction and persuasion. As distraction increases from low to moderate levels, the likelihood that a recipient will evaluate the merits for a recommendation decreases while retention of the message arguments remains high. The effect of this is to increase the attitude change found in response to weak arguments, but to decrease the attitude change engendered when there are meritorious arguments for a recommendation (Petty, Wells, & Brock, 1976). As distraction continues to increase, however, the attention to and encoding of the message arguments drops, and attitude change is reduced regardless of the merits of the arguments (Romer, 1979; see Petty & Brock, 1981; Petty & Cacioppo, 1981). Hence, it may be the case that hypnopaedic presentations of persuasive messages can increase or decrease persuasion depending upon the quality of the arguments supporting the recommendation and the recipient's ability to learn and elaborate on the message arguments that are presented.

Several Western studies do indeed suggest that a person's cognitive defenses against weak arguments for a recommendation are lowered during the transition from wakefulness to sleep and, therefore, may be susceptible to attack using hypnopaedic tutorials. Barber (1957) compared the suggestibility of people who were awake, drowsy (or in light sleep), and hypnotized. He found that subjects who were drowsy or sleeping lightly, and subjects who were hypnotized, were more suggestible than subjects who were awake. A report by one subject in Barber's (1957) study indicated that "I was just sleepy enough to believe what you were saying is true. I couldn't oppose what you wanted with anything else" (p. 59). In another study, attitude change (assessed using pre- and postattitude scales) was examined after subjects were exposed to a counterattitudinal message (favoring interracial marriage) during a state of wakefulness, drowsiness/light sleep, or deep sleep (Felipe, 1965). Attitude change in the state of wakefulness and deep sleep was negligible, whereas attitude change in the drowsy/light sleep state was significant. Finally, Budzynski (1976) reported several case stories in which he and his colleagues exposed clients to what could be considered persuasive (psychotherapeutic) messages while maintaining their clients' state of drowsiness/light sleep using biofeedback. In one case, Budzynski (1976) described a student with severe test anxiety who responded with large changes in EDA when "certain words from a list [were] read to him" (p. 377). A message was prepared in which it was suggested that the words and the situations they represented would no longer cause the person to feel anxious. The student recorded the message and twice listened to it during a drowsy/light sleep state. Afterward, the student was again exposed to the list of words, but this time no substantial deflections of EDA following the key words were observed. The student also reported a lessening of test anxiety. This research is suggestive, but far from conclusive. For instance, even if hypnopaedic presentations facilitate persuasion, there remains important questions regarding the persistence of the attitude change. The Soviet work in this area nevertheless has brought attention to these issues and, perhaps more importantly, has uncovered a number of the parameters that appear important for successful hypnopaedic tutorials (see Rubin, 1971).

Emotions

Western psychologists and psychophysiologists have done considerably more research on emotions than Soviet psychologists. Rahmani (1973) indicates that the sole chapter on emotions and feelings in the two-volume *Psychological Science in the USSR* lists only 56 papers and books in the area in contrast to bibliographies of many hundreds of works that can be found in chapters dealing with thinking and learning. Moreover, the study of emotions is one of the areas where the gap between Soviet and Western psychological study is widest.

In one interesting set of studies (Grimak & Ponomarenko, 1967), heart rate and respiration were recorded to determine the bodily reactions to emotional stress. In the first experiment, beginning parachutists were hypnotized, and a parachute jump was verbally recreated as they lay motionless on the floor. In a second experiment, experienced pilots were placed under actual flying conditions, and their automatic controls failed to operate when the pilots were ready to land their aircraft. (This latter stressor may not have been as excessive as it may initially seem, since pilots typically go on manual control prior to landing.) The analyses of the autonomic responses to these emotionally stressful situations revealed three distinct patterns of responding. One, which characterized the inexperienced more than experienced subjects, reflected a low level of responding before and during the critical moment and a flurry of "functional deviations" after the critical moment. (This pattern appeared to be similar to the pattern people sometimes display before, during, and immediately after an unexpectedly close call in an automobile.) The pattern is schematically displayed in the top panel of Figure 25-1. A second pattern, which was reported to be almost as frequent among the experienced as the inexperienced subjects, was characterized by an increased pulse and respiration rate at the critical moment (see the middle panel of Figure 25-1). This pattern of autonomic activity is similar to that found by Fenz and Epstein (1967) to characterize relatively novice parachutists on the day of a jump. A third autonomic pattern, which was exhibited more frequently by experienced than inexperienced subjects, was characterized by a rise in pulse and respiratory rate that reached peaks before the critical moment (i.e., during a period of anticipation) followed by a decline (see the bottom panel of Figure 25-1). This pattern is similar to that found by Fenz and Epstein (1967) to characterize experienced parachutists the day of a jump. Grimak and Ponomarenko (1967) reported that the type of reaction did not reflect

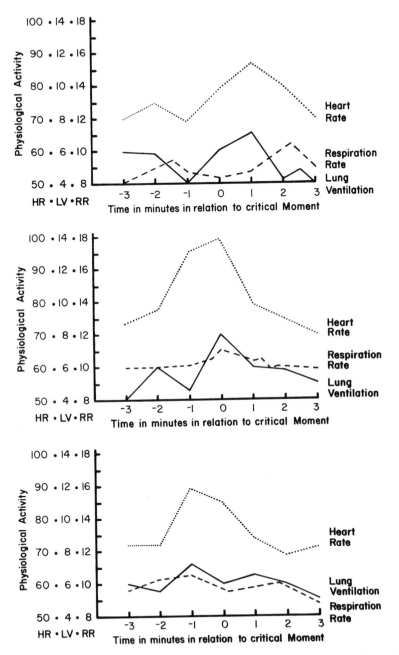

FIGURE 25-1.   Three temporal patterns of autonomic activity to emotional stress. A pattern characterizing relatively inexperienced subjects is displayed in the top panel, a pattern characterizing both inexperienced and experienced subjects is displayed in the middle panel, and a pattern generally characterizing experienced subjects is displayed in the bottom panel.

the quality of the subject's performance, but the sensitivity of their measure is unclear. It may be that when people know that a fearful event is impending they respond physiologically with greater activity in the autonomic nervous system (i.e., conditioned emotional response). With practice, people may develop means of coping with their physiological reactions to avoid its subjectively unpleasant effects or its debilitating behavioral effects (cf. Fenz & Epstein, 1967; Kagan, Haith, & Caldwell, 1971).

Grimak and Ponomarenko's (1967) study is not too dissimilar to studies conducted by Western psychologists studying the James–Lange theory of emotions (cf. Grings & Dawson, 1978). However, a tenet common to most Soviet theories of emotion is that the cerebral cortex acts as a coordinator, interpreting perceptual signals, monitoring proprioceptive and interoceptive signals, and commanding effectors to respond appropriately. Yet according to the concept of activity, which most Soviet models of emotion embrace, the emotion does not arise within a particular center of the body or brain, but rather the physiological substrates of emotions "are less their bases than they are the springboards for their subsequent development" (London, 1950, p. 88).

A description of a theory of emotion popular in Soviet psychology may be helpful. What would appear to be one of the more sophisticated Soviet theories of emotion has emanated from the work of Beritashvili (1969). Beritashvili has studied the emotional behaviors of animals following the removal of the neocortex (the most recently evolved, outer layer of the cerebral cortex) or the entire cerebral cortex. Beritashvili found that removal of the neocortex does not deprive the animals entirely of emotional reactions. For instance, when deprived of food, cats become restless, mew, and cry furiously; they act as if terrified when subjected to painful stimulation; and they enter a rage during irritation to the skin. Moreover, electrical stimulation to areas in the lower cortex (the archipaleocortex) can obtain these same types of reactions. Finally, a pairing of a neutral sound or light with such stimulation is often sufficient for conditioned emotional responding to develop. None of these emotional behaviors are observed, however, in the decorticate animal (i.e., following the removal of the entire cerebral cortex). Beritashvili (1969) has also noted that stimuli act on the archipaleocortex via the reticular formation and, independently, via nuclei of the diencephalon (i.e., part of the forebrain that includes the thalamus and hypothalamus—see Chapter 1). From these and similar observations, Beritashvili (1969) constructed the following model of emotions:

> It may be assumed that, during the first effective influence of a vitally important object on the organism, a perception by means of the neocortex as well as an emotional excitation by means of the archipaleocortex is produced. As a result of the coincidence of these neuropsychic processes, differential neural bonds are first formed between excited sensory complexes of the neocortex and the archipaleocortex by means of association

> pyramidal neurons. Therefore reproduction of an image of a given object should lead not only to orienting reactions via the neocortex but also to emotional excitation of the archipaleocortex with its subjective experience and overt somatovegetative expression. (p. 660)

Hence, in the tradition of Pavlov, emotions are viewed as the product of organismic–environmental interactions, regulated by the cortex, and expressed in somatic and autonomic changes. Note that, contrary to Schachter and Singer's (1962) cognitive–physiological model of emotions and the peripheralist views of James (1884) and Lange (1885/1922), the somatovisceral and the subjectively qualitative components of an emotion are viewed as independent consequences of the cortical regulation of the organism's activity in the environment. Beritashvili's model can be used to describe Grimak and Ponomarenko's (1967) data by postulating that experience alters the cortical regulation of organismic–environmental interactions—a postulate endorsed by Beritashvili (1969). It is somewhat more difficult, however, to derive specific predictions regarding how experience will alter emotional responding in complex circumstances such as those studied by Grimak and Ponomarenko (1967) and those broached by Leventhal and Mosbach (Chapter 12), Fridlund and Izard (Chapter 9), Hager and Ekman (Chapter 10), and Sackeim and Gur (Chapter 11) in this volume.

Inner Speech

Given the emphasis today in social psychology on cognitive (particularly verbal) mediators (cf. Berkowitz, 1978; West & Wicklund, 1980), it may be informative to review the Soviet research on inner speech. The Soviet theory of and research on inner speech suggest methods for assessing independently the presence of concentrated verbal thought in social psychological paradigms as well as new experimental paradigms for examining the role of inner speech in social processes.

Before proceeding to the Soviet research, however, let us examine the specific meanings given some of the key terms:

> The term "inner speech" usually signifies soundless, mental speech, arising at the instant we think about something, plan or solve problems in our mind, recall books read or conversations heard, read and write silently. In all such instances, we think and remember with the aid of words which we articulate to ourselves. . . . The elements of inner speech are found in all our conscious perceptions, actions, and emotional experiences, where they manifest themselves as verbal sets, instructions to oneself, or as verbal interpretation of sensations and perceptions. This renders inner speech a rather important and universal mechanism in human consciousness and psychic activity. (Sokolov, 1972, p. 1)

Although inner speech was at one time held to be identical to external speech minus sound, work particularly by Vygotsky (cf. Cole *et al.*, 1981) and Sokolov (1972) have promoted the view that inner and external speech are related through partially independent processes. External speech is graphically characterized by Sokolov (1972) as follows:

> A rather complex phonetic, lexical, and grammatical system, human speech is characterized by a sound envelope, its form, with which is associated a meaning, which comprises its objective content. Both become fixed in the course of the historical development of language, acquiring a relatively constant character, and are mastered by each individual in the process of his intercourse with other members of a given language community. In mastering the societally determined system of generalized and abstract signals of reality that is language, man masters all the logical forms and thought operations connected with it in its role as a (verbally) mediated reflection of real connections and relationships among objects. (p. 2)

These definitions imply an intimate link between inner speech and thought, and indeed a close relationship between the two is postulated. Inner speech and thought, however, are not equated, since the same thought can be expressed (even to oneself) in different words, different grammatical forms, or in different signal systems (e.g., mathematical, pictorial, crypto-graphic).

Theoretical Positions

The theoretical work on the interrelationships among external speech, inner speech, and thought can be traced to Sechenov (1973) and Vygotsky (Cole *et al.*, 1981), where the notion was advanced that thinking begins as the encoding of objective associations. For instance, a child learns about his or her environment by various movements that lead to concrete associations between these movements and visual, auditory, tactile, and other sensory impressions. Mastering external speech allows the child to express these associations symbolically, which sets the basis for the transformation of thought from concrete images and associations to complex abstractions and generalizations. The mastery of external speech was also thought to facilitate self-regulation (e.g., by internalizing the instructions of parents and engaging in self-instruction to guide behavior). Sechenov, for example, observed that children made great strides in inhibiting their motoric responses to stimuli (i.e., to regulate their own behavior) when they developed external egocentric speech (i.e., talking aloud to oneself). Subsequently, Sechenov suggested, the central inhibition of motoric responses spread to the external expression of egocentric speech as well, leaving the child with covert egocentric speech as a means of regulating his or her behavior.

Following Sechenov and Vygotsky, motivated and purposeful external speech has become viewed as consisting of several stages: programming (i.e., a goal and plan); implementation of the program; evaluation of the implementation with respect to the plan and goal, which involves obtaining feedback; and adjustments in programming and/or implementation to achieve the goal (e.g., Akhutina, 1978). Although feedback regarding complex speech movements may derive from auditory as well as proprioceptive sources, research by Bernshtein (1969) on the coordination of fine motor movements suggests that proprioceptive feedback alone is fast enough to contribute to the control of external speech. Hence, the kinesthetic sensations from the speech musculature was viewed as an important link between thought and external speech. Any of a variety of symbolic representations (e.g., sign language, gestures, facial expressions) of a message can be used to achieve social communication and self-regulation, but language is a particularly flexible and pervasive selection because sounds are more effective than gestures, especially in darkness or at distances.

To transmit a message effectively to another person using external speech, words must be selected that have a communal meaning. Either normatively endorsed words must be selected or idiomatic expressions must be supplemented by additional signals (not necessarily verbal) that together convey the intended message. Next, these symbols must be organized into a syntactic structure that conveys the subject and predicate (who is doing what to whom, how, and why). Finally, if verbal signals are chosen, the words must be articulated clearly.

In contrast to external speech, inner speech functions primarily to facilitate the development and communication of one's thoughts to oneself, as preliminary drafts of social speech, as a private voice for self-regulation, and as a workspace for formulating overt actions. Inner speech, therefore, can be greatly condensed, since there is nothing to be gained by retaining in inner speech many of the syntactic, semantic, and phonetic attributes of external speech. Vygotsky characterized the syntactic aspects of inner speech as more fitful, fragmentary, and abbreviated than external speech. There is a "simplification of syntax, a minimum of syntactic breaking down, expression of thought in condensed form, a considerably smaller number of words" (1956, p. 359). On the basis of Vygotsky's observations of children, he concluded that the abbreviated form of inner speech is accomplished by "the absolute and complete predicativeness of inner speech . . . it is never necessary for us to name that about which we are speaking, i.e., the subject. We always limit ourselves only to what is being said about this subject, i.e., the predicate. But this is precisely what leads to the dominance of pure predicativeness in inner speech" (Vygotsky, 1956, p. 366). The phonetic aspect of external speech is diminished, as well. "In inner speech we do not need to pronounce a word in its entirety. We understand, by virtue of our very intention, what word we wanted to say.

. . . Strictly speaking, inner speech is almost wordless" (Vygotsky, 1956, p. 368).

Finally, the semantic aspect of inner speech is viewed as being different than that of external speech. The semantic structure of inner speech is highly idiosyncratic, contextual, "and include[s] not only the objective meaning of words but all the intellectual and affective content connected with it" (Sokolov, 1972, p. 48). Related to the use of idiosyncratic phrases in inner speech is the grouping of semantic units, which reduces the phrases to new or hyphenated words in inner speech. Vygotsky notes that this reduction in phrases in inner speech subsequently leads on occasion to the emergence of new hyphenated words in external speech. In sum, external speech is internalized and transformed ("streamlined") during the development of higher psychological processes to form an efficient, idiomatic signaling system for thought and feelings (see Figure 25-2). The consequences of the development of inner speech include the growth of a "private" side of an individual and the reduction of impulsiveness.

Soviet theoretical work on inner speech since Vygotsky (1956) has led to a few revisions (cf. Akhutina, 1978; Sokolov, 1969, 1972). One of the most important revisions concerns the phonemic reduction in inner speech. Anan'ev (1960) holds that phonemic reduction in inner speech is accomplished primarily through the dropping of vowels. There were by this time observations indicating that inner speech typically included the initial sounds or letters of words and that it often was similar in form to the abbreviations of words used in the written language. (Recall, however, that we are speaking of the Russian written language. There are no comparable observations for the English language, for instance.) Finally, the *absolute* predicativeness of inner speech was rejected, as instances in which it was substantive were found. "Inner speech based on a certain concreteness of thought is predicative. When, on the other hand, an object is as yet not recognized and identified in perception, not outlined in thought, inner speech is substantive" (Anan'ev, 1960, p. 336).

Although other models of inner speech have been proposed (e.g., Komlev, 1980–1981; Leont'ev, 1969), the models reviewed above are classics in Soviet psychology and form the foundation for empirical work in this area.

The survey of differences between external and inner speech, which as we noted are based largely on the social nature of the former and the

FIGURE 25-2. Schematic diagram of Vygotsky's model of the development of an utterance. Adapted from Akhutina (1978).

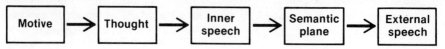

idiosyncratic nature of the latter, may appear a bit tedious from the view of a social psychologist or psychophysiologist. These differences are important to consider, however, if the postulated cognitive processes common in social psychological theories are to be assessed objectively using, for instance, electromyographic recording procedures. For instance, if the stream of reportable states is viewed theoretically as mirrored in a sequence of discrete electromyographic events, it should be difficult to find a normative or prototypical waveform that accurately characterizes different individuals' expression of a common thought or idea in inner speech since their condensed representation of the thought or idea is likely to vary. Moreover, the nature of the inner dialogue accomplishing a given sequence of thoughts may vary within individuals across situations because of contextual differences (e.g., different idioms may be selected). The task of extracting information about covert information processing, however, can proceed systematically once these factors are taken into account. For example, one implication is that it may be especially informative to include a "calibration signal" in experimental designs wherein the electromyographic patterns accompanying known psychological responses (e.g., responding to a personally relevant counterattitudinal communication) are recorded.[2]

Sokolov (1969, 1972) has contributed a great deal to this area, particularly to our understanding of what features of the stream of electromyographic signals accompany different aspects of inner speech. We turn next to Sokolov's electromyographic investigations of thought and inner speech.[3]

2. The inclusion of such a "calibration" signal is not new in Soviet studies. Recall that Putlyaeva (1980) reported that Soviet investigators using autonomic measures of emotional reactions determined their subjects' idiosyncratic heart rate response to positive and negative stimuli before proceeding.

3. Electromyographic recording is but one technique used to study inner speech. Other methods include auditory distraction (e.g., ordinal counting while listening to someone speak) and mechanical retardation of articulation (e.g., by clamping the lips and tongue between the teeth), both of which interfere with the normal dynamics of inner speech, and external articulation (e.g., reading aloud), which presumably facilitates the processes of inner speech (cf. Sokolov, 1969, 1972). Among some of the major findings obtained using these procedures is that the most important distinction between inner and external speech is not the "soundlessness" of the former, but rather its fragmentariness and its possible support through graphic representation. The results found using EMG recordings are representative and, in many instances, less artifactual (e.g., the distraction, distress, and apprehension subjects may experience when their tongue and lips are clamped between their teeth are avoided by the EMG recording procedure). Hence, we have restricted our summary of the empirical work on assessing objectively inner speech to that employing electromyography. The interested reader may wish to consult Akhutina (1978), Chuprikova (1972), Komlev (1980–1981), or Sokolov (1969, 1972) for more detail about the varieties of Soviet psychological analyses of inner speech.

EMG, Thought, and Inner Speech

In the research summarized by Sokolov (1969, 1972), surface electrodes for EMG recording are placed on the tongue and lower lip. Subjects, who ranged from students at Moscow University to scientific personnel and young schoolchildren, were tested while seated in a reclining position in an electrically shielded chamber. Subjects received preliminary training in what apparently amounts to progressive relaxation, and an adaptation period preceded the introduction of experimental stimuli. Task instructions were presented aurally; tasks included vocalizing or silently articulating words, performing mental arithmetic, reading to oneself, listening to someone speaking, memorization and recollection of verbal material, and mental manipulation of graphic material.

Vocalizing and silently enunciating letters (e.g., "O") and words (e.g., "one," counting from one to five) revealed that, when vocalizing discrete sounds, adults display action potentials in the perioral region (e.g., in the area of the tongue and lower lip) that precede phonation by approximately 350 to 700 msec. This latent period of phonation is slightly exaggerated in schoolchildren, lasting approximately 500 to 1000 msec. With repeated vocalization of the same phoneme or word, the latent period diminishes slightly, but the latent period is condensed most when a string of phonemes is vocalized. The speed of external speech, therefore, affects the form of the preliminary perioral EMG activity.

The phonemic structure of words silently enunciated was also found to alter the underlying perioral EMG activity. In experiments where subjects silently articulated labial and nonlabial Russian vowels, the degree and temporal characteristics of tongue and lip EMG activity were clearly distinctive when a rapid scanning rate was used (cf. McGuigan & Winstead, 1974). Specificity in electromyographic responding was found too when the activity at the hands was considered. Unlike perioral EMG activity, the EMG activity at the hands did not distinguish the phonemic attributes of sounds and words; moreover, an increase in EMG activity was observed when concentrated mental activity was "relatively prolonged" (Sokolov, 1972, p. 170—cf. Cacioppo & Petty, 1981b). Lastly, Sokolov (1972) compared the spectra of the action potentials of the perioral muscles when the same words were spoken aloud and silently. He found that the spectra for silently pronounced words was narrower than that observed in words spoken aloud or in a whisper (which resulted in similar spectra). This difference was especially notable for low-amplitude action potentials, while the bandwidth of the majority of the action potentials was stable and ranged between 30 and 200 Hz.

Analyses of EMG activity during mental arithmetic resulted in a number of additional findings that generalize to silent verbal processing as well. When a subject first begins to count silently, phasic EMG activity increases in the perioral region. Shortly thereafter, the subject's continued counting to himself or herself is accompanied by a return of perioral EMG activity to basal levels. Moreover, repeated counting is not accompanied by the same intensive burst of EMG activity that characterized its initiation. If the stereotypy of the counting is altered (e.g., decrementing by 3 rather than 1), an increase in perioral EMG activity is again noted.

In a related fashion, solving a mathematical problem (e.g., deriving the square root of 225) is not accompanied by a substantial increase in perioral EMG activity if the answer is already known to a subject. If the answer must be derived from the information provided in the problem, intermittent bursts of perioral EMG activity are evident, but particularly when the problem is being formulated, the calculations (i.e., manipulation of symbols) are being performed, and the final answer is being organized for presentation. These intermittent bursts of muscle action potentials appear in the integrated EMG as a clear waxing and waning of perioral muscular activity:

> Such intensity fluctuations of motor speech excitation represent a rather characteristic pattern of the neurodynamics of mental problem solving. This pattern may undergo considerable changes, depending on the complexity of the given task and the acquired habits of problem solving, but the main factor—the alternating waxing and waning of the level of motor speech excitation—is there whenever the task presented offers difficulties of any kind for the subject's reasoning capacity. (Sokolov, 1972, pp. 196–197).

When Sokolov analyzed the EMG activity exhibited by an individual who was slow as compared to one who was fast (but, apparently, no more accurate) at mathematical calculations, he found several interesting differences. The former individual, of course, took longer to perform a given mathematical problem, and the total EMG activity that was evinced during the calculation of the answer was greater for this individual than for the individual who performed mathematical calculations rapidly. When the amount of EMG activity that each individual displayed was expressed per unit time (e.g., microvolts per second that the individual calculated an answer), however, fewer significant differences in EMG activity were evident (cf. Cacioppo & Petty, 1981a). This, Sokolov (1972) contends, is attributable to the especially high variability in perioral EMG activity characterizing the slow problem solver. These findings are illustrated schematically in Figure 25-3.

Further tests using these and other subjects comparing the responses to complex and simple (almost automatized) tasks revealed differences in time of solution (the former took longer), intensity of perioral EMG activity (the former elicited more frequent and larger amplitude action potentials), and variability (the former appeared to be accompanied by a more extreme waxing and waning of perioral EMG activity). Sokolov (1972) drew several

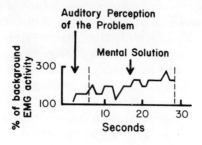

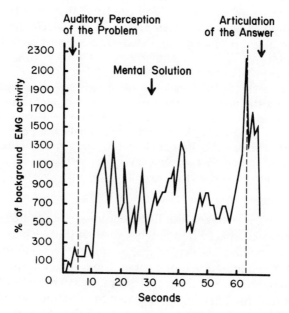

FIGURE 25-3. Graphic representation of the integrated EMG activity obtained over the perioral musculature during mental arithmetic [e.g., (23 × 13)/4]. The record of a subject who solved mathematical problems quickly is displayed in the top panel, whereas the record of a subject who solved mathematical problems slowly is displayed in the bottom panel. Adapted from Sokolov (1972).

inferences from his observations. He concluded that the intensity of localized perioral EMG activity is a direct function of the number of mental operations required to perform the task (p. 197) and of the number of "switchings to other operations required for solution" (p. 201), and that the intensity of perioral EMG reflects a "generalization of the excitatory process and its spreading to a broader region of the cerebral end of the motor speech analyzer" (p. 198).

It should also be emphasized that even when the automatism of mental operations is at a maximum, motor speech excitation does not disappear completely: it remains, as it were, on guard for protection of automatism, manifesting itself whenever the latter is disturbed and whenever there is transition to novel mental operations. (Sokolov, 1972, p. 202)

Finally, Sokolov argued that the mode of stimulus presentation exerts a strong influence on the intensity of perioral EMG activity. Audio presentations (i.e., a mathematical problem announced using a microphone) resulted in more intense perioral EMG activity than visual presentations (i.e., the same problem presented in written form). Unfortunately, the memorial requirements of the task were confounded with the mode of presentation (i.e., acoustically presented material had to be rehearsed if it was to be retained, whereas visually presented material was available for reinspection as needed). Hence, clear conclusions about the effect of the mode or presentation per se cannot be drawn.

Sokolov's (1969, 1972) analysis of perioral EMG activity during verbal processing, reading to oneself and listening to speech, revealed the same principles as outlined above for mental arithmetic. A brief mention of a few studies should be illustrative.

In one of the simpler studies, a subject was asked to "Try to figure out on what day of the week will September 1 of this year fall" (Sokolov, 1972, p. 182). While the subject developed an answer to the question, large increases in perioral EMG activity were observed. When 4 days later the same question was asked of the subject, there was no increase in perioral EMG activity. In another study, subjects silently read either a series of short Russian phrases (e.g., "There is not enough sunshine; The snow is everywhere; The trees are without leaves . . .") or complicated Russian sentences (e.g., "Whispering to one another, the boys stood beside the pipe into whose orifice Pet'ka had stuck his head"). The short phrases were generally unaccompanied by significant increases in perioral EMG activity, whereas the complicated sentences resulted in increases in perioral EMG activity. Reading a text in a foreign language (e.g., English), which was much more difficult for the subjects, was, as might be expected, accompanied by more intense perioral EMG activity. These and related findings are depicted schematically in Figure 25-4.

In yet another study, subjects were asked to listen to an excerpt from a fictional story, then to think of a title for the excerpt, and subsequently to "mentally reproduce the text." In each instance, perioral EMG activity appeared greater than basal levels, particularly during the latter two tasks.

Examination of perioral EMG activity during listening to another person speak revealed two instances in which activity deviated most (in the direction of greater excitation) from basal levels: "The moment of intense attention to the speaker's utterance and its fixation and whenever diffi-

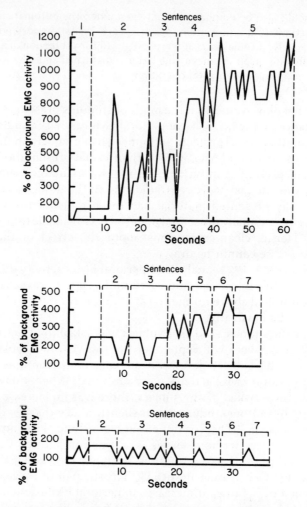

FIGURE 25-4. Graphic representation of the integrated EMG activity obtained over the perioral musculature during silent reading of text. The momentary halt in silent reading that occurred between each sentence is marked by vertical dotted lines. The record of a subject reading a foreign (English) text is displayed in the top panel, an initial reading of a text in the native language (Russian) is displayed in the middle panel, and a repeated reading of the Russian text is displayed in the bottom panel. Sokolov (1972) noted that following the production of the bottom record, a record as seen in the middle panel was again produced when the subject was instructed to "Reread it more attentively." Adapted from Sokolov (1972).

culties are experienced as regards comprehension of the speaker's utterance and its subsequent logical processing" (Sokolov, 1972, p. 179). The enhanced perioral EMG activity we have observed in response to counterattitudinal in contrast to neutral and proattitudinal communications (Cacioppo & Petty, 1979; see Chapter 3) is clearly in accord with the Soviet research on covert information processing.

Finally, investigations of perioral activity during visual problem solving have produced more conflicting results. Zinchenko, Nunipov, and Gordon (1973-1974) monitored lip EMG, EEG alpha blocking, and oculomotor responses during the performance of three types of visual tasks (i.e., maze, square, and compass tests). They found that as subjects worked on more difficult problems, external scanning diminished somewhat, whereas "internal scanning" (comparison of an image with a standard) increased in importance (as indicated by EEG and oculomotor changes). Perioral EMG activity, however, showed the same pattern for all the visual problems. This led Zinchenko *et al.* (1973) to suggest that "inner speech performed merely the function of planning activity and establishing the results obtained" (p. 86). In other words, perioral EMG activity did not reflect the manipulation of visual images or switching from one to another visual image. Sokolov (1972) found that constructing an image (e.g., of a ship) was unaccompanied by perioral EMG activity, although he did find evidence of increasing perioral EMG activity as subjects performed more and more complex maze tasks. Sokolov concluded, contrary to Zinchenko *et al.* (1973), that the localized EMG activity in the perioral region reflected the logical operations on concrete (visual) objects. This point, so far as we could tell, has remained unresolved in the Soviet literature.

CONCLUSION

Western social psychologists have been concerned with a broad range of topics dealing with human association. The demands of a discipline so wide in scope have led to such a specialization in social psychology that investigators from related areas of research (e.g., attraction, attitude formation) may be largely unfamiliar with each other's work (cf. Wyer, 1978). In addition, as was noted at the outset of this book, many of the theories in social psychology have either incorporated an almost entirely "conceptual" nervous system or ignored the influence of physiological processes altogether. To some extent, this is understandable given the demands of experimental social psychology as a discipline and the technology that existed in the past for investigating psychophysiological processes. However, as the contributors to the present book have demonstrated, psychophysiological technology has become increasingly accessible to researchers, and psychophysiological data are increasingly available to develop, assess, and refine the "conceptual" nervous systems in social psychological theories.

The Soviet psychological research bears on both the theoretical approaches taken and the methods employed in social psychophysiology. In this chapter we have reviewed a variety of specific procedures that might prove to be useful indices of social processes (e.g., perioral EMG activity; classically conditioned indices of attitudes), and we have surveyed the general, theoretical perspective advanced in Soviet psychology. It is interesting to note, though, that Soviet *social* psychology, which is still an emerging area within Soviet psychology, has apparently drawn some criticism for *not* delving deeper into the role of psychophysiological processes in human social behavior.

> Of course, contemporary psychological research provides more and more new evidence of the social factors that determine man's mental development. But at the same time, we have acquired a deeper understanding of the natural factors underlying this development. Over the past few decades our knowledge of the properties of the nervous system as the natural underpinnings of individual psychological differences has widened significantly. Hence to opt for any set of new facts in one area to the exclusion of all the others will yield only a one-sided solution to the question. Ultimately, of course, the only solution must lie in a dialectical approach in which new facts can be immediately fit into a unified theory and perceived in their interrelationships. (Budilova, 1973, p. 33)

It seems that in this regard Western social psychologists and psychophysiologists are beginning cooperatively to make significant, if not unique, advances in the scientific study of social behavior (Cacioppo & Petty, in press).

ACKNOWLEDGMENT

The research for and preparation of this chapter was supported by National Science Foundation Grants BNS-8023589 and BNS-8215734.

REFERENCES

Akhutina, T. V.   The role of inner speech in the construction of an utterance. *Soviet Psychology*, 1978, *16*, 3–30.

Anan'ev, B. G.   On the theory of inner speech in psychology. In *The psychology of century cognition*. Moscow: Academy of Pedagogical Science, RSFSR Press, 1960.

Anokhin, P. K.   Cybernetics and the integrative activity of the brain. In M. Cole & I. Maltzman (Eds.), *A handbook of contemporary Soviet psychology*. New York: Basic Books, 1969.

Barber, T. X.   Experiments in hypnosis. *Scientific American*, 1957, *196*, 54–61.

Beritashvili, I. S.   Concerning psychoneural activity of animals. In M. Cole & I. Maltzman (Eds.), *A handbook of contemporary Soviet psychology*. New York: Basic Books, 1969.

Berkowitz, L. *Cognitive theories in social psychology.* New York: Academic, 1978.

Bernshtein, N. A. Methods for developing physiology as related to the problems of cybernetics. In M. Cole & I. Maltzman (Eds.), *A handbook of contemporary Soviet psychology.* New York: Basic Books, 1969.

Bliznitchenko, L. Hypnopaedia and its practice in the USSR. In F. Rubin (Ed.), *Current research in hypnopaedia.* London: Macdonald, 1968.

Boring, E. G. *The history of experimental psychology* (2nd ed.). New York: Appleton-Century-Crofts, 1950.

Brown, J. S. *The motivation of behavior.* New York: McGraw-Hill, 1961.

Budilova, E. A. The relationship between psychology and physiology. *Soviet Psychology,* 1973, *11,* 23–34.

Budilova, E. A. N. G. Chernyshevsky and materialistic psychology. *Voprosy Psikhologii,* 1978, *5,* 29–30. (English summary)

Budzynski, T. H. Biofeedback and the twilight states of consciousness. In G. E. Schwartz & D. Shapiro (Eds.), *Consciousness and self-regulation: Advances in research* (Vol. 1). New York: Plenum, 1976.

Cacioppo, J. T., & Petty, R. E. Attitudes and cognitive responses: An electrophysiological approach. *Journal of Personality and Social Psychology,* 1979, *37,* 281–299.

Cacioppo, J. T., & Petty, R. E. Electromyograms as measures of extent and affectivity of information processing. *American Psychologist,* 1981, *36,* 441–456. (a)

Cacioppo, J. T., & Petty, R. E. Electromyographic specificity during covert information processing. *Psychophysiology,* 1981, *18,* 518–523. (b)

Cacioppo, J. T., & Petty, R. E. A biosocial model of attitude change. In J. T. Cacioppo & R. E. Petty (Eds.), *Perspectives in cardiovascular psychophysiology.* New York: Guilford, 1982.

Cacioppo, J. T., & Petty, R. E. Social processes. In M. G. H. Coles, E. Donchin, & S. W. Porges (Eds.), *Handbook of psychophysiology.* New York: Guilford, in press.

Cacioppo, J. T., & Sandman, C. A. Psychophysiological function, cognitive responding, and attitudes. In R. E. Petty, T. M. Ostrom, & T. C. Brock (Eds.), *Cognitive responses in persuasion.* Hillsdale, N.J.: Erlbaum, 1981.

Chuprikova, N. I. The completion of temporary connections through speech. *Soviet Psychology,* 1972, *10,* 276–302.

Cole, M., John-Steiner, V., Scribner, S., & Souberman, E. (Eds.). *L. S. Vygotsky: Mind in society.* Cambridge, Mass.: Harvard University Press, 1981.

Cole, M., & Maltzman, I. (Eds.). *A handbook of contemporary Soviet psychology.* New York: Basic Books, 1969.

Cooper, L. M., & Hoskovec, J. Personal communication, 1967. (Cited in F. Rubin, *Learning and sleep.* Baltimore: Williams & Wilkins, 1971.)

Corson, S. A., & Corson, E. O. (Eds.). *Psychiatry and psychology in the USSR.* New York: Plenum, 1976.

Cropsey, J. Karl Marx. In L. Strauss & J. Cropsey (Eds.), *History of political philosophy* (2nd ed.). Chicago: Rand McNally, 1972.

Felipe, A. *Attitude change during interrupted sleep.* Unpublished doctoral dissertation, Yale University, 1965.

Fenz, W. D., & Epstein, S. Gradients of physiological arousal in parachutists as a function of an approaching jump. *Psychosomatic Medicine,* 1967, *29,* 33–51.

Gergen, K. Social psychology as history. *Journal of Personality and Social Psychology,* 1973, *26,* 309–320.

Grimak, L. P., & Ponomarenko, V. A. Types of human autonomic shifts induced by emotional stress. *Zhurnal Vysshei Nervnoi Deyatel'nosti Imeni I. P. Pavlova,* 1967, *17,* 408–412. (Described in *Sleep learning in the USSR,* ATD Report No. 68-91-108-6. Washington, D.C.: Aerospace Technology Division, Library of Congress, February, 7, 1969.)

Grings, W. W., & Dawson, M. E. *Emotions and bodily responses.* New York: Academic, 1978.

James, W. What is emotion? *Mind,* 1884, *9,* 188–204.

Kagan, J., Haith, M. M., & Caldwell, C. (Eds.). *Psychology: Adapted readings.* New York: Harcourt, 1971.

Komlev, N. G. A linguistic interpretation of thought in relation to speech. *Soviet Psychology,* 1980-1981, *19,* 3-22.

Kornilov, K. N. Psychology in the light of dialectical materialism. In C. Murchison (Ed.), *Psychologies of 1930.* Worcester, Mass.: Clark University Press, 1930.

Krauss, R. M. Social psychology in the Soviet Union: Some comments. In S. A. Corson & E. O. Corson (Eds.), *Psychiatry and psychology in the USSR.* New York: Plenum, 1976.

Kurtsin, I. T. *Theoretical principles of psychosomatic medicine.* Toronto: Wiley, 1976.

Lange, C. The emotions. In K. Dunlap (Ed.), *The emotions.* Baltimore: Williams & Wilkins, 1922. (Originally published, 1885).

Leont'ev, A. A. Psycholinguistic units and the production of verbal utterances, 1969. (Cited in T. V. Akhutina, The role of inner speech in the construction of an utterance, *Soviet Psychology,* 1978, *16,* 3-30.)

Levy, C. M. Personal communication, 1969. (Cited in F. Rubin, *Learning and sleep.* Baltimore: Williams & Wilkins, 1971.)

Lomov, B. F. Sixty years of Soviet psychology. *Soviet Psychology,* 1978-1979, *17,* 68-82.

London, I. D. Theory of emotions in Soviet dialetic psychology. In M. L. Reymert (Ed.), *Feelings and emotions.* New York: McGraw-Hill, 1950.

Luria, A. R. The quantitative assessment of levels of wakefulness. *Soviet Psychology,* 1973, *12,* 73-84.

Luria, A. R., & Vinogradova, O. S. An objective investigation of the dynamics of semantic systems. *British Journal of Psychology,* 1959, *50,* 89-105.

Mackay, C. J. The measurement of mood and psychophysiological activities using self-report techniques. In I. Martin & P. H. Venables (Eds.), *Techniques in psychophysiology.* Chichester: Wiley, 1980.

McGuigan, F. J., & Winstead, C. L., Jr. Discriminative relationship between covert oral behavior and the phonemic system in internal information processing. *Journal of Experimental Psychology,* 1974, *103,* 885-890.

McLeish, J. *Soviet psychology: History, theory, content.* London: Methuen, 1975.

Merlin, V. S. The unique features of the galvanic skin parameter of a conditional response in the presence and absence of an orienting component. *Zhurnal Vysshei Nervnoi Deyatel'nosti Imeni I. V. Pavlova,* 1960, *10.* (Cited in L. V. Putlyaeva, The functions of emotions in the thought process, *Soviet Psychology,* 1980, *18,* 21-35.)

Moruzzi, G., & Magoun, H. W. Brainstem reticular formation and activation of the EEG. *Electroencephalography and Clinical Neurophysiology,* 1949, *1,* 455-473.

Ol'shannikova, A. E. Some physiological correlates of emotional states. In *Problems of differential psychology* (Vol. 4). Moscow: 1969. (Cited in L. V. Putlyaeva, The functions of emotions in the thought process, *Soviet Psychology,* 1980, *18,* 21-35.)

Oswald, I. *Sleep.* Baltimore: Penguin Books, 1966.

Pavlov, I. P. *Conditioned reflexes.* New York: Oxford University Press, 1927.

Petrovskiy, A. V. Some problems of research in social psychology. *Soviet Psychology,* 1971, *9,* 382-398.

Petty, R. E., & Brock, T. C. Thought disruption and persuasion: Assessing the validity of attitude change experiments. In R. E. Petty, T. M. Ostrom, & T. C. Brock (Eds.), *Cognitive responses in persuasion.* Hillsdale, N.J.: Erlbaum, 1981.

Petty, R. E., & Cacioppo, J. T. *Attitudes and persuasion: Classic and contemporary approaches.* Dubuque, Iowa: W. C. Brown, 1981.

Petty, R. E., Wells, G. L., & Brock, T. C. Distraction can enhance or reduce yielding to propaganda: Thought disruption versus effort justification. *Journal of Personality and Social Psychology,* 1976, *34,* 874-884.

Putlyaeva, L. V. The function of emotions in the thought process. *Soviet Psychology,* 1980, *18,* 21-35.

Rahmani, L. *Soviet psychology: Philosophical, theoretical, and experimental issues*. New York: International Universities Press, 1973.

Razran, G. The observable unconscious and the inferable conscious in current Soviet psychophysiology. *Psychological Review*, 1961, *68*, 81–147.

Romer, D. Distraction, counterarguing, and the internalization of attitude change. *European Journal of Social Psychology*, 1979, *9*, 1–18.

Rubin, F. (Ed.). *Current research in hypnopaedia*. London: Macdonald, 1968.

Rubin, F. *Learning and sleep*. Baltimore: Williams & Wilkins, 1971.

Schachter, S., & Singer, J. E. Cognitive, social and physiological determinants of emotional state. *Psychological Review*, 1962, *69*, 379–399.

Sechenov, I. M. *Biographical sketch and essays*. New York: Arno, 1973.

Shikhirev, P. N. Some aspects of methods used in social psychology research in the USA. *Soviet Psychology*, 1980, *19*, 73–92.

Simon, C. W., & Emmons, W. H. Learning during sleep? *Psychological Bulletin*, 1955, *52*, 328–342.

Sokolov, A. N. Studies of the speech mechanisms of thinking. In M. Cole & I. Maltzman (Eds.), *A handbook of contemporary Soviet psychology*. New York: Basic Books, 1969.

Sokolov, A. N. *Inner speech and thought*. New York: Plenum, 1972.

Strickland, L. H. *Soviet and Western perspectives in social psychology*. Oxford: Pergamon, 1979.

Strickland, L. H. Social psychology in the Soviet Union. *Personality and Social Psychology Bulletin*, 1980, *6*, 353–360.

Sviadoshch, A. N. The history of hypnopaedia. In F. Rubin (Ed.), *Current research in hypnopaedia*. London: Macdonald, 1968.

Vygotsky, L. S. Thought and language. In *Selected psychological investigations*. Moscow: Academy of Pedagogical Science, RSFSR Press, 1956.

Wertsch, J. V. *The concept of activity in Soviet psychology*. Armonk, N.Y.: Sharpe, 1981.

West, S. G., & Wicklund, R. A. *A primer of social psychological theories*. Monterey, Calif.: Brooks/Cole, 1980.

Wyer, R. S., Jr. Excerpts from letters received by Bibb Latane. *Personality and Social Psychology Bulletin*, 1978, *4*, 29–30.

Yaroshevskiy, M. G. I. M. Sechenov and the psychology activity. *Voprosy Psikhologii*, 1979, *4*, 107–108. (English summary)

Zinchenko, V. P., Nunipov, V. M., & Gordon, V. M. The study of visual thinking. *Soviet Psychology*, 1973–1974, *12*, 72–89.

AUTHOR INDEX

SUBJECT INDEX

Signs and Symptoms (MacBryde & Blacklow), 25
Situation Redefinition, 534
Skin conductance, 9, 146–148, 455, 655, 675 (*see also* Skin resistance)
and classical conditioning, 9
and extraversion–introversion, 400, 405, 408
and facial EMG, 266
and heart rate, 142
and social and political beliefs, 114–116
Skin resistance (*see also* Skin conductance)
and arousal, 142
and attitude measurement, 54–56, 59, 63
and empathy, 421, 422
and private mental effort, 43, 44
and signal processing, 650
and social facilitation, 445
spontaneous responses, 448, 449
SLDCH, 680
Sleep
patterns of, 710
sexual arousal in, 368
Smiling, 328, 329
spontaneous, 327–330
Snake phobia, 124
Sociability and extraversion–introversion, 391, 392
Social and political beliefs, 102–119
and arousal, 134
and classical conditioning, 107–111
cross-modal multiple indicator analysis of, 103, 104, 111–116
and discrimination, 107
and generalization, 107
and nonobtrusive measures, 116–118
and prediction, 103
and race, 111–119
and semantic generalization, 108, 109
and skin conductance, 114–116
Social communication, 370
Social event, definition of, 9
Social facilitation, 434–462
and arousal, 435, 436, 441, 443, 444, 452–455, 461
and attentional overload, 442, 443, 454
and central nervous system, 436n.
and cues, 440, 441
distraction/conflict hypothesis on, 440, 441, 454
and drive, 435, 436, 460
effects of social presence, 444–451
and electrodermal activity, 447–449

evaluation apprehension hypothesis on, 440
future directions for, 452–461
and heart rate, 443, 449
mere presence hypothesis on, 436–439
and misattribution, 459, 460
and multiple measurement strategies, 460, 461
and palmar sweating, 445, 446, 448, 451
parallel phenomena strategy in, 456–459
self-awareness theory on, 442
and vocal stress, 451
Socialization
and motivation, 417, 418
schema on, 551–553
sexual, 469
of symptom perception, 431
Social Psychology (McDougall), 353
Social psychology and psychophysiology, merger of, x
Social psychophysiology, overview of, x–xv, 3–32, 37–46
history, 5–10
evolution of perspective, 5–8
research strategies, 8–10
introduction, 3–5
prototypical example, 37–40
psychophysiological contexts, 42–44
selected concepts
bodily sensation and perception, 24–28
endocrine system, 28–30
habituation, 23, 24
interactive effects, 24
law of initial values, 22, 23
nervous system, 10–17
physiological arousal, 17–20
response patterns, 20–22
social psychological contexts, 40–42
social psychology and psychophysiology, 45–46
Society for Psychophysiological Research, 668
Sociobiology, focus of on adaptiveness of social behavior, xi
Sociopharmacology as a field, ix, x
Soviet Psychology, 697
Soviet psychophysiology, overview of
arousal and wakefulness, 700–706
on attitudes, 706–709
and consciousness, 694, 695
and dialectical materialism, 695
emotions, 712–715
on hypnopaedia and persuasion, 709–712